FUNCTIONAL ANATOMY AND HISTOLOGY OF THE LUNG

By

CHUZO NAGAISHI, M.D.
Emeritus Professor of Kyoto University

With the Collaboration of

NAOYUKI NAGASAWA, M.D. MASAYUKI YAMASHITA, M.D.
YOSHIO OKADA, M.D. NOBUO INABA, M.D.

from the Department of Thoracic Surgery,
Chest Disease Research Institute, Kyoto University

UNIVERSITY PARK PRESS

Baltimore and London

Library of Congress Cataloging in Publication Data

Nagaishi, Chuzo, 1907–
Functional anatomy and histology of the lung.

Bibliography: p.
1. Lungs. 2. Anatomy, Surgical and topographical. I. Nagasawa, Naoyuki. II. Title. [DNLM: 1. Lung—Anatomy and history. 2. Lung—Pathology. WF600 N147f 1972]
QM261.N34 611'.24 72–1241
ISBN 0–8391–0580–0

American edition, May 1972, published by UNIVERSITY PARK PRESS
Chamber of Commerce Building, Baltimore, Maryland 21202

Printed and Bound in Japan

To my respected teachers

Late Emeritus Professor TEIJI HOSHINO, M.D.

Emeritus Professor YASUMASA AOYAGI, M.D.

and

To my wife FUMIKO NAGAISHI

for her patience and devotion

FOREWORD

It is a great pleasure for me to learn that the publication of "Functional Anatomy and Histology of the Lung" is now being realized. This accomplishment represents a major landmark in the career of Professor CHUZO NAGAISHI.

As Professor NAGAISHI says in his preface, the important characteristic of his book lies in the point that this study of the structure of the lung has been carried out by an author who is preeminently a specialist in thoracic surgery; the book was developed and written taking into consideration various important clinical problems. Accordingly, there naturally is an understandable difference as compared with books written by professional anatomists; in this point, the volume assumes a unique position.

The well-known anatomist TIEDEMANN once said "Ärzte ohne Anatomie gleichen Maulwürfen; sie arbeiten im Dunklen und ihrer Hände Tagewerk sind Erdhügel" (Doctors who do not know anatomy are like moles; they work in the darkness only to make a heap of earth). His words are severe, but eternally meaningful. Supposedly, this saying by TIEDEMANN refers not only to anatomy but includes also the relationships of basic and clinical sciences in the broader sense; it is certainly true that a firm foundation in the basic sciences is the key to excellence in the clinical sciences and the practice of medicine.

In this regard, Professor NAGAISHI has had an excellent viewpoint; he has always insisted on the importance and necessity of the closest relationship between the clinical and basic sciences; more to the point, he himself is an exemplar of this attitude.

This book is the fruit of scholarly research carried out by Professor NAGAISHI and his associates during his many years as a very active and dedicated clinician. As I read this book, I am strongly impressed by his considerate and integrated attitude, and by his never-failing scholarly enthusiasm. Noteworthy in this book is the description of individual items, and without loss of an integrated attitude toward the entire subject. In recent years, research has tended to be analytic; this book contains ample examples of a healthy and desirable contrary trend.

Professor NAGAISHI was born in Kyoto in 1907. After graduating from Kyoto University, he entered the Department of Otorhinolaryngology where he studied particularly on the problems of tuberculosis of the larynx, under the direction of the late Emeritus Professor TEIJI HOSHINO. When the Tuberculosis Research Institute (presently the Chest Disease Research Institute) was founded at Kyoto University in 1941, Dr. NAGAISHI was transferred to the Institute to develop a program in thoracic surgery.

To prepare for this activity, he entered the Department of Surgery in the School of Medicine, and studied for five years under the direction of Emeritus Professor YASUMASA AOYAGI. Since then, Dr. NAGAISHI has continued his activity as Head of the Department of Thoracic Surgery. His academic and clinical philosophy has required that he concentrates not only on thoracic surgery, but also on morphology, physiology, pathology, chemotherapy, and on other related basic studies in the respiratory system.

He and his associates have reported a great number of fine works, and he has gradually cultivated deep friendship with a worldwide community of scholars.

Knowing Professor NAGAISHI, I must admire his originality, and testify to his indomitable spirit in overcoming difficulties. At the same time, he is a man of affection. He has a sincere and warm respect for his patients, and they cannot but be attracted by his personality.

When I look at the history of science, I well know that there is no end to the search for truth. The investigations of VESALIUS, of WILLIAM HARVEY, of SCHLEIDEN and SCHWANN, of VIRCHOW, of DARWIN, of MENDEL, of FLEMING, and of many other scholars, were all epoch-making achievements, and constituted splendid contributions to the development of science. However, from a strict scientific viewpoint, even their achievements were not complete, but required to be followed by concentrated efforts for attainment of further progress. In this sense, Professor NAGAISHI's studies reported in this book do not mean that they have been completed by this publication, but will have to be continued further by the author and others in Japan and abroad toward unstated and now unimaginable goals.

This book will surely be a memorable milestone in the history of science. I wish to express my highest esteem to Professor NAGAISHI for his painstaking work.

I am convinced that this book will warrant a favorable acceptance and warm welcome, at home and abroad.

February 1, 1971

KŌ HIRASAWA, M.D.
Formerly President and Professor Emeritus
Kyoto University
Member of the Japan Academy

FOREWORD

This impressive monograph summarizes a considerable part of the life work of a distinguished thoracic surgeon, Professor Emeritus CHUZO NAGAISHI of Kyoto University, who follows in the splendid traditions of scholar-surgeons represented more than a century ago by WILLIAM BOWMAN of England, and more recently by HARVEY CUSHING of America and WILDER PENFIELD of Canada. This book presents those aspects of functional pulmonary anatomy which have proved to be useful for the clinical thinking of a lung surgeon. It does not present the author's many advances in thoracic surgical technique, nor does it summarize his extensive contributions to understanding and management of chest diseases, particularly tuberculosis.

Surgeons come face to face with structural details as they carry out their procedures and develop rationale of management. A thorough understanding of structure and of its significance, then, becomes a necessity to a surgeon. HARVEY CUSHING thought it essential to master details of the gross anatomy of every part he was to invade, and, in addition, in order to improve his judgment as to the best procedure to follow, he made pioneering explorations into the microscopic anatomy and function of organs of surgical interest to him, such as the pituitary. In the same tradition, WILDER PENFIELD perceived that a neurosurgeon must understand the potentialities and characteristics of the several types of cells which can engender tumors of the central nervous system. These magnificent neurosurgeons pursued detailed, sustained, highly specialized microscopic studies of the hypophysis and of glial cells respectively, and in the course of their research, initiated to improve the rationale for surgical management, they made far-reaching innovative discoveries of general value to medicine and to science, as well as of specific value to surgery.

Professor NAGAISHI's name is rendered in Japanese by two Chinese characters which can be assigned the meanings, "long" and "stone", respectively. Though his name can hence be translated as "Longstone" in English, the first of the two characters often carries the significance of "chief" or "principal" or "leader" or "head person". Hence one can, without loss of accuracy, provide an alternative translation of the characters, as "chief stone", or "principal stone", conveying an idea often implied by use of the English term, "cornerstone". It is gratifying to see how Professor NAGAISHI's life work has conformed to this alternative rendering of the Chinese characters which express his name. For he has indeed made for us a cornerstone work on the anatomy of the lung. He perceived that a surgeon must be guided in his judgment by profound understanding of the structure and function of the organ towards which his surgical interests are addressed. He has carried out over the years many detailed descriptive and experimental studies of the lung. He mastered the relevant literature of the past and contributed substantially to that of his own lifetime. Like BOWMAN, CUSHING and PENFIELD before him, he grasped that surgical anatomy encompasses all the structural concepts of value to a surgeon in formulating rationale and judgments exercised in planning operations and regimen. Hence, to these scholars, surgical anatomy includes gross and microscopic anatomy, and to Professor NAGAISHI, includes ultrastructure and molecular anatomy as well. In extending surgical anatomy into the realm of ultrastructure, Dr. NAGAISHI and his associates have made skilful use of opportunities offered by recent technical advances in electron microscopes and in methods for utilizing these powerful instruments for studies of fine structural details of cells and tissues.

Professor NAGAISHI has been fortunate in living in a country which has pioneered in development of electron microscopes and electron microscopy and whose skilled workers, imaginative designers and well-organized manufacturers have created electron microscopes in considerable numbers and variety, of advanced design, with reliability and capability as good as any in the world. The author and his associates have taken excellent advantage of these movements, have mastered the necessary skills, and have included much of their handiwork for the benefit and enlightenment of readers of this book. Particularly interesting are the scanning electron micrographs of lung alveoli, showing communications between adjacent alveoli in accordance with the concepts of KOHN, which have been subject to considerable controversy. There are also included many fine transmission electron micrographs, presenting important details of cell relationships in various parts of the lung, and contributing substantially to understanding of lung function.

In 1957 and 1958 the author and his associates published in Japanese a forerunner of this present monograph, presenting in it the structure of the lung as conceived at that time. We welcome the present text in English, which makes available to scholars in all parts of the world a revised and up-to-date summary of the functional surgical anatomy of the lung.

April 5, 1971

H. STANLEY BENNETT, M.D.
Sarah Graham Kenan Professor of Biological and Medical Sciences
Professor of Anatomy
Chairman, Department of Anatomy
Director, The Laboratories for Reproductive Biology
University of North Carolina

FOREWORD

The history of the search for knowledge about the structure of the lungs, can be seen as a wonderful adventure, whose path has been unwinding over the course of several centuries. The attractive problems involved in this task have engaged the keen investigating minds of some of the most learned men. For millennia these problems remained obscure and without answer.

Primitive man; the poet of Homer's age; the bard of the ancient oriental civilization; each instinctively thought that the "breath of life" was derived from the chest and the lungs. Aristotle postulated the concept that breathing was a method of cooling the blood; the lungs, fulfilling this function, thus also "accidentally" were able to become the region for infiltration of air.

It is shortly after the first half of the seventeenth century, that the true story of lung structure begins. The initiators were two scholars belonging to the same epoch: MARCELLO MALPIGHI, Professor of Bologna University (Italy), and THOMAS WILLIS, Professor of London Medical College (England).

In the epistolae "De Pulmonibus" written in 1661 by MALPIGHI, as in the "Opera Omnia" of WILLIS, for the first time, the lungs were considered to be, not a solid, compact, fleshy mass, but rather a membranous, vesicular, canalized structure. It is from these early workers that the present-day rudimentary facts are derived. WILLIS and MALPIGHI realistically differentiated and gave a nomenclature to lobules, alveoli, bronchial ramifications, arteries and veins.

Based upon these very early fundamental elements that drew their origin from a finite period of time, 1661–1676, the bulk of ensuing knowledge has gradually developed.

Just how much has been recognized and discovered in these three-hundred years of journeying and exactly what is the present state of understanding of the fine structural components of the lungs, are illustrated in this book, with notable descriptive precision and superior systematic clarity.

It is with great honour and much pleasure that I introduce this impressive book; which also receives importance from the eloquent works of Professor CHUZO NAGAISHI, Head of the Department of Thoracic Surgery, in the Chest Disease Research Institute of Kyoto University, Kyoto, Japan.

Friendship of more than ten years binds us together; but, above all, I feel the highest appreciation for and deep admiration of his impassioned and discerning work as a scientist.

Sentiments, such as these, have been strengthened at each of our numerous encounters in Italy (Naples, Parma, Brindisi), in Japan (Tokyo, Kyoto), in Brasil (Bahia), in Denmark (Copenhagen), and in Switzerland (Lausanne).

At our meeting in this Institute at Kyoto, in September 1967, I first learned of his work and studied on the fine structure of the lungs. On that occasion, I saw the Japanese Edition (Vol. I, 1957 and Vol. II, 1958) of this book and I also learned then that he was in the process of preparing a new revised version in English.

He has now completed his book which surely will be of far-reaching interest and will receive well-deserved success.

Essentially, this is a work of systematic anatomy, however, not written by an anatomist, instead, it is an "exposé", by one of the most famous thoracic surgeons. For this very reason, the investigations and analyses, which have been undertaken in the various sections on the structure of organs are not only admirable from the point of view of morphology, but also remain firmly anchored to the requirements of physiology, pathology, clinical medicine and surgery. This is particularly valid for the bronchial anatomy, for the parts devoted to the lymphatic system and for the pulmonary and bronchial vascular systems.

The reader will also find, in the various chapters, many historical notes and there are noteworthy memories of the older pioneers, who studied the lungs from a morphological point of view; included, too, are recent contributions, and special mention is made of the achievements of electron microscopy.

The wonderful adventure continues, and to it, this book of Professor NAGAISHI, an eminent surgeon and an eminent anatomist, brings one of the most significant and outstanding contributions of modern times.

February 28, 1971

Professor ANTONIO BLASI, M.D.
Director, Tuberculosis Clinic and Graduate School of Respiratory Diseases
University of Naples

FOREWORD

This book is an encyclopedic survey of the detailed anatomy of the lungs involving all systems—broncho-alveolar, vascular, lymphatic, muscular, neural and pleural—ranging from the gross anatomical to the microscopic and ultramicroscopic, from clinical applications to experimental approaches, from the normal to the pathologic, from studies on man to those on experimental animals—the whole supplemented by comprehensive surveys of the literature, including historical aspects of the subject, and by detailed surveys of technical methods of investigation, many of them original.

It is indeed amazing that an active chest surgeon with administrative responsibilities could find the time to establish a Chest Disease Research Institute, such as the one in Kyoto, to work in it himself with his students, and finally to organize the first Asia Pacific Congress on Diseases of the Chest (APCDC, 1969) to which physicians from all over the world contributed.

From another standpoint this book fills a long-anticipated need. Western investigators, who for many years have been aware of the high quality of Japanese studies that have appeared in the German and English languages but who have not been able to read the many treatises in the Japanese language—such as the former edition of this book—will welcome this comprehensive survey of Japanese studies on the lung that have now been made available in the English language.

The only field not represented in this anatomical approach is the developmental side of pulmonary anatomy. But obvious this is a specialty in itself.

Finally, one wishes to pay tribute to the kindly personality of this scholar and surgeon. Those of us who have become acquainted with him through the International Congresses on Diseases of the Chest, and in the home of friends, have always found it a privilege to know this charming, gifted, cosmopolitan gentleman.

March 10, 1971

EDWARD A. BOYDEN, Ph.D. (Med. Sc.),
F.A.C.C.P. (Hon.)
Research Professor, Department of Biological Structure
School of Medicine, University of Washington

FOREWORD

Professor NAGAISHI has now added another scholarly achievement to his earlier two-volume work "The Structure of the Lung" and has greatly widened his audience by writing it in English. This new volume comes, quite appropriately, at a time when there is increasing interest in many old functions of the lung and discoveries of new functions. The discovery of pulmonary surfactant and its unique role in stabilizing alveolar volume and preventing atelectasis has led to examination of biosynthetic activities of cells lining the alveoli, alveolar ducts and terminal bronchioles. The discovery that the lung can actively take up substances (such as 5-hydroxytryptamine, some prostaglandins and bradykinin) present in mixed venous blood, can transform substances in mixed venous blood (*e.g.*, convert angiotensin I to angiotensin II) and can store and subsequently release chemical substances into the pulmonary venous blood, has led to renewed interest in the cells lining the pulmonary arteries, arterioles and capillaries.

The world-wide interest in air pollution has generated numerous studies on alveolar macrophages (that phagocytose foreign matter) and on sensory receptors in the bronchioles (that initiate bronchoconstriction in response to smog). And the Ciba Foundation Symposium (1968) on Breathing (marking the centennial of the discovery of the Hering-Breuer reflex) has led to much curiosity about receptors in the intrapulmonary airways that initiate the inflation and "deflation" reflex and may contribute to the sensation of dyspnea. And the possibility that surgical transplantation of the lung may soon be a reality has led physiologists to study the pulmonary nerves and lymphatics and the rate at which they regenerate after transsection.

Professor NAGAISHI in this volume combines his own rich experience with the gross and fine structure of the lung with a critical report on studies from many other laboratories and a valuable look at the classic literature of the 19th and early 20th century. Clinicians and basic medical scientists interested in the lung will benefit greatly from Professor NAGAISHI's integrated presentation of gross structure, of functional anatomy viewed by fluorescence microscopy, of fine structure examined by the light microscope and ultrastructure explored with both the scanning electron microscope and the transmission electron microscope. It is of particular value that this information is synthesized by an experienced thoracic surgeon who knows well the importance of basic knowledge to an understanding of clinical problems. It is almost unique that a thoracic surgeon has produced a definitive work on gross and fine structure; the sections dealing with the terminal bronchioles, alveoli, bronchial and pulmonary circulations and their interrelationships, lymphatics and nerves are covered with thoroughness not to be found elsewhere.

Professor NAGAISHI spent a sabbatical year at the University of California, San Francisco in 1959–60; subsequently a number of his very capable young staff have spent fellowships in this Institute. The interchange of ideas has been mutually beneficial and we regard the Institute in Kyoto as a sister Institute.

April 8, 1971

JULIUS H. COMROE, Jr., M.D.
Professor, Director, Cardiovascular Research Institute
University of California, San Francisco

FOREWORD

It was my pleasure to meet Professor CHUZO NAGAISHI in February 1963 when we were attending the Eighth International Congress on Diseases of the Chest in New Delhi, India. Later I was his guest in Kyoto where I had the opportunity of seeing his magnificent book on thoracic surgery. It was written in Japanese, of course, but its superb illustrations had English subtitles. Since then, Dr. NAGAISHI and I have met frequently in various parts of the world, and I have heard him speak on a wide variety of subjects including tuberculosis, carcinoma of the lung, and pulmonary embolism. No wonder that he has such an extensive bibliography on so many different scientific subjects.

Dr. NAGAISHI is not only an eminent thoracic surgeon but also an expert in the fields of anatomy, pathology, and cardiopulmonary physiology. He has held positions of leadership in the major societies in Japan which are devoted to the thoracic disciplines. He was President of the First Asia Pacific Congress on Diseases of the Chest in 1969 and was the principal organizer of this Congress. He has been active in the international activities of the American College of Chest Physicians and has served as a governor for Japan.

This volume, "Functional Anatomy and Histology of the Lung" is an outgrowth of the many years of painstaking research which Professor NAGAISHI and his capable associates have carried out. The original works were published in 1957 and 1958 and, of course, many advances in methodology have developed and numerous contributions to our knowledge of the anatomy of the lung have appeared since that time. Dr. NAGAISHI has been cognizant of the great importance of electron microscopy and its role in the understanding of the entire structure and function of the lung even to the cellular level. It should be emphasized that although he has utilized all of the extensive studies carried out by his research group at the Chest Disease Research Institute, Kyoto University, he is the sole author of this volume. To be sure he has been most generous in giving credit to his co-workers, all of whom have attained distinction in academic careers of their own. However, this monumental work is indeed the product of his own pen.

In the six chapters of this book, Dr. NAGAISHI has described the bronchoalveolar system, the vascular system, the lymphatic system, the nervous system, the muscular system, and the pulmonary pleura. In each chapter the world literature has been exhaustively reviewed. The historical aspects are thoroughly covered, and the important embryologic data are emphasized. The work of the morphology study group in Kyoto is described in detail, and the techniques of tissue preparation also are outlined. Particular emphasis has been placed on the recent studies of the fine structure of the lung and the great fund of new knowledge that electron microscopy has contributed.

Dr. NAGAISHI not only has provided us with an authoritative treatise on the anatomy and histology of the lung but also has correlated this information with clinical, pathologic, and physiologic problems; hence, this book should be of great interest to the practicing physician and surgeon. As a thoracic surgeon with a strong background in basic science he was well qualified to accomplish this task. It is indeed a fittting culmination to a distinguished career.

At my request, my colleague, Professor MATTHEW DIVERTIE, reviewed the manuscript. Dr. DIVERTIE has been involved in studies of the morphometry of the lung in various diseases for many years. Professor W. H. HOLLINSHEAD, Chairman of the Department of Anatomy of the Mayo Graduate School of Medicine, also has been kind enough to read the book. Both have expressed their admiration for the thoroughness of Professor NAGAISHI's work and the excellence of his presentation. With its encyclopedic approach to the subject, the book is certain to become a standard reference for all who are interested in the anatomy of the lung.

March 11, 1971

ARTHUR M. OLSEN, M.D.
Professor of Medicine
Mayo Graduate School of Medicine
University of Minnesota
Chairman, Division of Thoracic Diseases
Mayo Clinic and Mayo Foundation

FOREWORD

It is a personal honor to be invited to write a note of introduction to the author of this volume. I first enjoyed acquaintanceship with Dr. NAGAISHI during his stay in San Francisco as a visiting professor in 1959–60. Subsequent chances of fate made it possible to extend our relationship in Kyoto (1961, 1966), and again on several occasions in San Francisco, during his trips to attend various national and international conferences. Derivative from this more than casual relationship has been an increasing appreciation of Professor NAGAISHI's studies, and of his contributions to the anatomy, physiology, and surgery, of the chest and lungs. The anatomical studies were published (in Japanese) in 1957 and 1958, in two copiously illustrated and thoroughly documented volumes representing ten years of studies by the Professor and his group of younger followers and collaborators. These volumes summarized the multitude of studies then extant, particularly those in Japanese. Subsequently a whole new series of studies have been carried out in Japan, and in the author's laboratories, using newer modalities and techniques; these, in sum, have led Professor NAGAISHI to place on record a newer scanning of the structure of the lung. He has chosen to prepare this new publication in English, in order that references to previously unavailable or untranslated Japanese works may become available to workers in other countries. The results of this effort are here available in this comprehensive and thoroughly illustrated and documented monograph. Even the casual reader cannot but be impressed by the magnitude of the task and the care exhibited in its execution. For the first time, we have available a scholarly evaluation and critical interpretation of a particular segment of Japanese medical science. The work will stand on its merits; that it will contribute importantly to antiparochialism and to a breakdown of provinicalism in medical science is of transcendent importance.

The accomplishment of this objective is the work of a well trained and far sighted investigator. Dr. NAGAISHI graduated in Medicine from Kyoto University's Medical School in 1933, and after the usual prolonged postdoctoral training, became Assistant Professor and then Professor, Head (1953) of the Department of Thoracic Surgery of the Tuberculosis Research Institute, Kyoto University. He was appointed Director of that Institute in 1964, of its successor, the Chest Disease Research Institute (1966), and subsequently of its newly built Hospital (1968–1970). He became Emeritus Professor of Kyoto University on April 1, 1971. His authorship of this new volume marks a kind of reverse Festschrift, dedicated to his students and collaborators in memory of many years of endeavor. During his career, Professor NAGAISHI has attained a national and international reputation. He has been President of the Japanese Association for Thoracic Surgery (1955), of the Japan Society of Chest Diseases (1969), and he was President and Organizer of the First Asia Pacific Congress on Diseases of the Chest (1969). He has been an officer and member of distinguished Japanese societies of surgery, thoracic surgery, chest diseases, cancer therapy, lung cancer, anaesthesiology, circulation, organ transplantation, blood transfusion, bronchoesophagology, clinical cytology, etc., and he has held honorary memberships of clinical and investigative societies in Argentina, Brazil, Chile, and Germany. He has represented Japan at various international clinical congresses, and he has been a Governor of the American College of Chest Physicians for Japan, since 1964. Such recognition has been awarded to Professor NAGAISHI primarily for his extensive studies in tuberculosis and lung cancer. But honors such as these have accrued to a man who has created a school of followers who have become experts in morphology, physiology, pathology, and in clinical medicine and surgery. We have then an example, par excellence, of the skilful surgeon, schooled himself in all of the sciences basic to his art, who has made significant contributions to the teaching and learning of his subject, in all its diversities and complexities; in this respect, Professor NAGAISHI is a "compleat" physician. Further, he combines all of his scholarly accomplishments with charming and attractive qualities. How may

I forget the afternoons in Kyoto when, without notice, Dr. NAGAISHI would appear in my laboratory and announce that the time was immediately correct to view the blooming of the iris, the cherry blossoms, or the wisteria; and off we would go to the Heian Shrine to enjoy rare and unique displays. I remember well, and am grateful for those times.

The first anatomical dissection of the human body was carried out in 1754 in Kyoto in the presence of a physician, YAMAWAKI TŌYŌ. His description (of the chest viscera) was brief and rich with imagery—

> ". . . Through a tube someone blows through the airway, and then both lungs expand—a very beautiful color (purple brocade) like the opening of the cicada wing. The heart hung between the lungs, an as yet unopened lotus blossom. . ." ("Zōshi", 1759).

It is the belief of the undersigned that something of this poetic quality will also be evident in this scholarly work of Dr. NAGAISHI, a spiritual descendant of the pioneer anatomist, scholar and physician of Kyoto.

April 7, 1971

WILLIAM O. REINHARDT, M.D.
Professor of Anatomy and Associate Dean
School of Medicine
University of California, San Francisco

FOREWORD

Prof. NAGAISHI's book is dedicated to the study of all the structures of the lung with special reference to the finest elements of its constituent parts.

The work concerns the morphological study of the finest structures of the lungs, but being written by a clinician who has devoted many years of his life to thorough investigations of clinical aspects of specific and non-specific pulmonary diseases, this book acquires special significance and rouses special interest. The reader will find here a detailed description of the bronchoalveolar system, the vascular system, the lymphatic system, the nervous system, the muscular system and the pulmonary pleura.

Although this is a book on the anatomy and histology of the above-mentioned systems it differs from similar books written by anatomists. Prof. NAGAISHI's book will render an invaluable assistance to each researcher studying one or another aspect of pulmonary pathology.

At present, this book in which a detailed description of the elements of the lymphatic, nervous, and bronchoalveolar systems is given assumes still greater importance and value in the light of recent data on the pathogenesis of chronic pneumonia. The thorough consideration of the finest structures of the tracheobronchial tree, particularly of the tracheobronchial epithelium, helps us to understand more clearly the mechanism of bronchial drainage function impairment responsible for turnig an acute and protracted pneumonia into a chronic one.

The lymphatic system of the lung is circumstantially described which is of great importance for the clinicians-pneumonologs. The more we study pulmonary diseases the more often we are compelled to recognize the significant part the lymph nodes of the tracheobronchial tree play not only in keeping up certain respiratory system diseases but also in initiating them. Being an experienced clinician and ingenious diagnost Prof. NAGAISHI understands very well the role of the lymphatic system of the lung. He pays, therefore, particular attention to this system and suggests his own nomenclature of the bronchopulmonary lymph nodes.

The author describes in detail the nervous system of the lung. The whole Chapter IV is dedicated to this matter. There are very interesting findings obtained during histological investigations of nerve endings of the lung. This is of high significance for better understanding of the pathogenesis of a number of diseases, in particular of bronchial asthma. Only the study of the condition of the finest structures of the bronchial nerve endings can shed light on the nature of this severe disease which is very difficult for understanding.

The problem of relationship between pulmonary and bronchial vascular systems in certain lung diseases is extremely important. In the literature it is not elucidated at all. The study of this relationship will assist not only the clinician in better understanding of the mechanism of some symptoms in various diseases but also the surgeon-pneumonolog in choosing a rational approach to the management of certain lung diseases.

One could have told very much about the value of the book and its author speak for themselves. The subject shows the publishment of the book to be well-timed and utterly important. The author is well-known for his works on clinical aspects of lung diseases as well as on the anatomy and histology of the lung. These matters have been extensively and successfully investigated by Prof. NAGAISHI in cooperation with his collaborators during many years. In his present monograph the author sums up the results of the all enormous long-term work done by himself and his collaborators, and because of that the book acquires particular value.

The book will be read with great interest and benefit by a representative of theoretical and experimental medicine engaged in studying the lungs as well as by any clinician interested in deep investigation of one or another aspect of the pulmonary pathology.

This monograph is a fruit of many years' work of the prominent specialist in the field of the pulmonary surgery. It will undoubtedly win a high approval among all the clinicians, and particularly among the pneumonologs.

March 2, 1971

Professor Fedor G. Uglov
Member of the Academy of Medical Science of the USSR
Lenin Prize Winner
Director of the All-Union Research Institute of Pneumonology
Head of the Department of Surgery
1-st Leningrad Medical Institute

FOREWORD

Prof. NAGAISHI's experience and rich scientific background have enabled him to write this comprehensive treatise on the lung and its anatomic structure. During his busy professional life he has always been preoccupied with the structure, function and diseases of the lung as a whole. His research work was undertaken in view of trying to improve the method of diagnosis and therapy.

This document gives impressiveness to what he writes regarding his knowledge and research. With great confidence, the author leads the physician towards the fundaments of the anatomy of the respiratory organ, giving consideration to practical aspects of physiology and pathology. The thoracic surgeons from all over the world will especially welcome a thorough presentation of the macro- and microscopic observations of the structure, because diagnosis, indication, operative methodology and post-operative treatment depend greatly on the value of these observations.

As will be seen from the title of the book, Prof. NAGAISHI, as a thoracic surgeon, discusses the macro-microscopic anatomy of the tracheobronchial system and the pulmonary vessels in detail, referring to all the differences between the right and left sides. I am deeply impressed by the abundance of the contents and the orderly and elucidative presentation of the description and illustration.

The author has particularly been interested in the observation of the alveolar system, and therefore, in this book, this art is specially noted. By the descriptive presentation he brings the past and new phenomena into a harmonious unity, *i.e.* the state of knowledge of our time. The fine structures of the alveolar epithelium and the alveolar capillary are studied just as emphatically as those of the pulmonary vascular and the bronchial vascular systems.

The lymph vessels and their functional roles have been examined very carefully. For many decades, this separate circulatory system has played a role in the pulmonary and pleural diseases, and moreover, in the case of pulmonary tuberculosis, the elucidation of its pathogenesis was impossible without the knowledge of the lymphatic ways. With the development of the modern surgery of the bronchial carcinoma, the anatomy of the lymphatic system has gained a new significance, in deciding the operability in the open chest as well as the indication for a thoracotomy. Next to the anatomy and the microscopic structure of the lymph node and lymphatic system, the author is especially interested in the lymph flow and predisposing sites of metastases with regard to the pre-operative estimation of the operability with the aid of mediastinoscopy. By subtle scrutiny, Prof. NAGAISHI has succeeded in differentiating the common positional order of the groups of lymph nodes, and in doing so he has proposed a new theory for the topographic systematology, which deserves particular attention.

Among the functional systems examined by the microscopic observation I wish to remark upon the vegetative nervous system whose afferent and efferent courses are pursued to their endings in the bronchopulmonary tissues. Concerning present advanced anatomical knowledge, it may be stated that, in spite of all endeavours by many investigators in the past, the problem of the correlation to the function of the nervous system has been solved only to a limited extent.

The book can be considered as a compact and rich presentation of the macroanatomic and the fine-structured component elements of the lung, and by these characteristics it has the value of an encyclopedia on the morphology of the respiratory organ. Conceived out of the daily experience and the desire for learning in the clinical field, enriched substantially by operative observation and experience, this book was written with the intention of introducing specialized findings on the anatomy of the lung; thus the accomplishment of this piece of work should be considered as a contribution to science which has great and reliable value to the practical duties of the physicians, and the surgeons in particular: Prof. NAGAISHI is most successful in including various subjects into a wide and homogeneous basis whereby achieving a solid foundation which is equally important for both science and practice. Thus, besides feeling content with his competent piece of work the author can be assured of the deep gratitude of his colleagues, which he has earned.

March 31, 1971

Prof. Dr. KARL VOSSSCHULTE,
Direktor der Chirurgischen
Universitätsklinik Giessen

PREFACE

This is a book on the functional anatomy and histology of the lung written by a thoracic surgeon.

The description refers systematically and collectively to the results of our studies, and in the light of previous investigations.

Most of the illustrations are original, excepting for a very few which are indispensable to understanding the content. The inserted illustrations are clearly mentioned as to source.

It was in 1941, 30 years ago, that I resolved to devote myself to the development of surgery of the lung.

What had come to mind at that time was the decision to perform not only clinical but also basic studies of the systems concerned and by the chest surgeons themselves and within the same department, in order to build up chest surgery in as complete a form as possible.

Consequent on this decision, and after World War II, I organized three groups of my associates in research in the Department of Thoracic Surgery of the Chest Disease Research Institute of Kyoto University. Subsequently I have devoted myself entirely to the development of thoracic surgery on this basis to the present time.

In this book, the structures of normal lung, particularly its fine structures are described systematically from studies obtained by our morphology study group, which was organized in 1948. Chapter I–IV describe successively the bronchoalveolar system, the vascular system, the lymphatic system, the nervous system, the muscular system and the pulmonary pleura.

As will be seen from the above, this is clearly a book on anatomy and histology. However, we have endeavored to elucidate various problems not yet made clear by making use of new methods, and fresh materials, such as freshly resected lungs obtained by surgical procedures, comparatively fresh whole lungs from bodies after accidental death, fresh fetal and animal lungs; and throughout we have borne in mind various clinical problems relating to chest diseases. I therefore consider this book to be not precisely comparable to those that have been written by anatomists.

It will give great pleasure to the author if this book is of any assistance, not only to those scholars in basic research but also to chest physicians and chest surgeons.

In the years 1957 and 1958, I published a book on "The Structure of the Lung" (Vol. I and II, in Japanese), in cooperation with my associates Naoyuki Nagasawa, M.D., Masayuki Yamashita, M.D., Yoshio Okada, M.D., and Nobuo Inaba, M.D.

Since then, remarkable progress has been seen in methods of study. We refer to improvement in transmission electron microscopy, development of the scanning electron microscopy, rapid freezing methods, use of fluorescent method to demonstrate vegetative nerves, diffusion of the use of the flexible bronchofiberscope, and use of television in X-ray study, selective segmentography and selective angiography, etc. Thanks to these developments we have successively obtained many new data.

So, I decided to write another book in English, mainly about the fine structures of the lung, incorporating these newly obtained data.

Total pages of the Japanese Edition was 608 pages. However, the English Edition will be published in one volume of about half the pages of the Japanese Edition, considering the publisher's request.

Accordingly, I had to omit most of our studies on the surgical anatomy from the English Edition, except for the essential points of the macroscopic findings.

Thus, while the title of the Japanese Edition was "The Structure of the Lung", that of the English Edition is more appropriately entitled "Functional Anatomy and Histology of the Lung".

The collaborators who were in our department at the time of publication of the Japanese Edition now occupy responsible positions elsewhere.

Therefore, this whole volume was written this time by myself alone. However, this book still contains many data amassed by my associates in these past years. It is now the sincere wish of the author to enumerate the names of these researchers as collaborators again this time, in the memory of the days when I shared pleasures and pains with them.

In the text, the outline, history, methods of study, and the pathological, physiological and clinical problems relating to the normal structure of the lung are put in small types.

March 31, 1971

CHUZO NAGAISHI, M.D.
Professor, Head, Department of Thoracic Surgery
Chest Disease Research Institute
Kyoto University

ACKNOWLEDGEMENT

I wish to gratefully appreciate generous forewords by my respected senior Emeritus Prof. KÔ HIRASAWA, and my esteemed overseas friends, Prof. H. STANLEY BENNETT, Prof. ANTONIO BLASI, Prof. EDWARD A. BOYDEN, Prof. JULIUS H. COMROE, Prof. ARTHUR M. OLSEN, Prof. WILLIAM O. REINHARDT, Prof. FEDOR G. UGLOV, Prof. KARL VOSSSCHULTE (*in alphabetical order*), with full of compliments and praises which have added splendor to this book. I also wish to extend my respects and thanks to Prof. and Mrs. W. O. REINHARDT who kindly have taken care of correcting the English version, sharing their busy time. I am also indebted to Mrs. BETTY KELLY (The REINHARDTS' friend) who had stayed in Kyoto for three months for her many helpful advices and suggestions in the efforts of finishing the English manuscripts.

I am also grateful to my associates of the Morphological Study Group of our Department for their collaboration in the essential researches which built foundation of this book. As well, my thanks are also extended to Mrs. YOKO NOHARA who cooperated in English translation of the Japanese manuscripts. To my secretary, Miss TERUKO ONOGI I wish to express my appreciation for her sincere efforts in handwriting of the Japanese manuscripts, and preparing materials, having made overtime everyday since September, 1969. Lastly, I wish to thank as well to Igaku Shoin Ltd. who kindly accepted the publication of this book.

June 16, 1971

CHUZO NAGAISHI, M.D.
Emeritus Professor of
Kyoto University

CONTENTS

Chapter I. Bronchoalveolar System

The bronchoalveolar system denotes the part of the respiratory system which has conventionally been designated as the bronchial system; it may be divided into two principal parts, one possessing the character of an airway and the other having a respiratory character.

The former comprises the portions of the bronchial tree from the main bronchus, extending peripherally to the terminal bronchioles; the latter corresponds to what may be called the alveolar system or alveolar region, extending from the respiratory bronchioles to the alveoli.

It is no exaggeration, in this context, to state that the term bronchoalveolar system represents the lung both structurally and functionally and hence is properly designatory of the lung.

The achievements that have been made in the study of the lung are indeed numerous and diverse in content, the earliest reports having appeared some three hundred years ago.

The outline of the macroscopic structure of the system as yet is sparse in not a few respects, and it is for this reason that certain clinical and basic studies of the lung may seldom be satisfactory explicated by our current knowledge of the structure of the lung.

I. GENERAL SURVEY OF TRACHEA AND BRONCHI

A. External Appearance

The trachea is continuous with the larynx by way of the cricoid cartilage. Normally, it begins at the level of the seventh cervical vertebra, extending downward along the anterior wall of the esophagus to the fourth or fifth thoracic vertebra at which level it divides into the main divisions, the right and left main bronchi.

The level of the tracheal bifurcation usually corresponds to that of the second costal cartilage as projected to the anterior thoracic wall. In children, the bifurcation is at the level of the third cartilage.

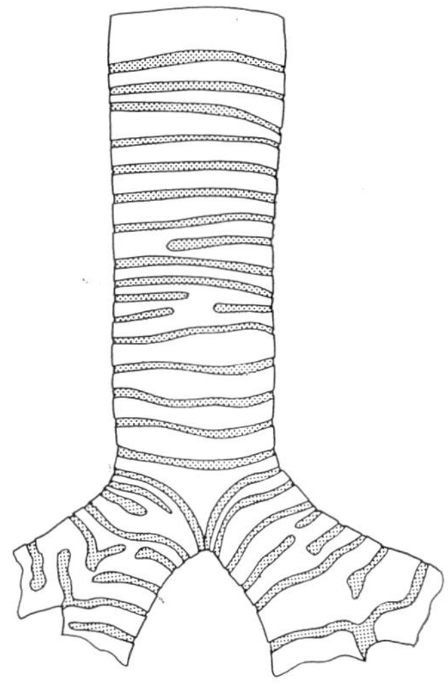

Fig. 1 Cartilages of the trachea and main bronchi.

The major part of the tracheal wall (Fig. 1) is formed by a series of sixteen to twenty horseshoe shaped hoops of hyaline tracheal cartilages; these are invested by annular ligaments which span the intervals between them. The hyaline cartilages, 3 to 4 mm in width, are arranged in a regular series, except that at times several adjoining cartilages are united, and in some instances individual cartilages are diversely bifurcated.

The posterior wall of the trachea, on the other hand, is composed of a flat membranous part devoid of hyaline cartilage. Between this part and the anterior wall of the esophagus there are loose connective tissues.

The trachea branches off into two main divisions, the right and left bronchi, at an angle of seventy to one hundred degrees. The right bronchus forms an angle of 20 to 40° with the vertical line, and the left bronchus forms an angle of 40 to 60°. The carina or keel is situated at the inside of the tracheal bifurcation.

The right bronchus is somewhat larger in caliber than the left but is conversely a little shorter in length. The right bronchus may appear as if it is an extension of the trachea; the left bronchus appears to be a branch of the trachea.

The left main bronchus divides into two lobar bronchi, upper and lower, and the right main bronchus into three lobar bronchi, upper, middle and lower.

On the left side, the region peripheral from the point where the upper lobe bronchus is divided from the main bronchus is regarded as the lower lobe bronchus. On the right side, NAGAISHI, et al. designated the region from the bifurcation of the upper lobe bronchus to the bifurcation of the middle lobe bronchus as the intermediate bronchus, and the region peripheral from the point of the bifurcation of the middle lower bronchus as the lower lobe bronchus.

The lobar bronchus, in turn, produces segmental bronchi to supply discrete areas of lung tissue termed segments, eight on the left and ten on the right.

The bronchial cartilages lose the typical horseshoe shape where the lobar bronchi begin and the membranous part disappears. With the progressive further ramification of the bronchus, the cartilaginous pieces in the bronchi are quite irregular in shape and are arranged like pavement or stepping stones. With further bifurcations of the bronchi in more peripheral regions, the cartilaginous pieces become more isolated, and finally the pieces appear to be scattered in various parts of the bronchial wall. Plates of cartilages are found, in general, at levels of bifurcation.

B. Tracheobronchoscopic and Flexible Bronchofiberscopic Findings

Endoscopically, the trachea is inclined somewhat to the left of the median line. The posterior wall is relatively flat, though at times slightly protuberant into the tracheal space. The anterior wall is rendered somewhat rigid, assuming an arch-like shape transversally by virture of the presence of the tracheal cartilages.

On extreme exertion, the trachea is pressed and flattened ventrodorsally. In infants, in particular, such a finding is encountered even on deep inspiration.

Because of pressure of the thyroid and of the aortic arch, the cross sections of the upper part and the part slightly above the tracheal bifurcation are ovoid internally. Pulsations can be seen endoscopically through the tracheal wall at the level of the aortic arch.

The trachea and the bronchi are quite elastic but loosely connected with the surrounding tissues, and can readily be moved at endoscopic examination.

Thus, remarkably flexible and movable, the trachea and the bronchi are constructed so as to permit a rather free bending against traction or pressure from the surrounding tissues, as well as in respiratory movements, in order to constantly concerve a sufficient airway.

Fig. 2 shows the endoscopic views of the trachea and bronchi as seen on flexible bronchofiberscopic examinations.

C. Normal Respiratory Movements

In company with the movement of the thorax and the diaphragm, the lung expands passively on inspiration and shrinks passively on expiration.

The thorax may be regarded as a cylinder supported dorsally by the vertebral column, somewhat narrowed at the upper end and opened widely at the lower end.

The upper part of the thorax consists of muscles and other soft tissues that are based on the first rib, manubrium of the sternum and body of the first thoracic vertebra. The movement of this part of the thorax, however, is rather modest and the respiratory movement of the lung encompassed by it is limited.

The lateral wall of the thorax is composed of the series of the ribs other than the first, by the costal cartilages and intercostal muscles, etc., permitting significant respiratory movements.

Situated practically parallel to the boundary line between the upper and middle lobes and the lower lobe of the lung anteriorly are the fifth rib or fifth intercostal space. The respiratory movements of the lung above and below this boundary line differ greatly in their features.

The thoracic movement is directly reflected in the upper and middle lobes and the upper part of the lower lobe of the lung, at inspiration. The greater part of the lower lobe, expanding *in toto* in

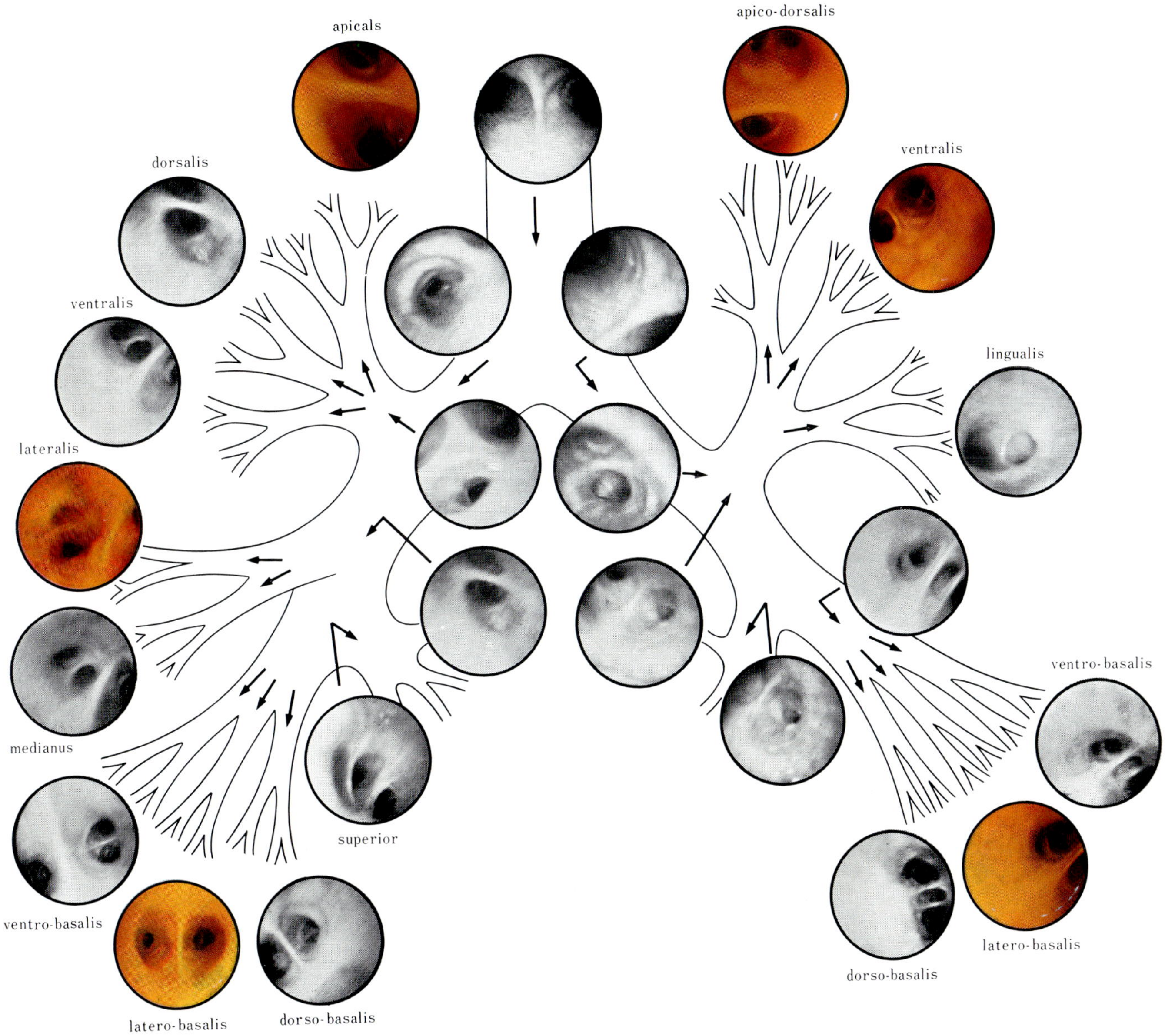

Fig. 2 Flexible bronchofiberscopic findings (S. IKEDA).

harmony with the movement of the thorax, expands and inflates downward and outward, in company with the descending movement of the diaphragm.

II. STRUCTURE OF TRACHEA AND BRONCHUS

A. Macroscopic Structure

1. Tracheal Cartilages and Membranous Part

The wall of the trachea is, as mentioned above, supported by a series of sixteen to twenty horseshoe shaped hyaline cartilages which are invested by annular ligaments; the latter spans the intervals between the cartilages and complete the tracheal wall dorsally.

The membranous part is composed of layers of smooth muscle, a flat, elastic membrane, an epithelial layer, and other cellular components. It extends to the level of the lobar bronchus, and is lacking in the segmental bronchi and in more peripheral bronchi. As can be seen (Fig. 3), the membranous part of the trachea adheres to the anterior wall of the esophagus by way of a small quantity of loose connective tissue.

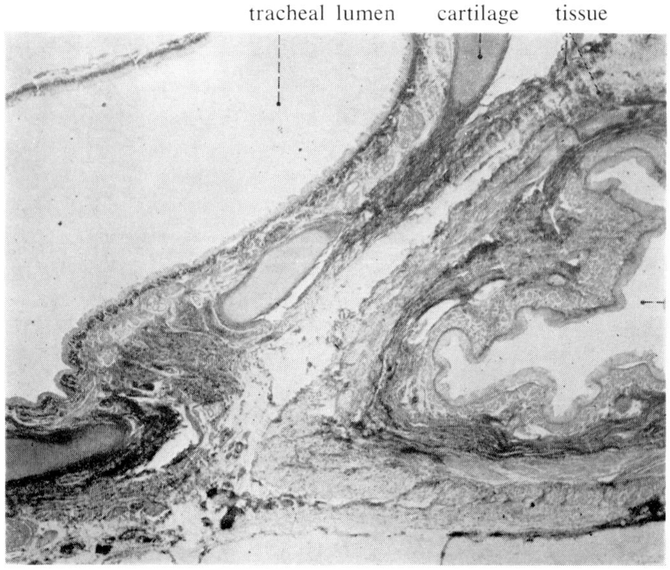

Fig. 3 Trachea and esophagus of the fetus.

Formalin-fixed specimens of the trachea usually exhibit marked contraction of the non-cartilaginous part. However, during life, the annular ligaments span the intervals between cartilages and render the tracheal wall somewhat rigid.

2. Tracheal Bifurcation

Situated at the level of the tracheal bifurcation, where the two main divisions of the trachea, the right and left bronchi begin, is the tracheal carina or keel.

The carina, comprising mainly cartilaginous elements and projecting into the interior of the windpipe, links and the anterior and posterior walls of the trachea at its bifurcation. HELLER and von SCHROETTER (1897) have described the tracheal carina as being composed primarily of three structurally distinct parts, cartilaginous, membranous and partly membranous.

The cartilaginous part of the carina, according to these authors, may be subdivided principally into two parts, tracheal and bronchial, depending upon whether the cartilage belongs to the trachea or to the bronchi.

The latter may be further divided roughly into two parts, right or left bronchial. In some instances, bronchial cartilages on both sides are found to occur in unity with each other to form a double-bronchial cartilaginous carina. Rarely, the tracheal cartilage and the bronchial cartilage are found united together to constitute a tracheobronchial carina.

Bronchial cartilages vary in shape. They rarely take a simple ring-like shape; in most instances, they are united together or various ramified.

The bronchi lose the horseshoe shape on merging with the lobar bronchi. The shape becomes round; the bronchial cartilages and membranous parts that have been supporting the horseshoe shape disappear. The cartilages then surround irregularly the circumference of the bronchus.

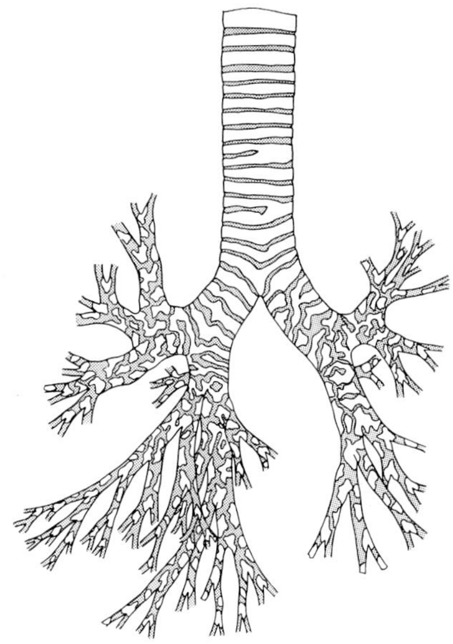

Fig. 4 Bronchial cartilages.

Fig. 4 is a schematic representation of the macroscopic distribution of tracheal and bronchial cartilages.

3. Blood Vessels

The networks of nutrient blood vessels distributed to the walls of the trachea and bronchi belong to the systemic circulation.

Bronchial arteries run along the adventitia which consists of connective tissues and covers the outer surface of the trachea. The main bronchial arteries usually accompany the bronchi bilaterally, proceeding toward the periphery, supplying the annular ligaments and membranous part with many small branches. These branches are further distributed to the perichondrium, to smooth muscles and to secretory glands. They pass through the elastic lamina of the trachea as well as the mucosal-muscular layers of the bronchi, to be distributed as capillary network in the mucous membranes. Bronchial veins proceed in the opposite direction and convey the blood into the azygos or hemiazygos vein.

The blood vessels distributed to the trachea and to the bronchi correspond to the extrapulmonary bronchial vessels that have been designated by M. YAMASHITA (1954). However, the direction and points of origin differ entirely from those of the intrapulmonary bronchial vessels described by YAMASHITA. Detailed accounts will be given in the chapter on the vascular system.

B. Fine Structure

The walls of the main bronchi and intrapulmonary bronchi are practically the same instructure as for the trachea, being comprised of mucous membrane, cartilages, muscular layer, adventitia, etc.

In the following part of this section, the general structure will be first described; accounts as to the differences between the various structural units of the bronchial system will then be given.

1. Mucous Membrane

a. Tracheobronchial Epithelium

The trachea and the bronchi are lined by a mucous membrane with ciliated epithelium upon its inner surface, and also containing goblet cells and basal cells. The epithelium appears as if in layers or stratified, but actually all the cells rest upon a common basement membrane. That is, as has already been described by SCHULTZE (1871), the tracheobronchial epithelium is composed of a single layer of ciliated cells with some germinal epithelial cells among them; there is no evidence of stratification of the epithelial cells that line the trachea and bronchi.

Fig. 5 is a schematic representation showing this relationship, and Fig. 6 exemplifies microscopic evidences in support of the view.

Ciliated Epithelium: The ciliated cells are columnar in appearance. They diminish gradually in height in the bronchial branches are not rather cuboidal in further peripheral areas.

As shown in Fig. 7, electron microscopic observation reveals the presence of numerous microvilli as well as a number of cilia at the free edges of these cells. The microvilli are projections of the cytoplasm.

As can be seen from Fig. 8, there exists at the center of each cilium a pair of central filaments

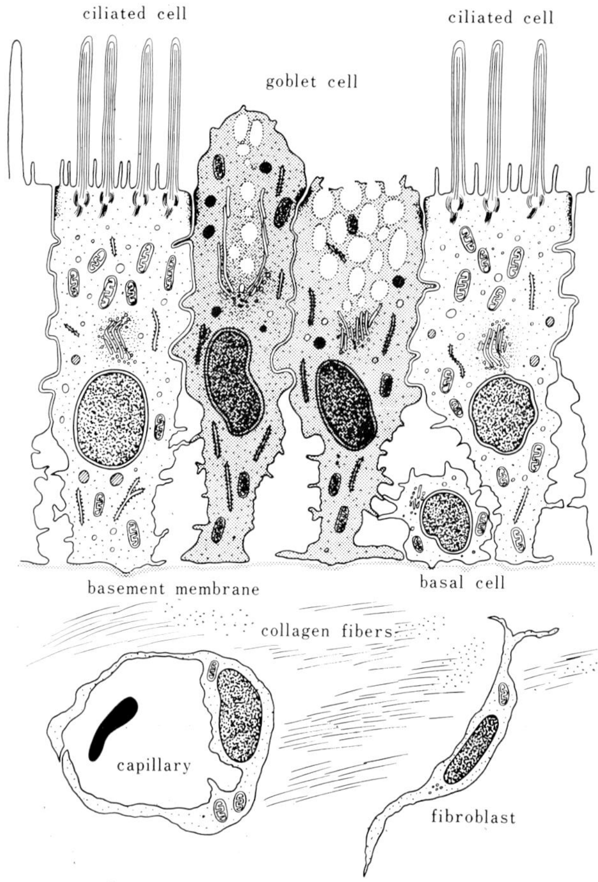

Fig. 5 Bronchial epithelial cells (schema).

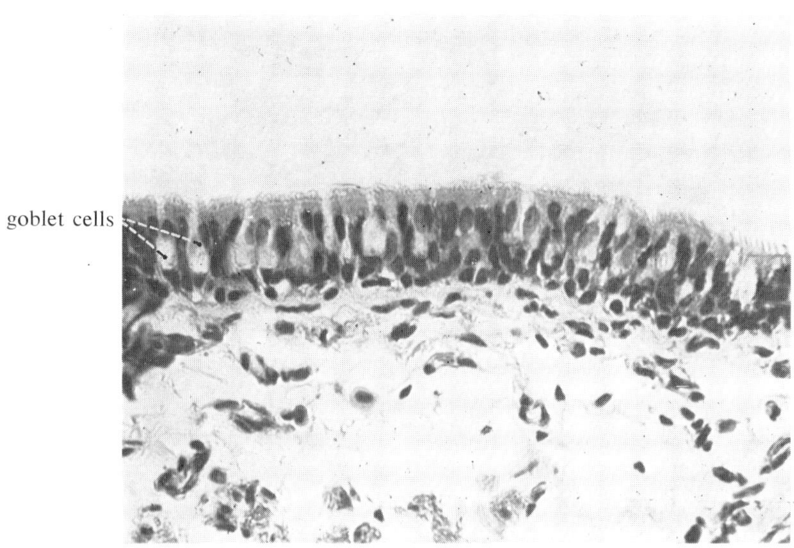

Fig. 6 Bronchial epithelium.

surrounded by nine pairs of peripheral filaments. The ciliated epithelium is generally believed to be regenerated from dividing cells.

The cilia extending from inside the cell into the respiratory passage penetrate the cuticles. These cuticles covering the surface of the ciliated cells correspond to ectoplasms, and are generally believed to have bearing functionally on the absorption of substances. The nucleus, round to ovoid, is usually situated centricellularly, though somewhat closer to the basement membrane. In normal states, mitotic figures are found infrequently.

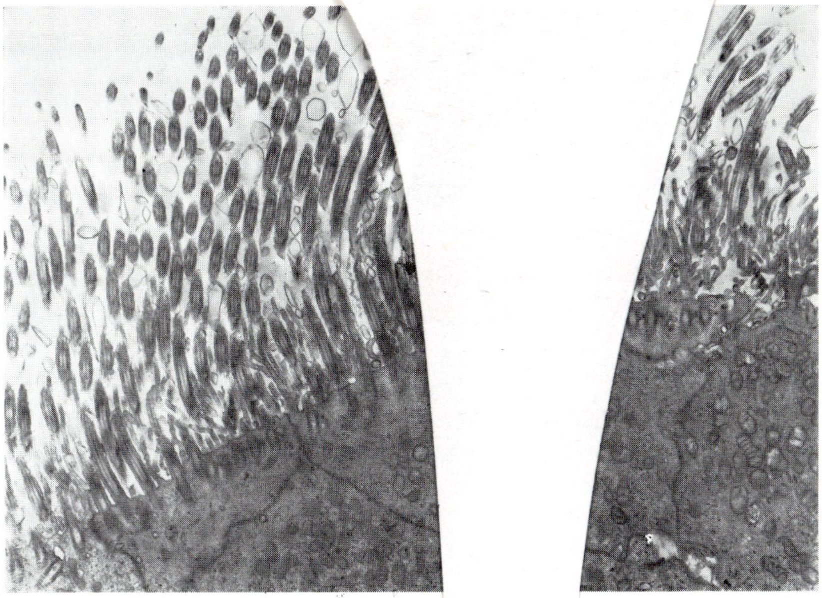

Fig. 7 Ciliated cells [obscured] us.

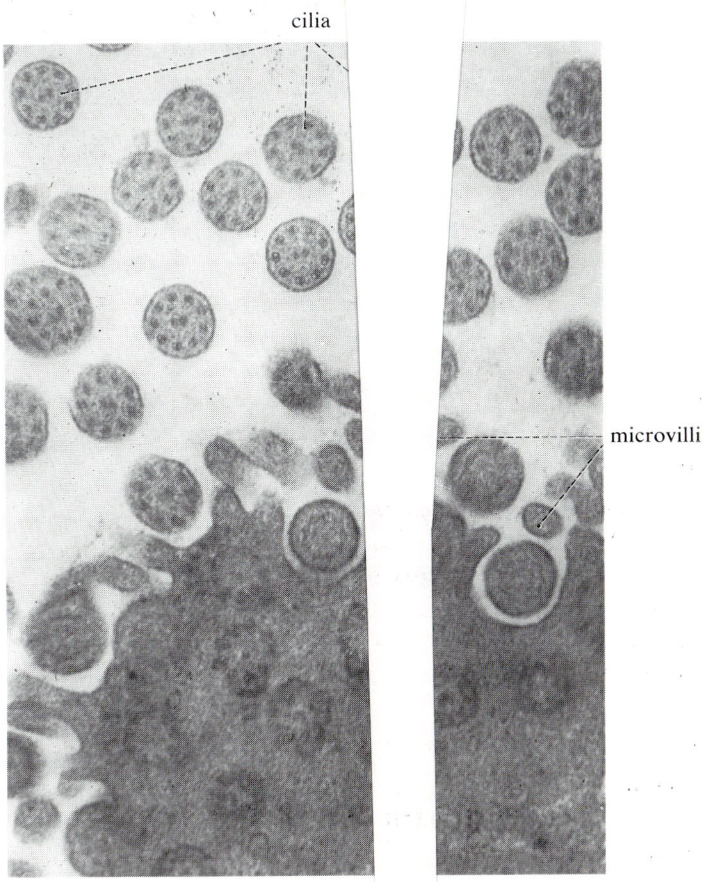

Fig. 8 Cilia of bronchia[obscured] elium.

MILLER (1937) reported on ciliated cells as occasionally possessing two nuclei, and BOCKENDAHL (1885) observed mitotic figures when investigating the regenerative process of the tracheal epithelium. The authors have not as yet encountered such microscopic findings.

The connection between adjoining ciliated cells, according to CHAMBERS and RÉNYI (1925), is not organic in nature, unlike the case of stratified pavement epithelial cells. Exfoliation of single cells, therefore, is generally considered to have no direct effect upon the neighboring cells.

Ciliated cells that have been detached from the epithelial sheet into the respiratory passage have free edges which are apparently wider than the opposite basal edges. Not infrequently these detached cells are devoid of cilias. In sputa, these cells are in many instances elliptical in shape and very poorly cytoplasmic, with hypochromic nuclei.

Goblet cells: Goblet cells are interposed between the ciliated epithelial cells; their longitudinal cross sections, as can be seen from Fig. 9, are usually barrel shaped.

When observed from the epithelial surface, the individual goblet cells are seen to be clear and round. The clear ovoid parts correspond to the cups of the goblets, from which abruptly narrowed cytoplasmic extensions reach the basement membrane beneath. The translucent parts are at times compressed and deformed by the neighboring ciliated epithelium. Nuclei are usually situated in the outer portions of the translucent parts of individual cells. The distance between the nucleus and the adjoining basement membrane is similar in all the cells.

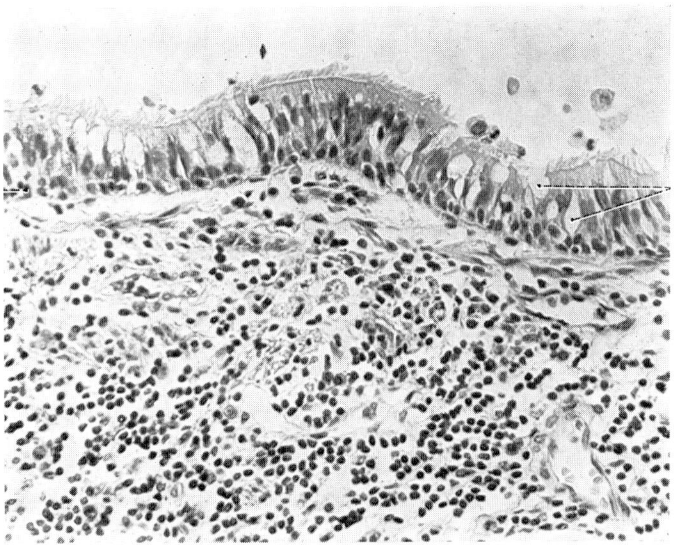

Fig. 9 Bronchial epithelium.

The number of goblet cells in the tracheobronchial tree varies; it is greater in the trachea than in the bronchi, and is virtually nil in the cuboidal epithelium of the peripheral parts of the bronchus.

Fig. 10 is an electron microscopic finding of a goblet cell.

WALLER and BJÖRKMAN (1882), MERKEL (1902), and KÖLLIKER (1854, 1881), described goblet cells as representing ciliated cells undergoing mucous degeneration, whereas DRASCH (1881), stated that goblet cells represent a transitional form between Keilzellen and ciliated epithelium.

Basal Cells: Basal cells rest immediately upon the basement membrane and are pressed on by the neighboring cells, thereby being quite variable in shape. The nucleus is normally basal in position; the cell body is usually tall, narrowly triangular or spindle-shaped and situated directly on the basement membrane. It is not rare that the cells extend almost to the epithelial surface.

Fig. 11 is an electron microscopic finding of a basal cell.

MILLER (1937), distinguishing the basement cells from replacing cells, has described the replacing cells as originating in basement cells including the Ersatzellen of Kölliker and the Keilzellen of Drasch.

Basement Membrane: The basement membrane, which constitutes a boundary between the epithelium and the lamina propria, is observed as a band of homogenous, amorphous material in sections stained with hematoxylin and eosin, whereas, after the silver impregnation, it is observed as a thin membrane composed of dense networks of slender argyrophilic fibers.

b. Lamina Propria and Elastic Longitudinal Bundle

The lamina propria is composed of connective tissues which are highly vascular, with networks of arterioles and capillaries which essentially are bronchial vessels. With silver impregnated tissue preparations, it is noted that the walls of these arterioles and venules are encircled by annular muscle cells. Nuclei of endothelial cells are also seen sporadically within this area. Capillary networks are distributed immediately beneath the basement membrane.

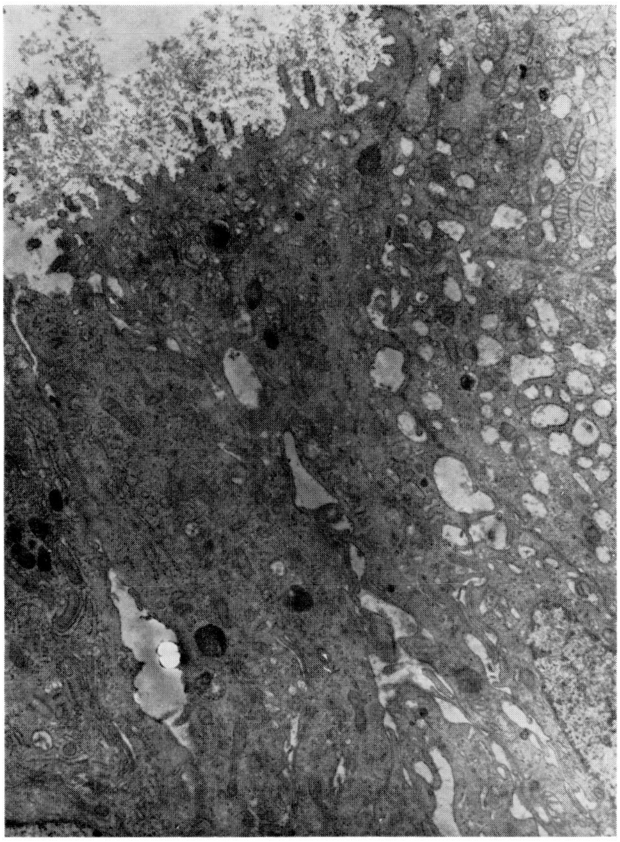

Fig. 10 Goblet cell of the bronchial epithelium.

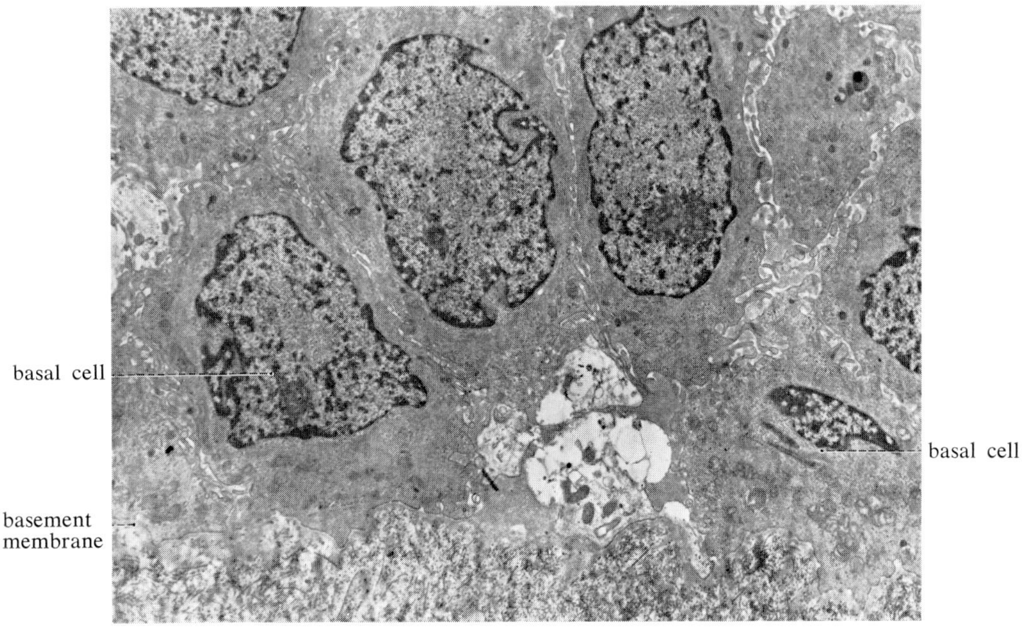

Fig. 11 Basal cell of the bronchus.

Embedded in the lamina propria are vessels, lymphatic tissues and nerve fibers. External to the lamina propria of the wall of the trachea, there is a well defined layer of longitudinal elastic fibers, the elastic longitudinal bundle, which is limited to the trachea (Fig. 12).

c. Submucous Coat

The submucous coat consists of a loose network of connective tissues in which bronchial vessels, nerve fibers, tracheal or bronchial secretory glands and adipose tissues reside. The secretory glands are relatively more abundant in the anterior wall.

The secretary elements essentially belong in the category of tubulo-alveolar glands.

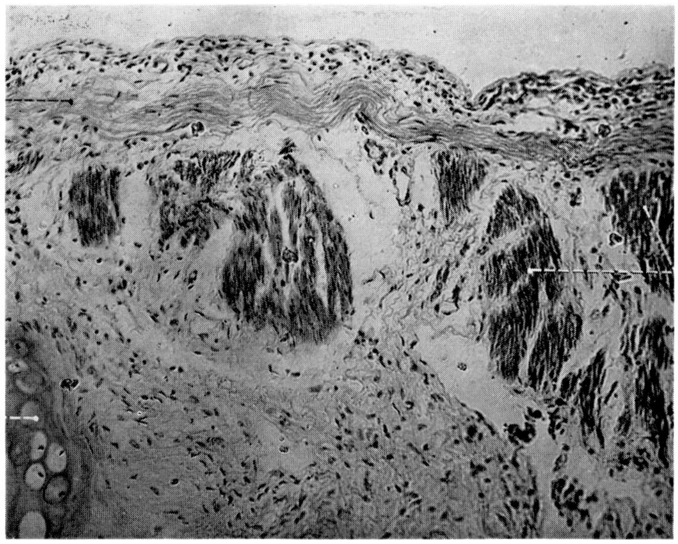

Fig. 12 Longitudinal elastic bundle of the bronchus.

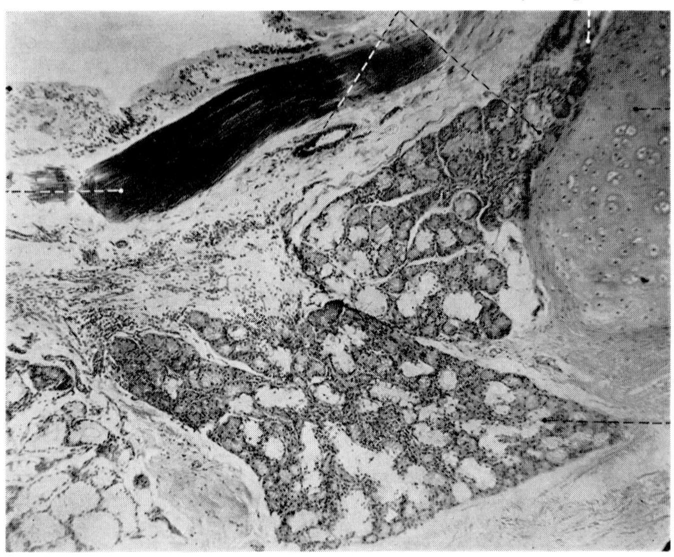

Fig. 13 Bronchial mucous gland.

In the membranous part, bodies of the glands are found external to the layer of smooth muscles. These glands are furnished with long excretory ducts which penetrate the muscle layer and open upon the surface of the mucous membrane.

Serous and mucous cells are the grandular cells contributing to the serous or mucous secretion; these two types of cells at times occur together to effect a mixed mucous and serous secretion. The mucous cells are translucent, whereas in the case of serous cells, the cell bodies are rather dark under the photomicroscope.

Fig. 13 shows the histological appearance of a bronchial mucous gland; Fig. 14 is an electron microscopic finding of a bronchial mucous cell.

2. Cartilage

The macroscopic structure of the tracheal and bronchial cartilages is as described above.

3. Muscular Layer

The intrinsic musculature of the trachea and the bronchi is composed, without exception, of smooth muscle.

External to the layer of muscles of the membranous part, which annularly encircle the tracheal tube, are longitudinal muscles which are present in a small quantity.

The muscular layer encircling the bronchi consists of spiral bands of smooth muscles, the distribution of which is demonstrably sparse. This layer, as well as related elastic fibers, undoubtedly serves to render the respiratory tract satisfactorily elastic.

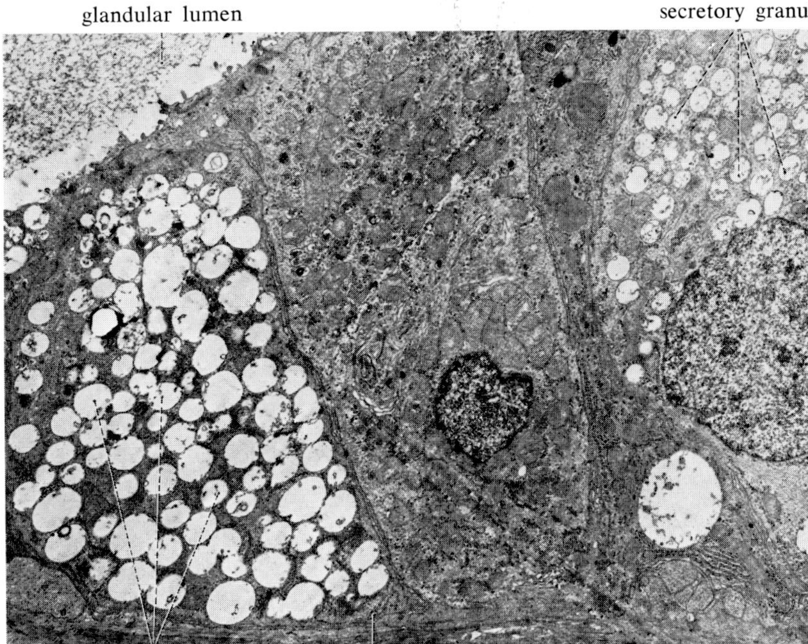

Fig. 14 Bronchial mucous gland (transmission electron microscopy).

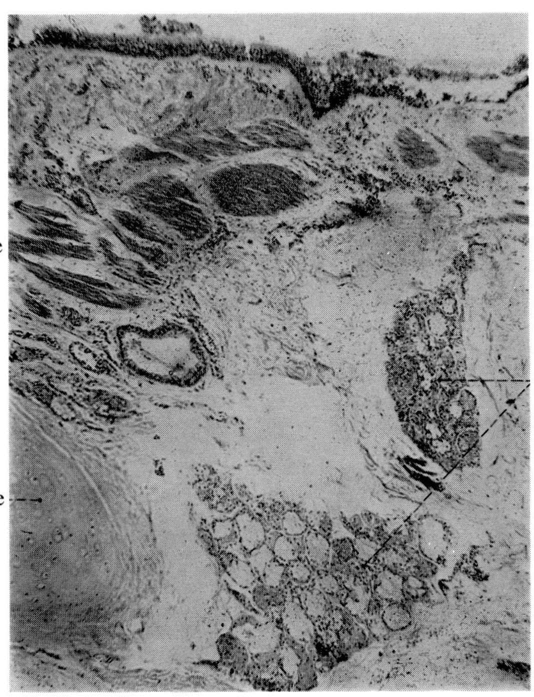

Fig. 15 Elements of the bronchial wall.

Shown in Fig. 15 is smooth muscle of the bronchial wall. The exact distribution and morphological characteristics will be described in detail in the chapter pertaining to the muscular system.

As for localization of the muscles in the bronchial and tracheal walls, there are two opposing views.

MILLER (1937, 1947) has quoted the theory of CUVIER (1805) that muscles are found outside the cartilage in the tracheal and bronchial walls of carnivora, consistently internal to the cartilage in the case of herbivorous animals, and in most cases internal to the cartilage in the human, but it is evident that the view does not have wholehearted support. MILLER claims that muscles are all connected with the perichondrium at some distance from the tip of the cartilages irrespective of their localization relative to the cartilage. On the other hand, VERSON (1871) and FRANKENHÄUSER (1879) describe that the lateral side of the muscular insertions connects with the intercartilaginous connective tissues.

4. Adventitia

The adventitia of the trachea and the bronchi is composed of connective tissue which contains small numbers of elastic fibers; the latter impart strength to the walls, and connect with adjoining organs and tissues. Particularly, the adventitia of the membranous part is joined by a layer of loose connective tissue to the esophagus.

III. INTRAPULMONARY BRONCHI AND BRONCHIOLES

A. Types of Bronchial Branching

Numerous studies have been published as to the mode of intrapulmonary branching of the bronchi.

Adopted conventionally, besides the usual anatomical approaches, are the methods whereby mercury, the metallic compound of WOOD, or other rapidly solidifiable, colored liquid materials are injected intrabronchially. In recent years, however, casting of the bronchial tree by the injection of synthetic rubber or resins has come to be most frequently applied.

While a review of classical literature concerning the intrapulmonary bronchial distribution or architecture will not be engaged in here, the question of whether bronchi diverge to give off successive generations monopodially or by dichotomy has been in controversy for many years.

FLINT (1907) and MILLER in (1937) attempting to establish standardization of the types of bronchial branching, described intrapulmonary bronchial branching as monopodial in the case of the main bronchi, but monopodial and dichotomous in the distal remainder.

The findings obtained by NAGASAWA, M. YAMASHITA and NAGAISHI (1952) in studies with acrylic resins which were introduced intrabronchially were as follows: The main bronchi branch off monopodially, whereas the small bronchi are predominantly ramified dichotomously, and (with exception of the branches in the neighborhood of terminal bronchioles) most of the small bronchi even in fairly peripheral regions failed to show regular dichotomous branchings, since one of each pair of branches was often found to be developed or enlarged out of all proportion to its counterpart.

Some of the respiratory bronchioles peripheral to the terminal bronchioles were monopodial, and alveolar ducts were found to be ramified mostly in a trichotomous manner.

Shown in Fig. 16 is a diagram of ramifications of the respiratory tree including the trachea, main bronchi and intrapulmonary bronchi.

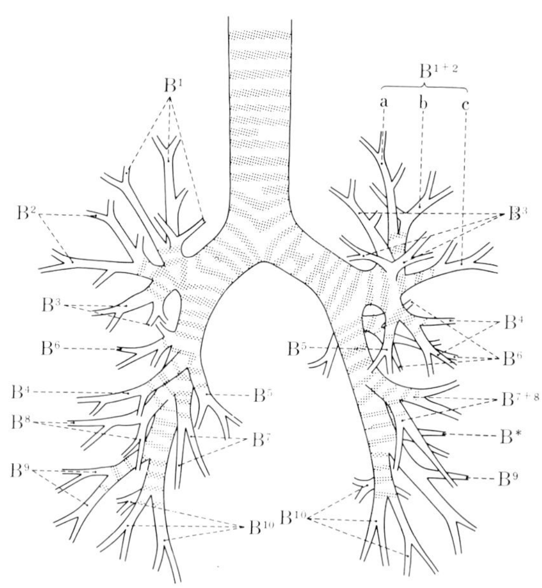

Fig. 16 Branching of the bronchus.

Supplement: Methods for Injection of Acrylic Resin into Bronchi and Blood Vessels

In as much as the methods for intratracheal or intrabronchial injection of acrylic resins have been employed frequently, not only in the above quoted studies of the mode of bronchial ramifications but also in the research studies on the bronchoalveolar system and the vascular system of the lung, the techniques will be described here. As for preparation of resin casts, there are the methods introduced by LIEBOW, and by several other groups of investigators. Here, the methods of the present authors (NAGAISHI, NAGASAWA and M. YAMASHITA, 1952) will be described.

Table 1 Injection material for making of resin cast

Method I		weight ratio	
i)	Methylmetacrylate (Polymer)	100.0	powder
	Benzoyl peroxide	3.0	
	Dibutylphthalate	20.0	
ii)	Methylmetacrylate (Monomer)	100.0	solution
	Dimethylanilin	2.1	
	Dimethylethanolamin	1.5	
iii)	Color dye		
Method II		**weight ratio**	
	Ethylacrylate (Monomer)	100.0	
	Methylmetacrylate (Polymer)	20.0	
	Benzoyl peroxide	0.5	

Method I

The method herein to be described is designed to provide an instant preparation of acrylic resins for intratracheal or intrabronchial injection, and an instant or rapid polymerization of the resins, and to effect resin casting of the lumina of even the most minute bronchial and vascular branches. It is also practicable with this method to fill the lymphatic vessels of the lung.

Consequently, not only does the method facilitate examination of necropsy materials obtained from laboratory animals, or of clinical specimens that have been resected surgically; it is also possible to inject resins at any time into autopsy specimens which come to hand without advance notice. Such are the practical advantages of the method.

Preparation of Injecting Material: Table 1 shows the composition of the injection material.

As can be seen, the principal components are methylmethacrylate monomer and polymers:

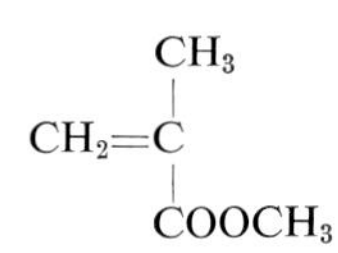

monomer

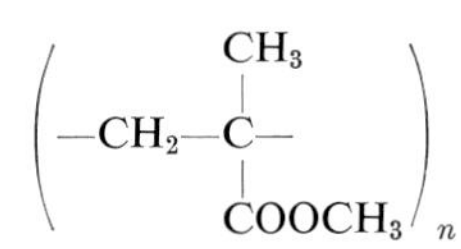

polymer

Benzoyl peroxide, dimethylanilin and dimethylethanolamin are used concomitantly as polymerization accelerators and dibutylphthalate as a plasticizer. In attempting to prepare roentgenographs of the injected specimens, the injection may be conveniently performed with the described casting material by adding five per cent bismuth subnitrate.

When it is necessary to distinguish between the bronchi and the blood vessels by colors, oil paints may be added to the injection mixture.

The kind and quality of oil colors substantially affect the condition of resin polymerization. Therefore, it is important to carefully investigate beforehand the condion of polymerization with the individual coloring materials to be added, before preparing the colored injection materials.

As a polymer the material should be in powder form and as fine as possible.

On theoretical grounds, mixtures containing polymers ranging in size from 100–200 mesh can be said to reach, upon injection, the extremities of the bronchioles but, in practice, polymerization is apt to progress inconveniently to an excess before the material reaches the outer-most peripheral spaces unless particularly fine polymers of around 300 mesh are used. Therefore, it is definitely advisable to use polymer powders of approximately 300 mesh whenever injection of the casting material into the terminal areas such as alveoli and capillaries is attempted.

As the composition shown in Table 1 is based on the data obtained as optimal for preparation of the injection material at a room temperature of 15°C, it is of import to vary or adjust the ratio of (i) to (ii) and the amount of benzoyl peroxide to some extent according to the room temperature at which the material is prepared and injected. This is because the temperature, the (i)–(ii) ratio and the amount of benzoyl peroxide to be added eventually affect the rate of polymerization to a considerable degree.

When the room temperature is about 15°C, the (i)–(ii) ratio should desirably be 1:5, whereas when the temperature is higher, it should advisably be 1:6 to 1:8, prior to preparation of the material, ingredient (ii) may be precooled in an ice-water bath for best results. If the room temperature is particularly low, the ratio may be reduced to 1:2 to 1:4.

It is also important to note that the amount of benzoyl peroxide to be added should be reduced to below 2 or above 4 when the room temperature at which the casting material is prepared and injected is higher or lower than the average respectively.

Irrigation: In injecting resins into the bronchi it is not necessary to irrigate the bronchi beforehand. However, irrigation of blood vessels with physiological saline is advisable before injection of the casting material into the vessels. For this, the specimen should desirably be as fresh as possible.

Fig. 17 shows the apparatus. The authors have devised it for irrigation of blood vessels.

The irrigation of pulmonary blood vessels can be done in two ways:

Irrigation from the pulmonary artery: If irrigation is to be performed with the lung remaining in the thoracic cavity, "d" in Fig. 17 is introduced into the right ventricle of the heart before initiation of the irrigation. If irrigation is to be undertaken with the lung removed from the thoracic cavity, "d" should be introduced into the central end of the pulmonary artery. The pressure suitable for irrigation of blood vessels is approximately 20 mmHg.

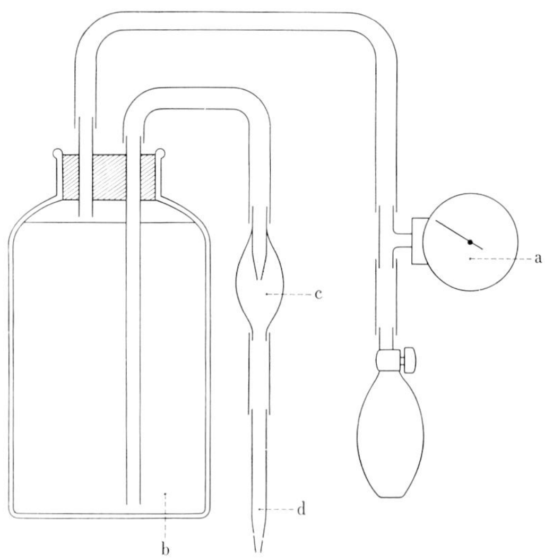

Fig. 17 Instrument for irrigation.
a: manometer, b: saline solution
c: drop bottle, d: pipe for instillation

Irrigation from the bronchial artery: Irrigation is initiated by introducing "d" into the base of the aorta after ligation of all such blood vessels as the common carotid artery, the subclavian artery, the innominate artery and the descending aorta, as well as intercostal arteries which may be ligated at positions peripheral to the branching of bronchial arteries.

The optimal pumping pressure of irrigation is about 120 mmHg. Caution should be exercised to hold the pressure below this level.

Irrigation is continued until the effluent irrigating solution from the pulmonary vein becomes completely cleared of blood macroscopically.

Injection of Acrylic Resin: The resins are injected by means of the apparatus shown in Fig. 18 which should be shaken constantly during the injection.

Intrabronchial injection of resin may be accomplished by means of a syringe.

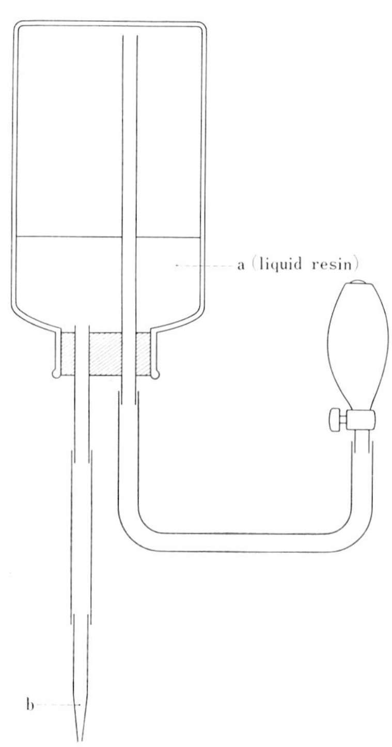

Fig. 18 Instrument for resin instillation.
a: liquid resin
b: pipe for instillation

When the pulmonary artery or the bronchial artery is to be filled with the resin, "b" in Fig. 18 is introduced into the base of the pulmonary artery or of the aorta respectively for injection just as in the case of irrigation.

When injecting into the blood vessels, a syringe may also be used as in the case of the intrabronchial injection, but the use of the syringe is often not desirable since excessive pressurization may result.

Polymerization of the Injected Resin: The injected acrylic resin undergoes polymerization spontaneously with the lapse of time at room temperature, and the specimen solidifies within a short space of time.

Corrosion of the Surrounding Tissues: After polymerization of the injected resin is completed, the hardened specimen is soaked in a 20 to 30 per cent caustic soda solution, which may be renewed at 24-hour intervals. The process, *i.e.* corrosion, is usually continued for about three days. The surrounding, unwanted tissues thus become corroded and the resin which is quite refractory to acids and alkalis, remains as a cast of the lumen of the vessels.

Rinsing of Resin Cast: The resin cast thus prepared is thoroughly rinsed in softly running water, with great care being taken to avoid breakage.

Observation of Resin Cast: The resin cast thus completed is examined macroscopically; portion or portions may be removed and observed under the microscope.

Photographs and photomicrographs of the cast may be taken and sketches made for detailed examination.

Method II

The method is particularly suited for preparation of resin casts and for microscopic observation of microtome sections, as in the case of the preparation of ordinary tissue sections for histological study.

Therefore, unlike Method I above, removal of the surrounding tissues by corrosive treatment need not be done, and the tissue, containing casts, are cut into sections.

The chief ingredients of the casting mixture to be employed in Method II are ethylacrylate monomer and its polymers:

$$CH_2{=}\overset{\displaystyle H}{\underset{\displaystyle COOC_2H_5}{C}} \qquad \text{monomer}$$

$$\left(-CH_2-\overset{\displaystyle H}{\underset{\displaystyle COOC_2H_5}{C}}-\right)_n \qquad \text{polymer}$$

which may be combined with other ingredients according to the composition shown in Table 1.

As can be seen, the purpose of Method II is primarily to make possible parallel microscopic examination of the architecture, both histologic and three dimensional, of the lumen of the respiratory tree and of associated blood vessels.

For this reason, in Method II, the tissue containing a resin cast is cut into halves with an encephalotome; one half is processed as in the case of Method I for removal of surrounding tissues by corrosion, and the other half is made into sections for microscopic examination without removal of the tissues by corrosive treatment with caustic soda.

In the latter case, the sections are fixed in alcohol, washed with water and embedded in carbowax. For clearing, the sections are treated with oliganum oil but not with xylol, since the injected acrylic resin is soluble in organic solvents such as xylol and benzene.

Disadvantages inherent in Method II are that ethylacrylate has a considerably more offensive odor, and the casts made by this method are fairly inferior in quality to those prepared by Method I. There is obviously room for further improvement of Method II.

B. Main Bronchi and Lobar Bronchi

As described elsewhere above, there are three lobar bronchi, *i.e.*, upper lobe, middle lobe and lower lobe, into which the right main bronchus divides; the left main bronchus gives off two lobar bronchi, the upper lobe and the lower lobe bronchi.

The mode of branching of lobar bronchi from main bronchi is monopodial.

Whilst, as is generally accepted, the mode of branching of the segmental bronchi is variable, it is indeed rare that the lobar bronchi display such variation.

The types of variation of main or lobar bronchial structure include: (1) absence of the normal lobar bronchus, (2) positional abnormalities, (3) excess of number, etc.

Since the lung has developed out of repeated bifurcations of tissues of entodermal origin into the mesoderm, a parallel relationship can always be seen between variations of bronchial architecture and those of the pulmonary parenchyma.

Reported variations include, for example, abnormalities in the direction of bronchial distribution, absence of portions of bronchi and associated lack of the middle lobe, formation of a part of the upper lobe as a result of branching-off of a bronchus which may be called an accessory bronchus from the right main bronchus, cystic or diverticular formatio of an abnormally small pulmonary lobe (which the normal lung lacks) and subdivision of the right upper lobe caused by excessive numbers of bronchi branching out immediately above the tracheal bifurcation.

Variations of the bronchial architecture are encountered with overwhelming frequency in the right lung, whereas in the left lung, they are extremely rare.

C. Segmental Bronchi and Pulmonary Segments

1. History

AEBY (1880), EWART (1889) and NARATH (1901) are the investigators who have gone beyond the confines of classical pursuit of study of the lung, and who have made great strides forward with modern views on the architecture of bronchial ramifications.

EWART (1889) first described the anatomy of segmental bronchi in detail and brought forth the concept of pulmonary segments. In "The Bronchi and Pulmonary Blood Vessels", EWART stated that there are portions of the lungs which form respiratory segments, each containing a variable number of lobules which are mutually independent from the viewpoint of source of air supply; thereby both the bronchi and the portions of the lungs into which they diverge (segments) bear corresponding names. It is unquestioned that with the advent of EWART's conception the present day study of pulmonary segments has been greatly facilitated.

With the development of bronchoscopy in the 1920's, and with the subsequent development of bronchographic techniques, studies on the architecture of the bronchial tree have flourished.

KRAMER and GLASS (1932) in the United Kingdom, for example, advocated their conception of bronchopulmonary segments; and later NELSON (1934), worked out a nomenclature of individual pulmonary segments, taking into account their respective topologic characteristics.

Hard on the heels of advances in these studies in Great Britain, HERRNHEISER and KUBAT (1936) of Germany gave specific names to pulmonary blood vessels after carefully reviewing published studies.

In all these studies, investigators have displayed a deep interest in pulmonary segmentation and in the mode of bronchial branching. Original views are reflected in the naming of bronchial branches, blood vessels and pulmonary segments. Even so, it appears that there are substantial differences in viewpoints.

Subsequently, in the United States, CHURCHILL and BELSEY (1939) reported on a segmental resection of the lingula of the left upper lobe for the treatment of bronchiectasis, thus taking the initiative in the application of segmental anatomy to thoracic surgery. And in 1943, JACKSON and HUBER published their nomenclature of the bronchi, based on the anatomical relationship of pulmonary segments.

As can be seen from Fig. 19, these latter authors advocated the advantage of designation of the tertiary bronchi (*i.e.*, secondary bronchi within the pulmonary lobe), using terms applicable to the pulmonary segments to which they belong. In naming these segments they adopted as far as possible the names that had conventionally been employed in the past, with the view of making the nomenclature convenient for practical, clinical use. The nomenclature of JACKSON and HUBER is characteristically simple and clear, having relatively few exceptions, and formulated by taking fully into account the needs and requirements of clinicians.

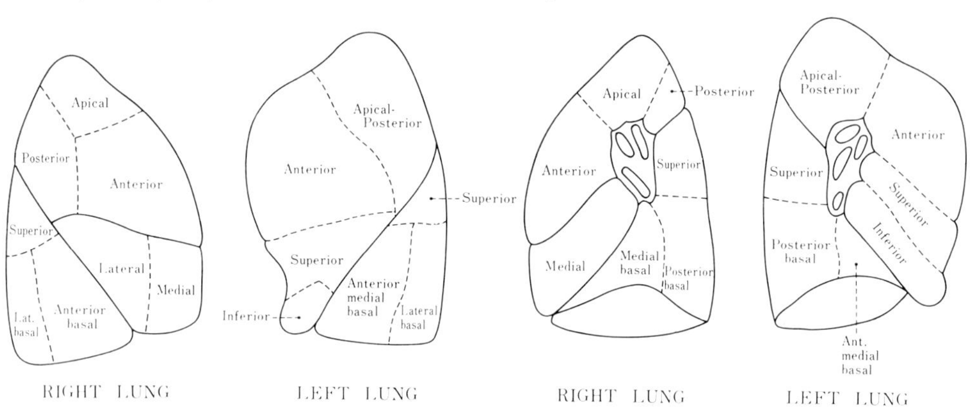

Fig. 19 The bronchopulmonary segments, shown in both lateral (left) and mediastinal (right) aspects. The terminology used in this illustration is the one the authors are suggesting (JACKSON-HUBER).

With the study of JACKSON and HUBER as the turning point and in response to the practical demands on the clinicians' side, assessment of the lung fields has come to be extensively pursued, especially from the standpoints of surgical anatomy and as having diagnostic importance in localization of pulmonary foci of disease.

Such studies may be exemplified by those published by BOYDEN and his associates (1945) in the United States and Appleton (1945) in the United Kingdom. In Japan, achievements have been made in this field by H. YAMASHITA and ISHIKAWA (1951), SHIOZAWA (1952), UJI-IYE (1952), T. TAKAHASHI (1952), and ISHIBASHI (1952).

All these studies are characterized by emphasis on clarification of the mode of normal as well as abnormal branching of the segmental bronchi, arteries and veins.

2. Conception

Pulmonary segments are also termed sublobes.

Each lobe is divided into two to six segments which vary in size and shape and according to position

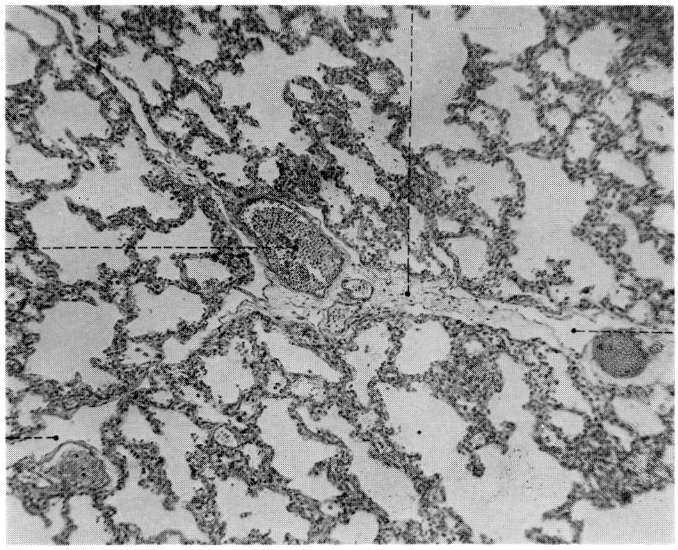

Fig. 20 Intersegmental connective tissue.

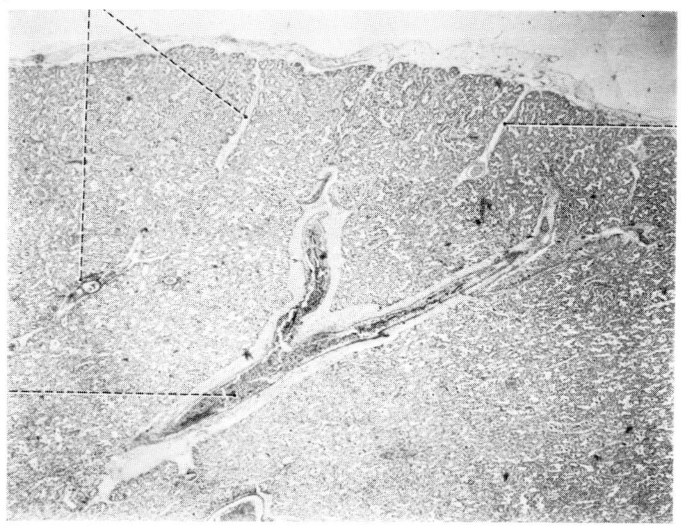

Fig. 21 Intersegmental septum of the fetus.

within the lobe. For example, if a particular segment is small, other segments within the same lobe may be relative larger. The shape of each segment, similarly, is influenced by that of adjoining segments in the same lobe. Pulmonary segments consequently are not necessarily uniform in shape and in size.

However, from the viewpoint of bronchial ramifications, pulmonary segments are somewhat polyhedral, with the bases of secondary bronchi of respective lobes as the apices. These segments are alike in that each has at least one of its faces exposed upon the surface of the lung.

Pulmonary segments, the main structural constituents of which are bronchi and pulmonary arteries and veins, contain bronchial arteries and veins, lymph vessels, nerves and other constituents that contribute to the structure of the pulmonary parenchyma.

Studies of comparative anatomy of the lung demonstrate clearly discernible intersegmental as well as interlobular borders in the sheep and cow, whereas in the dog the borders are quite indistinguishable. The human is in an intermediate position in this respect.

The intersegmental borders are in some instances clearly discernible on or through the pulmonary surface, although such instances are rather rare.

With the exception, therefore, of a few particular segments, for example, S^1 and S^2 in the right upper lobe, S^{1+2} and S^3 in the left upper lobe, S^4 and S^5 along the mediastinal margins of the middle lobe, and basal segments and B^6 in the lower lobe, intersegmental borders are usually not distinguishable.

Intersegmental septa are comprised of somewhat loose connective tissue, pulmonary veins, lymph vessels and small distal branches of the bronchial vessels, as shown in Fig. 20.

Interlobular septa are structurally similar to intersegmental septa as will be described later, although branches of the pulmonary vein in the intersegmental septa are larger than those in the interlobular septa.

As may be gathered from this anatomical characteristic, the role that may be played by intersegmental septa as a protective wall against pulmonary foci is not necessarily definitive or confining, and consequently, the possibility exists for direct invasion and extension of a focus in a segment to the neighboring healthy segment.

It is not rare that a clear, distinct line of demarcation is evident between a focus containing segment and an adjoining unaffected segment, as a result of active proliferation of intersegmental connective tissues, in cases of slowly and progressively enlarging foci in tuberculous lungs. By contrast, intersegmental septa usually fail to serve as a protective wall in the lung when infectious foci in two adjoining segments tend to fuse into one and enlarge. It is for this reason that large cavities extending across an intersegmental septum (or across septa between two or three neighboring segments) are encountered not infrequently.

Evident formation of intersegmental septa, as has been described by HATANAKA (1952) in his reports of histogenetical studies, is demonstrable in fetal lungs of three months of age, whereas interlobular septa are usually forming in the second fetal month.

Shown in Fig. 21 is a fetal lung of six months of age. In this lung, a line of intersegmental demarcation can be noted centrally on the left side of the pulmonary artery.

3. Nomenclature

The nomenclature of the bronchial branches and pulmonary segments of JACKSON and HUBER (1943) is still not entirely beyond question; the schema has been and is criticised and reassessed by investigators according to various viewpoints, depending upon whether they are anatomists, pathologists or clinicians.

Representative views are: 1. of KRAMER and GLASS (1932), and of NEIL (1939) who regard the lateral and medial subsegments of the anterior segment as two independent segments respectively. 2. Separation of the lingula of the left upper lobe from the upper lobe, hence three segments in the left upper lobe (BROCK, 1942–1944; SCANNEL, 1949). 3. Unification of the area of distribution of the lateral branch of superior segment and that of the horizontal branch of posterior segment, as a single independent pulmonary segment (BROCK). 4. Division of S^{1+2} and S^{7+8} of the right lung into two segments, respectively, and a similar division in the left lungs as well, hence a total of ten segments as proposed from a surgical point of view by ISHIBASHI (1952).

It has been claimed by BOYDEN that a part below S^6 which had not been considered by JACKSON and HUBER should be regarded as a subsuperior segment, S^*.

Subsuperior segments reportedly are present in the right lower lobe in 40 (H. YAMASHITA, 1951) to 60 per cent (BOYDEN, 1955) of the subjects studied, whereas they are less frequently seen in the left lower lobe, *e.g.* 30 per cent (H. YAMASHITA, et al., 1954).

In Japan, a committee on the nomenclature of bronchial branching was first organized in 1951 and, after much complication and discussion, agreement was reached to follow the plan of JACKSON and HUBER, for clinical purposes.

It was decided to adopt the plan of JACKSON and HUBER for segmental bronchi and to add to this the subsuperior segmental bronchus B^* and to designate this area under the name of the subsuperior segment.

Fig. 22 is the models made by the present author and his associates according to the nomenclature stipulated by the Japanese committee.

Right Lung

a. Upper Lobe

The right upper lobe bronchus divides into three segmental bronchi, B^1, B^2 and B^3 and, accordingly, the right upper lobe is divided into three segments, *i.e.* S^1, S^2 and S^3.

B^1......apical segmental bronchus	S^1......apical segment
B^2......posterior	S^2......posterior
B^3......anterior	S^3......anterior

As to the mode of branching of segmental bronchi of the right upper lobe, there are six different types.

According to SHIOZAWA (1955), type I (40%) is most commonly seen, where B^1, B^2 and B^3 branch out independently of each other. Type II (24%) is characterized by branching-out of B^2 independenly and that of B^1 and B^2 from a common trunk; type III (14%) is characterized by independent branching of B^3 and that of B^1 and B^2 from a common trunk. In type IV (10%), B^1 branching of B^3 and that of B^1 and B^2 from a common trunk. In type IV (10%), B^1 branches out independently and B^2

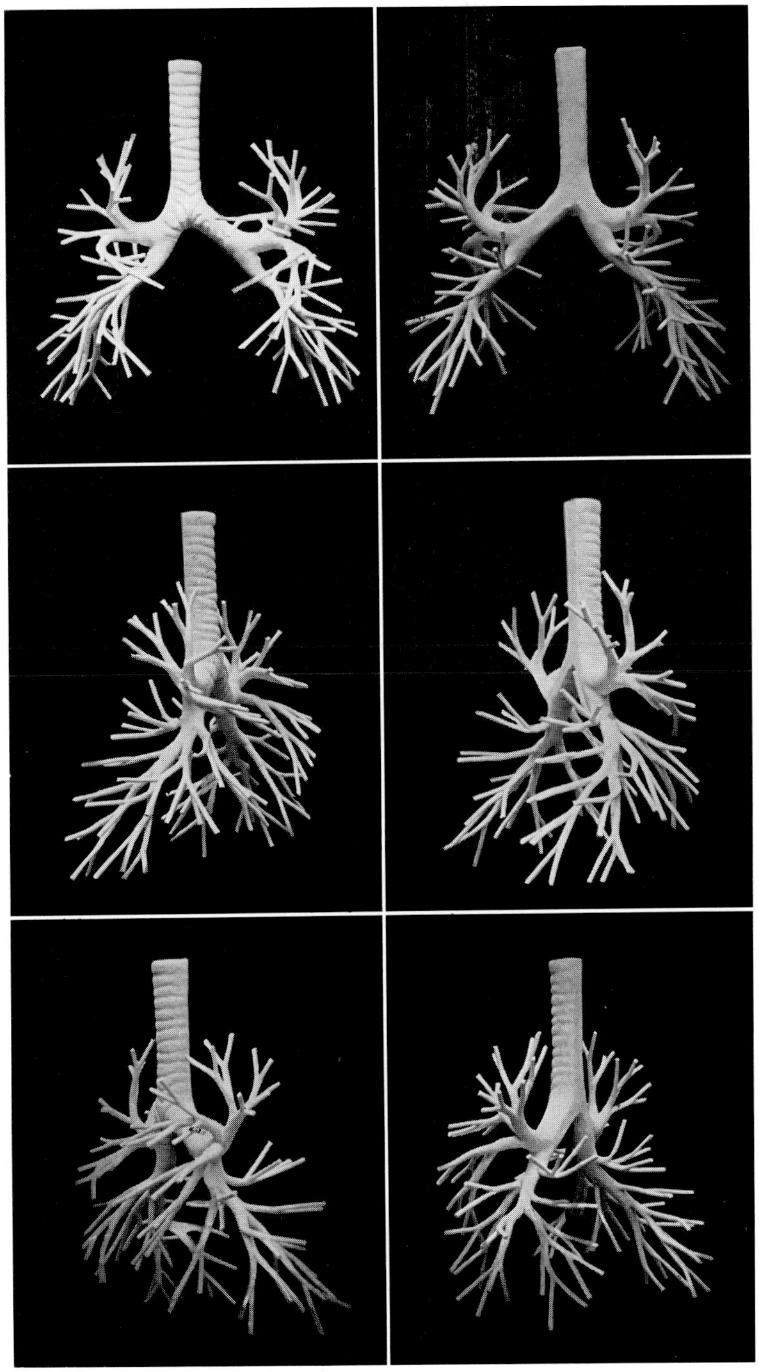

Fig. 22 Models of bronchial branching.

and B^3 come out of a common trunk. In type V (10%), B^2 is lacking and branches corresponding to B^2_a and B^2_b originate in B^1 and B^3 respectively. In type VI (2%), B^1 is lacking and branches corresponding to B^1_a and B^1_b come from B^2 and B^3 respectively.

These types of branching of segmental bronchi affect the size and extent of the lobes and segments which the bronchi supply. In type V, S^1 in particular, is small, and in type VI, S^1 often spreads extensively.

A selective bronchographic (segmentographic) study carried out, using a Métras' catheter and dionosil, by one of the associates of the author, LIN (1958), demonstrated that B^1 divides into B^1_a and B^1_b at the level of the dorsal fifth rib, the former chiefly supplying the apical region, the latter supplying the antero-inferior region of the apex.

The selective bronchograms also show that B^2 divides into B^2_a and B^2_b at the level of the fifth intercostal space as viewed ventrodorsally, and at the level of the sixth intercostal space as viewed dorsoven-

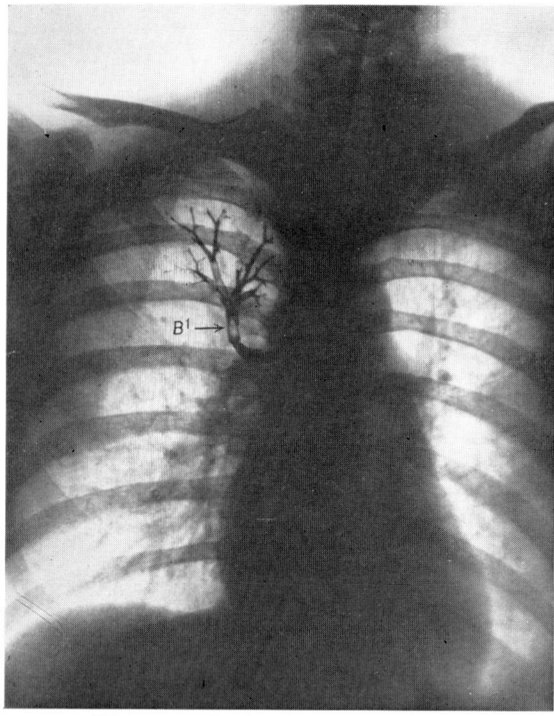

Fig. 23 Selective bronchogram of B¹.

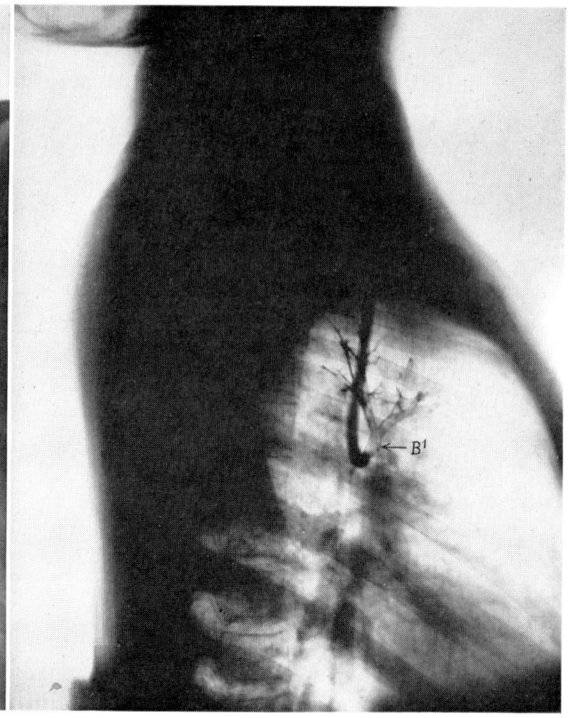

Fig. 24 Selective bronchogram of B¹.

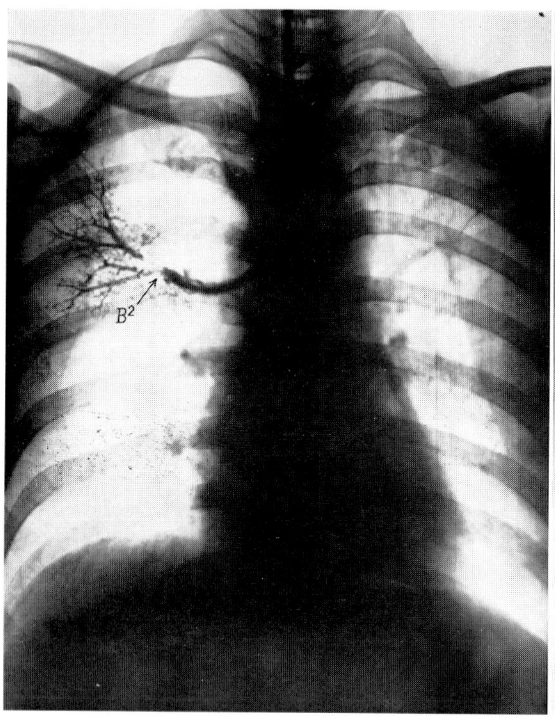

Fig. 25 Selective bronchogram of B².

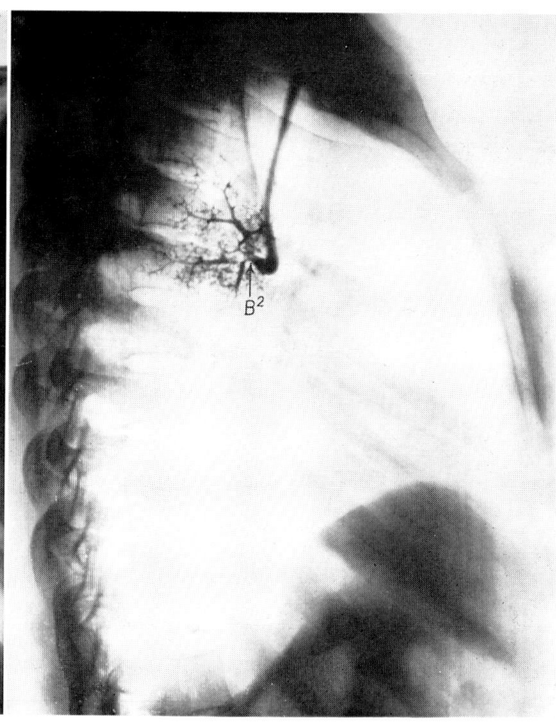

Fig. 26 Selective bronchogram of B².

trally, the former being distributed mainly to the posterosuperior region of the apex and the latter to the posterolateral region.

As can be known from alveographic analyses of pulmonary segments, practically no circumstances exist in which the projected medial border of S^2 is found extending over the mediastinal border.

B^3 divides into B^3_a and B^3_b at the level of the sixth intercostal space.

Fig. 23 is a roentgenogram of S^1 by dorsoventral segmentography of B^1, and Fig. 24 is its lateral projection. Fig. 25 and 26 show S^2, and Fig. 27 and 28 demonstrate S^3.

b. Middle Lobe

The middle lobe bronchus gives off two segmental bronchi, *i.e.* B^4 which extends anterosuperolaterally,

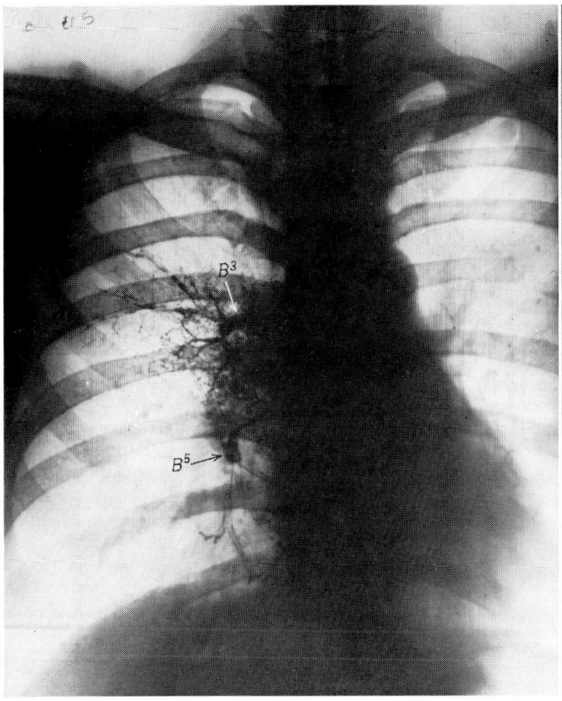

Fig. 27 Selective bronchogram of B^3 and B^5.

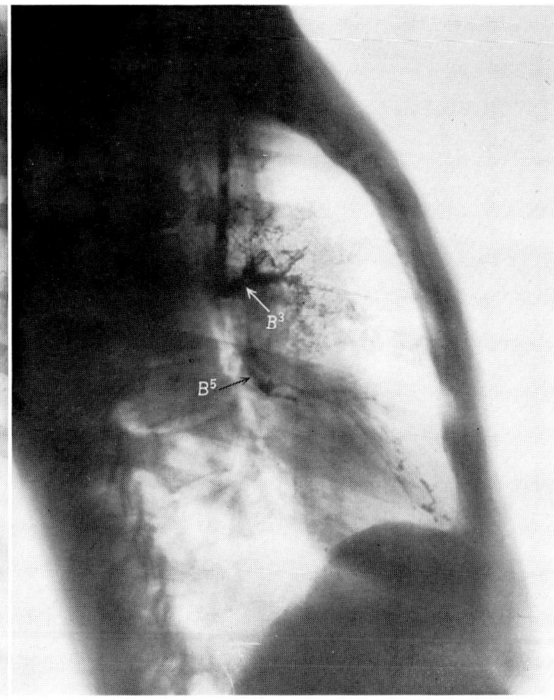

Fig. 28 Selective bronchogram of B^3 and B^5.

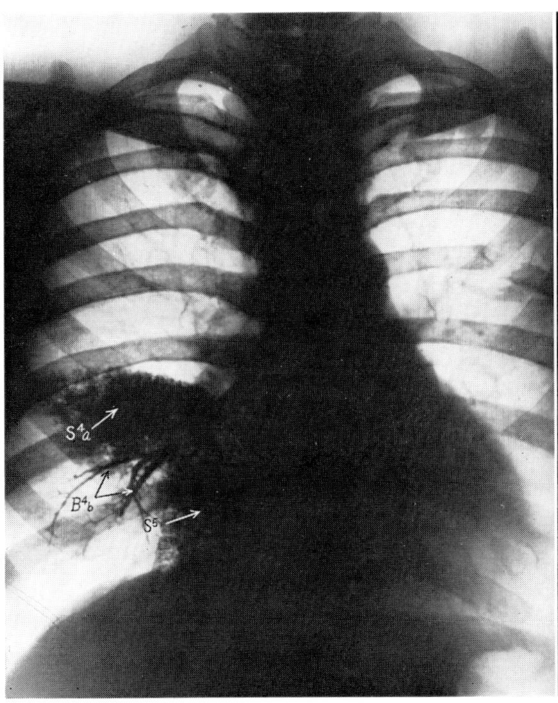

Fig. 29 Selective bronchogram of B^4 and B^5.

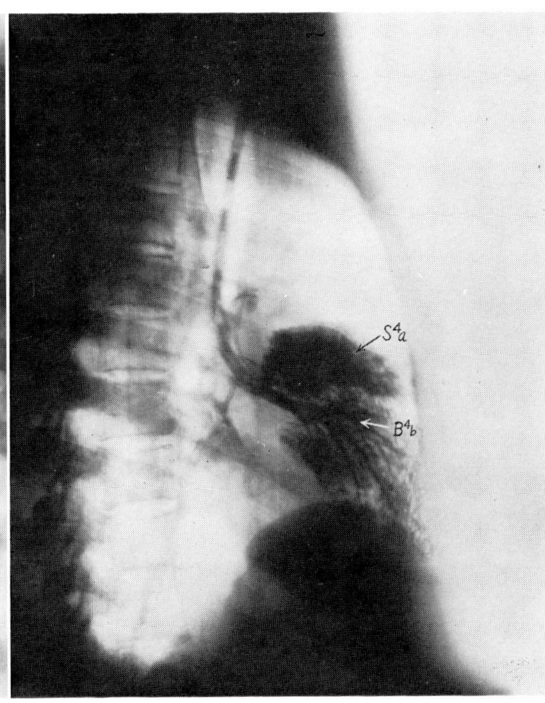

Fig. 30 Selective bronchogram of B^4.

and B^5 which reaches out anteromedially and inferiorly. The middle lobe, accordingly, is divided into two segments, S^4 on the lateral side and S^5 on the medial side.

B^4......lateral segmental bronchus	S^4......lateral segment
B^5......medial	S^5......medial

B^4 and B^5 are practially comparable in caliber to each other but, in some instances, the former is found to be smaller than the latter (SHIOZAWA, et al. 22% and BOYDEN 18%). In most of such cases B^4_a branches off from B^{4+5}. However, conversely, there are occasional cases in which B^4_b is found intruding into B^5 and, rarely, B^4 and B^5_a lie one upon another, as is the case in the left lung (SHIOZAWA, et al. 6% and BOYDEN 18%).

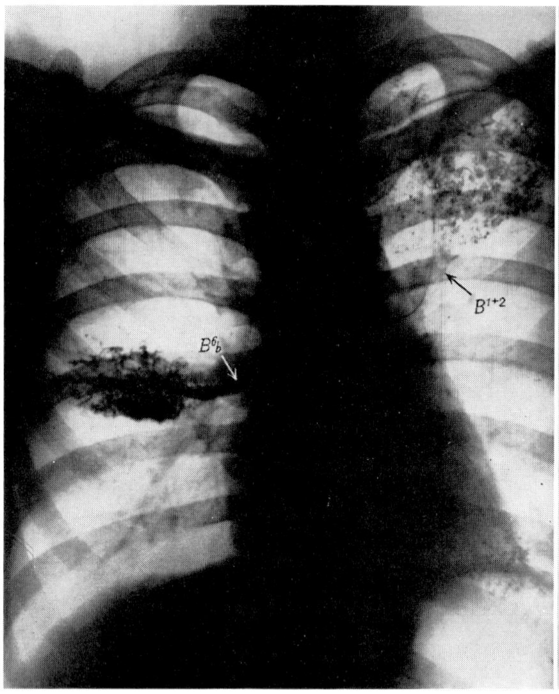

Fig. 31 Selective bronchogram of B^6 and B^{1+2}.

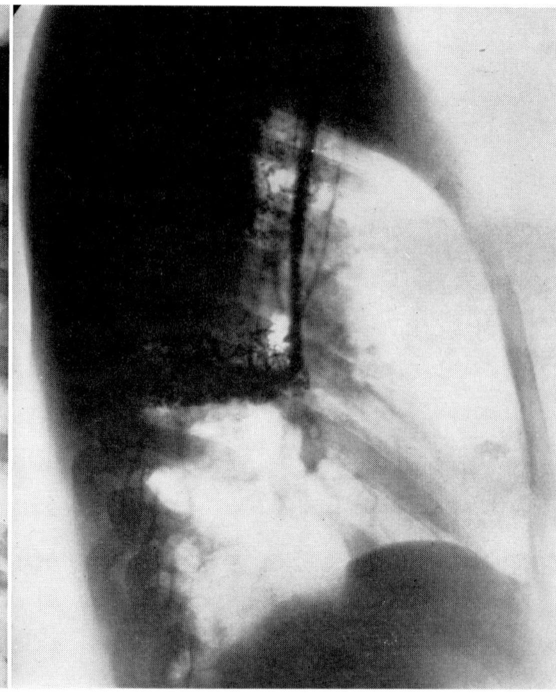

Fig. 32 Selective bronchogram of B^6.

Studies by selective segmentography carried out by LIN demonstrate that B^4 bifurcates to yield B^4_a and B^4_b at the level of the dorsal seventh intercostal space. B^5 departs from B^4 at the level of the dorsal eighth rib and successive generations run anteroinferiorly, thought in a slightly lateral direction, whereas B^5 divides into B^5_a and B^5_b and, the branches of which are distributed to the anteromedial region.

Fig. 29 and 30 are segmentograms of S^4 and S^5 as demonstrated by selective bronchography of B^4 and B^5.

c. Lower Lobe

In the right lower lobe, the bronchus diverges to give off a series of five segmental bronchi, B^6, B^7, B^8, B^9 and B^{10}, to divide the lobe into five pulmonary segments which are designated S^6, S^7, S^8, S^9, and S^{10}. In the lower lobes, as described above, B* and S* are often found to exist.

B^6......superior segmental bronchus	S^6......superior segment
B*.....subsuperior	S*.....subsuperior
B^7......mediobasal	S^7......mediobasal
B^8......anterior basal	S^8......anterior basal
B^9......lateral basal	S^9......lateral basal
B^{10}.....posterior basal	S^{10}.....posterior basal

B^6 arises from the posterior wall of the right lower lobe bronchus (occasionally from that of the middle lobe bronchus), and immediately divides into a series of the three segmental bronchi which are coded B^6_a, B^6_b and B^6_c respectively. Though extremely rare, two B^6 may rise from the right lower or middle lobe bronchus (SHIOZAWA, et al. 2%). S^6 corresponds to the apex of the lower lobe, thus largely representing the post-hilar portion of the lobe.

B^6_a, as seen by means of dorsoventral segmentography, arises at the level of the eighth rib, ascending to reach the apical region of the lower lobe; B^6_b runs lateroposteriorly to reach the interlobular pleural surface and the lateral surface of the costal pleura and adjoins S^8 and S^9.

B^6_c runs posteroinferiorly from its origin to reach the pleural surfaces adjacent to the vertebrae and posterior parts of the ribs.

B* is observed to be present in 44 (H. YAMASHITA) to 60 per cent (BOYDEN) of subjects, usually in the presence of a poorly developed S^6_c or of a combined poor development of B^9_a and B^{10}_a. B* may be a single bronchus (BOYDEN 48% and H. YAMASHITA 38%) or, in rare instances, two bronchi (BOYDEN 13% and H. YAMASHITA 6%).

Fig. 31 is a roentgenogram of S^6 taken by dorsoventral segmentography of B^6, and Fig. 32 is the relevant lateral roentgenogram of S^6.

B^7, arising at the level of the posterior part of the eighth rib, divides into B^7_a which extends postero-inferiorly, and B^7_b.

B^7 is always present in the right lung. The left lung is in most instances devoid of B^7. In the left lung, the place of B^7 is partly taken by B^6_c, B^8_c, B^9_a and B^{10}_a, although rarely, B^7 is present in the right lung (Boyden 10%, Ishibashi 6% and H. Yamashita 2%).

As mentioned above, Jackson and Huber, and Brock, et al. are of the opinion that S^7 and S^8 combined should represent at single independent pulmonary segment whereas Boydon, Appleton and Ishibashi claim that S^7 must be regarded as an independent pulmonary segment.

Of the branches departing from the lower lobe bronchus, segmental bronchi of the basal segments other than B^6, B* and B^7 diverge in the direction of the diaphragm.

B^8......anterior basal segmental bronchus	S^8......anterior basal segment
B^9......lateral basal	S^9......lateral basal
B^{10}.....posterior basal	S^{10}.....posterior basal

In both lungs, the most common type of branching is that in which B^8 arises most proximally from the lower lobe bronchus and subsequently (distally) the bronchus divides into B^9 and B^{10}, *i.e.* type B^8, B^9+B^{10}. The second most common type is that of B^8, B^9 and B^{10}; the last common type is B^8+B^9, B^{10} which is characterized by division into B^8 and B^9 to serve as common trunks, followed by B^{10} which serves as a terminal trunk.

The results of studies by Lin using dorsoventral selective bronchography indicate that B^8 arises at the level of the posterior part of the eighth rib and divides into B^8_a which extends anterioinferiorly, and B^8_b running downward in the direction of the diaphragm.

Fig. 33 is a roentgenogram showing S^9 and S^{10} as demonstrated by dorsoventral selective segmentography of B^9 and B^{10}, and Fig. 34 is the lateral roentgenogram.

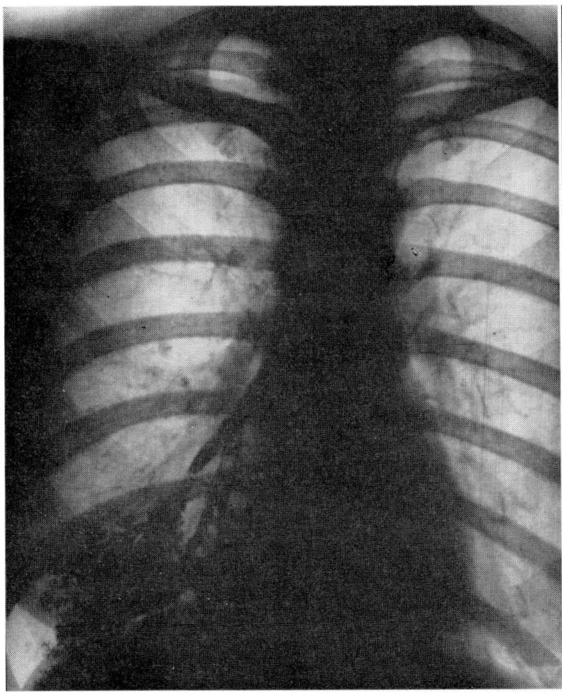

Fig. 33 Selective bronchogram of B^9 and B^{10}.

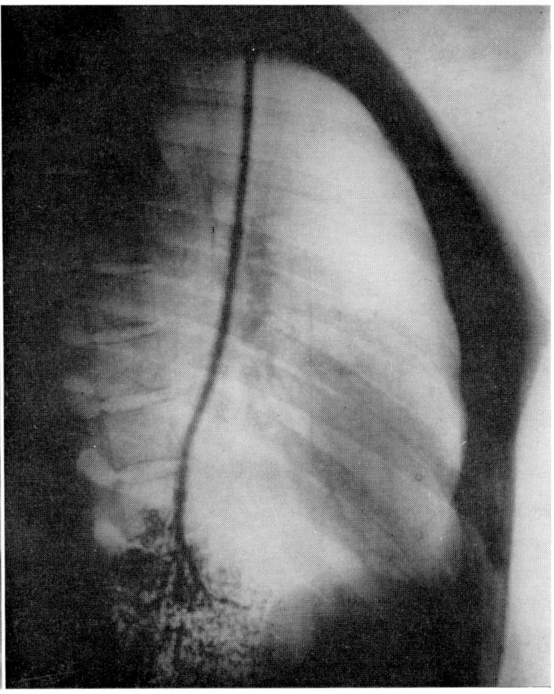

Fig. 34 Selective bronchogram of B^9 and B^{10}.

Left Lung

a. Upper Lobe

The left upper lobe comprises two main divisions, the upper and lower divisions corresponding respectively to the right upper and middle lobes. The latter also bears the name of the lingular division, because it resembles in shape a tongue.

The bronchial distributions are as follows:

Upper Division

B^{1+2}...apical-posterior segmental bronchus	S^{1+2}...apical-posterior segment
B^3......anterior	S^3......anterior

Lower Division

B^4......superior lingular segmental bronchus	S^4......superior lingular segment
B^5......inferior lingular	S^5......inferior lingular

However, in some countries, *e.g.* Germany, it is assumed that B^{1+2} is taken as two separate segmental bronchi, B^1 and B^2 and S^{1+2} accordingly are two separate segments S^1 and S^2.

B^{1+2} divides into three segmental bronchi, B_a^{1+2}, B_b^{1+2} and B_c^{1+2}. B_a^{1+2} mainly supplies the apex, B_b^{1+2} the posterosuperior and posteroinferior areas of the apex, and B_c^{1+2} the lateroposterior regions, respectively.

There are three distinct types as to the mode of branching of these segmental bronchi:

(i) B_c^{1+2} diverges most proximally, followed by branching-off of a common trunk for B_a^{1+2} and B_b^{1+2}; type B_{a+b}^{1+2}, B_c^{1+2}.

(ii) A common trunk for B_b^{1+2} and B_c^{1+2} branching away from B_a^{1+2}; type B_a^{1+2}, B_{b+c}^{1+2}.

(iii) B_c^{1+2} arises from B^3, apart from the common trunk for B_a^{1+2} and B_b^{1+2}; type B_{a+b}^{1+2}, B_c^{1+2}, B^3.

It has been described by SHIOZAWA that i represents the standard type, occurring in 62 per cent of cases studied; ii and iii are seen in 24 and 14 per cent respectively.

Dorsoventral roentgenograms, in a selective segmentography study by LIN revealed that B^{1+2} arose from the bronchus at a position comparable in level to the portion of the sixth intercostal space, thereby sending off B_a^{1+2} to the apex, and B_b^{1+2} to slightly lateral and posteroinferior regions of the apex, and B_c^{1+2} to lateral and slightly posterior regions of the apex respectively.

Similarly, B^3 was found to diverge from the bronchus at the level of the posterior portion of the sixth rib and gives off B_a^3 which runs lateroanterosuperiorly, B_b^3 which runs anteroinferiorly and B_c^3 which is distributed to the anterosuperior areas. In dorsoventral roentgenography S^3 in no instance goes above the level of the clavicle.

Fig. 35 and 36 show roentgenograms of S^{1+2}, dorsoventral and lateral respectively, as taken by selective segmentography of B^{1+2}.

Below S^3, the lower division of the left upper lobe is situated lateral to the heart. It is smaller than

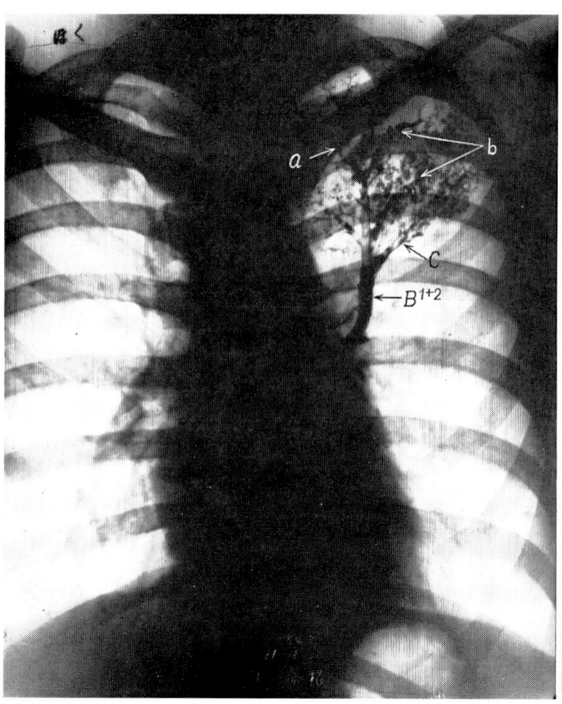

Fig. 35 Selective bronchogram of B^{1+2}.

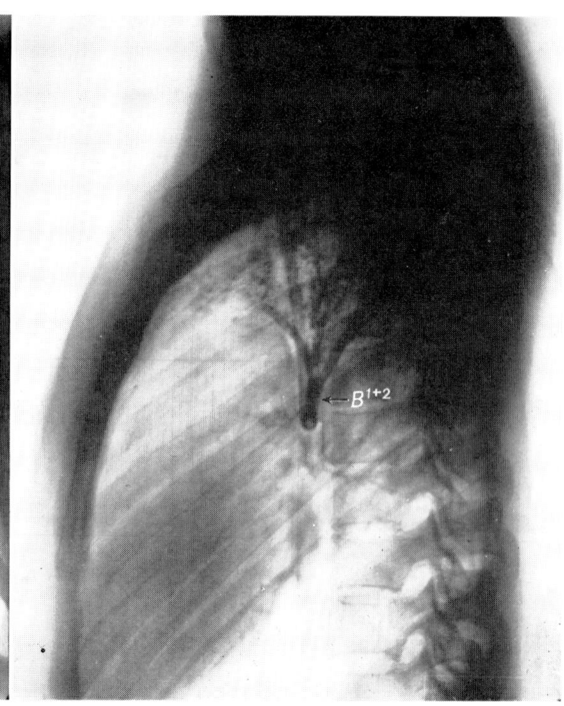

Fig. 36 Selective bronchogram of B^{1+2}.

the upper division, its size being dependent upon that of S^3.

According to the same selective segmentographic study by LIN, B^4 is usually found upon dorsoventral roentgenography to arise and depart from the upper lobe bronchus at the level of the posterior part of the eighth intercostal space.

B^4_a runs anterohilarly; B^4_b diverges into areas anteroinferior to the hilum.

B^5 arises at the level of the posterior part of the eighth intercostal space and diverges to yield B^5_a, which runs anteroinferiorly though slightly laterally, and B^5_b which runs anteroinferiorly.

Fig. 37 and 38 are roentgenograms of S^4 and S^5 taken by selective segmentography of B^5.

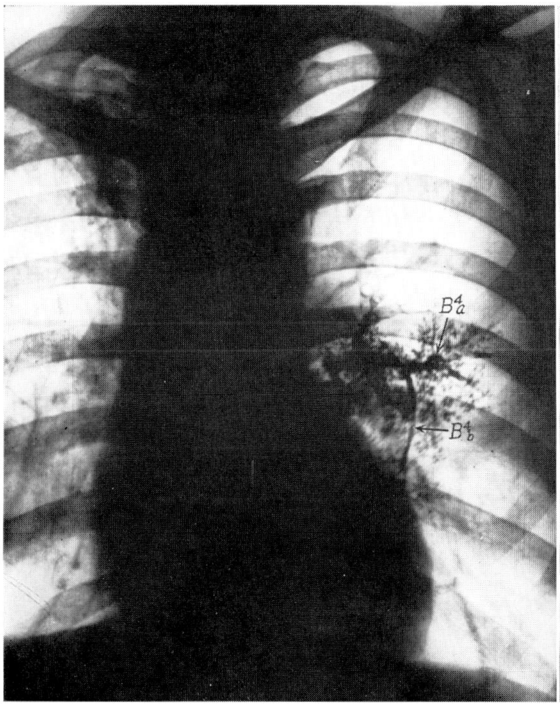

Fig. 37 Selective bronchogram of B^4.

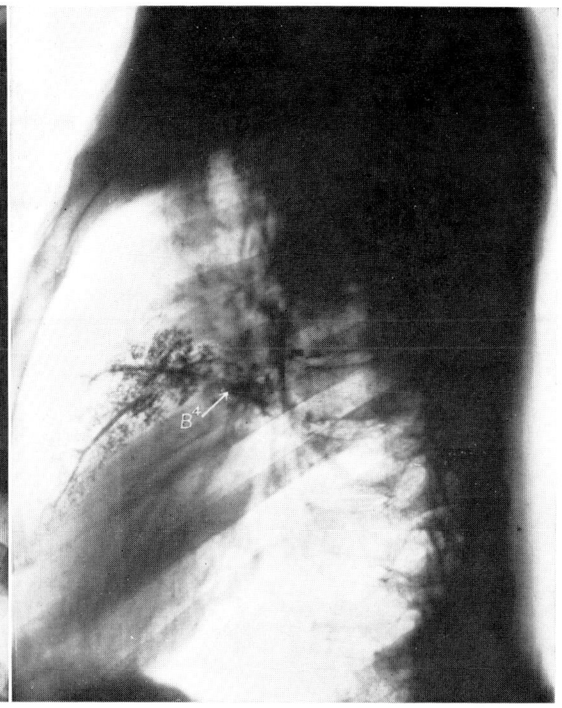

Fig. 38 Selective bronchogram of B^4.

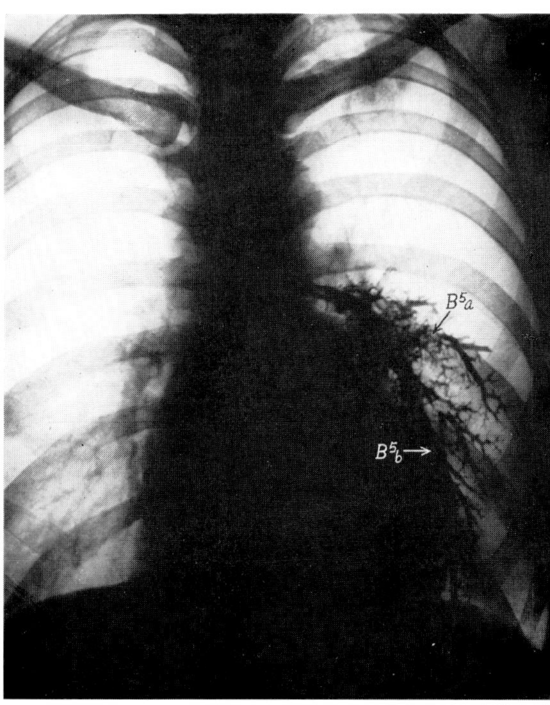

Fig. 39 Selective bronchogram of B^5.

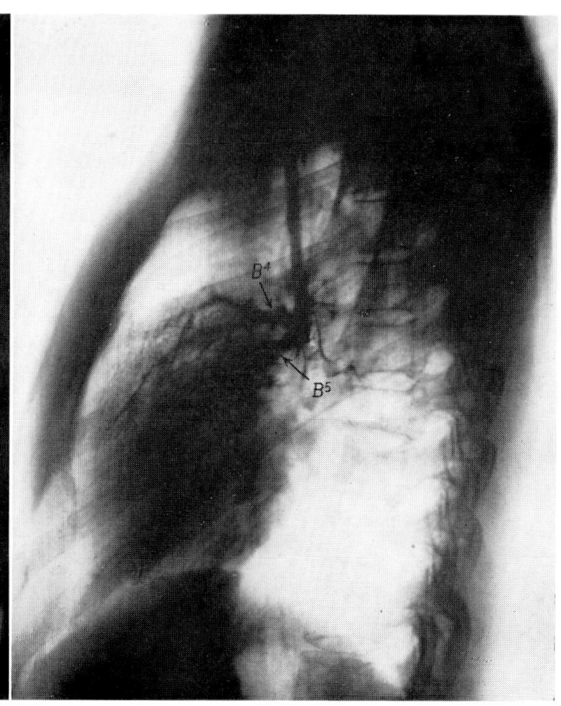

Fig. 40 Selective bronchogram of B^4 and B^5.

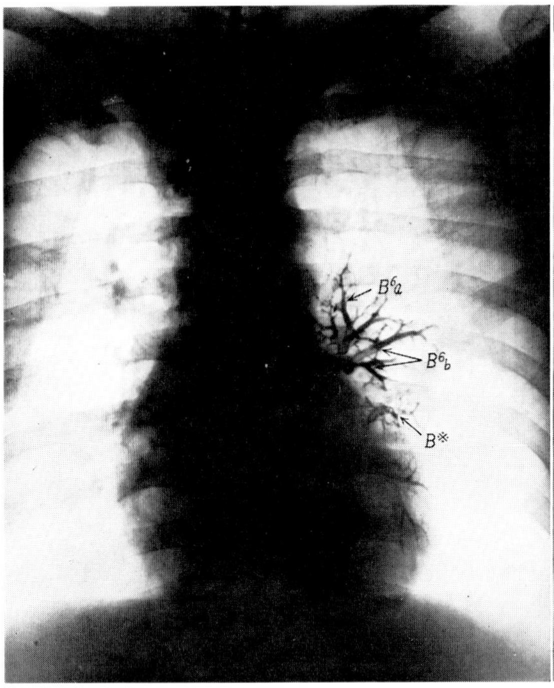

Fig. 41 Selective bronchogram of B^6 and B*.

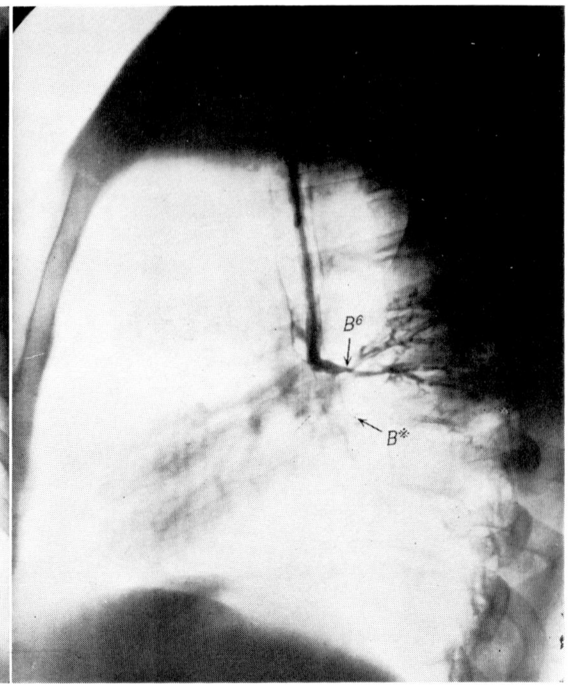

Fig. 42 Selective bronchogram of B^6 and B*.

b. Lower Lobe

The segmental bronchi B^6, B*, B^8, B^9 and B^{10} branch out from the left lower lobe bronchus. Accordingly, the five pulmonary segments S^6, S*, S^8, S^9 and S^{10} from the left lower lobe.

B^6......superior segmental bronchus	S^6......superior segment
B*.....subsuperior	S*.....subsuperior
B^8......anterior basal	S^8......anterior basal
B^9......lateral basal	S^9......lateral basal
B^{10}.....posterior basal	S^{10}.....posterior basal

B^6 as described by LIN is seen on dorsoventral roentgenograms taken by selective segmentography to branch out at the level of the posterior portion of the seventh intercostal space and to divide into three sub-branches, B^6_a, B^6_b and B^6_c which run posterosuperiorly, posteroinferiorly, and posteroinferiorly but slightly laterally, respectively.

B* is found to arise at the level of the eighth intercostal space, as revealed by dorsoventral selective segmentograms.

Fig. 41 and 42 are roentgenograms of S^6 and S* taken by selective segmentography of B^6 and B*.

B^8 arises at the level of the posterior portion of the seventh intercostal space, when viewed by dorsoventral selective segmentography, and divides into B^8_a which runs anterolateroinferiorly and B^8_b which descends toward the diaphragm.

B^9 arises at the level of the posterior portion of the eighth rib when seen on dorsoventral selective segmentograms and bifurcates into B^9_a which runs in a lateroposteroinferior direction and B^9_b which extends downward to areas adjacent to the diaphragm.

As an extension of the lower lobe bronchus, or as a terminal bronchus, B^{10} runs to areas posteroinferior to the lower lobe where, practically at the level of B^9, it produces B$^{10}_a$ which run in a posteroinferior direction and B$^{10}_c$ which goes in a direction toward the diaphragm.

D. Pulmonary Lobule

1. Conception of Lobule

The pulmonary lobule is a structural unit of the lung; in man, some five to ten acini constitute a lung lobule.

Interlobular borders are seen macroscopically as networks of demarcations, and these are frequently more prominent in male adults because of the overwhelmingly greater incidence of anthracotic deposits localized in the interlobular connective tissues. Fig. 43 shows a resected lung specimen from a male

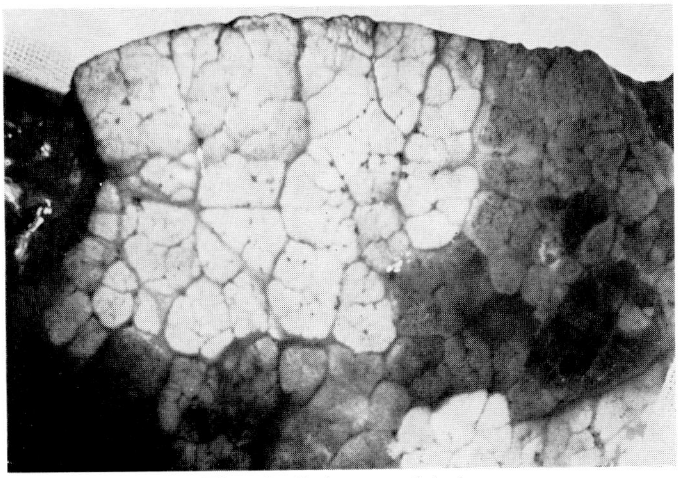

Fig. 43 Pulmonary lobules.

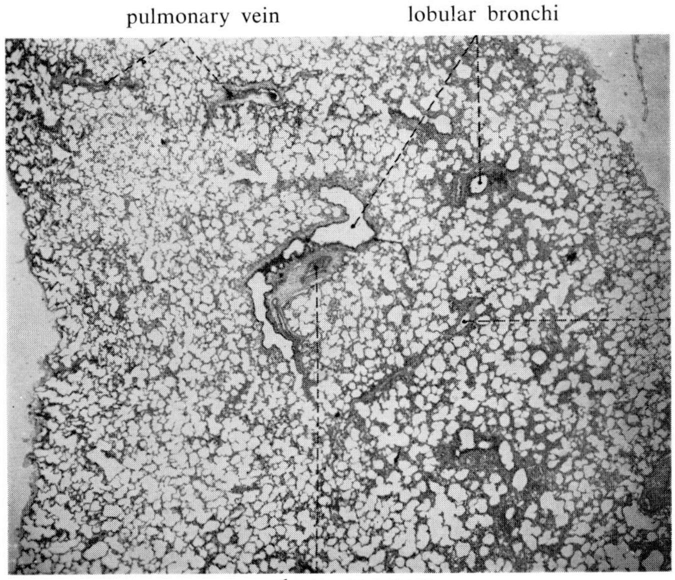

Fig. 44 Pulmonary lobules.

adult, as seen transpleurally, in which individual lobules appear as if demarcated perilobularly with fine dark lines (anthracosis).

Individual lobules are usually 0.5–2 cm in diameter though varying widely depending upon location. When seen from the surface of the lung, pulmonary lobules are irregularly polygonal; when viewed from the side, they are somewhat conical and converge to the central portion.

Fig. 44 is a photomicrograph showing a longitudinal section of a lobule; the pleural surface of the lobule is seen on the left and a central portion of the lobule is seen in the right and upper part of the section. As can be seen, a lobular artery and the accompanying bronchus enter the lobule from the pleural aspect and diverge toward the central portion.

The bronchial artery and its branches, in general, parallel the course and branching of the lobular bronchus, to be distributed to the capillary networks upon the alveoli; from these networks blood is returned by bronchial veins.

The interlobular border is composed of a thin layer of connective tissues in which interlobular veins, tributaries of the pulmonary vein, and accompanying lymph vessels are embedded.

The lobular bronchi correspond in most instances to the seventh to ninth bronchi when the lobar are taken as the primary (first-order) bronchi. Lobular bronchi of normal lungs in man usually range in caliber from 0.2 to 0.3 cm; their lumina can be seen macroscopically.

2. Arrangement

When air has gained entrance to the pleural cavity for one reason or another the lung collapses of its own elasticity. Associated with such collapse are diminutions in length and caliber of the bronchi and a

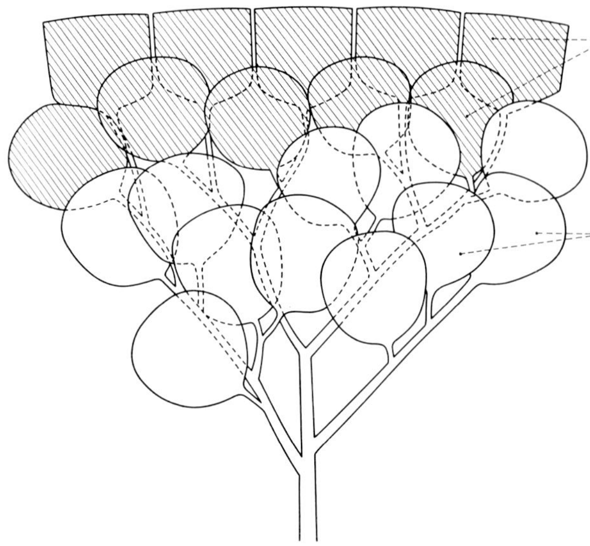

Fig. 45 Arrangement of pulmonary lobules.

consequent reduction in intrabronchial space. The magnitude of bronchial volumetric diminution varies with the location of bronchi and is usually most profound in the peripheral or distal portions.

Observations made in cases of artificial pneumothorax have revealed that the most profound collapses occur in areas three to four centimeters deep to the pleural surface.

Minimal pulmonary collapse usually is not accompanied by bronchial flexion and, on bronchography, contrast media may enter freely into the peripheral parts. Conversely, when collapse of the lung is extensive and marked, the bronchial tree in such an area coverges, to assume the shape of a half-furled umbrella, with diminution in bronchial caliber and in distances between branches. In such cases, contrast media may fail to fill the distal bronchial branches.

3. Classification

Pulmonary lobules, according to the resin cast study of N. Nagasawa and Nagaishi (1953) may be divided into two groups, superficial and deep.

The superficial lobules extend on inspiration to a depth of about 3 to 4 centimeters from the surface of the lung and are arranged in one to two layers as shown in Fig. 45. The deep lobules are situated in the central portion of the lung, enveloped with a girdle-like arrangement of superficial lobules. They form several lobular layers and retain their normal structure and function almost completely even in severe collapse of the lung.

On grounds that are not strictly anatomical, Macklin (1936) divided the lung structurally into two principal systems, the peripheral and the central, the former being post-terminal bronchiolar and the latter constituting areas proximal to the respiratory bronchioles. He stated that the former was chiefly involved in respiration, but having also some bearing on the transport of air and secreted materials, and that the latter had no bearing on respiration but was involved only in the transport of air and secretions.

Sauerbruch (1930) described the part actually involved in respiration as the "Lappenmantel" consisting of two layers of lobules, the outer layer of which corresponds to small bronchial branches of the third to fourth order. Sauerbruch further stated that the central portions of the lobe referred to by him as "Lappenkern" lack lobules and are connecteed with each other, being surrounded by connective tissues containing bronchi, blood vessels, lymph vessels and nerve plexuses and ganglia.

The "Lappenmantel" of Sauerbruch is thus considered to correspond to the superficial lobules of Nagasawa and Nagaishi. According to studies carried out by the latter investigators however, the Sauerbruch view that the layers forming the "Lappenmantel" can be construed as pulmonary lobules, and that small bronchial branches of the third to fourth order represent alveolar bronchi, is obviously misleading from the anatomical point of view. The view of Sauerbruch, with the hypothesis of "Lappenmantel" to which structural and functional importance is attached, nevertheless, is undoubtedly far sighted.

It is unquestioned that some physiologic differences exist between the superficial and the deep lobules. For example, there are differences in tonicity or expansibility of lung tissues as between the superficial and the deep areas; consequently it is also probable that superficial lobules differ from deep lobules in particular respect to caliber of capillary networks and in velocity of the circulating blood.

It is of interest that hematogenous metastases of malignant tumors of the extrapulmonary organs tend to localize mainly in subpleural areas or in regions adjacent to the pulmonary surface.

IV. PERIPHERAL PARTS OF BRONCHIAL TREE AND ALVEOLAR REGION

A. Division and Nomenclature of Peripheral Parts of Bronchial Tree

From the functional point of view, the lung may be said to comprise the respiratory tract or airway and the respiratory portion. The former consists in passages through which the inspired air comes in and the expired air goes out, whereas the latter takes an active part in gas exchange. The respiratory tract or airway consists of that portion of the respiratory tree extending to the terminal bronchioles; the remaining distal areas constitute the respiratory portion or alveolar region.

For the sake of convenience, these will henceforth be described collectively as the peripheral parts of the bronchial tree and the alveolar region.

These parts accordingly include the entire respiratory part or alveolar region and the terminal bronchioles which are in a sense extremities of the respiratory tract.

As for standardization of the nomenclature of this part of the respiratory tree, J.N.A. and B.N.A. terminologies are well known.

In J.N.A. terminology, these are designated bronchuli, bronchuli respiratorii, ductuli alveolares, sacculi alveolares, alveoli pulmonis, etc., whereas in B.N.A. terminology, these are designated bronchioli, bronchioli respiratorii, ductuli alveolares, sacculi alveolares, alveoli pulmonum, etc., respectively. Correspondent to these, the terms terminal bronchiole, respiratory bronchiole, alveolar duct, alveolar sac, pulmonary alveolus will be henceforth used in this text.

B. Fine Structure of Peripheral Parts of Bronchial Tree

1. Terminal Bronchiole

The terminal bronchiole is at times referred to simply as bronchulus.

Terminal bronchioles are the most distal portions of the bronchus that preserve the character of an air tract. Peripheral to these are the alveolar sacs which function to effect gas exchange. The terminal bronchioles are fine tubers having a relative abundance of smooth muscles, supported by connective tissues that contain elastic fibers; the walls of these bronchioles are not supported by cartilages.

Peribronchial lymph vessels, as will be described later, can be traced down to areas in which terminal bronchioles are distributed, but in areas distal they are no longer observed.

Fig. 46 is a photomicrograph showing a terminal bronchiole and the ensuing respiratory part or alveolar region. As can be seen, the wall of the terminal bronchiole is lined by a single layer of ciliated cuboidal epithelium.

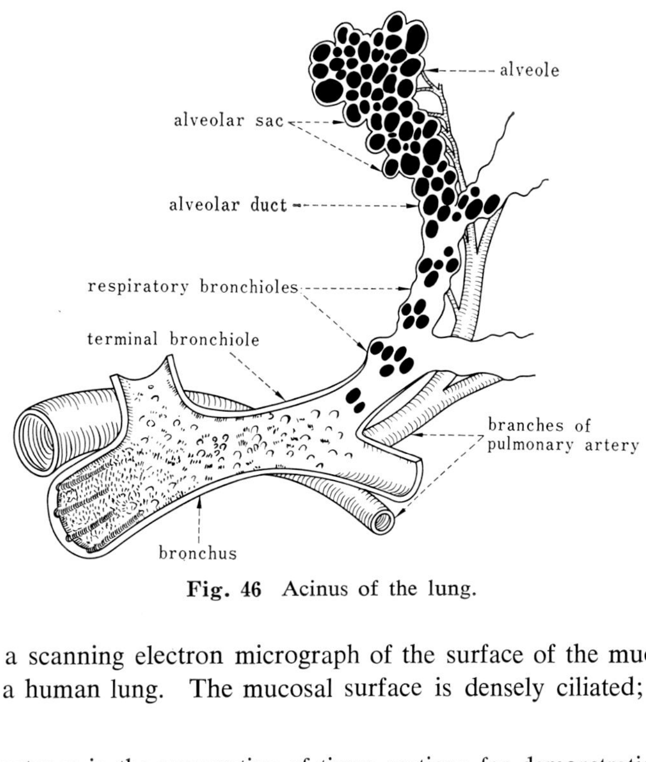

Fig. 46 Acinus of the lung.

Shown in Fig. 47 is a scanning electron micrograph of the surface of the mucous membrane of a terminal bronchiole from a human lung. The mucosal surface is densely ciliated; non-ciliated goblet cells occur sporadically.

Of great practical importance in the preparation of tissue sections for demonstration of the structure of the

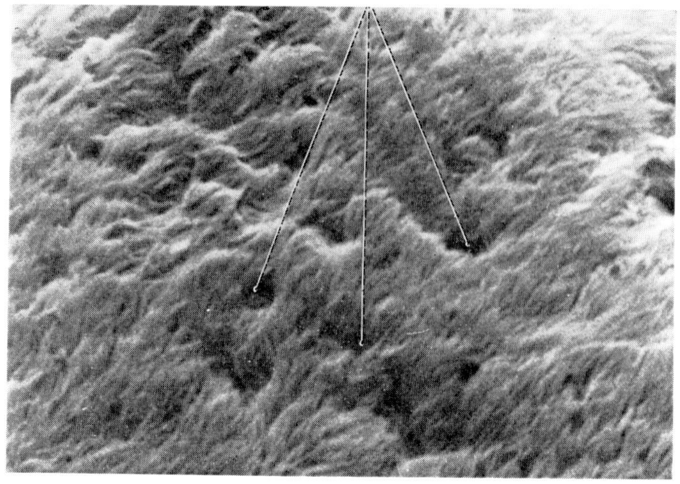

Fig. 47 Cilia of the bronchus (scanning electron microscopy).

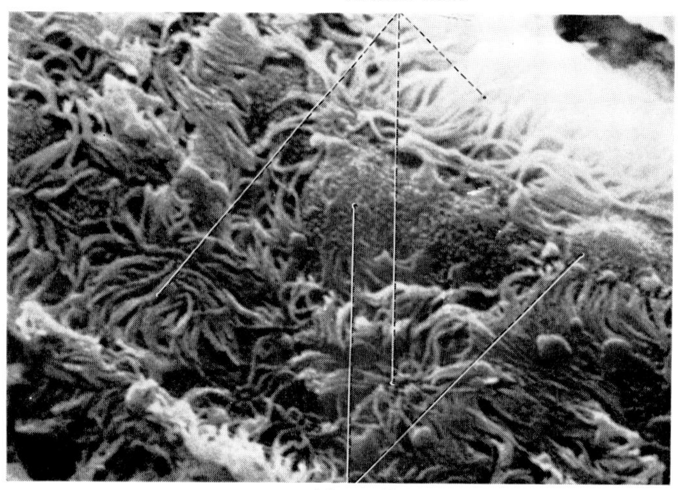

Fig. 48 Ciliated and goblet cells of the bronchus.

mucous membrane of these regions is pretreatment by thorough washing with trypsin-containing physiologic saline to eliminate the abundance of mucus with which the mucosal surface is usually covered.

Fig. 48 shows the mucosal surface of the terminal bronchiole of a specimen obtained from a guinea pig lung. A clear distinction is evident in this section as between ciliated epithelial cells and goblet cells, the free surface of the latter being devoid of cilia but furnished with numerous, fine projections.

The extremities or the most peripheral or distal ramifications of the bronchial tree were first characterized by WATERS (1860) and figuratively described as being "terminal", *i.e.*, terminal or ultimate bronchial tubes.

2. Respiratory Bronchiole

Terminal bronchioles ramify to produce yet smaller branches termed respiratory bronchioles whose walls differ in structural feature from those of the more proximal tubes; these respiratory bronchioles bear outpocketings which are called alveoli.

Based on a study of resin castings of specimens obtained from the lung of man, NAGASAWA and NAGAISHI concluded that there are two distinct types or modes of branching of respiratory bronchioles from terminal bronchioles.

Presented in Fig. 49 is diagram of ramifications of a terminal bronchiole.

Type I: This is considered to represent the standard type. A single terminal bronchiole divides into two primary respiratory bronchioles, each of which in turn produces two secondary respiratory bronchioles, forming a total of our (secondary) respiratory bronchioles.

Type II: From a single terminal bronchiole two primary respiratory bronchioles arise; one of these two primary respiratory bronchioles yields two secondary respiratory bronchioles, forming a total of

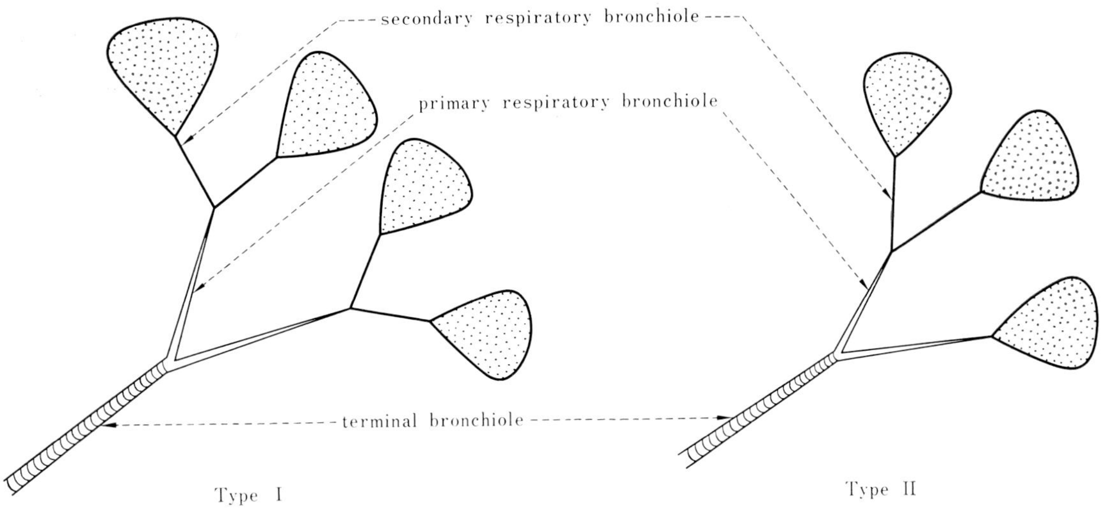

Fig. 49 Branching of peripheral part of the bronchoalveolar system.

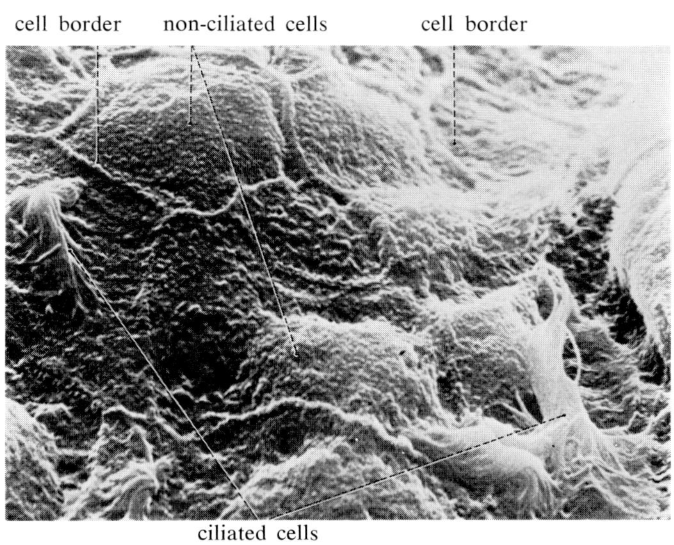

Fig. 50 Ciliated and non-cliated cells of the terminal bronchiole (scanning electron microscopy).

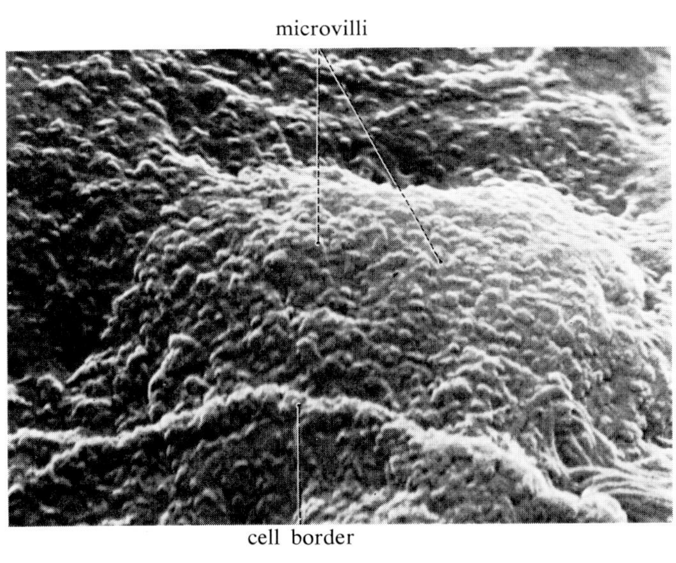

Fig. 51 Surface of the non-ciliated cell of the terminal bronchiole (scanning electron microscopy).

three secondary bronchioles. MILLER (1937) has noted that formation of tertiary respiratory bronchioles is very rarely seen. Studies carried out by NAGASAWA, et al. (1957), however, could not find such a formation.

All of the portions of the respiratory tree referred to in this section are contained in the pulmonary lobule, thereby constituting the structural units of the lobule.

Extending from the peripheral part of the terminal bronchioles to the respiratory bronchioles the non-ciliated epithelial lining gradually and progressively increases in extent.

Fig. 50 is a scanning electron microgram of a peripheral part of a terminal bronchiole of a resected human lung specimen.

Fig. 51 is a higher magnification of this portion.

Here, evident distinction can be drawn between the ciliated and non-ciliated cells.

These microscopic features are remarkably consistent with those described by BARBER, et al. (1968) in a study of the structure of olfactory mucous membranes.

Somewhat roughened surfaces of mucous membranes are seen occasionally in areas extending from the terminal bronchiole to the respiratory bronchiole of lung specimens from guinea pigs and mice as shown in Fig. 52. Fig. 53 is a higher magnification of this area.

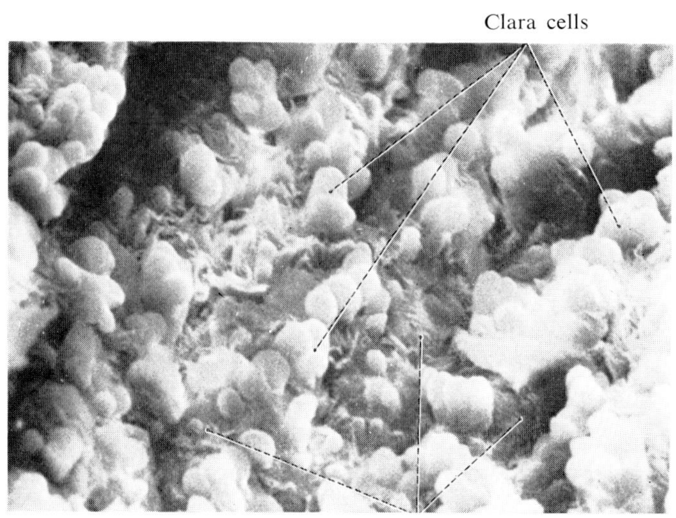

Fig. 52 Clara cells (scanning electron microscopy).

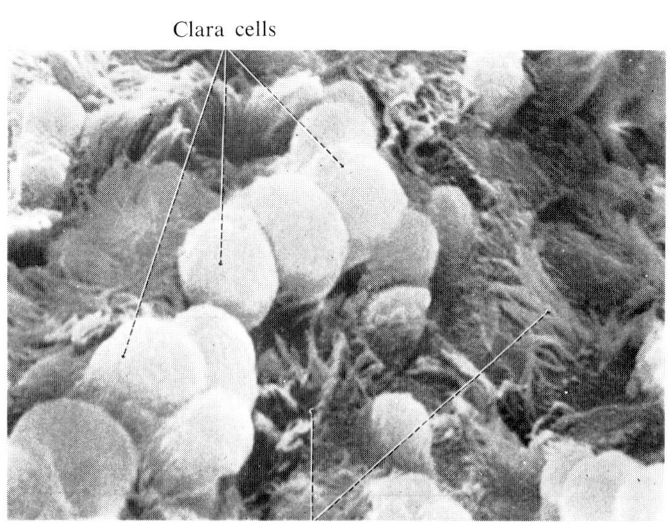

Fig. 53 Clara cells (scanning electron microscopy).

The mucosal surfaces appear somewhat roughened because of the presence of a number of Clara cells which occur as papillary or club shaped projections.

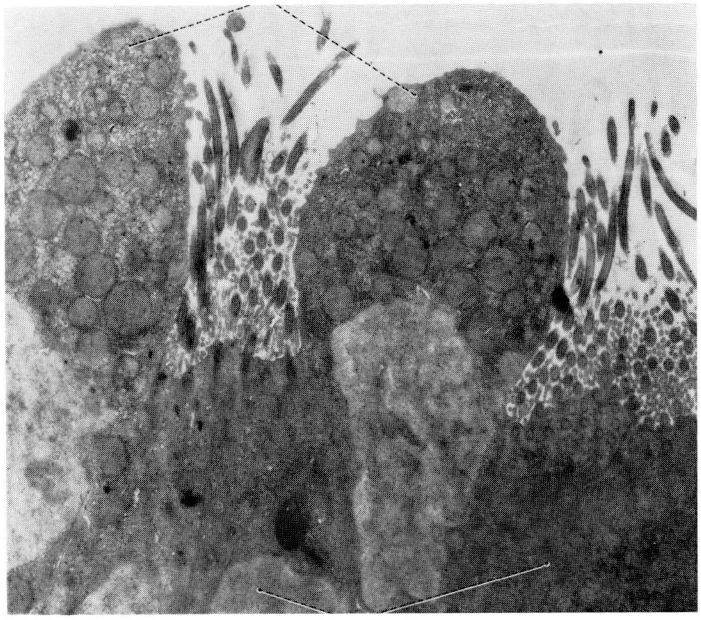

Fig. 54 Clara cells (transmission electron microscopy).

The non-ciliated bronchiolar epithelial cells were first described by KÖLLIKER (1881) as being present in the epithelial lining of terminal bronchioles. In later years more detailed acounts were given by CLARA (1936).

As can be seen from Fig. 54, Clara cells protrude into the bronchiolar space, as contrasted with the free edges of ciliated epithelial cells. It is for this reason that Clara cells are seen as papillary projects in scanning electron micrographs. These findings were obtained by OKADA and NAGAISHI (1969) in their scanning electron microscopic studies. The ultrafine structure of Clara cells has been studied in detail by transmission electron microscopy by KARRER (1956), KISCH (1958), NIDEN, et al. (1966 and 1967), and by GMELICH, et al. (1967).

Particularly characteristic of Clara cells is the presence of an abundance of small smooth-surfaced endoplasmic reticulum and large rounded mitochondria distributed extensively in the cytoplasm. The former often occur as small, cylindrical or minute reticulate formations and tend to be localized collectively

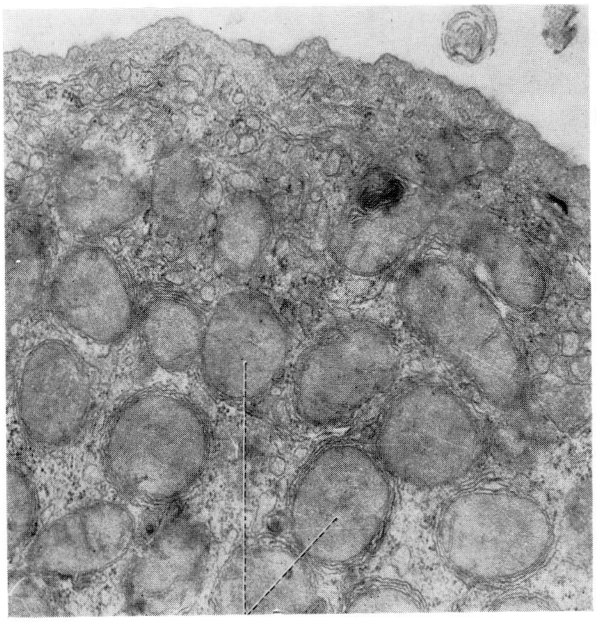

Fig. 55 Mitochondria of the Clara cell (transmission electron microscopy).

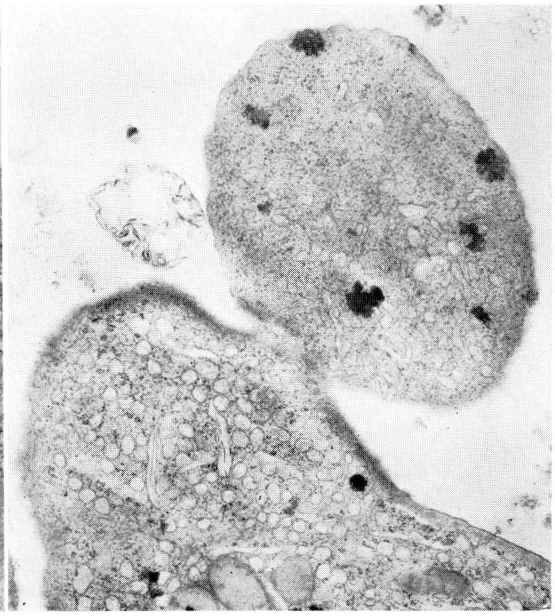

Fig. 56 Cytoplasmic projection of the Clara cell (transmission electron microscopy).

near the free margin of the cells. It is also a frequent finding that lamellar endoplasmic reticula concentrically encompass the mitochondria. Mitochondria of the Clara cells contain crista which are characteristically few in number in comparison to other epithelial cells, as shown in Fig. 55.

Microscopically, there are occasional cytoplasmic compressions along the free margins of Clara cells as shown in Fig. 56.

Such a finding suggests that a portion of the cytoplasma is about to be liberated into the bronchiolar space as an apocrine secretion. The portions severed are slightly more electron dense than the cytoplasmic matrices of Clara cells, and contain numerous fine smooth-surfaced endoplasmic reticula, but in no instance do they contain mitochondria.

It is generally accepted among investigators that Clara cells function as apocrine secretors.

HAYEK, et al. (1953) described Clara cells as producing a mucous secretion; whereas NIDEN (1966, 1967) and AZZOPARDI (1969) reported that these cells essentially secrete lipoproteins which serve as a source of alveolar surfactant material.

It is perhaps premature to conclude that Clara cells produce the surfactant material merely from the finding that they are active in lipoprotein secretion. Inasmuch as the type B alveolar epithelial cells which will be described later are found to be existent in the lungs of all vertebrates, it seems to be permissable to regard this type of cell as a main secretor of the alveolar surfactant material, in the absence of evidence to the contrary.

Meanwhile, according to observations of OKADA and NAGAISHI (1964, 1969), osmiophilic lamellar intracytoplasmic inclusion bodies are rarely demonstrated in Clara cells, as shown in Fig. 57.

These inclusion bodies apparently differ from fat granules and from phagosomes or autolysomes but bear great resemblance to the osmophilic bodies that are usually seen in type B alveolar epithelial cells.

It is not necessarily inconceivable that Clara cells produce an apocrine secretion and at the same time synthetize lipoprotein to take part in the production of alveolar surfactant material, but we would like to hold this conclusion in abeyance, pending further accumulation of experimental data.

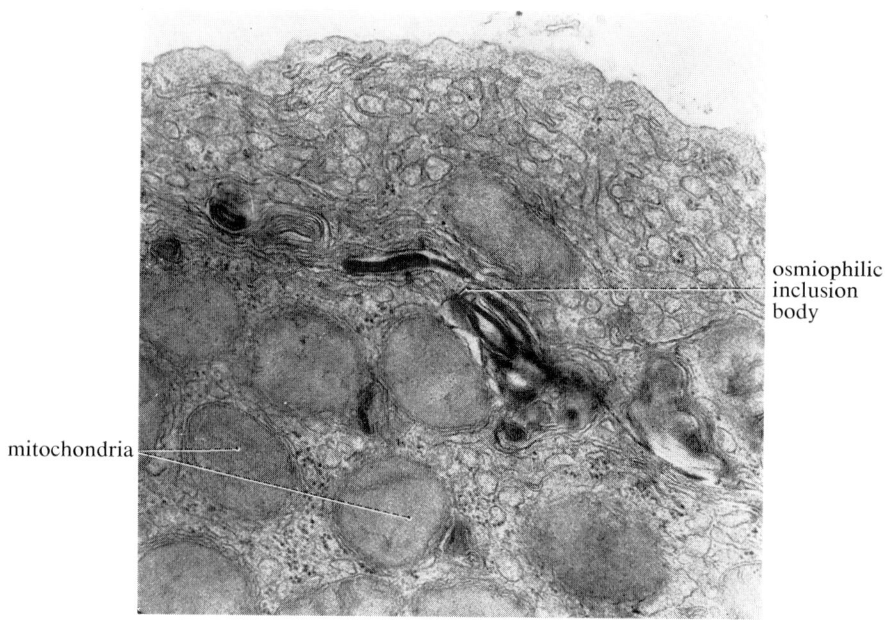

Fig. 57 Osmiophilic inclusion body of the Clara cell.

3. Alveolar Duct

Three elongated alveolar passages or ducts diverge from each respiratory bronchiole.

As described earlier, the mode of bronchial branching is mainly monopodial or dichotomous in bronchi to the level of the respiratory bronchioles; trichotomous branching, however, occurs almost exclusively in alveolar ducts.

Alveolar ducts are also called alveolar passages. The term "Alveolargang" was introduced by SCHULTZE (1871) as a general term for respiratory bronchioles and alveolar ducts. This term bears at present a definition somewhat different from the original. As pointed out later by KÖLLIKER, the lining epithelium is structurally different between the respiratory bronchiole and the alveolar duct.

Shown in Fig. 58 are photomicrographs of the state of distribution of elastic fibers in the walls of terminal bronchioles, respiratory bronchioles and alveolar duct. As can be seen, an immense abundance of elastic fibers is present in the lamina propria of the terminal bronchiole and in the adventitia; the elastic fibers diminish in quantity as the branches proceed peripherally.

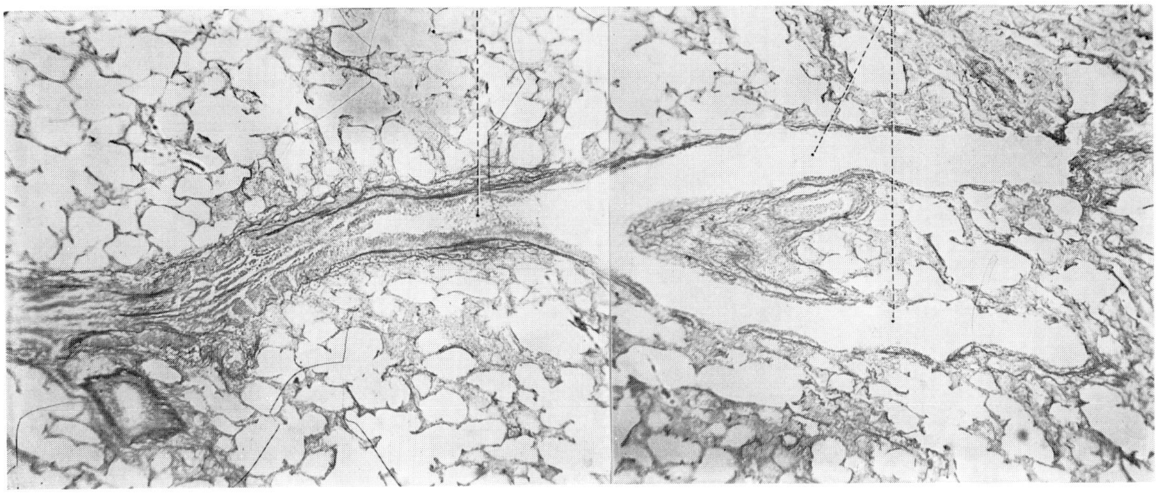

Fig. 58 Distribution of the elastic fibers.

4. Alveolar Sacs

Each alveolar duct terminates in one or more, usually three, alveolar sacs which form irregular projections arising from the extremities of the alveolar duct, each sac bearing numerous terminal alveoli.

In addition to the structural elements and terminal ramifications of the respiratory tree just noted, MILLER (1937) has described an element that is interposed between the alveolar duct and the alveolar sac, namely the atrium. From the extremity of each alveolar duct, three to six semicircular, cylindrical structures called atria arise, each individual atrium communicating with an alveolar duct and opening into a number of irregularly shaped alveolar sacs. Numerous alveoli project out of the walls of individual alveolar sacs and atria. MILLER based his conclusions on a series of studies using lung specimens obtained from a male adult (47 years of age), from a 9 week old infant, and from lungs of dogs and cats. Microscopic observations of serial sections of the lung led to reconstruction of the understanding of the architecture of the terminal ramifications of the respiratory system. MILLER stated, however, that the atria are difficulty visualizable under the photomicroscope in the usual thick collodion impregnated specimens, inasmuch as they are essentially concealed by the alveolar sacs which arise therefrom. The presence of atria is as yet a matter of some debate, however.

Based on studies of the comparative anatomy of the lungs of vertebrates, OGAWA (1920) found no basis for a particular structural separation of what has been termed the atrium in the human lung.

As for structural interrelations between the alveolar duct and the alveolar sacs, a number of earlier investigators presented a variety of views.

The earliest report is that of ROSSIGNOL (1846) who designated the very extremity of each lobular bronchus as the infundibulum, based on studies of the lungs of reptiles and amphibians.

The infundibula, forming small cysts or cones at the very end of the lobular bronchi, as described by ROSSIGNOL, bear numerous alveoli which thus partition the inner surfaces of the infundibular chambers and

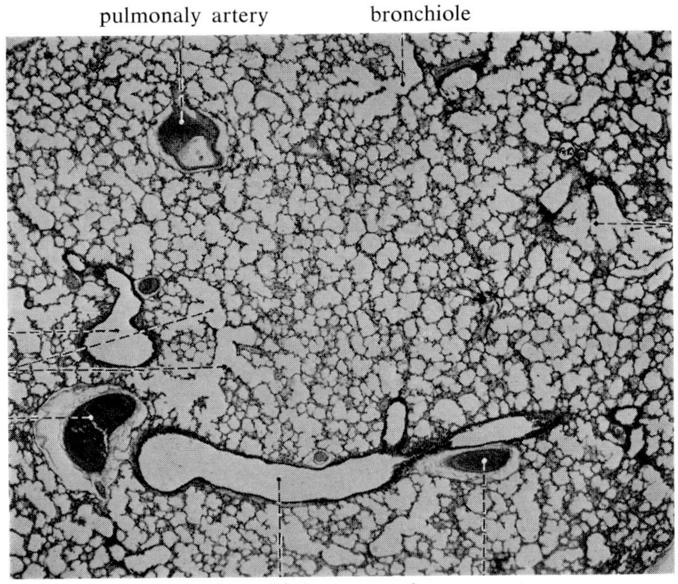

Fig. 59 Peripheral part of the bronchoalveolar system.

communicate with the external air through single openings. ROSSIGNOL regarded the infundibula as functionally important portions of the structure of the lung.

ADRIANI (1847) also used the term infundibula, in agreement with the view of ROSSIGNOL. The terminology of ROSSIGNOL was also employed by SCHULTZ (1850) and KÖLLIKER (1854).

Abrupt changes in structural features occur in areas distal to the alveolar ducts; numerous alveoli occur and, on expansion of the lung, the volume of their inner space increases remarkably, thereby rendering it rather difficult to understand the total picture of their three-dimensional architecture. It is probable, in this context, that divergences in the results of observation occur, depending upon the tissue specimens used as well as the methods of study employed.

As shown in Fig. 59, recurrent alveolar sacs come out parallel with alveolar ducts and fully occupy the interspace between neighboring peripheral bronchi.

Such a recurrent tendency is also seen with respiratory bronchioles and with alveolar ducts.

The walls of alveolar sacs, as described by MILLER, are composed of capillary networks, elastic fibers, reticulum, collagenous fibers and epithelium; the elastic fibers are situated in general in the center of the alveolar wall.

5. Alveole

Alveoli arise along respiratory bronchioles and distal branches. Those alveoli arising from respiratory bronchioles or alveolar ducts are relatively sparse and occur as hemispherical bulgings direct from bronchiolar walls. Interalveolar communications in these regions are effected by way of the lumina of bronchioles and alveolar ducts.

Respiratory bronchioles and alveolar ducts differ greatly in morphologic features from alveolar sacs, in that the former possess the character of air passages as is the case for proximal portions of the respiratory tree, whereas the latter assumes the shape of respiratory sacs, consisting of groups of alveoli.

There is nevertheless, in our studies, no evidence of substantial differences in the morphology of the alveoli of respiratory bronchioles and of alveolar ducts and those of Miller's atria or alveolar sacs.

Detailed accounts of the fine and ultrafine structures of the alveoli will be given later.

C. History of Studies on Peripheral Parts of Bronchial Tree

Numerous studies have been published concerning the architecture of the peripheral parts of the bronchial tree.

The published views on this subject may be briefly summarized as follows:

WILLIS (1676): Minute bronchial branches being embedded in layers of connective tissue occupy a certain portion of the intrapulmonary space. At the very end of each branch is a small air bladder. These individual small air bladders occur quite independently of each other and hence lack mutual intracommunication.

MALPIGHI (1679): The pulmonary parenchyma, composed of fine connective tissues, forms rounded and tortuous small air bladders (small air cells) which mutually communicate to render the parenchyma cellular.

REISSEISEN (1808): Examination by intratracheal insufflation of Hg reveals that the Hg column displays perfectly regular and successive bifurcations or divisions, the number of which progressively increases, and therefore the branches become denser as the divisions progress. Each bronchus terminates in cylindrical endings.

LEREBOULLET (1838): Numerous terminal capsules exist in alveolar regions, the capsules occurring mutually independently. These small bronchial branches conjoin to constitute a pulmonary lobule; the pulmonary lobules in turn conjoin to form a lung.

BAZIN (1832): Each bronchus terminates in a "cul-de-sac" by way of short branches. These terminal structures can be seen dilated only when the lung expands and, consequently, save been called cells or vesicles by a number of anatomists. He agreed with Reisseisen who had described the cellular or vesicular tissues as representing nothing more than the branches arising from bronchi.

These are descriptions from classical literature about the peripheral parts of the bronchial tree. Diagrams and figures in these articles seem to provide evidence in support of the views of REISSEISEN and of BAZIN. Their views are supported by GIRALDES (1839), as well.

The following studies add to our understanding of alveolar structure.

MALPIGHI (1679): He described small air bladders as being demonstrable not solely at the extremities of bronchioles, but along the walls as well, the latter being named lateral vesicles.

MOLESCHOTT (1845): He supported the description of MALPIGHI.

ADRIANI (1847): He claimed that even in healthy lungs there exists communication between two adjoining alveolar ducts. The report of ADRIANI is the first to describe alveolar pores, the presence of which is yet the subject of continuing controversy. The subject will be discussed later in detail.

SCHULTZE, (1850): He called alveoli situated at the blind end of each infundibulum "terminal alveoli"; all others were called "lateral or parietal alveoli".

MANDL (1857): His views are rather consistent with those of SCHULTZ, in that terminal alveoli are regarded as communicating with lateral alveoli only through the mediation of a bronchus common to each.

D. Acinus

1. History of Studies

An acinus constitutes the sublobular unit of lung tissue in man. The following is a brief historical review of the study of the acini.

KÖLLIKER (1854): He referred to the finest bronchial twigs and distal areas as primary lobules. Judging from his diagram of the lung of the newborn, his term "primary lobule" corresponds to the region peripheral to what is now referred to as the respiratory lobule.

TODD and BOWMAN (1859): Each primary lobule is composed of groups of alveoli belonging to a single common terminal bronchiole. The region now referred to as a pulmonary lobule was designated by them as the secondary pulmonary lobule.

WATERS (1860): He used the term terminal or ultimate bronchial tube to describe the ending branches of the bronchial tree. Air sacs occurring at one bronchial termination demonstrably had no conjunction at all with those occurring at other neighboring bronchial terminations. Individual air sacs were arranged to form what WATERS called a miniature of the lung, a little lobule or lobulette.

GERLACH (1860): Under the photomicroscope, bronchial terminations can be visualized. Each bronchial branch continues to a primary lobule which occurs in the shape of a short corn with the branch as its stalk. Bases of primary lobules are seen distinctly over the surface of the lung of infants whereas over the pulmonary surface of adults they are seen as polygonal areas, each comprising a few to several primary lobules. Regularly arranged pigmentations are evident in these areas.

According to GERLACH, the finest bronchi measured 0.1125 mm in diameter, and the bases of primary lobules 0.45 to 0.675 mm. The base of each secondary lobule measured from 1.8 to 2.7 mm. It thus followed that what was referred to as a secondary lobule represented portions of the lung that were by far smaller than what now is referred to as a pulmonary lobule.

RINDFLEISCH (1872): The term acinus was first used by him in describing the fine structure of the lung; a clear conception of acinus was thus formed. He said that both the acinus and the lobule constitute the units of lung tissues in man, and that the former is invariable whereas the latter varies in size.

For example, one lobule may be composed of two acini; others may consist of twenty to thirty acini, thereby the lobules vary in size accordingly to numbers of acini.

In a secondary lobule, stated RINDFLEISCH, the bronchus divides into seven branches which in turn divide into two short sub-branches respectively. Each of these bronchioles extends dendriformly, producing three to five alveolar ducts and, out of each Alveolargang, an acinus in formed.

TURNER (1877): He, too, pointed out the presence of what are practically the same as the primary lobules of KÖLLIKER, referring to the terminal bronchial tubes distributed to the infundibula and areas peripheral to them as primary lobule.

CHARCOT (1887): He took a view on the acinus differing from that of RINDFLEISCH. The term acinus is used here to denote those belonging to the "Alveolargang" of SCHULTZE and those corresponding to the lobulette of WATERS.

LAGUESSE (1898): The pulmonary parenchyma divides into lobules, and primary or simple lobules are seen to be situated at the surface of the lung. The secondary lobule of GERLACH, et al. is referred to here as a primary lobule.

In LAGUESSE' definition, each bronchus opened into acini or bronchiole acinuse, terminating in short chambers furnished with numerous alveoli; each of these chambers corresponds to the acinus of RINDFEISCH and CHARCOT.

BERDAL (1903): The sublobular bronchus is in line with the axis that links the center of the lobular base with the lobular vertex. The sublobular bronchus forms intralobular bronchi which in turn yield intralobular bronchioles, and these bronchioles form short tubular parts called acinar bronchi. These bronchial branches, by way of short passages, form bell shaped tubes called vestibules, each of which terminates in three to five alveolar ducts.

The primary lobule was said to consist of such an alveolar duct and one to several infundibula opening out from it. Four to five such primary lobules constituted a chamber called an acinus, and fifteen to eighteen such acini constituted a secondary lobule, according to BERDAL.

LOESCHCKE (1921): The lung acinus was cleverly diagramed by this investigator. The acinus was said to be composed of a bronchiolus verus terminalis which divided into two bronchioli respiratorii, each of which in turn subdivided into two to three branches (Alveolargänge), each of which terminated in a sacculus alveolaris.

HUSTEN (1921): The portions peripheral to the primary respiratory lobule, *i.e.* secondary and tertiary bronchioles and alveolar ducts and respiratory sacs which belong to them, as well as blood vessels which accompany them, constitute the unit of lung tissue and are referred to as acini.

BRAUS (1924): Taking the acinus as the morphological unit of lung tissue and, with reference to diagrams published by LOESCHCKE, he dexterously schematized the structure of lung tissues. Twelve to eighteen acini form a lobule and each of such lobules is surrounded by interlobular septum.

The lobule of Braus therefore corresponds to what is now generally referred to as the secondary lobule. It is extremely difficult to systematically consolidate these complicated and divergent series of studies.

MILLER (1937): A consistent approach to these subjects has been pursued by MILLER. He set forward the anatomy of the lung by methods developed by himself; the resulting extensive achievements are collected in his lifework "The Lung" which contains descriptions not only of the bronchial system but also of the vascular, lymphatic, and nerve supply to the lung. Although descriptions on the innervation of the lung are scarce, MILLER's text has generally established a firm footing as basic literature in this field of study. Of particular note are a number of beautifully prepared diagrams of the bronchial system, especially of "air space", that afford a better and clearer understanding of the subject.

The views of MILLER on the bronchial system may be briefly summarized:

Each terminal bronchiole divides into two respiratory bronchioles which are usually subdivided into primary and secondary respiratory bronchioles and, in some cases, also into tertiary respiratory bronchioles.

Respiratory bronchioles individually bifurcate to yield two alveolar ducts which in turn divide to produce alveolar sacs. Between the alveolar duct and the alvolar sac, an irregular chamber called the atrium is interposed.

Alveolar ducts, atria, alveolar sacs and alveoli together with accompanying blood vessels, lymphatic vessels and nerves, were designated collectively by MILLER as the primary lobule. He said that each secondary lobule was composed of a number of such primary lobules and that there was a fibrous septum and marked pigmentations in between neighboring secondary lobules.

He also stated that the lobule and not the acinus constituted the unit of lung tissue.

2. Author's Conception of Acinus

Studies with acrylic resin casts of the broncho-bronchiolar tree as conducted by NAGASAWA and NAGA-

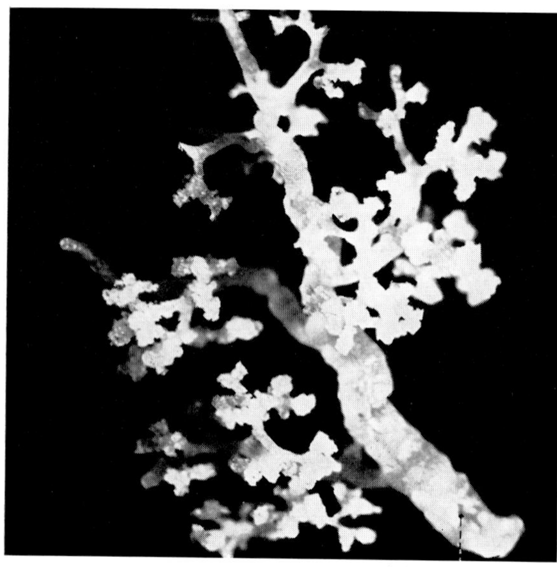

Fig. 60 Resin cast of the peripheral part of the bronchoalveolar system.

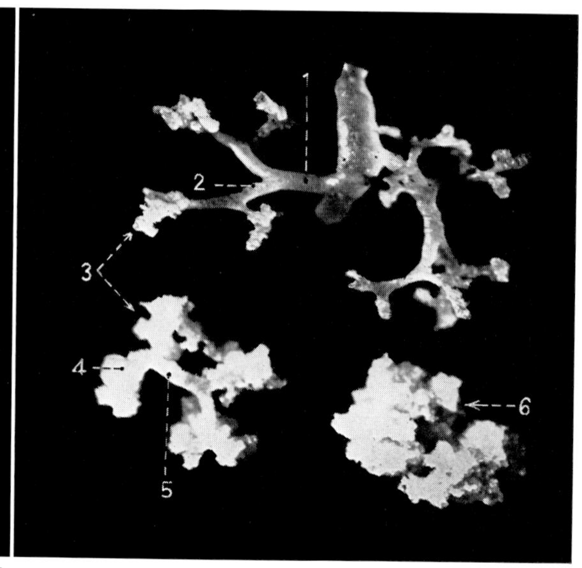

Fig. 61 Resin cast of the peripheral part of the bronchoalveolar system.

1: terminal bronchiole
2: primary respiratory bronchiole
3, 4: acini
5: secondary respiratory bronchiole
6: acinus

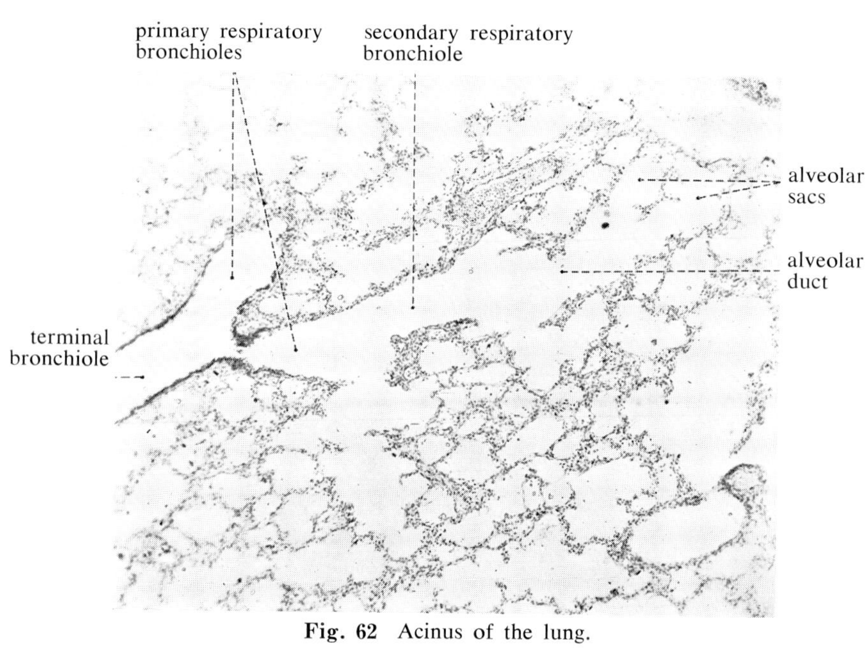

Fig. 62 Acinus of the lung.

matter of concern to many investigators. KIYONO (1914), SAKAMOTO (1917), NAKANOIN (1917), TOMITA (1918), MAJIMA (1929), and HAYAKAWA (1928) stated that histiocytes were recognizable in nucleated cuboidal cells as well as in the epithelial cells, as will be described later.

In Europe and in the U.S.A., FOOT (1919–1927), PERMER (1920) et al. supported the above view. However, KIYONO and a number of other researchers were definitely on the side of an epithelial covering to the alveolar wall.

In summary, the current conception is that histiocytes are cells which are quite abundant in the alveolar region, but are not the main constituents of covering epithelia of the alveolar wall.

3. History of Electron Microscopic Studies

The first electron microscopic observation of covering tissues of the alveolar wall was conducted by LOW (1953), and with definite support for the existence of an epithelial alveolar wall covering.

Somewhat later, similar observations were made by SWIGART and KANE (1954), and by NAGAISHI and ITAGI (1954).

LOW and SWIGART agreed that the endothelial cell of the alveolar capillary does not lie naked on the alveolar wall, but that a certain substance intervenes between the alveolar air and the capillary. However as to the question whether the substance was epithelial or mesothelial the authors were of opposite opinions.

The following is a brief summary of their views.

LOW (1953): The cytoplasm of the epithelial cells lies upon the basement membrane facing the alveolar space. Epithelial cells were observed quite commonly but some portions were so thin that it was somewhat difficult to designate them as continuations of epithelial cells. The epithelial cells were extremely thin and barely visualized even by electron microscopic observation. In particular preparations the thickness of the cell process was less than 0.2 μ. The same findings were obtained on rabbit, guinea pig, dog and man, but this did not suffice to disprove the existence of a non-nucleated plate.

The substance forming a septum between alveoli consisted of a basement substance of a fibrous nature which was not observed in endothelial cells or epithelial cells, and which somewhat resembled reticulum. This substance was sustentacular tissue filling the space between capillaries and appeared to be situated between the alveolar space and septum. In some instances it was observed as a discontinuous membrane lining the alveolar wall. Since the membrane was extremely thin, keen observation was required; otherwise it could be erroneously concluded that capillaries were uncovered in the alveolar space.

The findings by NAGAISHI's group at that time were similar to those of LOW, and will be described later in detail.

In the years 1953–54 no highly efficient electron microscope had been developed. Therefore, the results of all the electron microscopic findings were rather incomplete.

Thereafter, remarkable progress was made in the development of apparatus, in techniques of preparation of specimens, and in investigational methods. Further precise studies were carried out by various authors, such as POLICARD, et al. (1957), KISCH (1958), SCHULZ (1959), CAMPICHE (1960), HATTORI (1965), KIKKAWA, et al. (1965), BROOKS (1966), NIDEN (1966 and 1967), YAMADA (1969), and others.

Since 1954, the transmission electron microscope has been used by ITAGI, N. NAGASAWA, OKIDA, ISHIKO, Y. SENDA, DAIDO and NAGAISHI, and observations were made on peripheral parts of the bronchi and alveoli. After 1967 OKADA and NAGAISHI demonstrated the ultrafine structure of bronchi and alveoli, using the scanning electron microscope as well.

Preceding further details, the apparatus, material and method of study adopted by the author and his colleagues will briefly be given.

Supplement: Apparatus, Materials and Methods for Transmission and Scanning Electron Microscopies

1) Apparatus: Japan Electron Optics Laboratory Co., Ltd., Model JSM-7 for transmission electron microscopy, and Model JSM-S for scanning electron microscopy.

2) Materials: Specimens of lung from man, dog, cat, rabbit, guinea pig and mouse; hens, cocks and pigeons; toads and newt; striped snake, gecko and tortoise were used.

Specimens were taken from quite fresh materials. In man, a normal portion of freshly resected lung was taken immediately after thoracotomy, in order that the tissue would not be damaged by subsequent surgical procedures.

3) Methods of Study

a) Transmission Electron Microscopy

When the transmission electron microscopy was used, the specimen was processed by glutaraldehyde double fixation or by osmium fixation, followed by epon embedding. However, for reference purposes, methacrylate embedded specimens, made about 1954, were also used in the early stages of the study.

Ultrathin sections were pretreated by simple staining with lead or by double staining with lead and uranium salts.

b) Scanning Electron Microscopy

The scanning electron microscope is an apparatus used to examine the surface of an object. The secondary radiation from the surface of the object is registered photographically.

The material to be studied must be quickly (preferably instantaneously) prefixed, dried in a vacuum, and then shadow cast with metal. Adequate dehydration is most important. Up to the present the most commonly used methods have been freezing or dehydration with acetone.

PEASE, et al. (1966) and BLÜMCKE, et al. (1967) have employed freezing methods.

The method adopted by OKADA and NAGAISHI (1967), when using mouse, guinea pig or rabbit tissues, employed liquid nitrogen which is injected into the pleural space, respiration being controlled under intratracheal anesthesia; the lung is instantly frozen and is left in this condition until sufficiently dried.

Using this method, tissues in the body can be kept in comparatively good condition, excepting for the mucous membrane. Because this membrane is covered with mucous observation of the surface of the bronchi or alveoli is consequently rather difficult at the level of magnification desired.

Dehydration with acetone requires preliminary fixation of the material in formalin glutaraldehyde or osmium; the specimens are then rinsed with water and processed into acetone solutions in the usual manner.

After the last immersion in pure acetone is finished, the material is dried by vacuum pumping.

Because of the adequate preservation of the material and the fine results obtained, the latter method has been approved by BARBER, et al. (1968) and TOKUNAGA, et al. (1969).

In order to investigate the actual surface of the mucous membrane, it is desirable to remove the mucous before fixation. The surface can be washed with saline solution, containing 0.1% trypsin.

Carbon and metal are preferably used for the surface coating of the material. The carbon coated specimen is further coated with metal. However, in many instances, a single coating with metal is enough. The authors, in fact, use the specimen coated with gold.

Table 2 summarizes the above methods.

Table 2 Preparation of Specimens for Scanning Electron Microscopy.

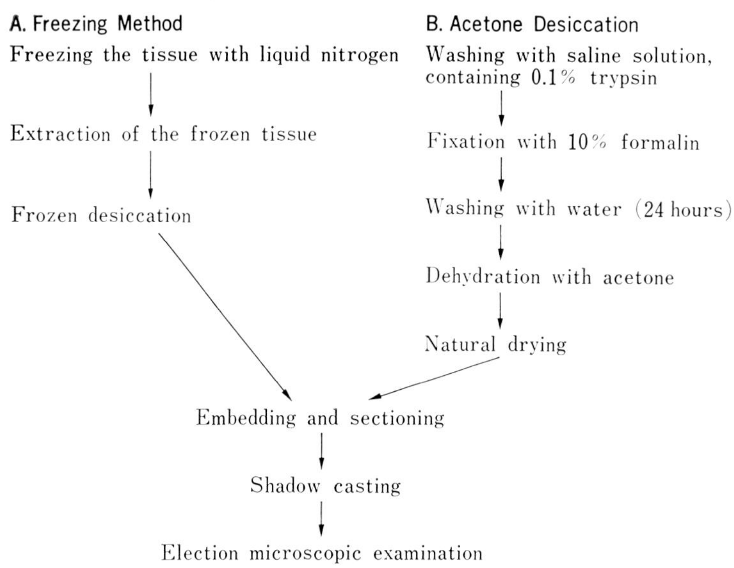

B. Ultrafine Structure of Alveolar Region

Hereinafter, transmission electron microscopic as well as scanning electron microscopic findings and the views of the author's group about the ultrafine structure of alveoli will be related, and, as appropriate, optical microscopic findings will also be referred to.

1. Alveolar Epithelium

As shown in Fig. 63, the alveolar wall in mammals is lined continuously by a layer of epithelium, with two types of cells which are morphologically different.

It is quite appropriate to consider that these two types of cells are of epithelial origin since they each have basement membrane immediately beneath. This observation has been confirmed, phylogenetically and ontogenetically, by ISHIKO, SENDA, OKADA, and NAGAISHI (1956 and 1964).

In one of the two types of alveolar epithelial cells, there is a nucleus in the center and the cytoplasm stretches out in disc shape along the surface of the alveolar wall.

Fig. 64 and 65 present examples of this type of alveolar epithelial cell in the human lung, as seen by transmission electron microscopy.

In this type of epithelial cell, a somewhat thick cytoplasm is observed in the nuclear region; the cytoplasm stretches out in thin wing-like processes to cover and hence form in part the alveolar wall. The cytoplasm actually covers the entire surface of the alveolar capillaries and septal interstices. The thinnest part of the cytoplasma has a thickness of about 0.1 μ. In some instances it is about 0.07 μ, *e.g.* in the guinea pig.

No microvilli are observed on the surface of this type of cell.

The thinnest part of the alveolar wall is the region between two adjacent alveolar spaces. The thickness of the basement membrane in these regions is about 0.02–0.04 μ. Therefore, the total thickness of the wall will be about 0.2 μ including the processes of cytoplasm of the two alveolar epithelial cells and their respective basement membranes, and including minute amounts of interalveolar substances.

Gas exchange is performed in the exact region where the capillaries are immediately deep to these cytoplasmic processes. This part forms the air-blood barrier. The cells were simply designated as alveolar epithelial cells until some ten years ago; in recent years other types of cells have been defined. The former are referred to by various names.

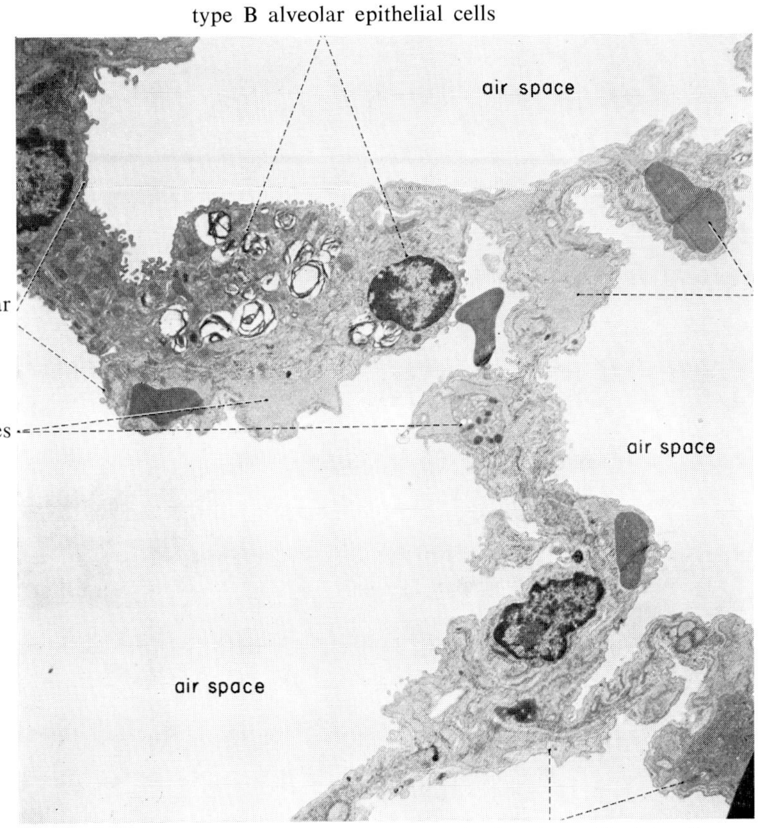

Fig. 63 Ultrafine structure of the alveolar region.

They are: Alveolar epithelial cell (NAGAISHI, ITAGI, 1956), Type A alveolar epithelial cell (TAKAGI and YASUDA, 1958), Type I alveolar epithelial cell (CAMPICHE, 1960), and small alveolar cell (POLICARD, et al., 1957, 1962).

The other type of alveolar epithelial cell which covers the alveolar wall is mostly cuboidal in form; microvilli are seen on the free surface, but the cells are devoid of laterally extending thin processes of cytoplasm. Osmiophilic lamellar bodies inside the cytoplasm are particularly characteristic of this cell.

This cell also tends to bulge into the alveolar space.

Fig. 66 shows a typical cell of this type.

This cell was termed the alveolar wall cell by ITAGI and NAGAISHI (1954), and until recent years this name has been widely used in Japan.

At that time, it was not yet clear whether this cell was of epithelial or mesenchymal origin, but in order to distinguish it from the alveolar epithelial cell, it was provisionally named the alveolar wall cell.

Later became evident, from the studies of the author and other researchers, that this cell is also of an epithelial origin; it is therefore called by various names: Type B alveolar epithelial cell (TAKAGI and

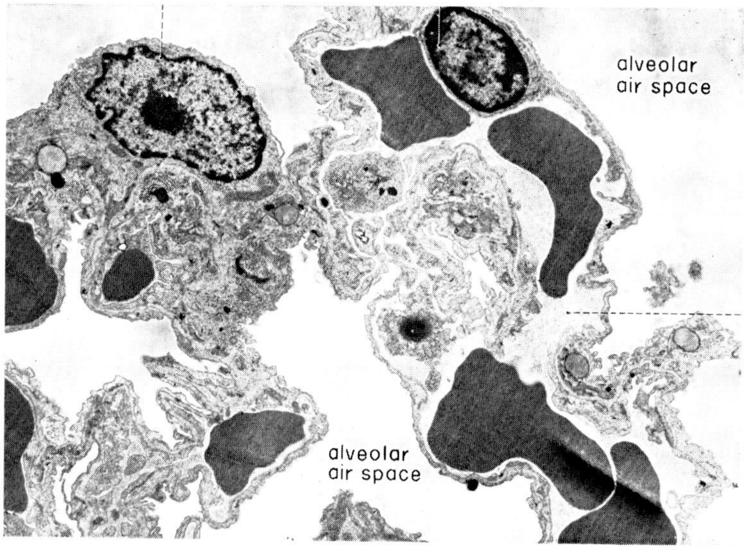

Fig. 64 Type A alveolar epithelial cell (human lung). (transmission electron microscopy)

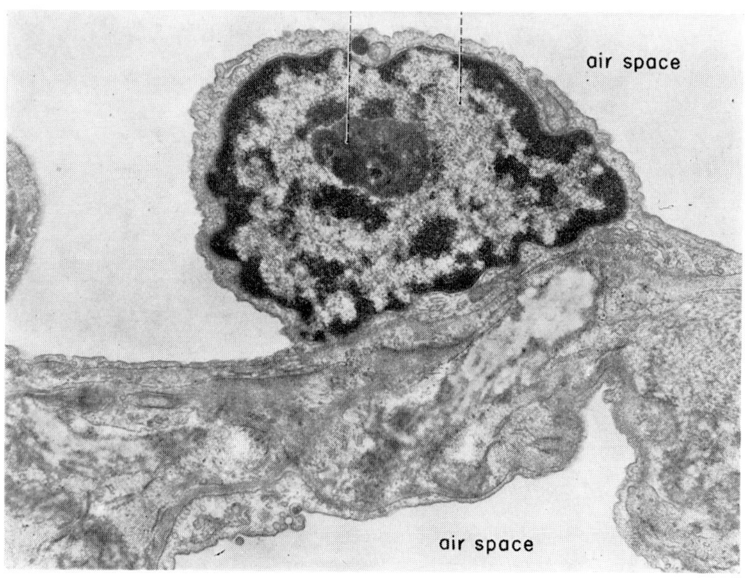

Fig. 65 Type A alveolar epithelial cell.

YASUDA, 1958), Type II alveolar epithelial cell (CAMPICHE, 1969), large alveolar cell (POLICARD, et al., 1957, 1962), or granular pneumocyte (BENSCH, et al., 1967).

In July 1969, YAMORI suggested (at a symposium held in Kyoto on the theme of "Ultrafine Structure of the Lung and Lung Diseases", held under auspices of the Japan Society of Chest Diseases) that the two types of epithelial cells which cover the alveolar wall should be designated as the squamous lining and the cuboidal secretory type, respectively.

YAMORI's suggestion was based on the idea that function as well as form must be taken into consideration. However, if the designation is to be made from this standpoint, the present author recommends the terms squamous gas exchange and cuboidal secretory types to be more in accord with the functional-morphological situation.

BROOKS (1966) suggested adoption of the term type A and type B alveolar epithelial cell designated by TAKAGI and YASUDA as general terms.

Hereinafter, the terms type A alveolar epithelial cell (squamous gas exchange type) and type B alveolar epithelial cell (cuboidal secretory type) will be used.

In short, the alveolar wall is continuously lined with epithelial cells, types A and B, excepting for the openings of the respiratory bronchioles and Kohn's alveolar pores.

The type B alveolar epithelial cell (cuboidal secretory type) exhibits microvilli on its free surface, facing the alveolar space, and has osmiophilic lamellar bodies in the cytoplasm, as shown in Fig. 67.

The inclusion bodies are characteristic in this cell and are called by various names as follows:

capillary

osmiophilic lamellar bodies

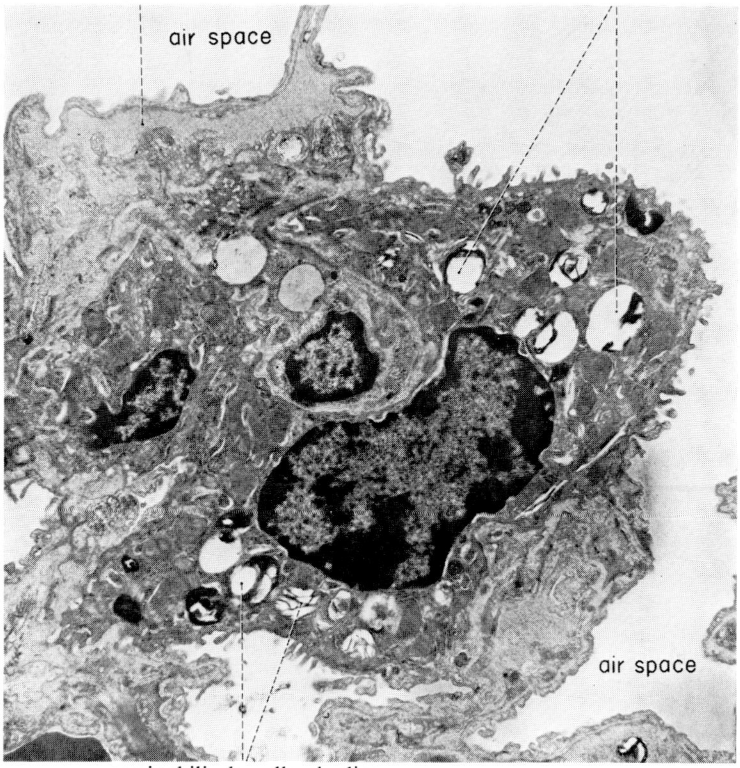

osmiophilic lamellar bodies

Fig. 66 Type B alveolar epithelial cell.

osmiophilic lamellar bodies

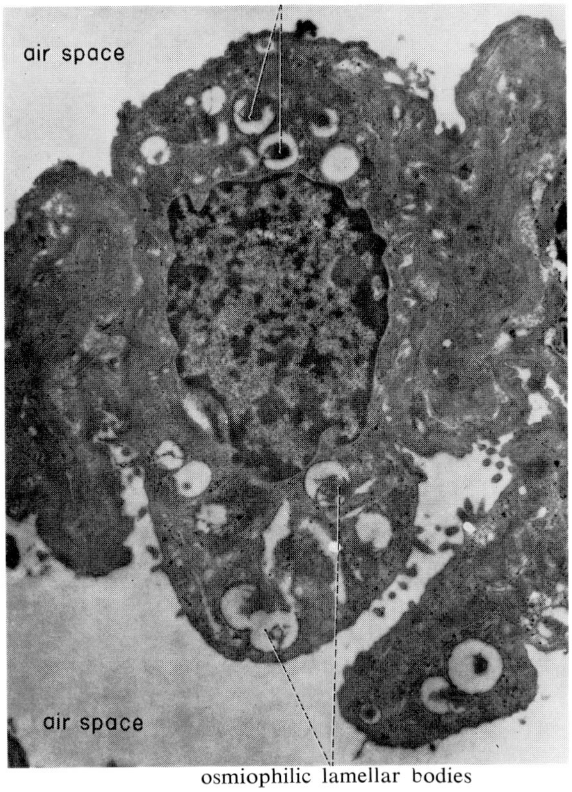

osmiophilic lamellar bodies

Fig. 67 Type B alveolar epithelial cell.

Osmiophilic body (ITAGI, 1956 and ISHIKO, 1959) Osmiophilic inclusions, lamellar transformations, osmiophilic bodies (POLICARD, et al., 1957), plasmasomes (KISCH, 1958), lamellar forms, mitochondrial transforms, lamellar inclusions, osmiophile Einschlüsse (BARGMANN, et al., 1956).

The term osmiophilic lamellar body is to be used hereafter.

2. Comparative Anatomic and Phylogenetic Studies on Alveolar Epithelial Cells

The following is a report of the studies performed by ISHIKO, OKADA, and NAGAISHI, et al. (1959, 1964).

Amphibia: In toad, frog and newt, thin processes extending from the cytoplasm are seen in both A and B type cells as shown in Fig. 68(a) and (b). Osmiophilic lamellar bodies are observed in the cytoplasm.

However, further detailed observation shows that the cells are of two types, one resting immediately over the processes of the alveolar capillary projecting into the alveolar space, the other occupying the narrow region between two neighboring capillaries.

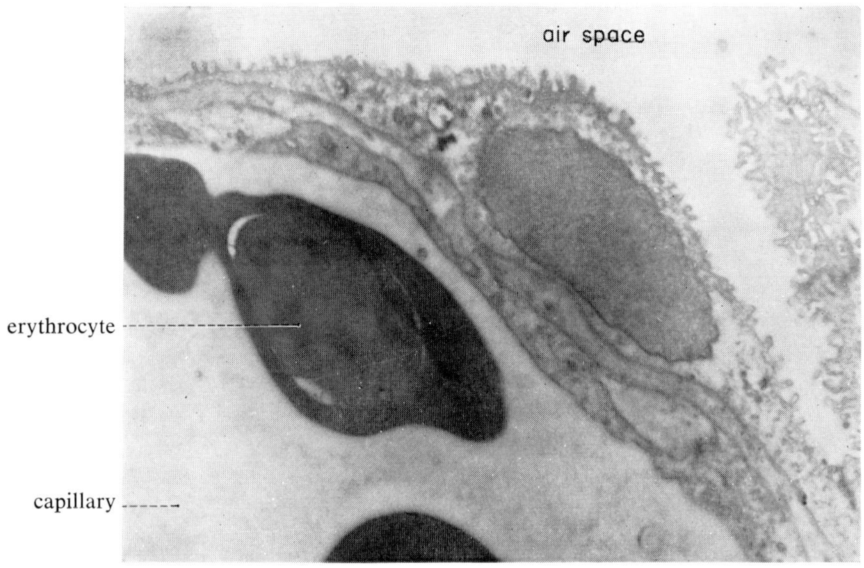

Fig. 68 a Type A alveolar epithelial cell (frog lung).

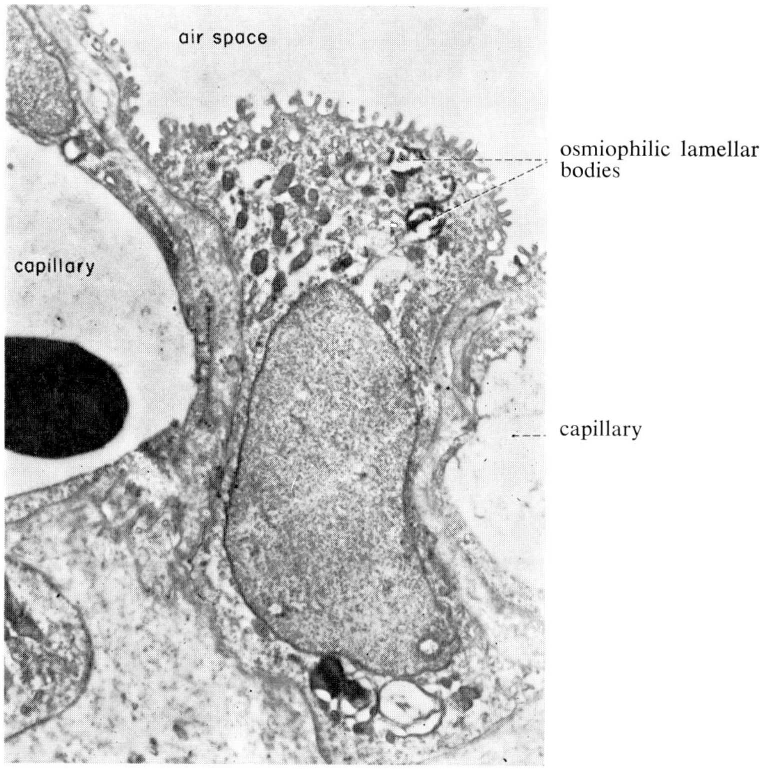

Fig. 68 b Type B alveolar epithelial cell (frog lung).

These cell types correspond to type A and B, respectively.

As was pointed out by Ishiko (1959), the differentiation of type A and B in the alveoli of amphibias may be incomplete, the two cells presenting similar fine structures.

Reptiles: Differentiation of types A and B cells is more evident in reptiles such as the striped snake, gecko and tortoise.

In particular, the type A cell of the tortoise resembles that of mammals, and osmiophilic lamellar bodies in the extended thin cytoplasma are not observed. Type B cells have osmiophilic bodies in addition to the thin processes of cytoplasm observed in type A. But as shown in Fig. 69, type A cells of snakes are quite similar to those of mammals.

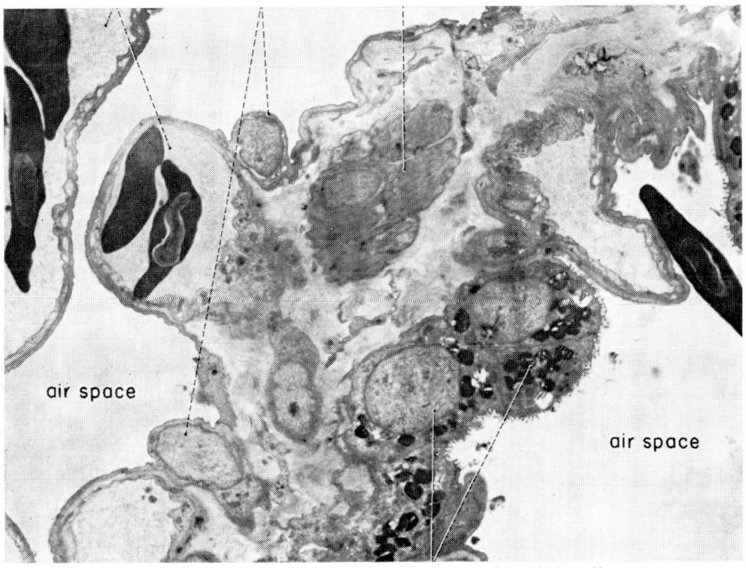

Fig. 69 Ultrafine structure of the alveolar region (snake lung).

Moreover, type B cells have osmiophilic lamellar bodies and are devoid of the thin processes of the cytoplasm.

Type A and B cells of the snake are quite similar to those of mammals in that the two types are completely differentiated.

Birds: The alveolar epithelial cells of birds such as the hen, cock and pigeon are somewhat different when compared to those of amphibia, reptiles, and mammals.

In birds, the parts corresponding to the alveolar regions are lined with type A cells, as shown in Fig. 70; type B cells are not found in this part. The same findings were reported by Bargmann, et al. (1961) and Policard, et al. (1962).

As shown in Fig. 71, type B cells are observed to form a continuous lining over the those regions closer to the origin of the bronchioles.

Thus, in birds, not only the form but also the distribution of type A and B cells differ.

Fig. 72 is the schema representing the phylogenetic progression from amphibia to mammals, as described as above.

The observations on birds give the impression that the type B cells resemble, in their structure, the bronchial epithelial cells.

The author considers that the above impression is further corroborated by the fact that in mammals, type B cells are observed to be most numerous in the transitional part of alveoli and bronchioles, whereas in reptiles, type B cells are found intermingled with the ciliated cells of the bronchioles.

3. Ontogenetic Studies of Alveolar Epithelial Cells

In the human fetal stage, it is difficult to distinguish type A and type B epithelial cells morphologically. Fig. 73(a) and (b) show the similarity of types A and B.

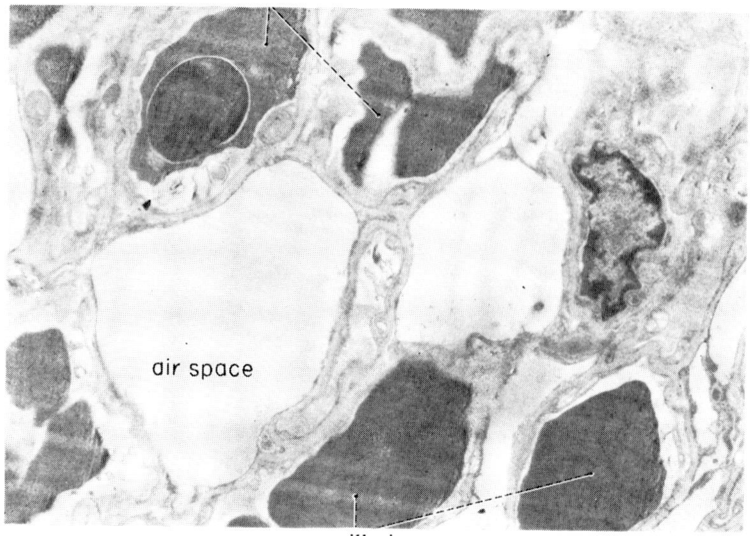

Fig. 70 Ultrafine structure of the alveolar region (bird lung).

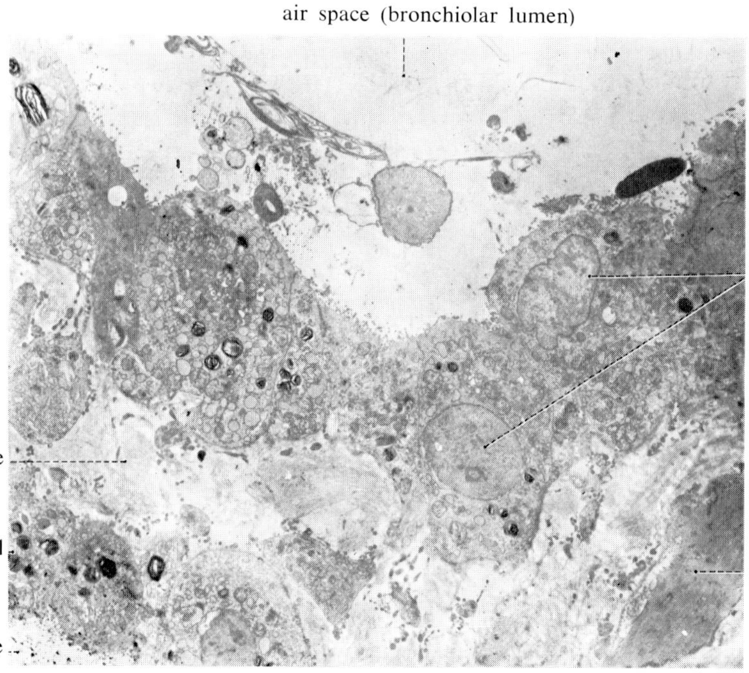

Fig. 71 Ultrafine structure of type B alveolar epithelial cell (bird lung).

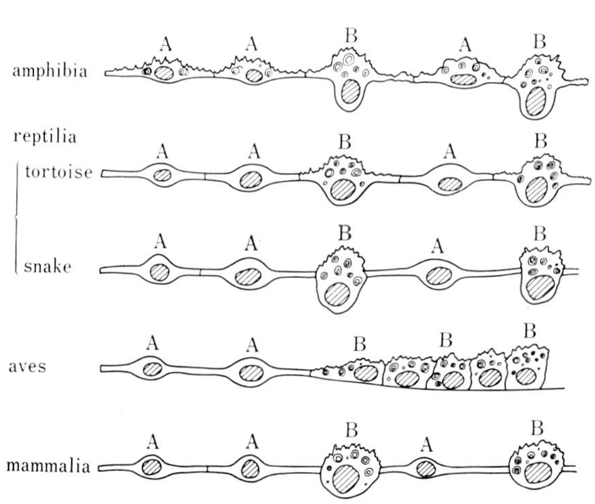

Fig. 72 Comparative morphology of the alveolar epithelial cells in vertebrate lung.

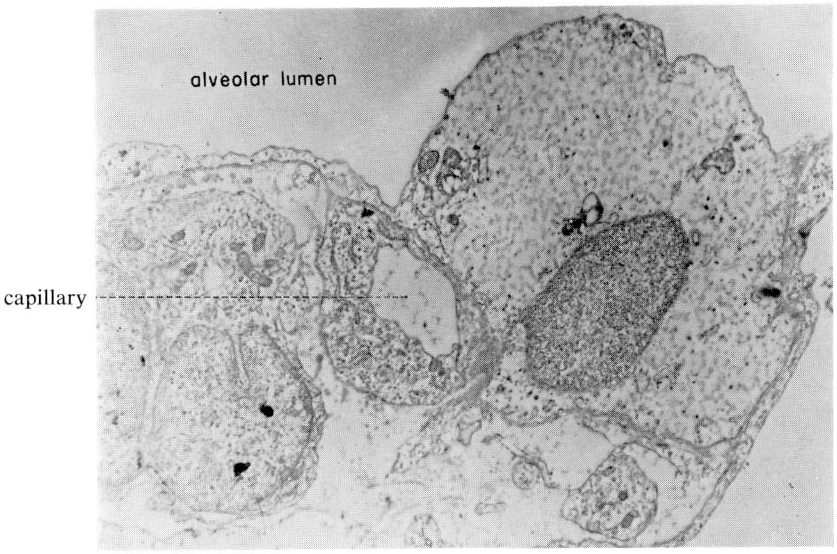

Fig. 73 a Type A alveolar epithelial cell of the fetus.

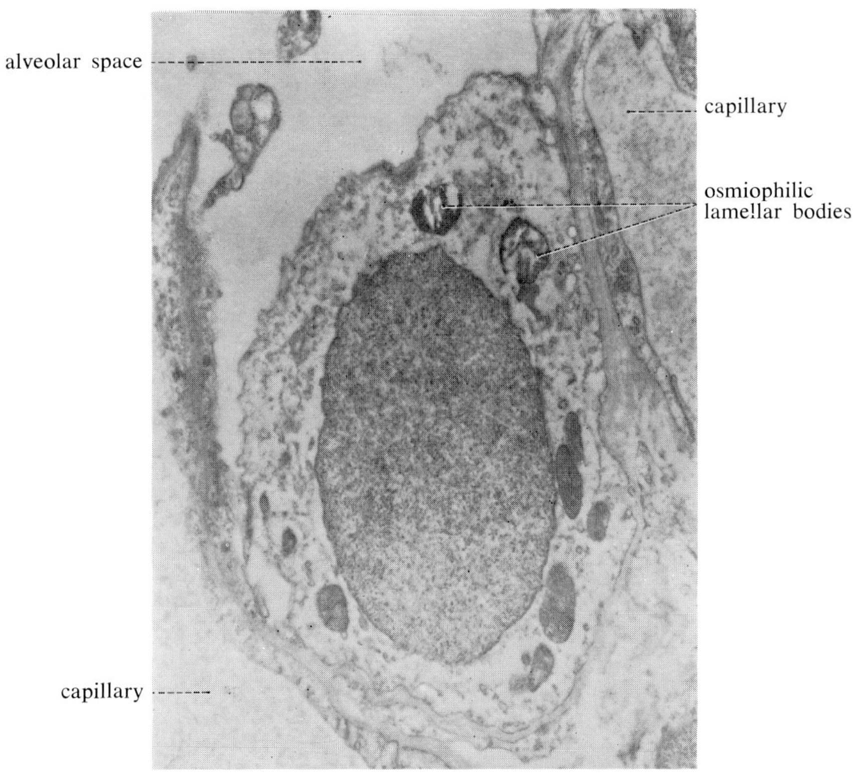

Fig. 73 b Type B alveolar epithelial cell of the fetus.

4. Type B Alveolar Epithelial Cell (Cuboidal Secretory Type); its Relation to Alveolar Surfactant

In the early stage of electron microscopic studies of alveoli, the osmiophilic lamellar bodies specifically noted in the cytoplasm of type B cells were considered to be transformed mitochondria; however, in recent years, BUCKINGHAM, et al. (1966) and many other authors have denied this relationship. For instance, KIKKAWA, et al. (1965) stated that these bodies had a close relationship to Golgi's apparatus.

Fig. 74 is an example of an electron micrograph of this cytoplasmic inclusion body.

These osmiophilic lamellar bodies are rich in phosphatide. Accordingly, the attention of investigators has been concentrated on their function as main sources of origin of alveolar surfactant.

Alveolar surfactant is in general phosphatidic; its main component is considered to be dipalmitoyl lecithin.

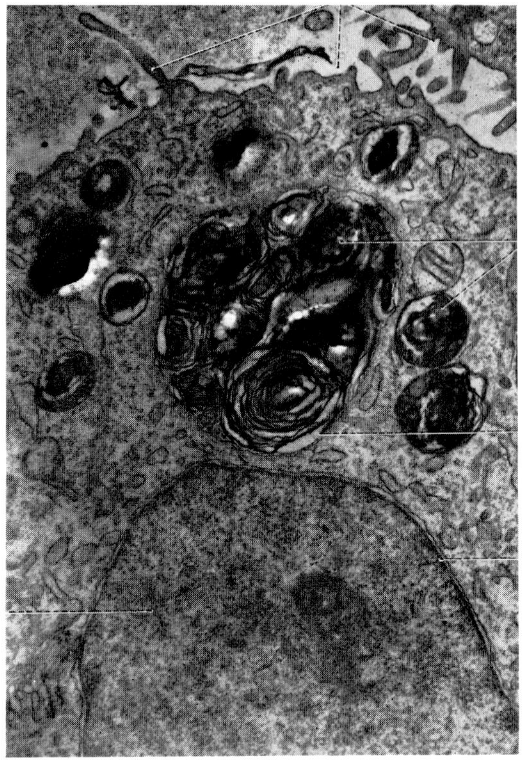

Fig. 74 Osmiophilic lamellar bodies of the Type B alveolar epithelial cell.

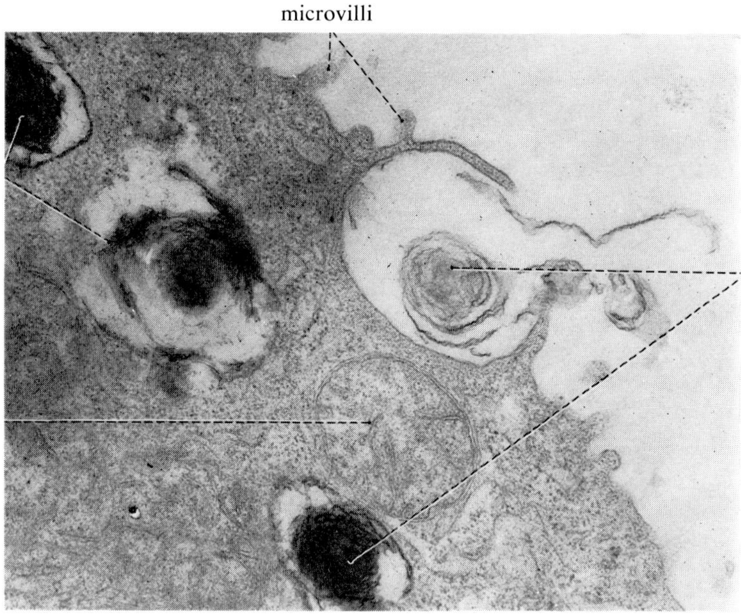

Fig. 75 Secretion of the osmiophilic lamellar body.

According to KIKKAWA, et al. (1965), the development of osmiophilic bodies parallels the increase of lecithin.

BUCKINGHAM, et al. (1966) stressed the role of type B cells in the production of surfactant. In their experiment they gave palmitate-^{3}H to rabbits and showed a rapid uptake by type B cells.

Morphologically, as shown in Fig. 75, osmiophilic lamellar bodies which have been released from type B cells into the alveolar spaces have been often observed. Osmiophilic lamellar bodies seem to be released into the alveolar spaces by merocrine secretion (HATASA, et al., 1966).

It is known that the released or extruded osmiophilic lamellar bodies lose their concentric and circular arrangement and form lattices or flat board-like shapes (HATTORI, et al., 1965, 1969; WEIBEL, et al., 1966).

As regards the nature of the osmiophilic lamellar bodies, HATTORI (1969) has made extensive and detailed investigations.

Regarding their systematically arranged lattice-like ultrafine structure, there is an idea that the alveolar surfactant is not simply lipid, but is in the form of a lecithin-protein complex (KIKKAWA, et al., 1965; WEIBEL, et al., 1966).

According to OKADA (1969), in the case where osmiophilic bodies are released from type B cells, the release is said to be made by holocrine-like secretion. Fig. 76 shows such a finding.

osmiophilic lamellar bodies

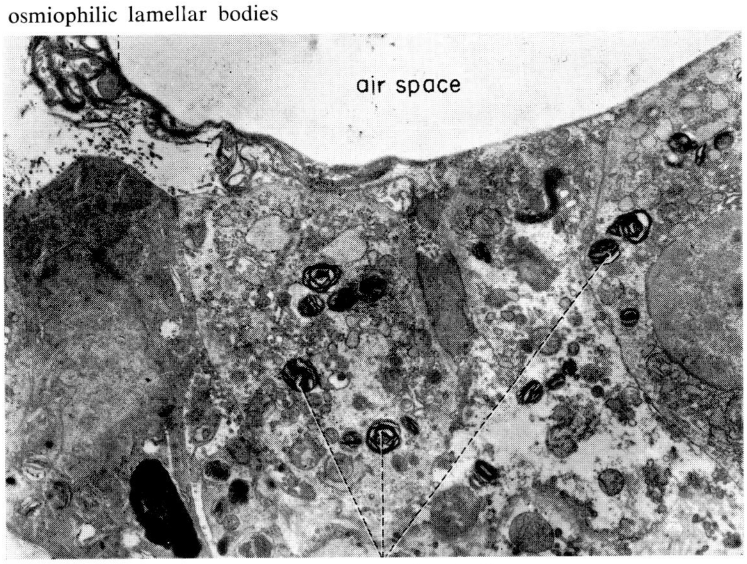

osmiophilic lamellar bodies

Fig. 76 Secretion of the osmiophilic lamellar bodies in the bird lung.

In the lungs of birds, as described earlier, the type B cells lie close to each other in the region corresponding to bronchioles, and when they collapse and detach themselves a large number of osmiophilic lamellar bodies is said to be released into the bronchiolar spaces. The released osmiophilic lamellar bodies become disentangled and arrange themselves in a straight lamellar form. As TYLER, et al. (1969) state, they may transit into the alveolar space.

By optical microscopic observation (BOLANDE, et al., 1964) and by electron microscopic observation (PATTLE, 1963; GRONIOWSKI, et al., 1964 and 1966; WEIBEL, et al., 1968), existence of a substance adjacent to the alveolar space which is considered to be surfactant has been proved.

However, as between the biochemical and morphological studies on alveolar surfactant there exists a deep gap, even today.

As mentioned by N. SENDA, et al. (1967), there are many questions about the alveolar surfactant (as well as its clinical significance) to be answered by further studies.

5. Role of Type B Alveolar Epithelial Cell in Adenomatous Hyperplasia

An exuberant repair mechanism consequent on inflammatory changes may result in adenomatous hyperplasia of the alveolar epithelium.

Such changes are very important in discussing the pathology of development of cicatricial cancer of the lung and of other diseases of the lung, as reported by OKADA, DAIDO and NAGAISHI (1967), but there still remain many questions about these cells which have such an important role in the course of diseases.

Transmission electron microscopic observations were made by OTSUKA, OKADA and NAGAISHI (1960 and 1966) on tissues resected from lung cancer patients after preoperative irradiation by ^{60}Co.

The following are observations on patients who received varying amounts of ^{60}Co irradiation.

In ^{60}Co irradiated regions, the first change is seen as degeneration and detachment of type A cells (Fig. 77).

Sloughing of epithelium caused by detachment of type A cells, as shown in Fig. 78, causes the basement membranes, fibroblasts, and interstices of the alveolar septum to protrude nakedly in to the alveolar spaces.

Subsequently the number of cuboidal cells on the surface of the alveolar wall undergoes proliferation forming a continuous lining, *i.e.* so-called adenomatous hyperplasia is formed.

Fig. 79 is a schema of the various changes noted above.

The typical adenomatous hyperplasia, formed as mentioned above, exhibits cuboidal cells which, as shown in Fig. 80, present a striking similarity to type B alveolar epithelial cells.

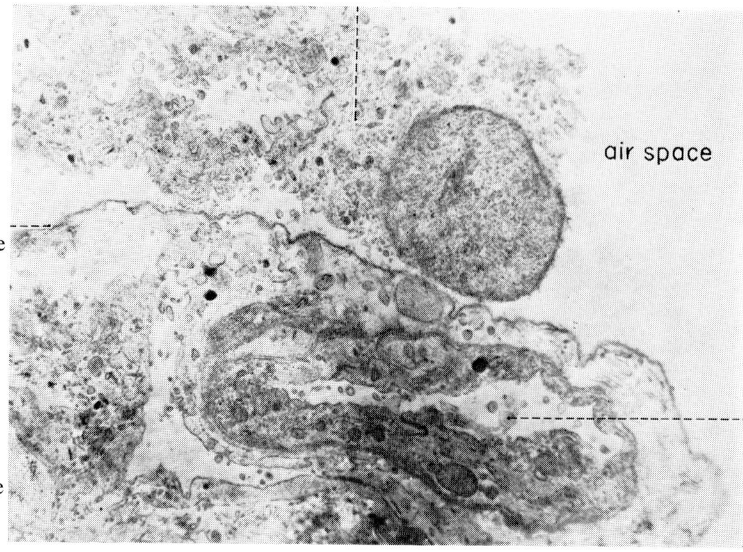

Fig. 77 Degeneration of type A alveolar epithelial cell.

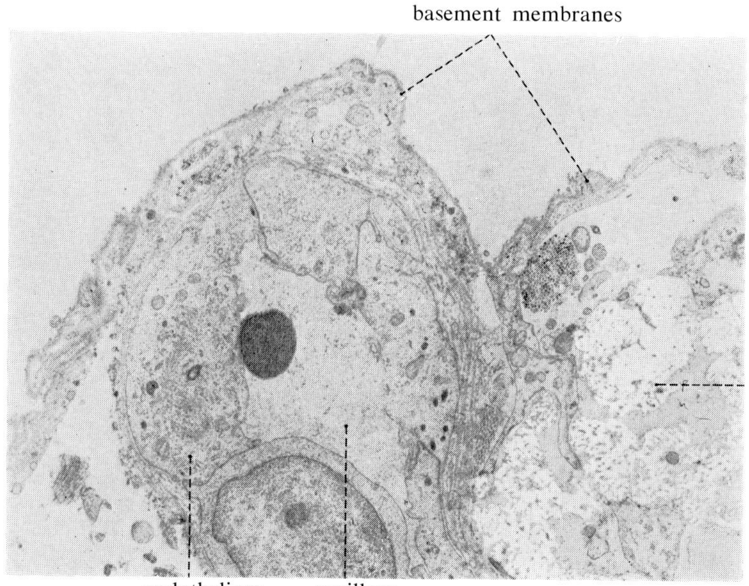

Fig. 78 Alveolar septum of the fibrotic lung.

Namely, the cells are cuboidal in shape, are devoid of cytoplasmic processes and typical osmiophilic lamellar bodies are found in their cytoplasm.

The number of osmiophilic lamellar bodies varies in each cell, some cells having scarcely any.

From the findings mentioned, the author considers that type A alveolar epithelial cells are easily damaged, whereas type B cells are resistant to radiation injury; one of their functions is apparently to replace the denuded regions from which type A cells have been detached.

Thus, type B cells are considered to play a role as a reserve source for epithelial cells.

The cuboidal epithelial cells lying in bronchioles have been also regarded as a source of reserve cells. However no data is available as to this point from the our present studies. This problem will be described in the following paragraph, based on a report by EBE (1969). Thus, the regeneration or hyperplasia of epithelial cells in the alveolar region is thought to have some relation to the mechanism of development of bronchiolar carcinoma or alveolar cell carcinoma. In addition to the above, the relationship of the pulmonary adenoma of the mouse (caused by urethane intake) to type B alveolar epithelial cells was examined by electron microscopy by KLÄRNER, et al. (1960), OKADA, et al. (1962), SVOBODA (1962), HATTORI, et al. (1965), and by DAIDO (1966), and it was shown that type B cells have a strong regeneratively activity.

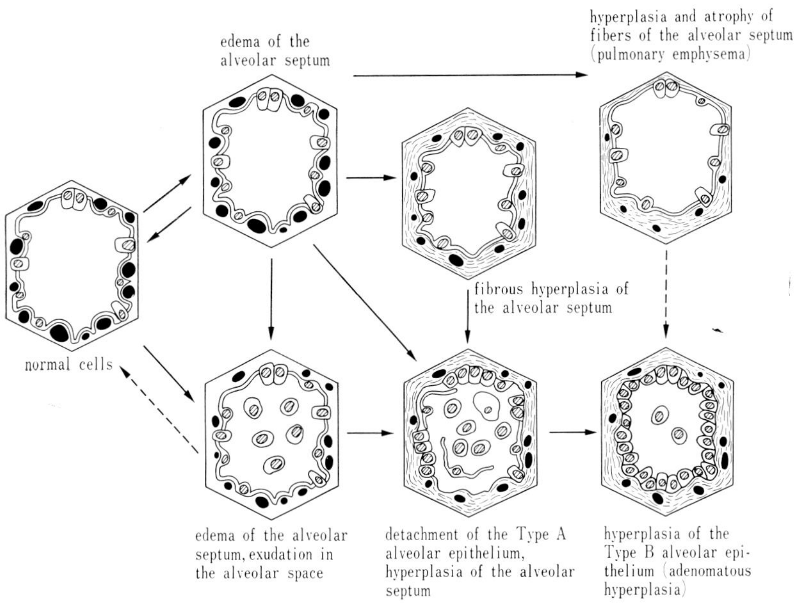

Fig. 79 Changes of the alveolar septum in the fibrotic lung.

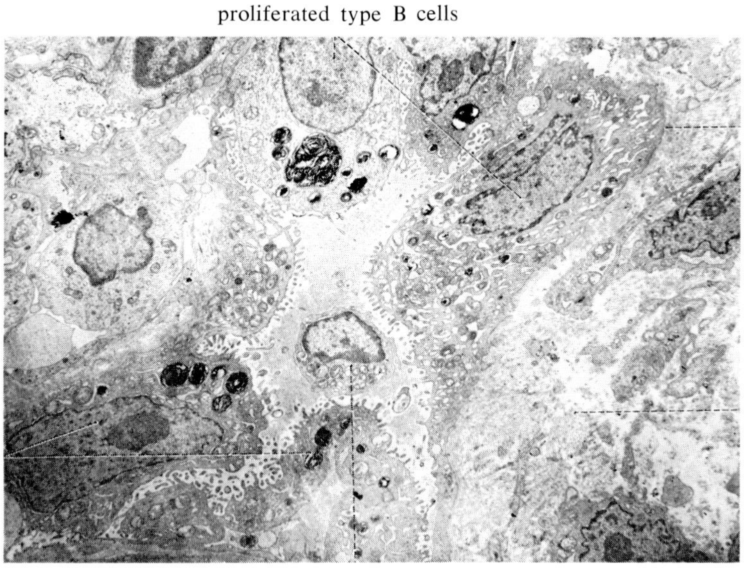

Fig. 80 Ultrafine structure of the adenomatous hyperplasia in the alveolar region.

6. Regeneration of Alveolar Epithelium, particularly of Type A Alveolar Epithelial Cell (Squamous Gas Exchange Type)

From what cells and in what way are type A alveolar epithelial cells regenerated? It is inconceivable that one cell remains unchanged throughout life, from birth till death, without being replaced by a new cell of the same type.

It is rather difficult to follow the phases of replacement or regeneration of the type A cells.

As already described in the preceding section, the regions in which type A alveolar epithelial cells exfoliated after radiation, were repaired by type B alveolar epithelial cells. Quite a number of such findings have been reported, but there are few descriptions of repair by type A cells. Regarding transformation of type B to type A cells there are no verified reports.

Guieyose-Pellissier (1920): Inhalation of poisonous gas caused rapid hyperplasia of alveolar epithelial cells in rats. Amitotic figures were observed in many parts, and there were very few mitotic figures.

Bertalanffy and Leblond (1953): Though they were quite few in number mitotic figures were observed in some cases.

However, the fact is that when these reports were issued it was not yet evident that the alveolar wall was covered with two types of epithelial cells. Therefore the reports do not disclose evidence of a kind sufficient to confirm that the division of type A alveolar epithelial cells had occurred.

EBE (1969) reported interesting experiments on the regeneration of type A and B alveolar epithelial cells.

His experiments were conducted with the purpose of investigating further details about the so-called "agricultural drug pneumonitis", as reported by KINOSHITA, and OGIMA, et al. (1968).

EBE's experiments were made on rabbits. A solution of blasticidin-S (hereafter called BC-S), one of the agricultural drugs, was insufflated intratracheally into the lung of rabbits with the aim of producing pneumonitis. The progress of the condition and of its therapy was followed by optical and electron microscopies.

According to his experimental plan, if the alveoli were severely damaged, this would cause a collapse of the cells; regeneration of alveoli would be evidenced by the replacement of detached cells.

EBE briefly divided the whole processes into five stages.

The first stage occurred one or two days after the insufflation of BC-S. In this stage the main changes were seen as pulmonary edema and local bleeding.

At 3–5 days after insufflation of BC-S, in the second stage, inflammatory cells infiltrated the alveolar wall and hyperplasia of the non-ciliated epithelial cells in the peripheral portion of respiratory bronchioles was observed.

At 6–10 days, in the third stage, alveoli were progressively destroyed, epithelial cells in the region of respiratory bronchiole proliferated and adenomatous constructions formed.

At 12–30 days after insufflation of BC-S, in the fourth stage, the epithelial cells in the adenomatous constructions differentiated into type A and type B alveolar epithelial cells. At the same time, air-blood barrier reconstruction occurred in company with the regeneration of capillary networks. Thus the destroyed lung tissues are partially regenerated. Epithelial buds will then expand and form new alveoli.

The fifth stage is 60 days after insufflation of BC-S. Almost complete alveoli will have been formed by this stage, leaving cicatrized tissues sporadically.

The development of the lung in its embryonal and fetal stages is briefly divided into the adenoid, tubular, and alveolar stages. A similar sequence of development is thus to be recapitulated in the regeneration of alveoli after injury.

EBE stated also that the regeneration of alveoli starts from non-ciliated cuboidal cells situated in the peripheral portion of respiratory bronchiole; from this cuboidal mother cell type A and type B alveolar epithelial cells are differentiated.

But the non-ciliated cells mentioned by EBE were apparently different from Clara cells; they were considered to be immature cells that might grow into either type of alvoelar epithelial cells.

In short, EBE considered the non-ciliated cuboidal cell to be the reserve cell for the two types of alveolar epithelial cells.

According to EBE this reserve cell is cuboidal in shape and with a large nucleus, but it is a small cell. In its cytoplasm mitochondria, Golgi apparatus, rough-surfaced endoplasmic reticulum, osmiophilic bodies and glycogen granules are observed.

Should EBE's understanding be correct, there may be a type of regeneration wherein type B cells replace type B epithelial cells, in addition to the regeneration leading to type A and B alveolar epithelial cells.

This author has had many opportunities to observe the regeneration of type B cells in repair of the regions showing type A exfoliation. We interpret this as hyperplasia of type B cells, but some of them may have been regenerated from a mother cell in the respiratory bronchiole, as reported by EBE.

In any case, it is an interesting question and future studies are necessary.

Regarding the regeneration of alveoli, findings are reported by MONTGOMERY (1944), ROMANOVA (1960), SHIMADA (1963), KLEINERMAN (1964), and others.

7. Aging Phenomena

It is known that in the aging process, elastosis, *i.e.* degeneration of elastic tissues, may be seen in the alveolar region. This may be of importance in lowering the compliance of the lung.

HATTORI and TAKENAGA, et al. (1969) carried out detailed investigations on elastosis using transmission electron microscopy. These authors considered the term "elastosis" to represent such situations as increases of elastic fibers, injury and degeneration of elastic fibers, and hyperplasia of collagenous fibers as seen by electron microscopy.

The changes associated with aging of alveoli may have some correlation with senile emphysema, and may progress even further in correlation with arteriosclerosis or other general phenomena associated with aging.

Furthermore, studies have been made on the aging phenomena as related to the structure of the surfactant which is indispensable to maintaing the surface tension of alveoli. Studies have also been made on the osmiophilic lamellar bodies which bear a presumed relation to the surfactant, and on the type B alveolar epithelial cells (cuboidal secretory type) which are considered to secrete surfactant. No definite conclusions have been reached at this stage.

8. Kohn's Alveolar Pores

A new direct interalveolar passage was described by KOHN (1881, 1893).

Kohn's pores have been studied by HAUSER (1894), NICOLAS (1898), HANSEMANN (1900), ZIMMERMANN (1900), OGAWA (1917), BRAUS (1924), MACKLIN (1936), and LOOSLI (1937), using optical microscopy.

Conflicting opinions have been reported, *e.g.*: 1) alveolar pores are artifacts (EBNER, 1899; MERKEL, 1902; OPPEL, 1905); 2) alveolar pores have not been found in young animals (MILLER, 1950); 3) alveolar pores are pathological, and are not observed in the normal lung (HENLE, 1871; TOLDT, 1881; RIBBERT, 1894; MILLER, 1950).

The existence of Kohn's pores was presumptive from a physiological standpoint; for example, ALLEN (1932) has reported on the phenomenon of collateral respiration. However, according to investigations made by the author's group in 1954 and 1955, using optical and transmission electron microscopies, the existence of Kohn's pores could not be confirmed in the human lung.

As a result, although Kohn's pores were demonstrated in the lung of the cat, we have been dubious bout their existence in the human lung. Recently, OKADA (1969) of the author's group, succeeded in roving their existence in human as well as in animal lungs, using scanning electron microscopy.

However, whether the pores remain open in resting respiration, or are in a closed condition, covered membranous surfactant, or closed on expiration is not yet known. In any case, it seems that air passes rough the openings, being regulated by fluctuations in intraalveolar pressure, or by other mechanisms yet undescribed.

Fig. 81 is a scanning electron micrograph of the alveolar wall in the mouse lung. These were normal ing animals and there is little doubt that the pores in this figure are similar to those described by Kohn. Moreover, it is evident that the number of pores in each alveole is much greater than might have been ected.

ig. 82 shows alveolar pores and fenestras in the aged human lung. In general, the pores are larger 1 those seen in the mouse. Whether those are original Kohn's pores or whether they are windows or stras produced by aging changes cannot be definitely stated. Regarding Kohn's pores evident differ nces are seen in the number and size according to kinds or ages of animals, or owing to extent and ee of pulmonary emphysema.

compared to the pores of the normal aged lung, the pores of the alveolar wall in an aged patient with ysema differ in that they are larger and have more of a window or fenestra appearance.

m this point of view, atrophy and degeneration of the alveolar wall in the senile or emphysematous lung esumed to be correlated with an expansion and increase in Kohn's alveolar pores.

ther words the destruction of the interalveolar septum in the senile or emphysematous lung is in many es presumed to be found following enlargement of Kohn's pores, and fusion after enlargement is caused rease or degeneration of elastic fibers, hyperplasia of collagenous fibers, etc.

rding to investigations carried out by KUNO and STAUB (1968), on artificial alveolar pores, changes in of such pores are in proportion to change in volume. Surface tension on expansion of the lung was

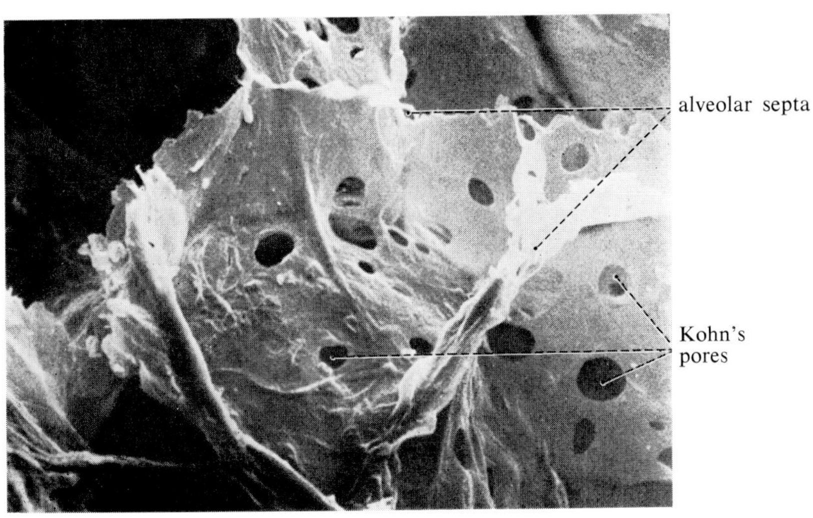

Fig. 81 Alveolar wall and Kohn's pores (mouse) (scanning electon microscopy).

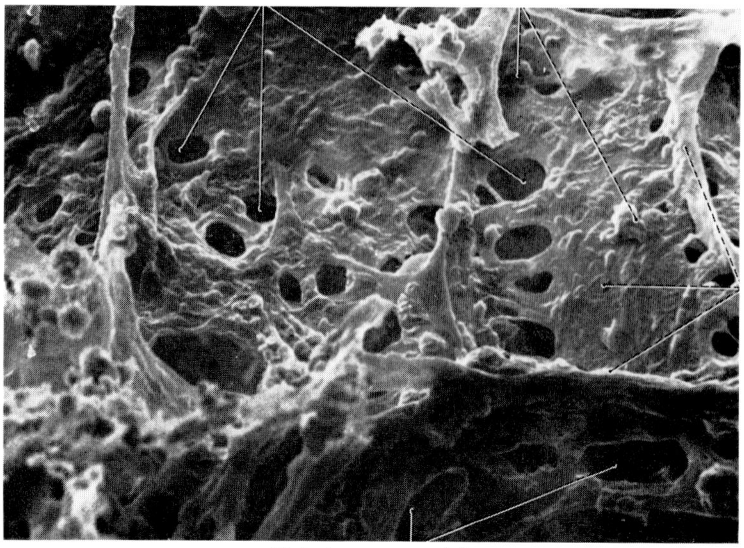

Fig. 82 Alveolar wall, magnifying Kohn's pores and fenestras (aged human lung).

said to be higher on the edges of pores than on those portions of the alveolar walls without pores.

The results of their studies and the author's morphological investigations have been carefully and thoroughly considered. We believe that in cases of over-expansion of lung, coupled with decrease of resistance in the alveolar wall, damage in the alveolar wall is most likely to take place at the location of the alveolar pores. Gradually this damage extends, finally forming a large window or fenestra, as in cases of emphysema.

9. Alveolar Capillaries

As is generally known, the pulmonary artery runs parallel to the bronchus. The arteriolar-capillary transition occurs in the region of the respiratory bronchiole.

NISHIMARU (1952) stated that the arteriole will transit into the venule through the sequence of branching capillaries, reticular capillaries, collecting capillaries, and venous capillaries.

NAGASAWA, YAMASHITA and NAGAISHI (1952) reported on the same observations, having examined resin castings made by injecting methylmethacrylate into pulmonary artery and veins.

The author will now describe the vessels which form the definitive capillary network of the alveolar wall.

Fig. 83 is a transmission electron micrograph of an alveolar capillary, and of its endothelial cells.

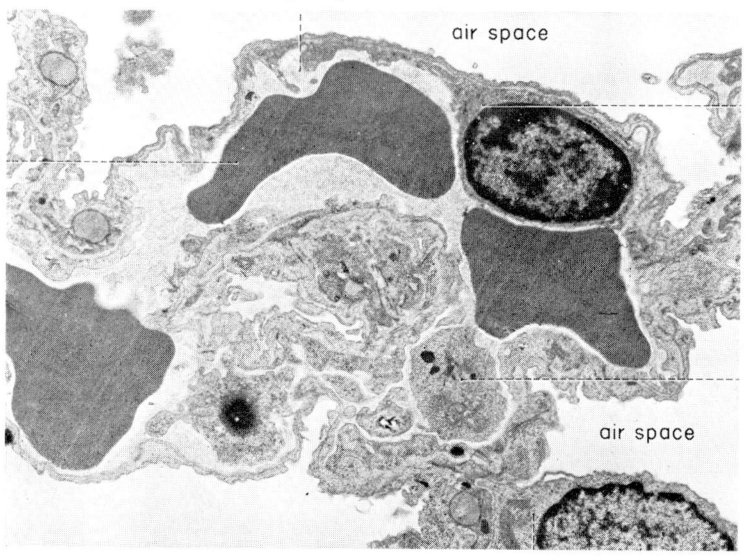

Fig. 83 Alveolar capillary.

The endothelial cells of the alveolar capillary bear a striking resemblance to type A alveolar epithelial cells (squamous gas exchange type). It is quite interesting that these two cell types participating in gas exchange resemble each other so closely.

The cytoplasm of endothelial cells is thicker in the region of the nucleus, but in the region surrounding the nucleus it is a thin membranous extension, lining continuously the capillary wall.

Immediately beneath the endothelial cells there is a layer of basement membrane.

In a back-to-back position on the basement membrane proper the basement membrane of the epithelial cells is observed. Thus, the basement membrane is composed, by union, of two basement membranes, as shown in Fig. 84.

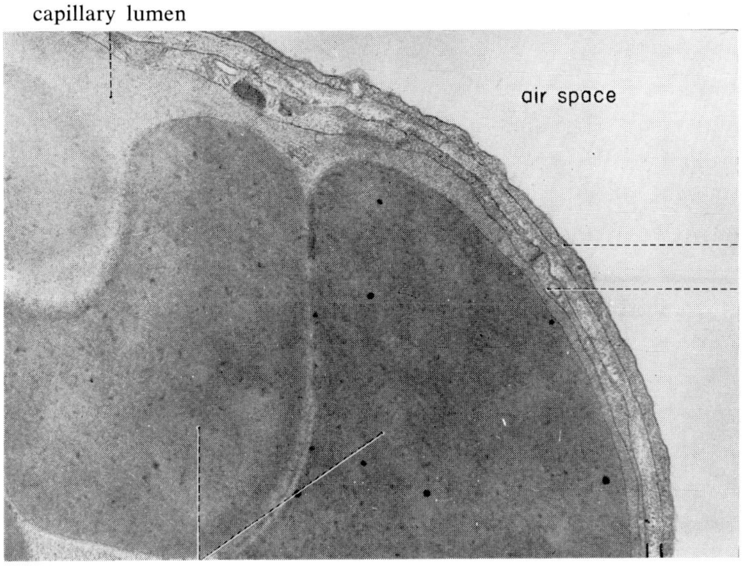

Fig. 84 Air-blood barrier of the alveole.

Muscle fibers are not observed in the capillary wall.

The air-blood barrier is thus composed of the thin processes of type A alveolar epithelial cells (squamous gas exchange type), the thin processes of the capillary endothelial cells and the basement membranes of the epithelial and endothelial cells. The thinnest part is approximately 0.15 μ in total thickness.

The fine structure in the air-blood barrier is critical to a speedy exchange of gases.

DIVERTIE and BROWN (1964) share this opinion.

A further detailed description of the alveolar capillaries will be given in Chapter II, Vascular System.

10. Connective Tissue

The connective tissue in the alveolar region is an extension of the tunica propria of the bronchial wall; its function is to support and to fill tissue interstices as well as to participate in regulation of the volume of the bronchoalveolar system.

These connective tissues consist of various cells, fibers and interstices, fibers being regarded as a part of the interstitium.

The fibers and interstices are of mesodermal origin, and are formed much later than epithelial tissues.

Nutrition of connective tissues in the alveolar region is mainly controlled by intrapulmonary bronchial vessels.

Interstice (Ground Substance): The interstice consists of interstitial fibers and cells. By electron microscopic observations, interstices are found to be filled or occupied by fine granules or net-like substances of comparatively low electron density, as shown in Fig. 85.

Muscular Fiber: For the sake of convenience muscular and connective tissues will be described together. Various opinions have been reported since olden times about the existence of muscular fibers in the alveolar region of mammals.

According to the examinations made by INABA, NAGASAWA, OKADA and NAGAISHI (1957), observations in animals show considerable individual differences.

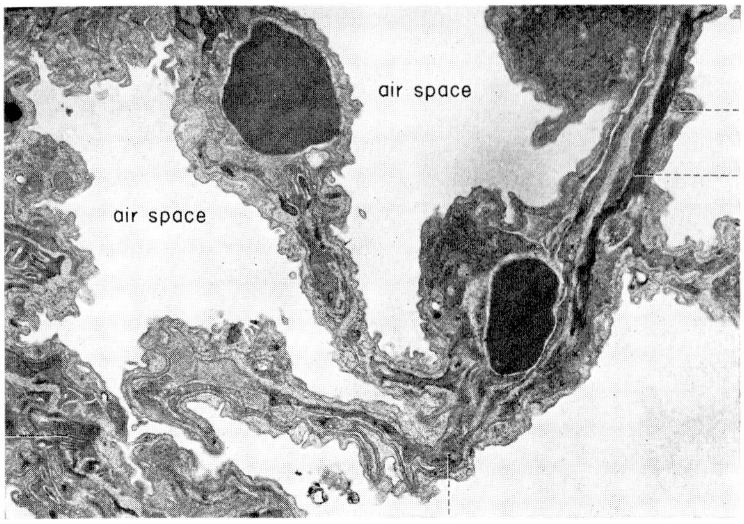

Fig. 85 Fibrous elements of the alveolar septum.

According to the literature, SCHULTZE (1871) showed muscular fibers in the alveolar ducts of mammals, and EBNER (1902) in the alveolar ducts of man. They stated that muscular fibers run annularly in the vicinity of the branching of alveolar ducts.

Against this, Prenent and BORIN (1911) stated that muscular fibers were not found in the peripheral parts of the alveolar duct of mammals, and STÖHR (1915) stated that muscular fibers were not observed in terminal capsules of man.

OGAWA (1917) reported that the extent and location of muscular fibers differed from one kind of animal to another.

Muscular fibers were always observed at the entrance of alveolar ducts in the lungs of guinea pig, rabbit, goat, dog, cat and man.

Two or three annular bundles of muscular fibers were found surrounding the entrance of the alveolar duct, the number of bundles decreasing toward the periphery and in some instances leaving only one bundle.

In the case of the guinea pig muscular fibers were sometimes not found in parts peripheral to the entrance of alveolar ducts. In cats, as stated by MÜLLER (1907), muscular fibers are more evident; dozens of fibers jointly form muscle bundles which are in evident annular arrangements, extending to the peripheral parts.

Entrance to Alveoli: KÖLLIKER (1881), EBNER (1902), and HAYEK (1953) showed the existence of muscular fibers at the entrance of the alveoli of man. SCHULTZE (1891) said that such muscular fibers were not found in mammals.

OGAWA (1917) reported that muscular fibers were observed in rabbit and goat, but in man and dog annular muscular fibers were less clearly observed. As to the cat, muscle fibers branched out from bundles surrounding the entrance of the alveolar duct, ran along the duct wall longitudinally and latitudinally, and joined annular muscular fibers at the entrance to the alveoli.

Alveolar Wall Region: According to studies carried out by INABA, NAGASAWA, OKADA and NAGAISHI (1957) in man, muscular fibers were observed in the region from the alveolar duct to the region of the alveolar wall; these were all smooth muscles in which many vegetative nerve fibers were distributed. They were presumed to have a role, together with elastic fibers, in preventing over-extension of the alveolar wall.

According to his reports, MÜLLER (1861) showed that muscular fibers were present in the alveolar walls of sheep and cow, and PISO-BORME (1867) verified this for the walls of cattle and man.

OGAWA (1917) stated that in the alveolar wall of cat, dog and man, fibers prolonged from muscular fibers at the entrance of the alveoli are found in some instances, but are not seen in other animals.

On the other hand, KÖLLIKER (human lung, 1854, 1881), SCHULTZE (mammalian lung, 1871), and EBNER (human lung, 1899), deny the existence of muscular fibers.

Elastic Fiber: The elastic fibers of the alveolar wall in man form a most delicate network, and in general the arrangements of fibers are the same as that of other mammals.

Fig. 86 shows the elastic fibers of the alveolar region (Weigert staining).

Of the elastic fibers which radiate from the annular fibers surrounding the entrance to the alveoli or the entrance of the alveolar duct, one or two bundles of particularly large caliber fibers are found. The alveolar wall is surrounded by thin elastic fibers which branch out from these large fibers.

These thin fibers unite again to form larger fibers which join the annular fibrous bundles in the opposite alveolar entrances.

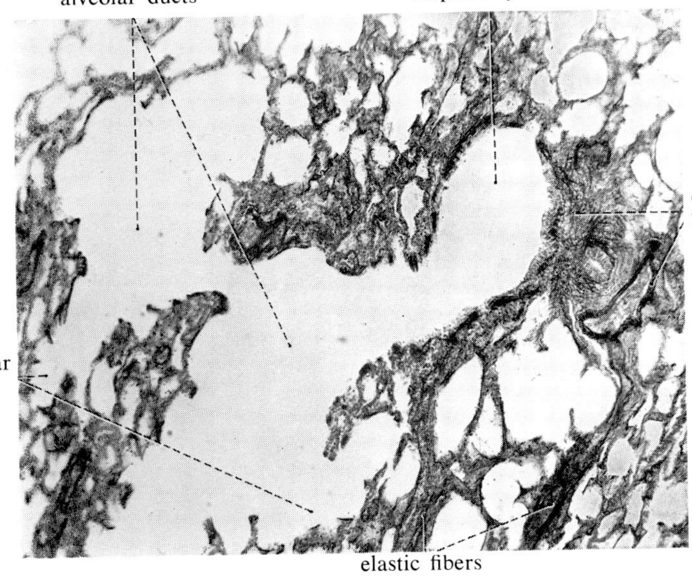

Fig. 86 Elastic fibers of the alveole.

As to the elastic fibers in man, LINSER (1900), MILLER (1906), ORSÓS (1907), and OGAWA, et al. (1917) report in detail.

MILLER (1906): From the alveolar duct to the entrance to the alveolus, the region is surrounded by complicated long belt-like elastic fibers. From these individual fibers are subdivided, some of them anastomosing with each other, forming networks. In view of the nature of the network, the fibers can stretch out in any direction in the alveolar region, but by their long-belt type or annular-like elastic bundles, the parts are maintained in a certain form. In the respiratory bronchiole or the entrance of the alveolar duct the elastic fibers, in company with muscular fibers, are arranged annularly to prevent over-distention.

LOW (1953): From the result of electron microscopic observations elastic fibers in the alveolar region are found bending in irregular shapes and small foramina are seen in not a few cases.

GROSS (1949): Investigations were made on the ultrafine structure of elastic fibers.

In elastic fibers obtained from the air-bladder of carp, from the ligamentum nuchae of cow, and from the aorta of a five year old child, filaments, 7 mμ in width, united in to a spiral to form fibrils; these fibrils were interwoven to form elastic fibers.

Morphologically, elastic fibers are considered to resemble collagenous fibers and are somewhat structureless. However, GROSS (1949) reported that these fibers have a certain structure.

Fig. 87 shows the elastic fibers of connective tissues.

Lattice Fiber and Collagenous Fiber: The arrangement of lattice fibers, as shown in Fig. 88, bears close resemblance to that of elastic fibers.

The lattice fibers of the respiratory bronchioles connect with the fibers of the alveolar duct, and at the entrance of the alveolar duct they are disposed in an annular shape.

At the entrance of the alveolus, fibers of the alveolar duct branch out and form a fibrous ring. From this ring several small fibers stretch out to the alveolar wall.

This lattice fiber spirals along with the capillary, bending and waving, subdividing and anastomosing, and terminates by forming a fine network, as shown in Fig. 89.

RUSAKOFF (1909): The lattice fibers of the alveolar wall in man were said to be the same as the fibrous ground substance of a secretory gland.

OKAJIMA (1933): The lattice fibers resembled collagenous fibers, but were composed of a younger precollagenous substance. Generally, they are argyrophilic fibers, forming a network around blood vessels, gland tubes, gland bodies, or their interstices.

OKAZAKI (1952): He examined mesenchymal fibers after silver impregnation and stated that these fibers were of various types:

Type I: This type has a distinct contour and forms a typical fiber network, which he called lattice fibers. Such fibers were mainly observed in hematopoietic organs.

Type II: This type has the form of a basement membrane and was mainly observed around blood capillaries, gland tubes, cardiac and striated muscle.

In such a basement membrane, extremely fine argyrophilic fibers are closely packed. In some cases, the membranes are so elaborate that no interstices can be found.

Type III: Mesenchymal argyrophilic fibers do not belong to either of the above two types but have comparatively distinct contours. The fibers stretch out individually and irregularly, sometimes appearing as clusters or arborescences.

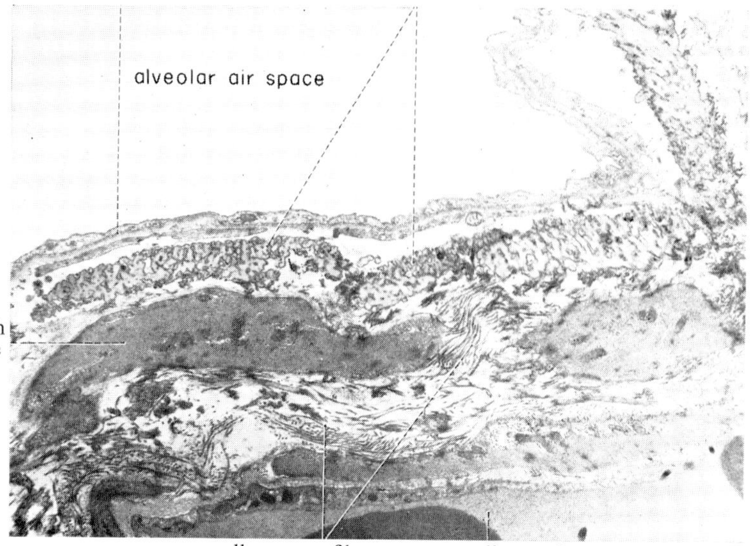

Fig. 87 Interstice of the alveolar region.

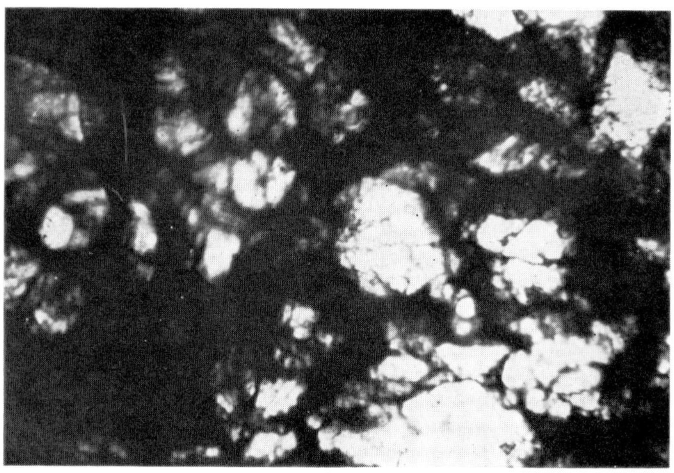

Fig. 88 Lattice fibers of the alveolar wall.

Transitional forms ranging between the above types and collagenous fibers are said to be reported.

As is well known, there are various classifications or terms for connective tissue fibers, *e.g.*, elastic, collagenous, argyrophilic lattice, etc.

Furthermore, according to size, they are divided into fibers and fibrils. In recent years, with the development of electron microscopy, fine fibrils about 1000Å (100 mμ) in width and protofibrils about 560Å in width are distinguishable. Between these fibrils a felt-like ground substance is observed.

Continuing investigations are being carried out on collagenous fibers.

Fig. 90 is an electron micrograph of collagenous fibers (Cr-shadowing) in the alveolar region. In the upper part of the picture electron dense basement membranes lined with epithelium are seen.

GROSS and SCHMITT (1949): They performed shadowing on sections made from the corium of human skin and obtained electron micrographs of collagenous fibers. 100 mμ-wide fibers were found in this section. In these fibers, regular lateral stripes are observed at 50–60 mμ intervals.

SASAKAWA, et al. (1951): They made electron microscopic observations on collagenous fibers obtained from the Achilles' tendon of man, rabbit, and toad, and found fine fibrils of 20–30 mμ width, at 40–60 mμ intervals, which were quite different from those of GROSS and SCHMITT. These fibrils were named ultraprotofibrils. Several ultraprotofibrils join and form a 100 mμ-wide fibril, as noted by GROSS and SCHMITT. These fibrils show a regular lateral stripe structure.

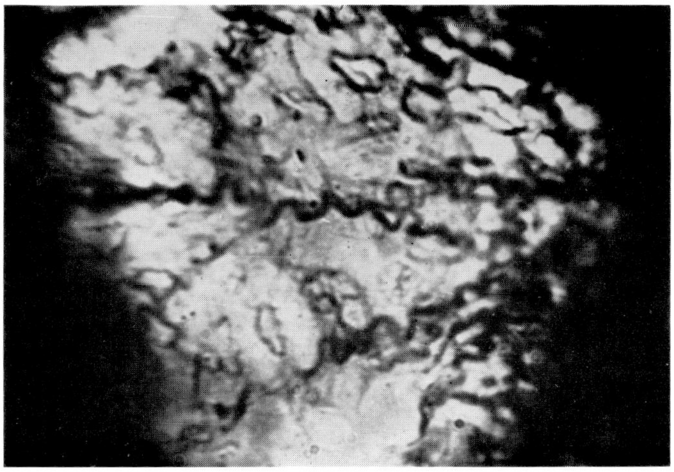

Fig. 89 Lattice fibers of the alveolar wall.

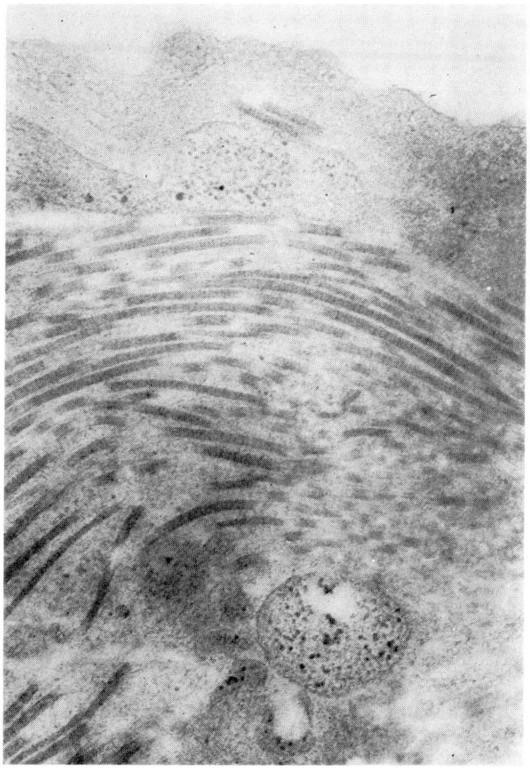

Fig. 90 Collagenous fibers of the alveolar septum.

11. Alveolar Connective Tissue Cells

In the connective tissues of the alveolar region the following cells are observed: namely, fixed, granular, and wandering.

Fixed Connective Tissue Cells: Fixed connective tissue cells originate from mesodermal cells and are called fibrocytes or fibroblasts.

Among the comparatively large cells lying in the collagenous fibers a small number containing stainable granules are observed. The nucleus of these cells are ovoid, egg or kidney shaped and contain little chromatin. These cells are also found in the connective tissues of the alveolar region.

Fig. 91 and 92 are electron micrographs of connective tissue cells from the alveolar region.

Möllendorf (1926, 1933): Fibrocytes may undergo metaplasia and transform into other types of cells.
Maximow (1926): Opposing Möllendorf's view, he said that the fibrocyte is a cell which has already undergone differentiation.

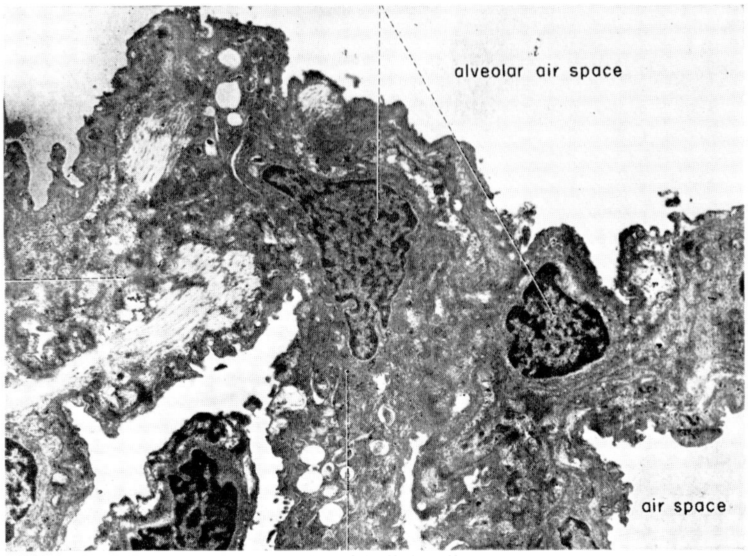

Fig. 91 Interstitial cells of the alveolar septum.

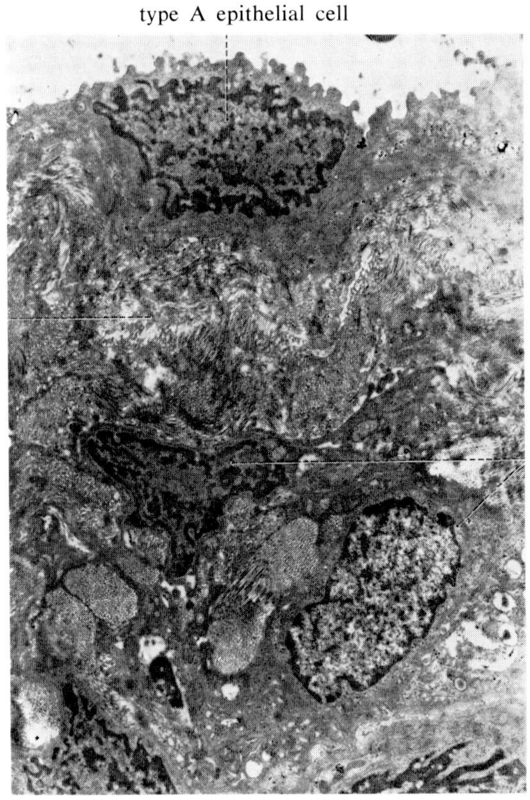

Fig. 92 Cellular and fibrous elements of the alveolar septum.

The following is a historical review of various other types of cells, not specific to or characteristically found only in the alveolar region.

ASCHOFF (1924, 1926): A specific cell group of mesodermal origin was found which was characterized by a phagocytic function. This cell group was named the reticuloendothelial system (ASCHOFF-KIYONO).

KIYONO (1933): Histiocytes and reticuloendothelium were collectively called the histiocytic system.

As it is well known, histiocytes are found extensively in connective tissue in a fixed or free state. The cells exhibit phagocytosis and a wandering locomotion in the tissues. The reticuloendothelium was mainly observed in hematopoietic organs.

Extensive investigations have been carried out on the reticuloendothelial or histiocytic system. Regarding the reticuloendothelial system, in particular, the differentiation of histiocytes and monocytes has been the subject of heated discussions.

However, the application of supravital staining (neutral red or janus green) in cytological examination has drastically changed former viewpoints.

AMANO (1948): Various cytological examinations were carried out applying supravital staining, which assisted in the differentiation of monocytes from other blood or reticulum cells, and the existence of an independent cell system (the monocyte series) was revealed. Up to this time the reticuloendothelial system was considered to have the primary role in reacting against inflammation; it then became clear, however, that the monocytes also played an important role.

AMANO (1949): He separated histiocytes from the reticuloendothelial system and identified the histiocyte system. He stated that, in form and function, histiocytes identify with reticulum cells, although from the embryological point of view they are not unitary.

AKAZAKI (1952): Although AKAZAKI held that cytologically there was no essential difference between reticulum cells and histiocytes, he differentiated reticulum cells from histiocytes on the basis that the former cells, together with their argyrophilic fibers, formed the reticulum. However, when the histiocytes were subjected to the same conditions as reticulum cells they tended to assume the same form as the reticulum cells.

Although belonging to the reticuloendotelial system the reticuloendothelium must be definitely differentiated from reticulum cells, both embryologically and cytologically; in reality, however the essential difference resides in the phagocytic function.

Therefore, AKAZAKI proposed the necessity for a new and revised classification of the reticuloendothelial system. This classification contains two divisions, one consisting of reticulum cell and histiocytes in the general connective tissues, the other consisting of reticuloendothelium and endothelium, the latter exhibiting a marked phagocytic function.

Granular Cells: Various granular cells are found in the alveolar region; they are as follows:

Mast Cells: These cells are not uniform in shape and in many cases have processes on the surface; the nuclei are comparatively small. An abundant number of coarse granules are observed which are water soluble, easily stained with basophil pigment, and often show metachromasia.

Plasma Cells: In many instances, these cells are round or ovoid, sometimes irregular in shape, and move slowly. The nuclei of the cell are round, comparatively small, and of the so-called radial shape. In most cases the nuclei are slightly eccentric in position; in the vicinity of the nucleus a clear plasma halo is observed.

Resting Wandering Cells: These cells are also called fragmentation cells, Klasmatozyten, polyblasten, adventital cells or macrophages. They are deformed in shape and have processes; on lateral view the cells are spindle shaped and the nuclei are darker in tone as compared to those of fibrous cells. The cellular function of phagocytosis is visualized experimentally using particles of trypan blue, pyrrol blue, lithium carmine or India ink. The cells show a marked response to stimuli such as inflammation, or in response to foreign bodies. When these cells absorb such a particle, they may become distended and spherical in shape and remain in position, in effect cease their wandering.

Eosinophil Cells: As with similar cells in the blood, these are spherical, containing segmented nuclei and coarse granules. The cells are comparatively large; the granules are deeply stainable with eosin or other acidic aniline dyes. The cells are often observed in the interstices of the lung increasing in number in case of inflammation.

Wandering Cells: In the alveolar region, wandering polymorphonuclear cells and lymphocytes are often observed. The percentage of wandering cells increases at the time of inflammation and differs markedly depending on the type and stage of inflammation.

Fig. 93 is a schema of the fine structure of the alveolar wall as elucidated above.

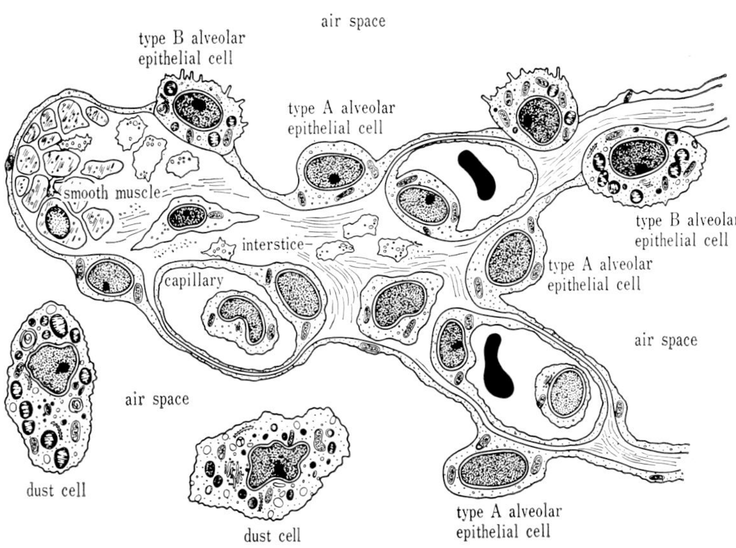

Fig. 93 Ultrafine structure of the alveolar region.

12. Free Cells in Alveolar Space

The cells observed and interpreted as being free in the alveolar space are generally called dust cells, alvolar phagocytes, large exudate cells, or heart failure cells. These cells are quite large; their longest diameter is about 12 μ. DIVERTIE and BROWN (1964) stated that the structure and origin of these cells are not yet clear.

According to transmission electron microscopic observations made by ISHIKO, OKADA and NAGAISHI (1959), two types of cells were usually noted in the alveolar space of the normal lung.

One type showed an abundant number of osmiophilic lamellar bodies in the cytoplasm, the other type exhibited a typical Golgi's complex but lacked the mentioned osmiophilic lamellar bodies.

Fig. 94 is an example of the former; in view of its inner structure it is considered to have originated in type B alveolar epithelial cells (cuboidal secretory type).

However, since the lamellar bodies of this cell can be also considered to represent phagocytosed particles, the origin of this cell is still in question.

Fig. 95 is an example of the latter, and it is considered to have its origin in the monocytic system. In this picture, phagocytosis (many particles of dust) is evident.

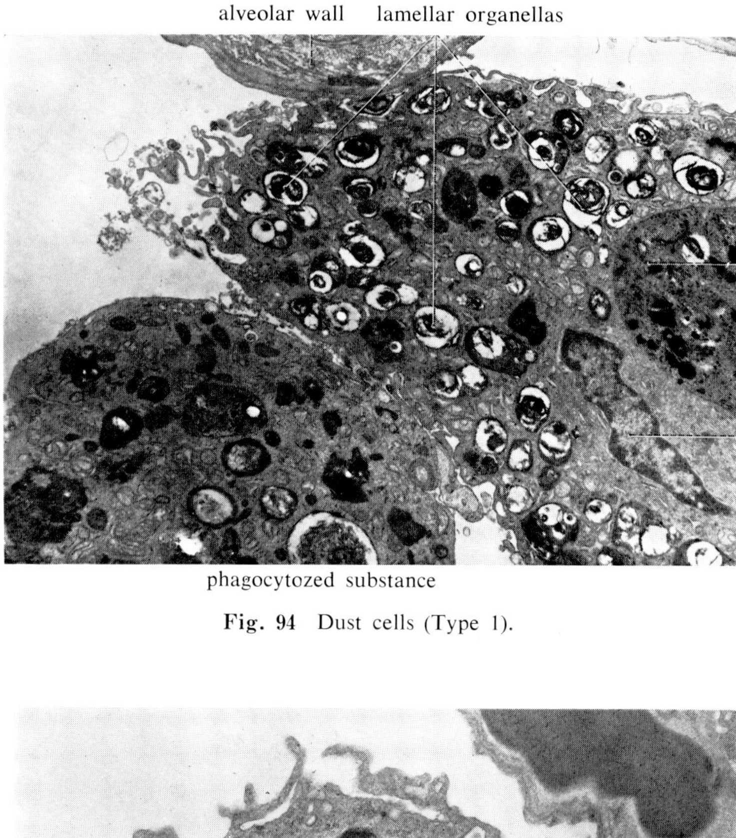

Fig. 94 Dust cells (Type 1).

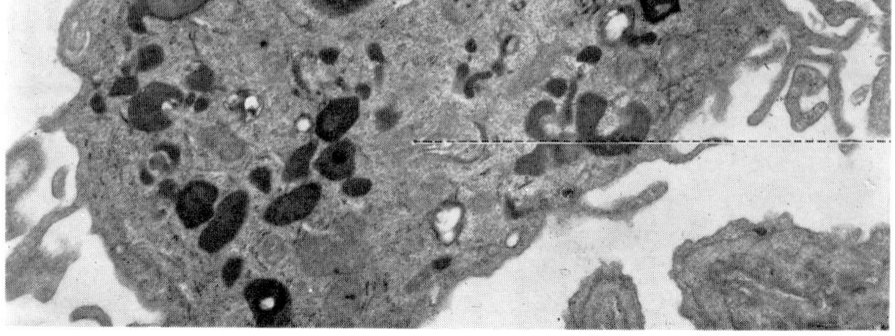

Fig. 95 Dust cells (Type 2).

Fig. 96 represents an example of a phagocytic cell of the monocyte system. This electron micrograph shows the phagocytosis of tubercle bacilli.

tubercle bacilli

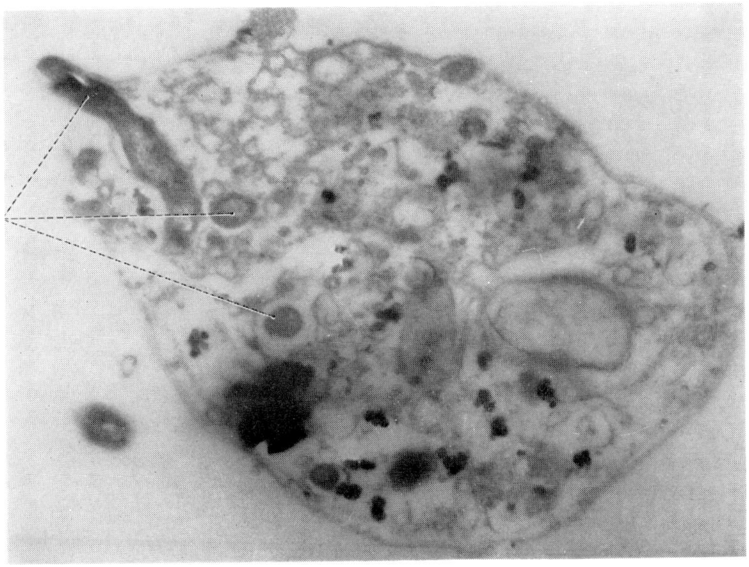

Fig. 96 Tubercle bacilli phagocytozed by type 2 alveolar dust cell.

Opinion is divided as to whether or not the lining cells of the alveolar wall are phagocytic. According to the experimental examinations carried out by Ishiko (1959) of the author's group, phagocytosis could not be found in either type A or type B alveolar epithelial cells.

The macrophage is the cell which shows an initial response to foreign substances insufflated via the tracheo-bronchial route, for example charcoal dust, pigment for vital staining and bacteria; neutrophil leucocytes respond secondly. The former are considered to be cells of monocyte system origin.

The degree of reaction differs depending on the nature and amount of foreign material. However, in the reaction thusly caused we cannot find essential differences in terms of the reaction to specific kinds of foreign bodies; in other words regardless of the nature of the foreign material, the cellular reaction appears to be non-specific, at least in initial phases.

Chapter II. Vascular System

The vascular system of the lung is divided into the pulmonary and the bronchial systems.

The former are blood vessels which regulate gas exchange; the latter serve as nutrient vessels. However, according to the studies performed by Nagaishi and M. Yamashita, et al. (1950–1969), the pulmonary vascular system is also considered to play a nutrient role in the alveolar region, but these observations have not been confirmed.

The bronchial vascular system is an extension of the systemic circulation, whereas the pulmonary vascular system forms an independent and specific circulation in the lung. Both anatomically and physiologically, the two systems exhibit quite different characteristics.

Compared with the systemic circulation, the pulmonary circulation is shorter in length and its blood pressure is far lower.

In the peripheral portions of normal lungs, both the systemic and the pulmonary circulations form complicated anastomoses. This creates many problems in the study of chest diseases and pulmonary physiology.

I. PULMONARY VASCULAR SYSTEM

The pulmonary vascular system is arranged in the order of artery, capillary and vein; in some instances, some branches of the pulmonary artery may directly connect with branches of the pulmonary vein. In such cases, the existence of functional arteriovenous shunts has been discussed by several researchers. According to anatomical investigations performed by Nagaishi and M. Yamashita (1957), and Weibel (1958), such shunts were not observed in normal lungs. Rink (1970), in his book "Lungenzirkulation", states that this is a question which definitely required further study.

The pulmonary artery carries venous blood from the right ventricle to the periphery of the lung; the pulmonary vein carries oxygenated blood from the capillary nets to the left atrium.

Accordingly, the character of blood in the pulmonary circulation is entirely opposite to that of the systemic circulation.

A. Pulmonary Artery and Vein in Mediastinal and Hilar Regions

1. Artery

As shown in Fig. 97, the pulmonary trunk arises from the conus arteriosus of the right ventricle, runs superiorly at the side of the root of the aorta, and bifurcates at the level of the fourth thoracic vertebra into right and left trunks which distribute to the right and left lungs.

In the region of bifurcation, Botallo's ligament (ligamentum arteriosum) is observed; this ligament connects the pulmonary artery with the inferior aspect of the aorta.

Botallo's duct (in fetal stages) transforms into the ligament after birth.

The right branch of the pulmonary artery is longer than the left; it extends to the posterior aspect of the ascending aorta and superior vena cava immediately beneath the aortic arch, and reaches the pulmonary hilum, passing anterior to the right main bronchus.

Then, at the level of the right upper lobe bronchus it runs parallel with and passes the ventral aspect of the bronchus at the level of the bifurcation of the upper lobe bronchus.

In view of its positional relation with the pulmonary artery, the right upper lobe bronchus is also called the eparterial bronchus.

The left pulmonary artery extends from the bifurcation, at an angle of 45° to the frontal plane, and rides over the left main bronchus where it bifurcates, to be distributed to the upper and lower lobes. In view of its positional relationship to the pulmonary artery, the left upper lobe bronchus is also called the hyparterial bronchus.

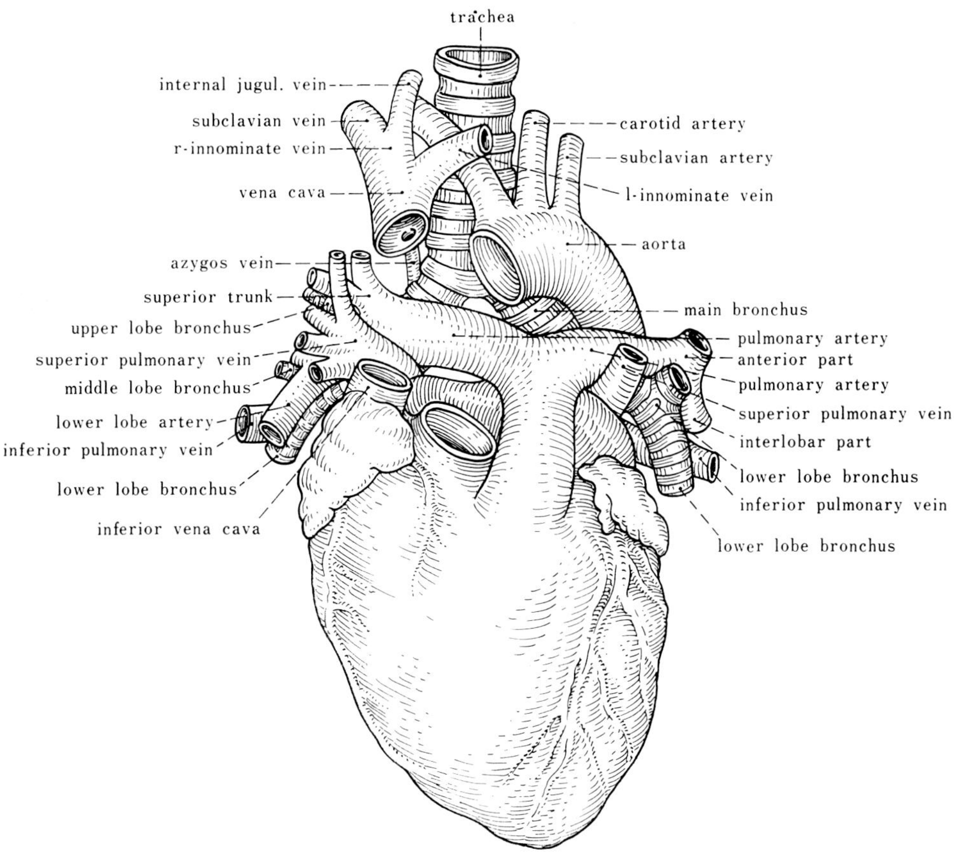

Fig. 97 Pulmonary artery and vein.

Figs. 98 and 99 are angiograms of the pulmonary arteries of the right and left lungs.

2. Vein

Differing from the artery, the venous outflow is in general, carried by the superior and inferior pulmonary veins which connect directly with the left atrium. In short, there are four veins opening into the left atrium.

Positional relationships of these veins in the pulmonary hilum are; the superior pulmonary vein which lies on the ventral side of the pulmonary artery and the bronchus, in each lung, and is easily seen from the anterior view; similarly the inferior pulmonary vein, on each side, is situated lowermost, and is most easily seen from the posterior aspect.

Clinically, these are referred to as left or right, superior or inferior veins. The right veins are slightly longer than the left.

Furthermore, there are examples wherein the number of branches of the pulmonary vein is equal to the number of lobes; namely, three on the right lung and two on the left. There are also instances wherein some divisions of upper lobe veins are united with those of lower lobe veins.

Regarding the segmental anatomy of the pulmonary vein BOYDEN (1945, 1955), GOMEZ OLIVEROS (1950) and M. YAMASHITA (1957) of the authors' group carried out detailed investigations.

Particularly, GOMEZ OLIVEROS (1950) published the valuable monograph "Veins of the Lungs" in which he described individual branches, and the frequency of the variation of these branches.

B. Pulmonary Artery and Vein in Pulmonary Segments

The patterns of distribution of pulmonary arteries and veins exhibit many individual variations.

As to the morphology of blood vessels, ADACHI (1931–1933) performed detailed investigations, from the viewpoint of the anthropologist. His achievements were published in two detailed volumes titled "Arteriensystem der Japaner" and "Venensystem der Japaner". These have received deserved international appreciation.

However, after World War II, coincident with rapid progress in the development of lung surgery, more detailed investigations of pulmonary blood vessels became necessary.

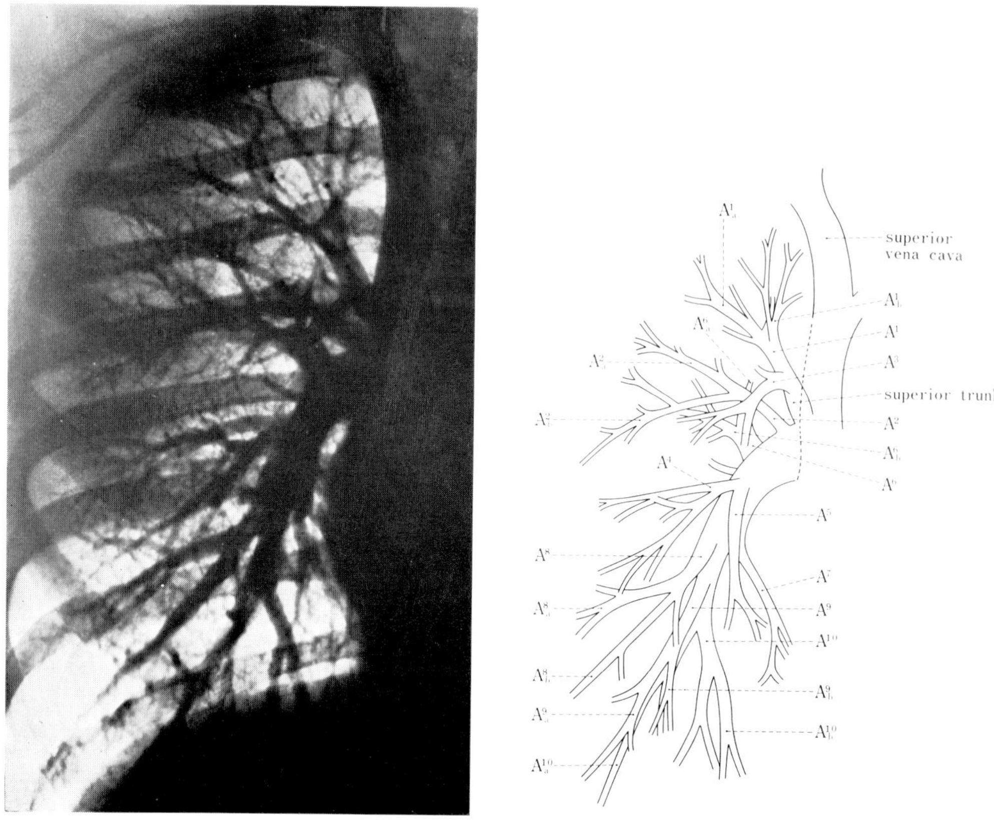

Fig. 98 Angiogram of right lung.

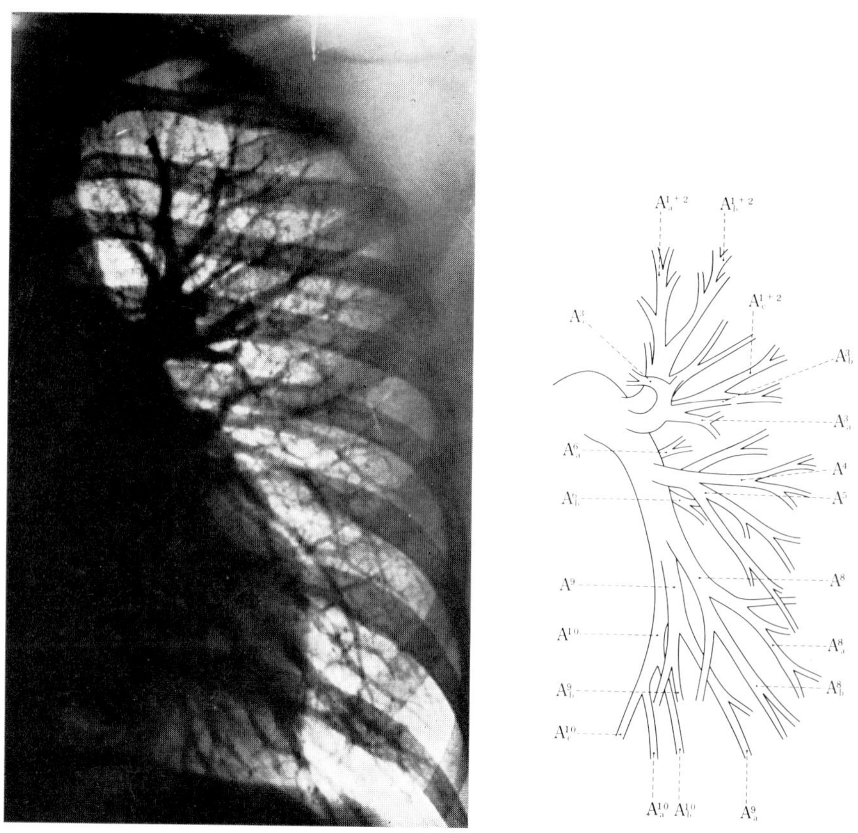

Fig. 99 Angiogram of left lung.

Regarding this matter, various reports were issued by authors such as APPLETON (1944), BOYDEN (1945, 1954), ISHIBASHI (1953, 1954), H. YAMASHITA (1953, 1954), SHIOZAWA (1955) and M. YAMASHITA and and NAGAISHI (1956, 1957). In particular, BOYDEN (1955), published a valuable book on the "Segmental Anatomy of the Lung".

All these studies are devoted to description, classification, and to designation of the branching of arteries and veins, and from the viewpoint of pulmonary segments and segmental bronchi.

The branches of arteries and veins are named to correspond to the designation of the respective pulmonary segments and subsegments. However, designations of the pulmonary blood vessels are not as uniform as for the bronchi.

In a number of instances, branches of blood vessels of a segment may intrude into the neighboring segment. These are called accessory branches, and are designated by an "X".

On surface projection, a pulmonary segment appears to occupy the shape of an irregular cone with the surface of pulmonary pleura as the base, and the root of the segmental bronchus as the apex, the central region of the segment being called the segmental hilum.

In the central part of the segment, as shown in Fig. 100, the segmental bronchus and segmental artery run close together, and in parallel.

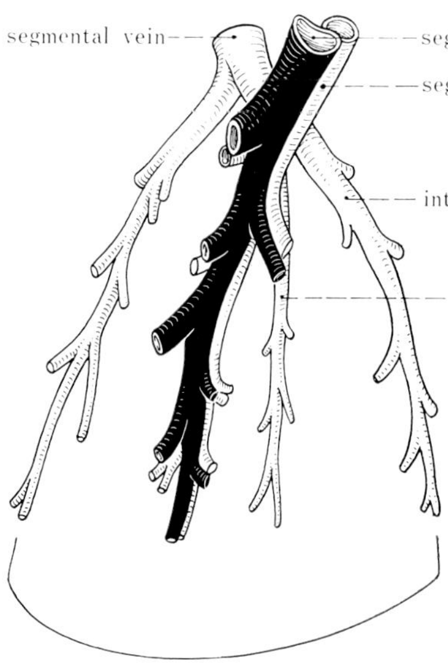

Fig. 100 Segmental bronchus and vessels.

The pulmonary veins are formed by: 1) central veins which run inside the pulmonary segments, and by intersubsegmental veins which drain subsegments; 2) intersegmental veins which surround pulmonary segments, collect the smaller veins, and run along segmental planes. The anastomoses of these veins usually occur in a region peripheral to the hilum of the segment.

The term segmental plane designates the border of two adjacent pulmonary segments. However, these segments are not separated by specific membranes; intersegmental veins and accompanying intersegmental lymph vessels occupy the extremely thin connective tissues extending from intersubsegmental or interlobular septa.

The surgical technique for segmental resection is based on this topographic anatomy.

In the pulmonary subsegments, the above relationships are similar.

1. Right Upper Lobe

Branches of Pulmonary Artery: The right upper lobe is divided into three segments, S^1, S^2 and S^3; the corresponding three segmental arteries being designated as A^1, A^2 and A^3.

The arteries to the right upper lobe, shown in Fig. 101, arise from two sources, one the anterior mediastinum and the other the interlobar region of the upper and lower lobes. One branch is called the superior trunk, and the other is an ascending artery.

The superior trunk is the first branch which arises from the right pulmonary artery; in many cases it is composed of the roots of A^1, A^2a and A^3

The ascending artery is, in many cases, composed of A^2b.

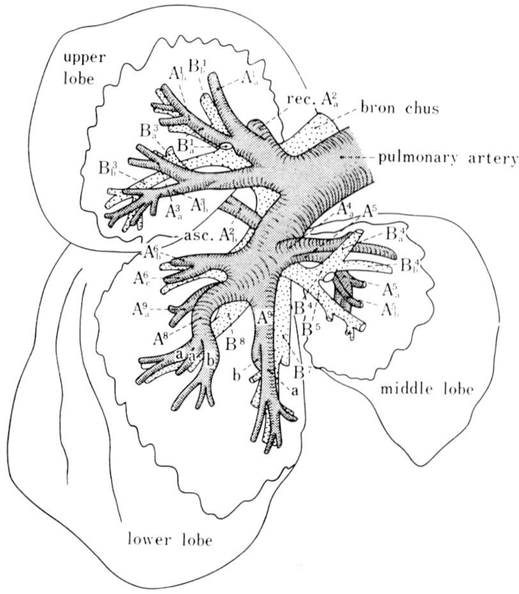

Fig. 101 Branching of right pulmonary artery.

A^1 is divided into A^1a and A^1b, A^2 into A^2a and A^2b, A^3 into A^3a and A^3b. They are distributed in the respective segments and subsegments.

As to the artery of the right upper lobe the following points are to be noted.

Of the types of branching of the right upper lobe artery, the most frequently observed is the type in which the superior trunk arises from the right branch of the pulmonary artery, shortly bifurcates A^2a and A^1.

A^2a, called the recurrent artery, descends surrounding the bronchus, and distributes in S^2. The recurrent artery occasionally stems from A^1a at a point peripheral to the difurcation of A^1a and A^1b.

The ascending artery, becoming A^2b, is distributed, as mentioned earlier, in S^2b, but occasionally becomes a part of A^2a or A^3, and is distributed in the region of S^2 or a part of S^3.

Both the ascending and recurrent arteries are mainly found to distribute in S^2 in a reciprocal relationship, *i.e.* when one is of larger caliber and supplies a larger area, the other is smaller in caliber and distributes in a more restricted area.

Branches of Pulmonary Vein: The vein of the right upper lobe receives blood from V^1, V^2 and V^3. Prior to emptying into the left ventricle, the vein is, in many instances, connected to the vein of the middle lobe. The veins of the right upper lobe and of the middle lobe are designated collectively as the superior pulmonary vein.

V^1 is the uppermost of the superior veins and receives blood from V^1a and V^1b.

V^1a is found immediately under the pulmonary pleura on the surface of the mediastinum, crosses A^3 posteriorly, passes along the borders of S^1a and S^1b, and receives blood from V^2d.

V^2, the interlobar terminal vein, is the largest and receives blood from V^2a, V^2b, V^2c and V^2d.

V^2 has two courses: one, passing under B^3, extends along the interlobar pleura to the hilum from the posterior side; the other, passing the borders of S^2b and S^3, courses to the hilum from the posterosuperior side.

The latter is called the central vein, distributing in the deep part of the lung.

As to V^2 the following points are to be noted.

In some instances, V^2 is not in the form of the interlobar terminal vein, nor does it have the central vein. When it is devoid of the central vein a branch of V^1 distributes as VX^2 in the region where usually V^2a is found to distribute, or VX^6 is found to arise from the trunk of V^2. When VX^6 is observed it is found that blood from V^6 empties into V^2.

V^3 receives blood from V^3a and V^3b. The former passes the borders of B^3b and B^3b2, the latter the borders of S^3 and S^4 of the middle lobe.

In some cases, V^3a empties into V^1, V^2b into V^2, and V^3 into the middle lobe vein. Thus, V^3 has more variations than other veins.

2. Middle Lobe

Branches of Pulmonary Artery: The middle lobe is divided into two segments, namely S^4 and S^5; the corresponding two segmental arteries are designated as A^4 and A^5.

Both of them stem from the inferior trunk (interlobar part) of the right pulmonary artery at about the same level as A^6.

In some cases, A^4 and A^5 join together and stem out as one branch, in some cases they stem out independently as separate branches. The ratio is, according to BOYDEN (1955), 48:52.

Branches of Pulmonary Vein: The vein of the middle lobe is composed of V^4 and V^5. In many cases, they completely empty into the lowermost edge of the superior pulmonary vein, but sometimes they empty into the left atrium independently.

3. Right Lower Lobe

Branches of Pulmonary Artery: The right lower lobe receives blood from the inferior trunk of the right pulmonary artery.

The right lower lobe is divided into S^6 and four basal segments. The corresponding five segmental arteries are designated as A^6 and four basal segmental arteries. In some cases A^* is observed.

The basal segmental artery is frequently divided into either A^{7+8} or A^{9+10}. Stemming from the inferior trunk of the right pulmonary artery, the former courses toward the anteromedial side and the latter courses toward the posterolateral side. Both of them run along the bronchus and almost parallel to it.

Branches of Pulmonary Vein: The vein of the right lower lobe is composed of five segmental or intersegmental veins, similar to the bronchi, and is called the inferior pulmonary vein. The inferior pulmonary vein is divided into V^6, which receives blood from S^6, and the common basal vein which receives blood from the basal segments. The latter is further divided into the superior and inferior basal veins.

4. Left Upper Lobe

Branches of Pulmonary Artery: The left upper lobe is divided into four segments, S^{1+2}, S^3, S^4 and S^5; the corresponding four segmental arteries are designated as A^{1+2}, A^3, A^4 and A^5.

The types of branching of the bronchus are somewhat different from that of the right side, and therefore the types of branching of the pulmonary artery also differ from those of the right side. This side is devoid of a branch corresponding to the superior trunk of the right side.

A^3 arises near the surface of the anterior mediastinum, as shown in Fig. 102. The other segmental arteries arise near the surface of the interlobar pleura or the posterior mediastinum.

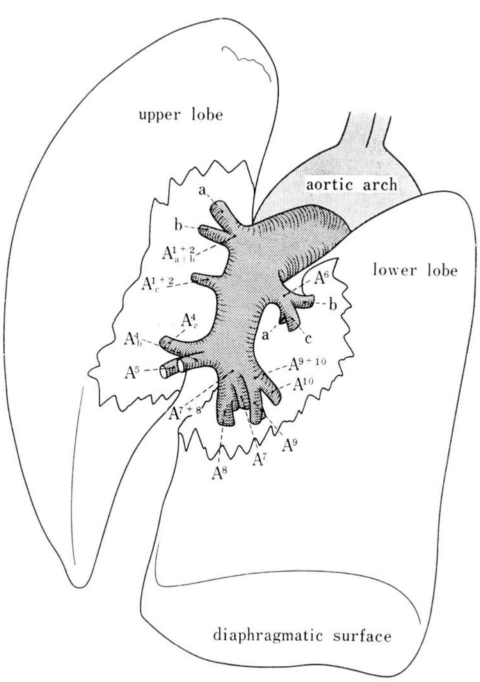

Fig. 102 Branching of left pulmonary artery.

Unlike the right side, B^1 and B^2 are not divided distinctly on the left side, and the corresponding segments are designated as S^{1+2}.

Therefore, segmental arteries are in many cases divided into three branches, $A^{1+2}a$, $A^{1+2}b$ and $A^{1+2}c$, or into two, $A^{1+2}a+b$ and $A^{1+2}c$. Sometimes $A^{1+2}a$ and A^3 have a common trunk.

Branches of Pulmonary Vein: The vein of the left upper lobe is divided into V^{1+2} (V^1 and V^2), V^3, V^4 and V^5. These are arranged in a vertical line near the surface of the anterior mediastinum. On the right side veins lie in the deep region of the lung; in the superficial region on the left side. Frequently, two to four veins compose the superior pulmonary vein.

V^{1+2} occupies the uppermost part of the superior pulmonary vein; Boyden (1955) divided it into V^1 and V^2.

V^1 receives blood from V^1a and V^1b, V^1a receives blood from $S^{1+2}a$, V^1b, passing the borders of $S^{1+2}a$ and S^3, becomes a part of the intersegmental septum.

V^2 receives blood from V^2a, V^2b and V^2c. V^2a passing between S^3a and S^4a, V^3b between S^3b and S^4b, and V^3c between S^3b and S^3c.

V^{4+5} is located at the lowermost of the superior pulmonary veins, becoming one branch in the majority of cases, but sometimes V^4 and V^5 are observed independently. V^{3+4}, V^{5+7} or V^4 are connected to the superior pulmonary vein, V^{4+5} or V^5 to the inferior pulmonary vein.

5. Left Lower Lobe

Branches of Pulmonary Artery: The left lower lobe is divided either into four segments, S^6, S^{7+8}, S^9 and S^{10}, or five segments, S^6, S^{7+8}, S^9, S^{10} and S^*; the corresponding four or five segmental arteries are designated as A^6, A^{7+8}, A^9, A^{10}, or A^6, A^{7+8}, A^9, A^{10} and A^*.

A^6 is further divided into three subsegmental arteries, A^6a, A^6b and A^6c.

The types of branching of the basal segmental artery on the left side are nearly like those of the right lower lobe. Frequently, however, B^7 and B^8 are observed as B^{7+8} on the left side. In this relation, H. YAMASHITA (1954) reported that in the branching of the artery the most frequently observed types is A^8; A^{9+10}, 54%, followed by A^{8+9}, A^{10}, 26%, $A^8 \cdot A^9 \cdot A^{10}$, 10%, $AX^7 \cdot A^8 \cdot A^{9+10}$, 6% and AX^7 arising from A^9, 4%. All these branches arise from the interlobar portions.

Branches of Pulmonary Vein: The vein of the left lower lobe similar to the right side, is composed of V^6 and the common basal vein, the latter being composed of the superior and inferior basal veins.

According to BOYDEN (1955), the most frequently observed type is $V^8 \cdot V^{9+10}$, 40%, followed by $V^{8+9} \cdot V^{10}$, 32%, V^6 being independent in many cases.

C. Pulmonary Artery and Vein in Pulmonary Lobule

As shown in Fig. 103, the arrangement and distribution of the pulmonary artery and vein in the pulmonary lobule and acinus are similar to that in the pulmonary segment.

In short, the arrangement and the distribution of pulmonary blood vessels in the pulmonary lobule

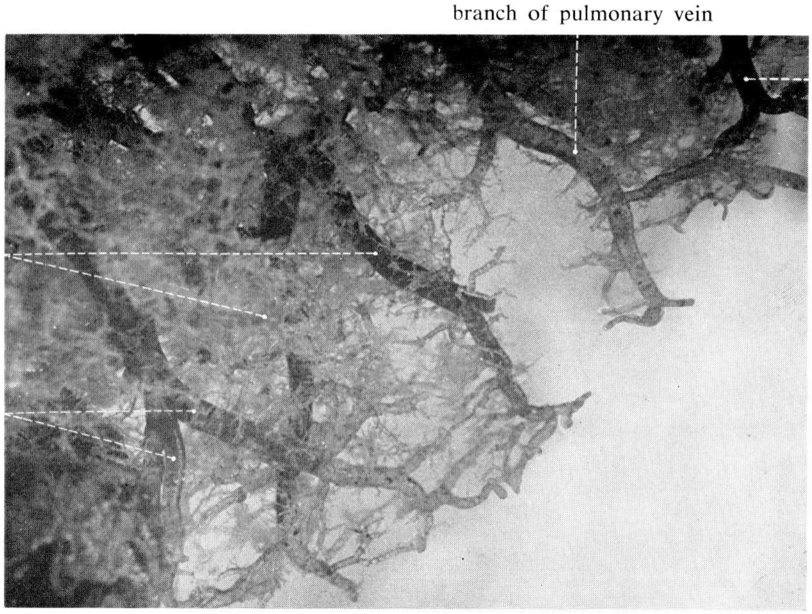

Fig. 103 Pulmonry arteries and veins.

and acinus are similar to that of the pulmonary segment but on a smaller scale.

In the central portion of the lobule, the lobular artery runs along the lobular bronchus and then ramifies into capillaries in the peripheral region. The lobular vein draining the capillary network becomes larger in caliber, and proceeds to the more peripheral portion of the pulmonary lobule where the interlobular vein is formed.

Each lobule receives the blood from its respective artery; each lobular vein receives the blood from two (or three) adjacent lobules.

D. Alveolar Capillaries

Resin castings disclose the alveolar wall capillary network, as shown in Fig. 104 (a), (b).

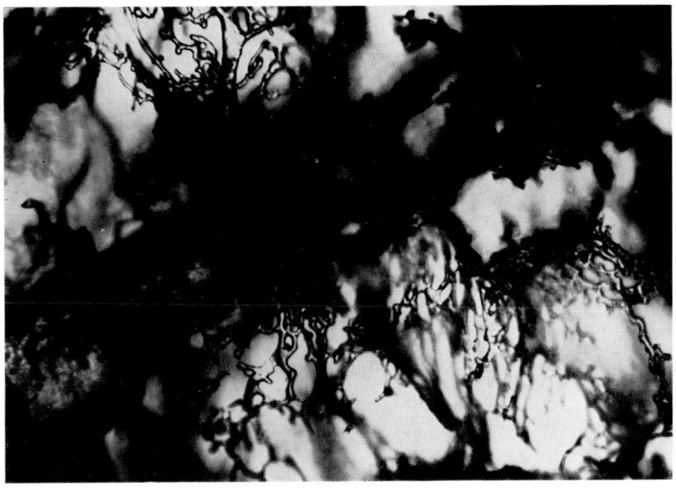

Fig. 104 a Capillary nets of the alveolar walls.

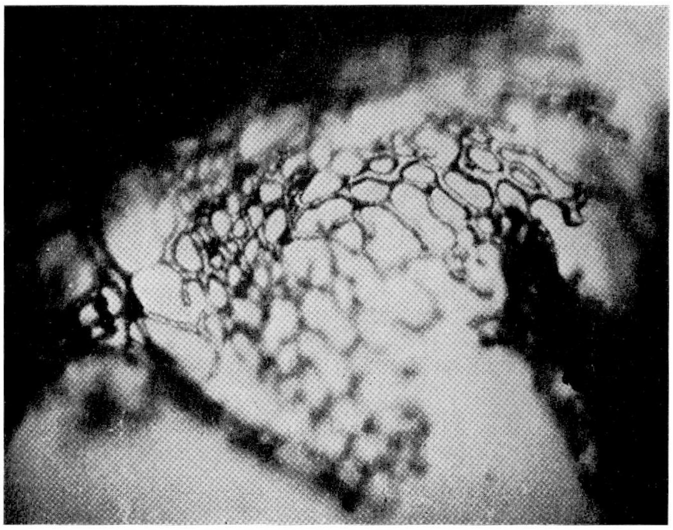

Fig. 104 b Capillary net of an alveolar wall.

The networks are composed of an abundant number of vessels of almost the same size; as a whole, the nets are in the shape of a half-cage.

The average diameter (ca 12–15 μ) of each of these capillaries is larger than for capillaries in other regions of the body.

According to WEIBEL (1963) the capillaries of the lung number about 300 billion.

The fact that the capillaries in the pulmonary vascular system are comparatively large in caliber and form anastomoses on the alveolar wall, coupled with the fact that the capillaries are situated immediately beneath the thin extensions of type A alveolar epithelial cells, and also that the capillary net projects inwardly toward the alveolar space, is the basis for the maximal expansion of the total capillary surface area.

The lung is thus constituted in such a way that it effectively fulfills its function in gas exchange.

Incidentally, as shown in Fig. 104, the capillaries located on each alveolar wall may be supplied with blood from two or three adjacent arterioles. The pulmonary alveolar capillaries are differentiated morphologically from the capillaries derived from the intrapulmonary bronchial systemic artery.

Table 3 shows a comparison of the capillaries derived from the pulmonary and bronchial vascular systems.

Table 3 Comparison with pulmonary and bronchial vascular systems.

		Capillary of pulmonary vascular system	Capillary of bronchial vascular system
distribution		alveolar wall	bronchial wall, pulmonary vascular wall and pulmonary parenchyma except alveolar wall
form		similar size, regularly	various size, irregularly
thickness		thin	thick
caliber of capillary		larger	smaller
character of blood	arterial side	venous blood	arterial blood
	venous side	arterial blood	venous blood

E. Pulmonary Blood Flow in Living Animals

Microscopic observations of blood flow in living animal have been recorded since olden times.

As to the pulmonary vascular system, such investigations have been carried out by MALPIGHI (1967), HALES (1733), COHNHEIM and LITTEN (1875), HALL (1925), ROEDER, et al. (1932), MACGREGOR (1934), and JOANNIDES, et al. (1930), on frogs, rabbits, cats and dogs.

Recently, two or three reports have been issued on this subject.

NAKATA (1953) developed a biomicroscopic apparatus with a long focusing condenser, and RAMOS (1954) invented a microscopic viviperception apparatus using a crystal red, studying blood flow in various organs. Their methods seem to have high practicality in view of their technically simple operating methods.

Following are observations by WATANABE (1959), of the author's group, on the lung of rabbits, carried out by adapting NAKATA's method.

The blood from the right ventricle flows to either the right or left trunk of the pulmonary artery and its segmental artery → subsegmental artery → lobular artery → acinar artery → arteriole → capillary → venule → acinar (interacinar) vein → lobular (interlobular) vein → intersubsegmental vein → intersegmental vein → lobar vein → pulmonary vein. The portion suitable for microscopic observation in the living body is generally the transitional zone between arterioles and venules.

The larger vessels are difficult to observe directly since they lie in the deep portion of the lung.

The blood flow in the pulmonary artery is in general pulsatile, and the portions with continuous flow are comparatively few.

Fig. 105 shows microscopic observations of blood flow in arterioles and capillaries, and in venules and capillaries.

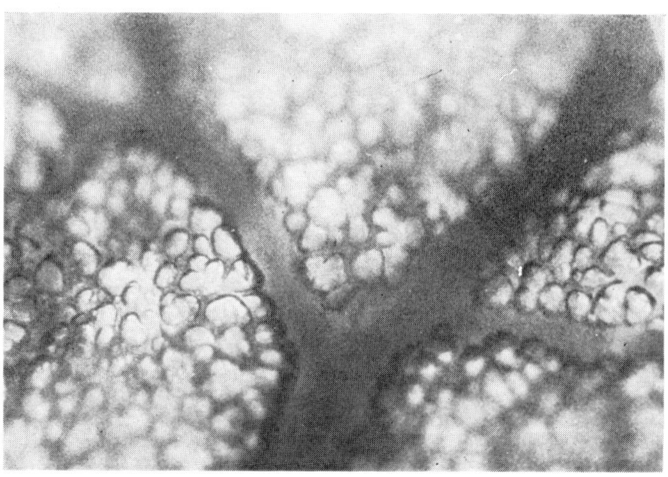

Fig. 105 Capillary nets of the alveolar wall.

Discernment of arterioles and venules is facilitated by observing the direction and distribution of blood flow. Vessels of this size may with difficulty be defined as arteriolar or venular on the basis of observed wall structure.

Generally, it is considered that blood in the arterial system flows from hilum toward pleural surfaces, in the opposite direction in venous tributaries. In the branches of the pulmonary artery blood flow is, as a rule, intermittent and pulsatile.

1. Blood Flow in Arterioles and Venules

Velocity of Blood Flow: The velocity of blood flow in the branches of pulmonary artery and vein varies according to vessel size; in the same vessels the velocity is seen to change from time to time.

In most appositional branches arising from the same blood vessel, considerable fluctuation in the velocity of the blood flow may be observed.

Suspension Phenomenon: Complete momentary cessation of the blood flow is frequently seen in branches of pulmonary arteries and veins.

The phenomenon is observed not only in the arterioles and venules, but also in fairly large vessels such as lobular arteries or veins.

If an arteriole ramifies in three branches, one branch may exhibit pulsatile and rapid blood flow, while the blood flow in the other two branches may be suspended for a little while.

The temporary suspension of the blood flow is not limited to a small portion of the lung, but is frequently seen sporadically and scatteringly in the whole lung.

When this phenomenon occurs in lobular arteries, the blood flow in the lobule may be temporarily completely suspended. Sometimes this phenomenon may involve as many as ten (or more) lobular arteries at one time.

The duration of the suspension of blood flow is quite variable.

Velocity of Erythrocyte Perfusion: The velocity of erythrocyte perfusion does not necessarily coincide with the velocity of blood flow.

In some instances, although the flow of the liquid component is comparatively rapid, the velocity of erythrocyte perfusion varies, and in the branching portions of blood vessels the perfusion of the erythrocytes may actually be suspended.

Aggregating and disaggregating phenomenon are also observed.

Erythrocytes may aggregate in some vessels to the extent that the plasma component is barely observable; in other vessels the liquid component is obviously flowing but erythrocytes are rarely observed.

The conditions leading to these phenomenons are constantly changing, even in the same regions.

2. Blood Flow in Alveolar Capillaries

Capillaries of the alveolar wall, as shown in Fig. 106, are reticular in form, and composed of four to nine (average six) small branches of arteriolar origin, and have many branches communicating with each other.

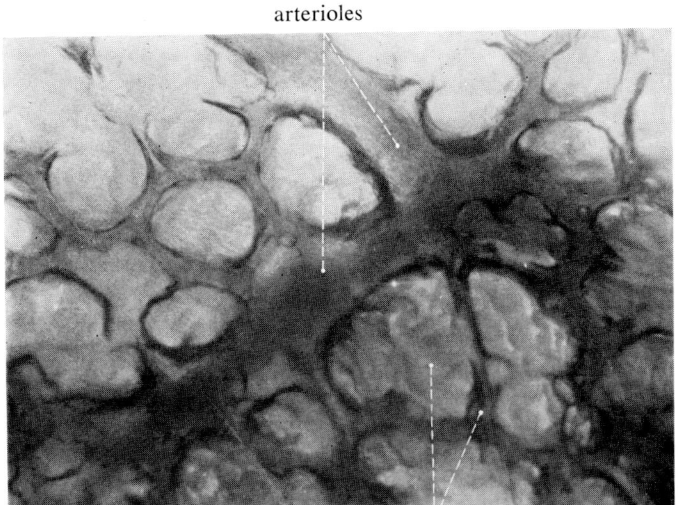

Fig. 106 Capillary nets of the alveolar wall.

The inside diameter of each capillary is so small that one or two erythrocytes can barely pass through.

3. Influence of Respiration on Alveolar Blood Flow

Compared with extrathoracic (systemic) blood vessels, the pulmonary vascular system is directly affected by the influence of respiration, the length and diameter of the vessels changing in relation to expansion and contraction of the lung.

The caliber and the length of the pulmonary artery decrease in the expiratory phase, and the blood flow tends to become pulsatile and slower in velocity.

On inspiration, the caliber and the length of the artery increase, the blood flow becomes less evidently pulsatile and of greater velocity.

Momentary cessation of blood flow is noted upon expiration, rarely on inspiration.

In the pulmonary vein and its tributaries the phenomenon is quite in contrast to the above.

4. Influence of Intratracheal Pressure on Blood Flow

In the pulmonary vascular system, blood flow is also markedly influenced by alterations in intratracheal pressure.

If the pressure is increased gradually, the velocity of blood flow will decrease and will cease. If the pressure is then decreased gradually, the blood flow will return to normal velocity in a short time.

This point must be noted on the occasion of performing high pressure respiration during intratracheal anesthesia.

5. Influence of Position of Body on Blood Flow

The blood flow in the pulmonary vascular system is also affected by the position of the body.

If the leg or head of an animal is lifted from a face down position, the blood flow in the alveolar capillaries gradually reduces velocity and in some portion almost ceases, but when the lifted part is returned to the former position, the blood flow returns to normal.

As explained above, the blood flow in the pulmonary vascular system is labile and ever-changing, even in the normal lung.

F. Structure of Pulmonary Vascular Wall

The course of blood circulation and the structure of the vascular wall differ in the fetal stages and after delivery. Before birth nutrition of organs and tissues of the body (including the lung) is regulated by blood reaching the fetus through the umbilical artery. Coincidentally, the structure of the fetal vascular wall differs from that of adults.

1. In Fetus

The pulmonary artery and vein in the fetus exhibit differences in the density, quantity and arrangement of the elastic fibers, and in the arrangement of smooth muscles as compared with the same vessels in the adult.

Elastic Fibers: Elastic fibers are observed earlier than the third month of the fetal stage in the pulmonary arterial wall, but those of the pulmonary venous wall can only be observed after the fourth month. The time of the development of the latter is about the same as for elastic fibers in the neighboring bronchi.

The density, quantity and arrangement of elastic fibers in the fetal stages are clearly different in the pulmonary artery and in the vein.

In the former, in the fourth month of the fetal stage, arrangements almost similar to those extent after the delivery are observed. In the latter, particularly in the vessels of larger caliber, the development of elastic fibers is relatively poor.

In the regions in which the caliber of the blood vessel is somewhat larger, and closer to the hilum, the elastic fibers of the pulmonary artery show better development than in the vein; on the other hand, in the peripheral portion where the calibers are somewhat smaller, the development of elastic fibers are better in the pulmonary vein than in the artery.

At the end of the fetal period the development of elastic fibers in the artery remains fixed, but in the pulmonary vein development progresses; by the 10th month of fetal life elastic fibers are observed in fairly large veins.

Particularly in the media, an even and dense arrangement is observed.

In the pulmonary vein, contrary to the artery, even in the last month of fetal life the differentiation of the internal and external elastic membranes is not yet evident.

As to the especially small blood vessels, the elastic fibers of the 10-month old fetus are arranged regularly in the pulmonary artery as internal and external elastic membranes.

In the more peripheral regions, the pulmonary artery is devoid of internal elastic membrane, and only the external elastic membrane is observable, while in the pulmonary vein the elastic fibers are well developed and have a highly stainable nature.

As explained above, in the fetal stages, the arrangement of elastic fibers in the pulmonary artery differs from that of the pulmonary vein; this, together with the difference in the arrangement by regions, makes discrimination of artery and vein quite simple.

Smooth Muscle: As shown in Fig. 107, the arrangement of smooth muscle in the pulmonary artery after the fourth month of fetal life is quite similar to that of adults. The quantity and size are almost the same as in the adult, that is, the main elements, elastic fibers and smooth muscles which compose the vascular wall are fully developed around the fourth month of fetal life.

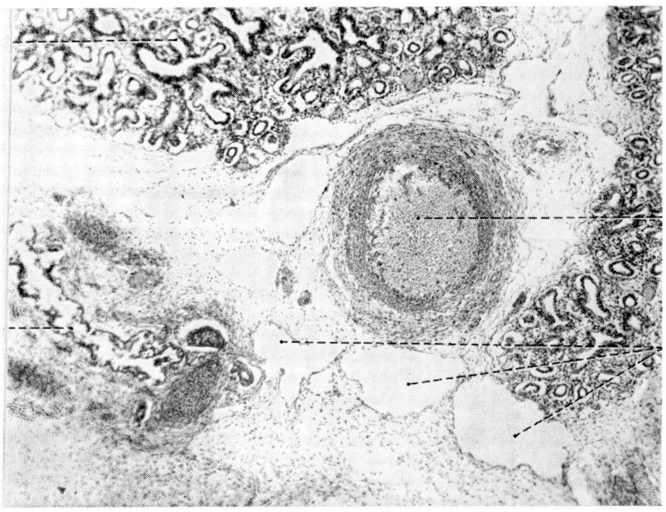

Fig. 107 Pulmonary artery of the fetus.

In the pulmonary vein, smooth muscle is developed in the second month of fetal life in vessels of comparatively large caliber near the hilum, and in the third month, is observed in somewhat smaller blood vessels. But at this age, the extent of development is minimal as compared with that of the pulmonary artery.

After the fourth month of fetal life, development of connective tissue cells occurs, and is accompanied by hyperplasia of smooth muscle. In the 10th month, the pulmonary vein develops to almost the same extent as the pulmonary artery.

Fig. 108 (a) and (b) show the central and peripheral portions of the pulmonary artery of a 4-day-old baby.

In general, smooth muscle cannot be observed in the pulmonary artery of the fetus in vessels smaller than 20–30 μ external dia., or in pulmonary veins smaller than 50–80 μ external dia.

Since the pulmonary artery and vein exhibit different contraction rates in the process of preparing the specimen, it is difficult to compare exactly the point at which the smooth muscles in both vessels can no longer be found by measuring the contracting rate.

Although there is some measurable difference between the vessels when one considers the pattern of vascular branching, among other things, the smooth muscle is found to disappear at about the same point in both pulmonary artery and vein.

2. In Adult

The arterial pressure of the pulmonary circulation is 8–25 mm Hg which is far lower than the mean value of arterial pressure of the systemic circulation, which is 80–120 mm Hg.

In view of the above, the vascular wall of the pulmonary artery is thinner than that of the bronchial artery.

The walls of pulmonary arteries and of arteries of the systemic circulation are composed of three layers: intima, media and adventitia; however, the media of the former is thinner than that of the latter.

The structure of the surrounding tissue of the blood vessels differs in the pulmonary and the systemic

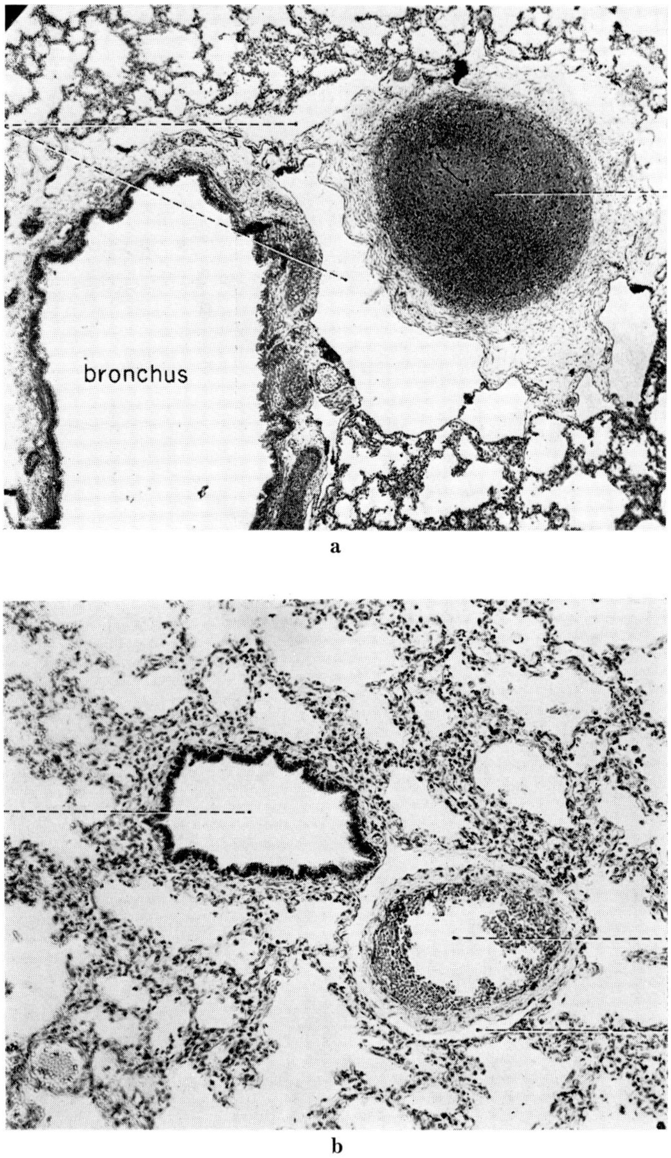

Fig. 108 Pulmonary arteries of a new-born baby.

circulations, the surrounding space being generally larger in the pulmonary circulation.

The tissues surrounding the pulmonary blood vessels are mainly composed of lymph vessels and loose connective tissues; these serve to accommodate the requirements of mobility and elasticity of the blood vessel. As a result, the perivascular loose connective tissues play the role of a buffer zone, permitting expansion and conraction of the lung.

In general, pulmonary tissues have rich elasticity, but the expansion and contraction degree of the pulmonary vascular system and the bronchial vascular system are substantially different.

As to the structure of the vascular wall itself (not to mention the difference between artery and vein but even among the arteries and the veins), the size or location accounts for obvious differences in structure.

Generally speaking, elastic fibers are well developed in the pulmonary artery, whereas in the pulmonary vein, and bronchial artery and vein, smooth muscles are more highly developed.

In general, in the normal lung, the pulmonary artery and vein, and bronchial artery and vein, communicate through their respective capillaries, the capillary networks being quite different.

Pulmonary Artery: The structure of the wall of the pulmonary artery varies from origin to peripheral portions.

In the portion immediately after bifurcation, the smooth muscles of the vascular wall are not observed. However, in the region of the hilum, the existence of the muscles is definitely seen, increasing toward the periphery.

Whereas the nerve endings are observed to be fairly abundant at the root of the pulmonary artery, the volume of muscle decreases gradually near the hilum. In the peripheral portion, *i.e.* in the so-called muscular artery region, the nerve endings are few, in contrast to the increase of smooth muscles on the vascular wall.

In other words, in the root of the pulmonary artery and also in the peripheral portions, the volume of smooth muscles and the nerve endings are in inverse relationship.

The external elastic lamina is observed in the arterioles. The internal elastic lamina decreases markedly in the peripheral portions. The internal and external laminae join together at the point where arterioles reach the size of about 50 μ, and at this point they are devoid of the media.

Pulmonary Vein: In the pulmonary vein, unlike the artery, elastic fibers are found evenly in the large caliber portions and peripheral areas and therefore it is easy to distinguish the external and internal laminae.

In the pulmonary vein, the media are mostly smooth muscles, and can be observed in the portions up to the postcapillary. However, in the pulmonary artery, in the portion smaller than about 50 μ caliber, the smooth muscle layers, *i.e.* the media, are rarely observed.

Unlike the veins of limbs, the pulmonary vein is devoid of venous valves; and instead, a muscle prominence projects into the vascular lumen.

The muscle prominence is composed of the annular and longitudinal muscles, and the intima. The development of the prominence is remarkable at the peripheral portion. The muscle prominence is contractible, but essentially differs from the venous valve.

II. BRONCHIAL VASCULAR SYSTEM

Galen was probably the first to report the distribution of the systemic blood circulation in the lung.

This was denied by Colombus (1559), whereupon this observation by Galen was neglected for another century, until again advanced by Marchettis (1656).

Later, Ruysch (1732) designated the systemic vessel as the bronchial artery. As the designation was first made by him, it is today believed that the bronchial artery was discovered by Ruysch.

Reisseisen (1808, 1822) and Sömmering (1808) claimed that the bronchial artery was a nutrient vessel.

Regarding the bronchial artery and the bronchial vascular system, further investigations were carried on by: Colberg (1863, 1866), Zuckerkandl (1881, 1883), Ghoreyeb (1913), Konaschko (1926), Barry (1931), Omochi (1937), Miller (1947), Schmidt (1947), Cauldwell (1948), Liebow (1949, 1950), Nagaishi and M. Yamashita (1950–1957), Marchang (1950), Manabe (1951), Hayek (1953), Matsuo (1954), Nakayama (1954), Aoki (1954) and Nakamura (1955, 1957). As to details, the above authors' opinions are diverse.

Since 1950 the authors (Nagaishi, M. Yamashita, N. Nagasawa and U. Takahashi, et al.) have been conducting detailed investigations into the structure of the vascular system, in order to clarify the role of the bronchial vascular system in lung surgery, in chest diseases, and in pulmonary pathophysiology.

A. Bronchial Artery

As will be described, bronchial arteries may arise from the descending aorta, the intercostal, subclavian or internal mammary arteries.

According to the region of distribution, the arteries are classified as extrapulmonary and intrapulmonary.

The extrapulmonary bronchial artery gives off small branches to the esophagus, to mediastinal tissues, and to hilar lymph nodes, before entering the territory of the lobar bronchus; other branches may anastomose with branches of the same arterial system which are distributed to neighboring regions.

The intrapulmonary bronchial artery distributes to the various structures of the bronchial wall, to pulmonary pleura, to lymph nodes, to walls of the pulmonary artery and vein and to nerves.

A more detailed outline of the bronchial artery follows.

1. Origin

Cauldwell (1948) and others have reported on the origin of the bronchial artery.

As already described, the bronchial artery may arise from the descending aorta, the intercostal, the left subclavian or the internal mammary artery, and has quite different relationships on the right and the left sides.

According to Cauldwell (1948), the origin of the bronchial artery is classified into nine major types, as shown in Fig. 109, individual variations being observed with high frequency. Even the most frequent type (I) is found in less than 50% of the observations.

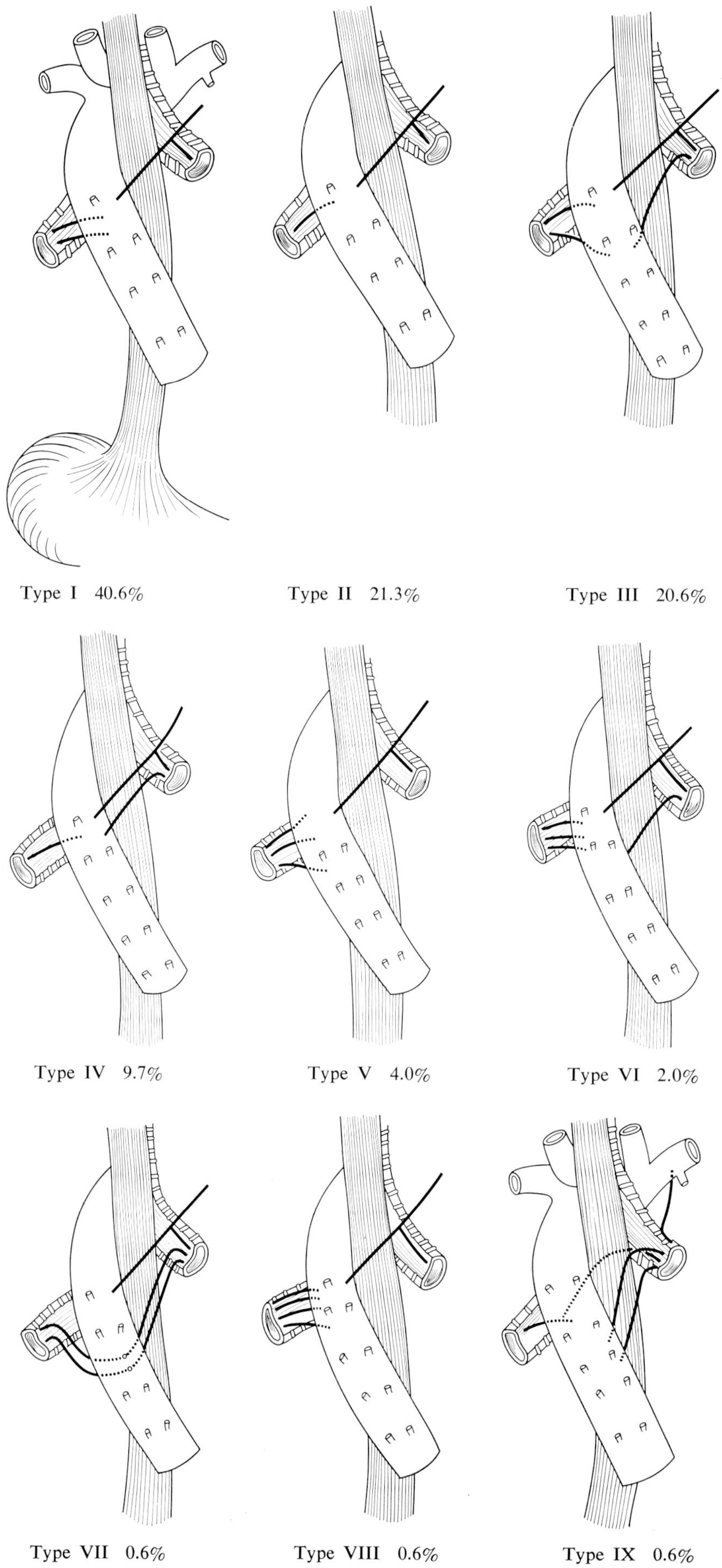

Fig. 109 Various types of origin of the bronchial artery (Cauldwell, 1948).

The principal arterial stem gives off two to five branches; it ramifies at the level of the second to fourth intercostal arteries as these branch out from the aorta.

The caliber of the arterial root is about the same as that of an intercostal artery. Figs. 110 (a), (b) show angiograms of the root portions of the bronchial artery of the dog.

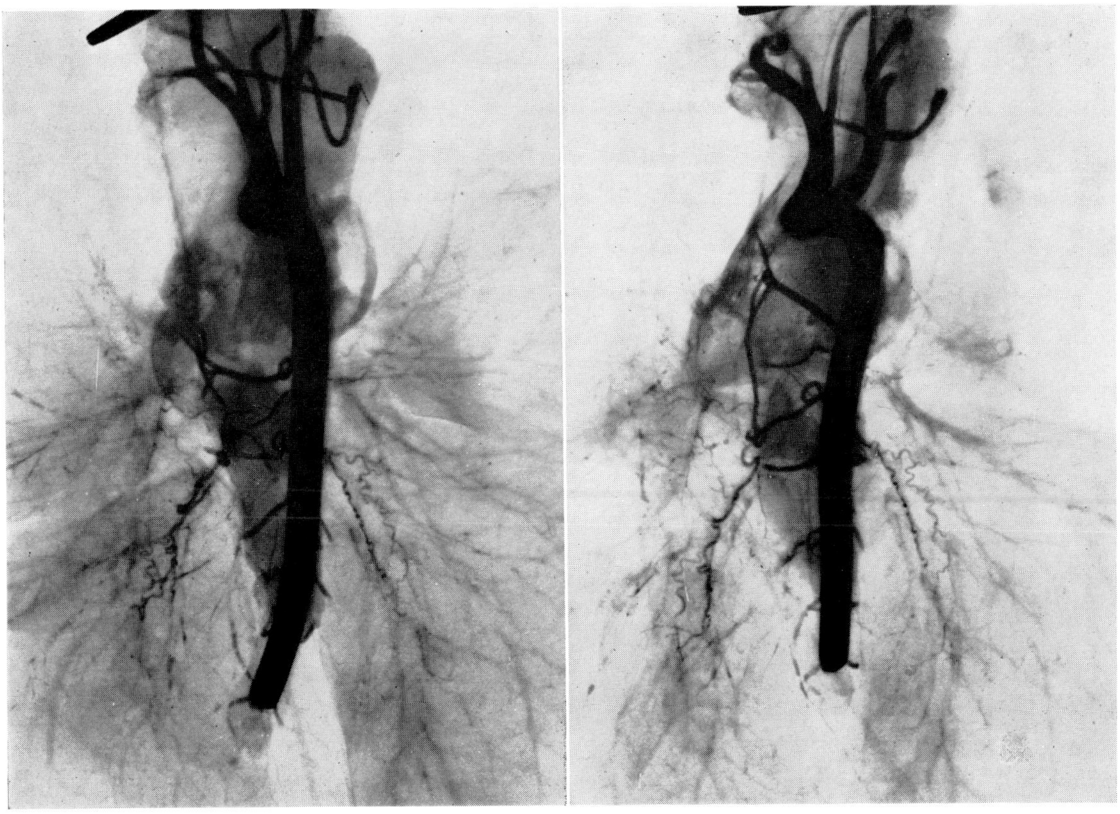

a b

Fig. 110 Bronchial artery of the dog (angiogram).

2. Distribution and Course

The bronchial artery ultimately distributes in the mucous membrane of the bronchial wall, in muscular layers and fibrous tissues and supplies secretory glands, perichondrium, pulmonary pleura, lymph nodes, walls of the pulmonary artery and vein, and nerves.

It gives off small branches to the wall of the esophagus, as shown in Fig. 111.

Table 4 is a simplified classification of the bronchial artery as reported by NAGAISHI and M. YAMASHITA (1952).

Classification I: The bronchial artery divides into two branches in the region of the hilum: to be more specific, into an extrapulmonary bronchial artery on the central side of the second order bronchus, and into an intrapulmonary bronchial artery on the peripheral side of the second order bronchus.

The blood flow of the extrapulmonary bronchial artery empties into the right atrium via the following route: extrapulmonary bronchial artery → capillaries → extrapulmonary bronchial vein → azygos or hemiazygos vein, or intercostal vein → superior vena cava → right atrium.

The blood flow of the intrapulmonary bronchial artery empties into the left atrium via the following route: intrapulmonary bronchial artery → capillaries → intrapulmonary bronchial vein → pulmonary vein → left atrium.

This classification is significant not only from the viewpoint of topographic anatomy but also for evident pathophysiological reasons.

Classification II: The bronchial artery is divided into superior and inferior bronchial arteries on the left side, and superior, middle and inferior bronchial arteries on the right side, according to the lobes supplied.

CUDKOWICZ (1951): Branches of the bronchial arteries distributed to the pulmonary pleura were designated by him (according to area supplied) as 'hilar pleural', 'lateral pleural', 'left oblique fissure', 'right horizontal

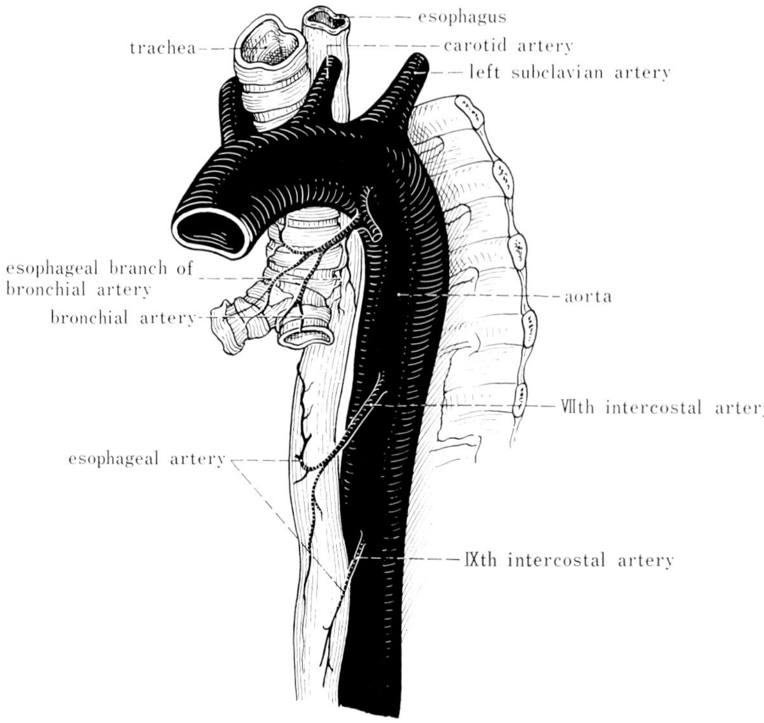

Fig. 111

Table 4 Classification of bronchial artery.

I. Classification according to distribution and course of venous drainage.
   1. extrapulmonary bronchial artery: through extrapulmonary bronchial vein to azygos or hemiazygos vein, or intercostal vein, and to right ventricle.
   2. intrapulmonary bronchial artery: through intrapulmonary bronchial vein to pulmonary vein, and to left atrium.

II. Classification according to pulmonary lobes
   1. right upper, middle or lower bronchial artery
   2. left upper lower bronchial artery

fissure' branches, etc. In particular, the blood vessel distributed to the apical pleura was claimed to be of great importance, having much to do with apical pulmonary disease processes.

Fig. 112 shows an example of Classification II.

1. Extrapulmonary Bronchial Artery: Before entering the lung, the extrapulmonary bronchial artery ramifies into many small branches to supply esophagus, mediastinum, and hilar lymph nodes as mentioned above, and to anastomose with other vessels distributed in the region.
2. Intrapulmonary Bronchial Artery: Compared to the extrapulmonary bronchial artery the intrapulmonary bronchial artery distributes to large portions of the lung. It is not a terminal artery as is the case with the pulmonary artery; its branches are connected to each other by a number of communicating branches.

Bronchial Artery of Bronchial Wall: Bronchial arteries anastomose with one another in the region posterior to the hilum immediately before entering to supply the lobar bronchi, and then ramify to their respective bronchi. The branches which run in the adventitia are largest in caliber, as shown in Fig. 113.

The main trunk and its branches run as shown in Fig. 114. They are classified into four types, *i.e.* arborescent, straight, bending and recurrent. They are in various forms, either running independently or intermingling with one another.

Of the branches which run in the inner layer of the bronchial wall, those in the muscular layer are generally small in caliber, those distributed in the mucous membrane being particularly fine.

Branches perforate the bronchial walls and form intramural networks immediately under the ciliated epithelium.

In its course along the bronchial wall the bronchial artery follows the bifurcation of the bronchial branches. In general, the artery bifurcates on the hilar or peripheral sides rather than at the exact point of bronchial bifurcation.

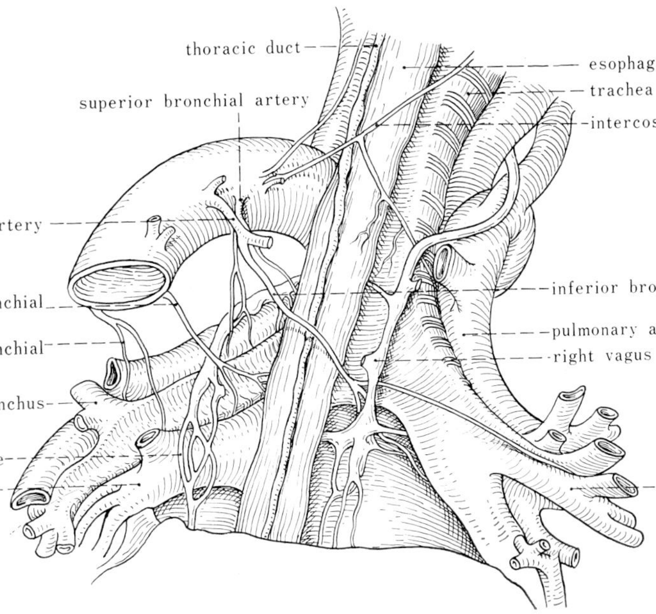

Fig. 112 Origin and branching of the bronchial artery.

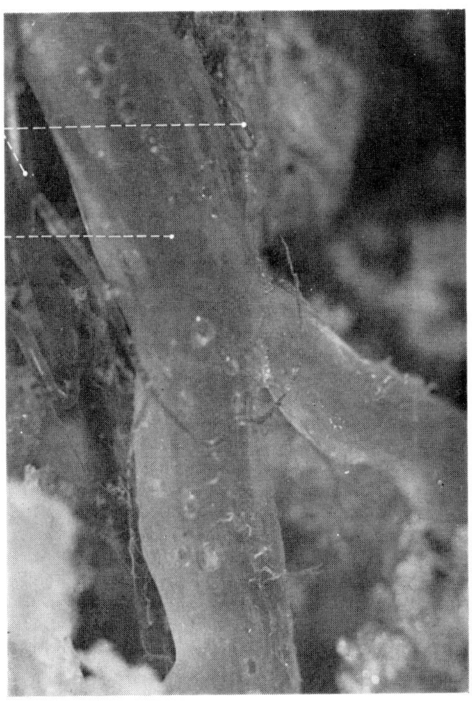

Fig. 113 Bronchial arteries in the adventitia of the bronchus.

As mentioned earlier, the artery runs toward the periphery, adjacent to the bronchial wall. No artery is found to run regularly along the membranous part of the bronchus.

Bronchial Artery of Perichondrium: The bronchial artery distributing in the periochondrium of the bronchial cartilages runs annularly, after branching out in an almost perpendicular line, along the borders of the bronchial cartilages.

When each cartilaginous ring is examined, the blood vessels in the peripheral portions are found to be larger than those on the hilar side. Both vessels give off fine arterioles to form a capillary network over the perichondrium.

Bronchial Artery to Bronchial Secretory Gland: Branches of the bronchial artery distribute also in the bronchial secretory gland, as shown in Fig. 115. From this point of view the bronchial artery is considered to have an important relation to the secretory activity of the bronchial glands, as well as in forming the nutrient blood vessels of these glands.

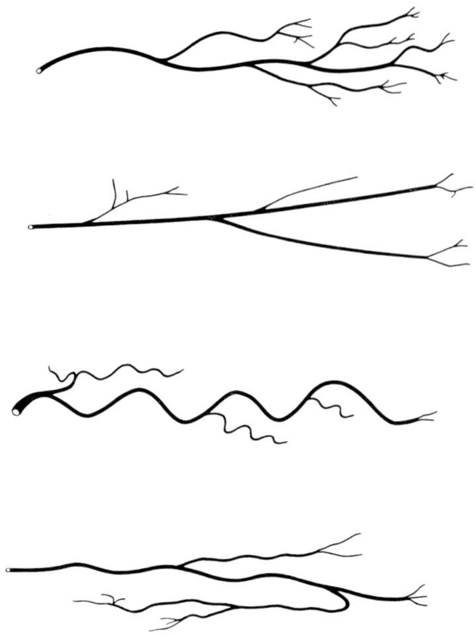

Fig. 114 Various types of the branching of the bronchial artery.

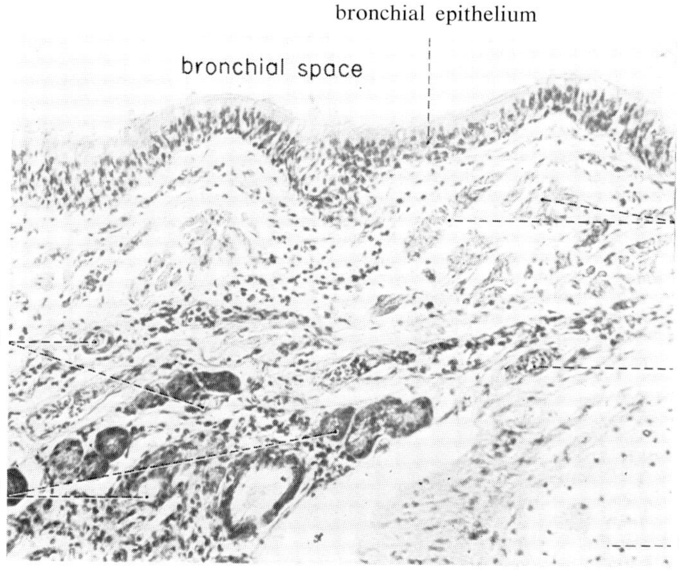

Fig. 115 Bronchial arteries in the bronchial wall.

Bronchial Artery of Pulmonary Pleura: HAYEK (1953) claimed that pulmonary arteries supply the pulmonary pleura, and that bronchial arteries distribute only in the proximity of the hilum. However, according to investigations made by M. YAMASHITA (1954), it was shown that the blood vessels distributing widely to normal pulmonary pleura are branches of bronchial arteries.

Some bronchial arteries to the pulmonary pleura run from the hilum to a region immediately beneath the pleura as shown in Fig. 116; others emerge from the hilum, run to the bronchial wall, to intersegmental or interlobular septa, and then appear on the surface of the lung to distribute in the pulmonary pleura.

The former can clearly be observed on the mediastinal surface of the pulmonary pleura, in a radial arrangement, with the hilum in the center.

As Figs. 117 and 118 indicate, those branches distributed to the borders of interlobar fissures, to apical pleura, to subpleural veins and to the pulmonary lobe are the largest in caliber.

Intercommunication of neighboring bronchial arteries is not as evident on the pleural surface as on the bronchial walls. Individual bronchial arteries appear to run, bend and wave slightly in their course.

In the event of collapse of the lung, stenosis of the bronchial artery and vein is not as evident as in the case of the pulmonary artery and vein. The vessels show bending but no change is seen in the length,

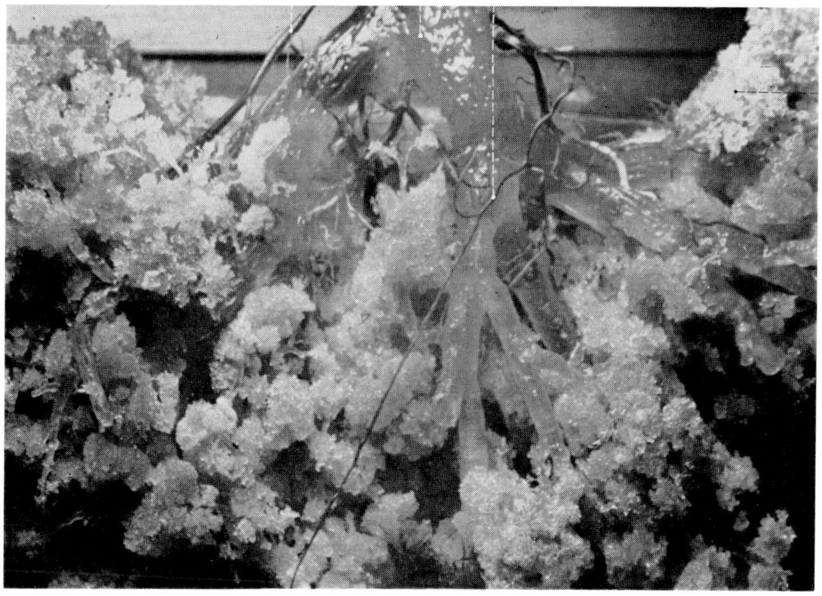

Fig. 116 Peribronchial and subpleural branches of the bronchial artery (resin cast).

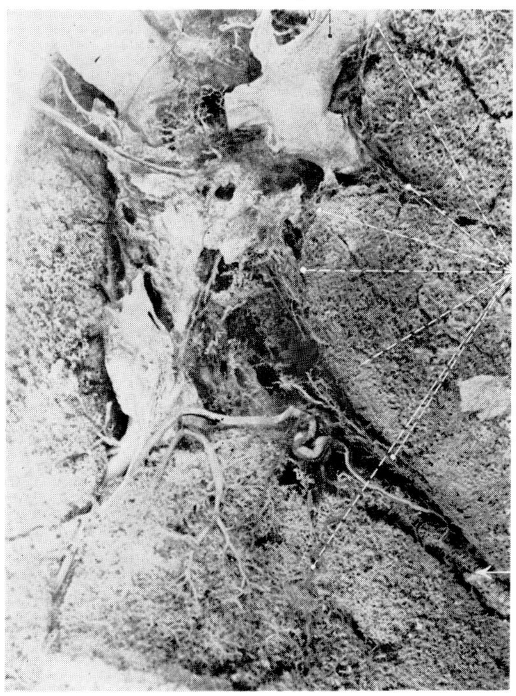

Fig. 117 Bronchial arteries.

because the bronchial artery and vein have a higher blood pressure than the pulmonary artery and vein.

As shown in Fig. 119, capillaries of the pulmonary pleura are sparse as compared to the richness of intrapulmonary capillaries, particularly those of the bronchial wall. The normal pleura is generally extremely thin; a few blood vessels suffice to provide nourishment. However, the diseased pleura may be accompanied by a variable to marked proliferation of blood vessels, as shown in Fig. 120.

Arterial Supply to Walls of Pulmonary Artery and Vein: Bronchial arteries course on the walls of pulmonary artery and vein, and are functionally vasa vasorum. They are not as dense as on the bronchial walls, and cannot be easily observed macroscopically on the walls of smaller vessels.

Fig. 121 shows an example of a resin casting in which the bronchial artery runs parallel with the pulmonary artery in the region close to the wall of the pulmonary artery. Branches of the bronchial

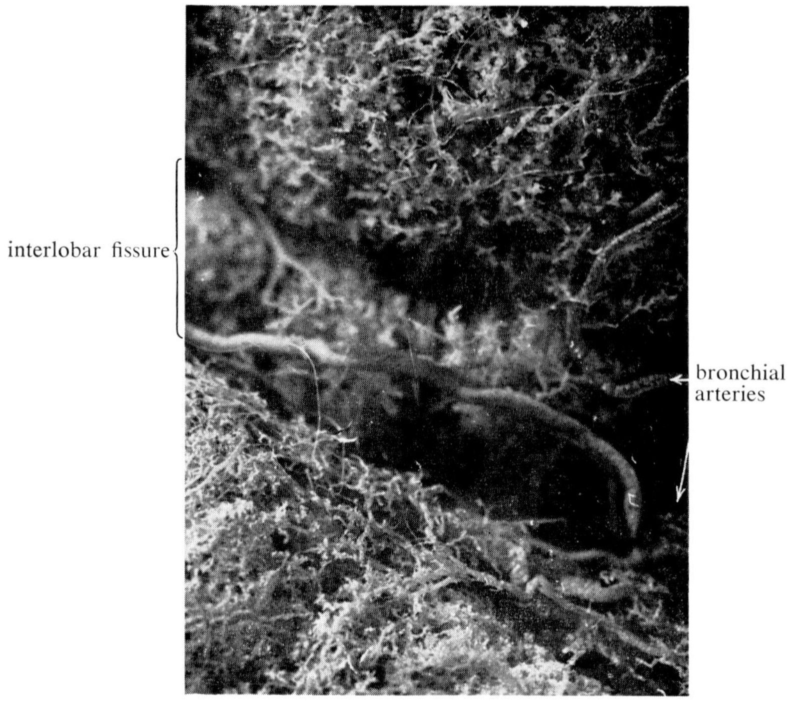

Fig. 118 Bronchial arteries in the interlobar fissure (resin cast).

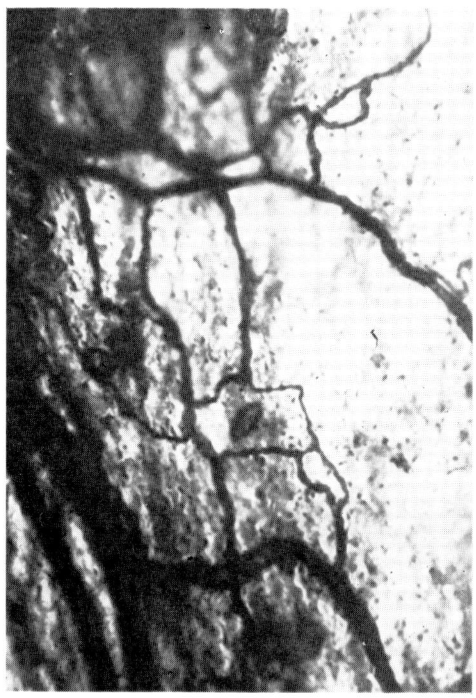

Fig. 119 Bronchial arteries of the pulmonary pleura (Bielschowsky's method modified by SUZUKI).

artery to the walls of the bronchus and the pulmonary artery may form abundant anastomoses, as shown in Fig. 122.

Bronchial Artery of Lymph Node: The arterial vessels supplying the hilar and intrapulmonary lymph nodes are bronchial arteries. Distribution to the hilar and intrapulmonary nodes is somewhat different. Small and direct branches of the aorta supply the lymph nodes adjacent to the trachea or main bronchus, but the arterial supply to lymph nodes adjacent and peripheral to the lobar bronchi may originate in branches of the bronchial arteries to the bronchial walls.

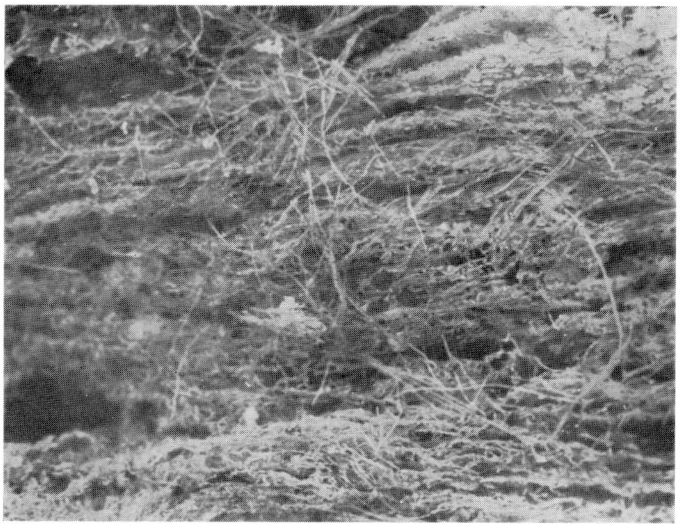

Fig. 120 Proliferated bronchial arteries of the pleura (resin cast).

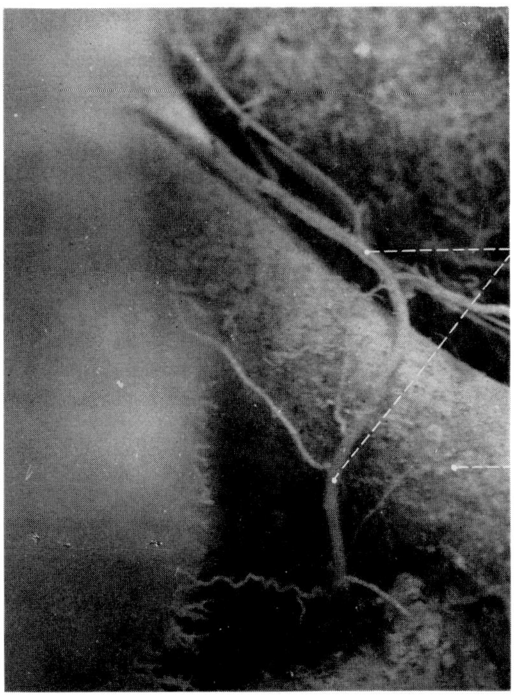

Fig. 121 Bronchial arteries in the wall of the pulmonary artery (resin cast).

B. Bronchial Vein

A definitive description of the bronchial vein has not yet been found, although a few investigations have been reported.

MILLER (1925) stated that the bronchial vein exists only in the hilum and in the region proximal to the hilum; its blood flow runs into the right atrium via the superior vena cava through azygos or hemiazygos vein, or intercostal vein.

MARCHAND (1950) stated that the small venous tributaries joining the pulmonary vein must also be called 'bronchial vein', in addition to the bronchial vein mentioned by MILLER.

NAGAISHI and M. YAMASHITA, et al. (1952) on the basis of studies of normal or nearly normal specimens, using perfusion or resin casting methods, classified the bronchial vein as extrapulmonary and intrapulmonary, as in the case of the bronchial artery.

The blood flow of the extrapulmonary bronchial vein empties into the right atrium via the azygos or hemiazigos, or the intercostal vein, and the superior vena cava; the blood flow of the intrapulmonary bronchial vein empties into the left atrium via the pulmonary vein as mentioned earlier. Table 5 presents a comparison of previous and current studies of the bronchial vein.

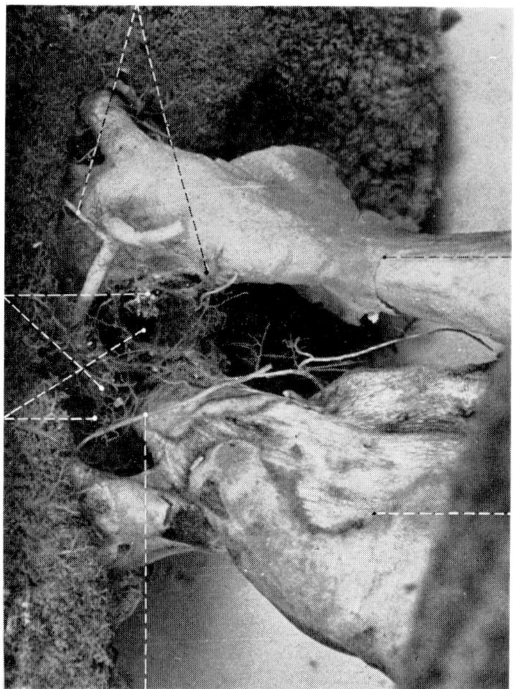

Fig. 122 Bronchial arteries in the peribronchial and the perivascular tissues (resin cast).

Table 5 Classification of bronchial vein.

NAGAISHI and M. YAMASHITA	MILLER	MARCHAND
extrapulmonary bronchial vein	bronchial vein	extrapulmonary bronchial vein
intrapulmonary bronchial vein		
superficial: long branch / short branch	pulmonary vein	
deep: long branch / short branch		intrapulmonary bronchial vein

The region which was designated by the present authors as the intrapulmonary bronchial vein was interpreted by Miller as a part of the pulmonary vein.

Among the extrapulmonary bronchial veins designated by Marchand, the veins which drain on the subpleural tissue and hilar tissue belong partly to the extrapulmonary bronchial veins, but include also a part of the intrapulmonary vein, as designated by the authors.

1. Extrapulmonary Bronchial Vein
   The extrapulmonary bronchial vein distributed in the hilar region originates in the extrapulmonary bronchial artery in the second order bronchus, *i.e.* the lobar bronchus. The blood flow of the extrapulmonary bronchial vein finally empties into the right atrium as mentioned earlier.
2. Intrapulmonary Bronchial Vein
   The intrapulmonary bronchial vein originates in the intrapulmonary bronchial artery in the bronchial wall peripheral to the second order bronchus, i.e. the lobar bronchus.
   The blood flow of the intrapulmonary bronchial vein finally empties into the left atrium as mentioned earlier.

From its appearance, the intrapulmonary bronchial vein is conveniently divided into long and short branches; from location it may be divided into the superficial bronchial and deep bronchial veins. The former is located in the pleura, the latter is in the lung.

Therefore, in a variety of combinations, the intrapulmonary bronchial veins can be classified as the long and short tributaries of the superficial and of the deep bronchial veins.

Long Branches of Superficial Bronchial Veins: Fig. 123 shows an example of a resin casting of the left lung, showing the course and distribution of the superficial long bronchial vein. As can be seen, such

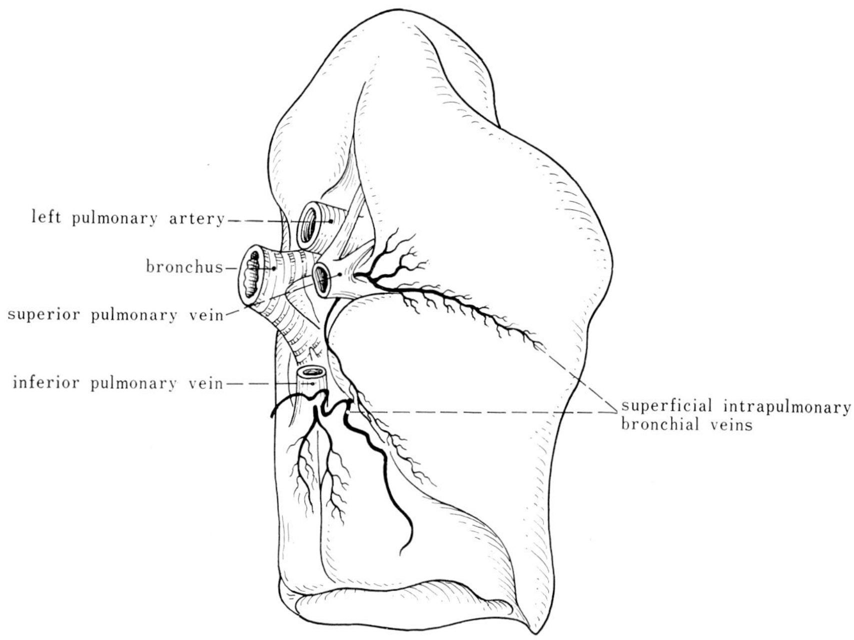

Fig. 123 Long branches of the superficial bronchial vein.

veins are located on the mediastinal surface of the pulmonary pleura and in general are arranged in a radial shape around the hilum. Forming anastomoses, tributaries run to the hilum where they anastomose with bronchial veins stemming from the walls of the pulmonary blood vessels, and then join the pulmonary vein.

Figs. 124 and 125 show the bronchial veins originating in the pulmonary pleura near the hilum; these connect with intersegmental pulmonary vein in the hilum after anastomosing with the bronchial veins of the bronchial wall.

The course and distribution of these branches in the pulmonary pleura are different from that of the pulmonary vein, and these branches are the long branches of the superficial bronchial vein.

The course of these bronchial vessels is similar to that of the subpleural pulmonary veins of the interlobar pleura and the mediastinal surface of the pulmonary pleura.

Short Branches of Superficial Bronchial Veins: These distribute on the surface of the pulmonary pleura, and join the interacinar and interlobular pulmonary veins.

Long Branches of Deep Bronchial Vein: Fig. 126 shows a resin casting which illustrates the relationship of the bronchus, pulmonary vein and the long branches of the deep bronchial vein in the hilum of the right lower lobe.

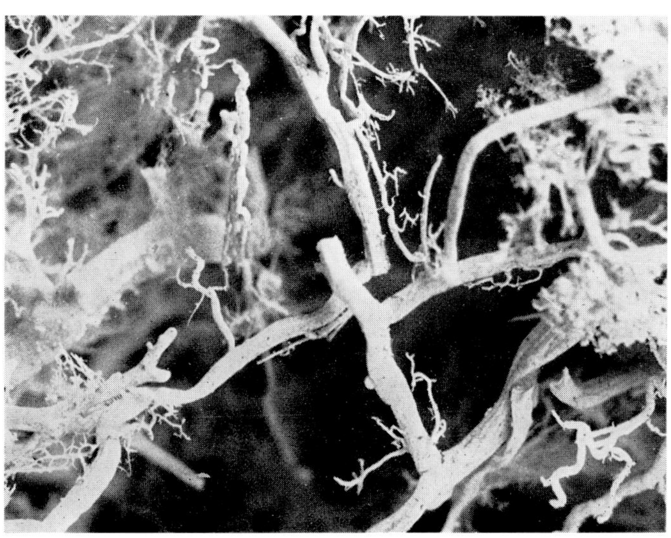

Fig. 124 Bronchial veins (resin cast).

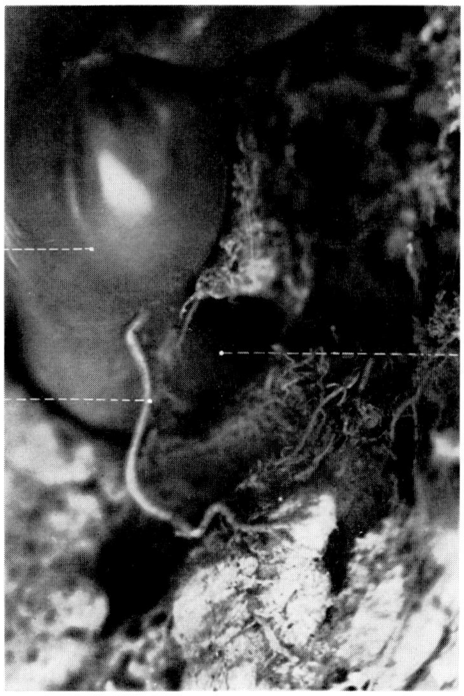

Fig. 125 Long branch of superficial intrapulmonary bronchial vein (resin cast).

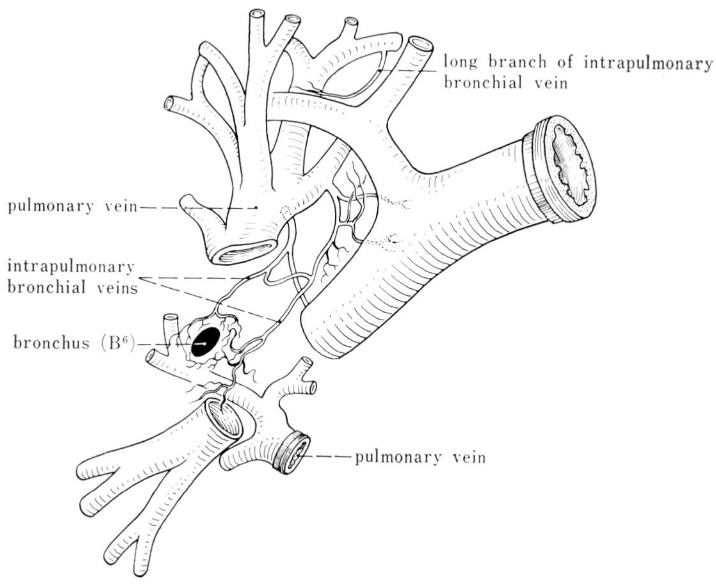

Fig. 126 Pulmonary vein and intrapulmonary bronchial vein.

In this specimen, acrylic resin was insufflated in the pulmonary vein and the bronchial artery to the peripheral regions, and also high viscosity resin was insufflated into the large bronchus, thus illustrating the relationship of the pulmonary vein to the bronchial vein.

In Fig. 127, a specimen shows a bronchial vein originating near the wall of the subsegmental bronchus of the lower lobe, ascending and joining the pulmonary vein of the upper lobe near the wall of the lobar bronchus. Only two of twelve cases were similar to the specimens shown in the above figure, in which the origin of the bronchial vein and juncture with the pulmonary vein occurred in different lobes.

Fig. 128 shows a long branch of another intrapulmonary bronchial vein of the same specimen. The bronchial vein runs along the fourth order bronchus in S^2, *i.e.* from the wall of B^2a to the third order bronchus, i.e. the wall of B^2, then changes its direction, bending in the shape of "<" and runs along the third order bronchus S^1, *i.e.* the wall of B^1, reaches the peripheral portion of the bronchus, and then joins the pulmonary vein.

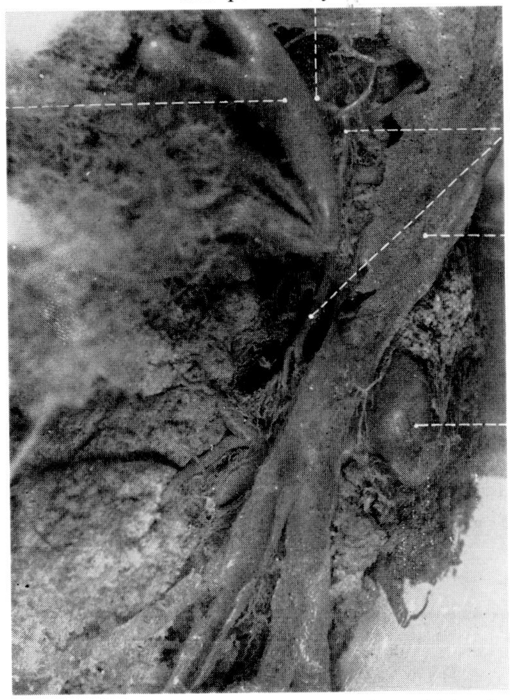

Fig. 127 Pulmonary vein and intrapulmonary bronchial vein (resin cast).

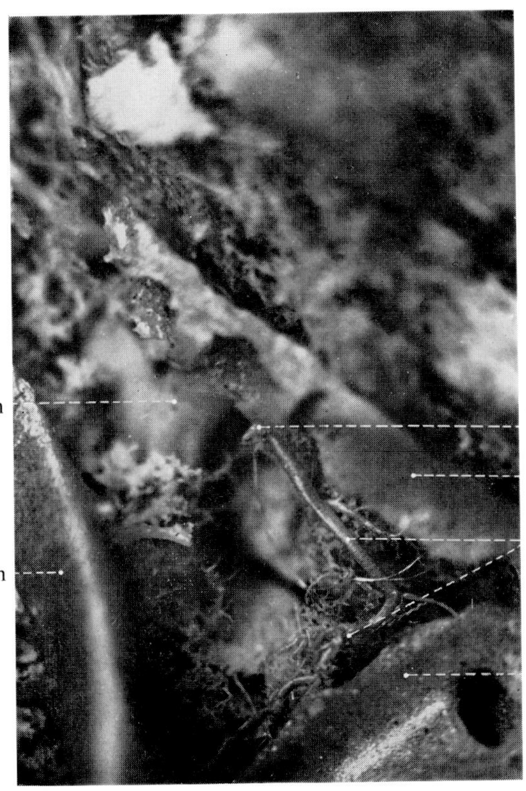

Fig. 128 Pulmonary vein and intrapulmonary bronchial vein (resin cast).

As is seen in this case, vessels which at first run toward the hilum and then change direction and run toward the periphery are observed in the bronchial vein, but none is observed in the pulmonary vein.

In the case of the pulmonary vein, the course is, as shown in Fig. 129, always central.

Several anastomoses are seen between the bronchial vein and small branches of the pulmonary vein which distribute near the alveolar wall.

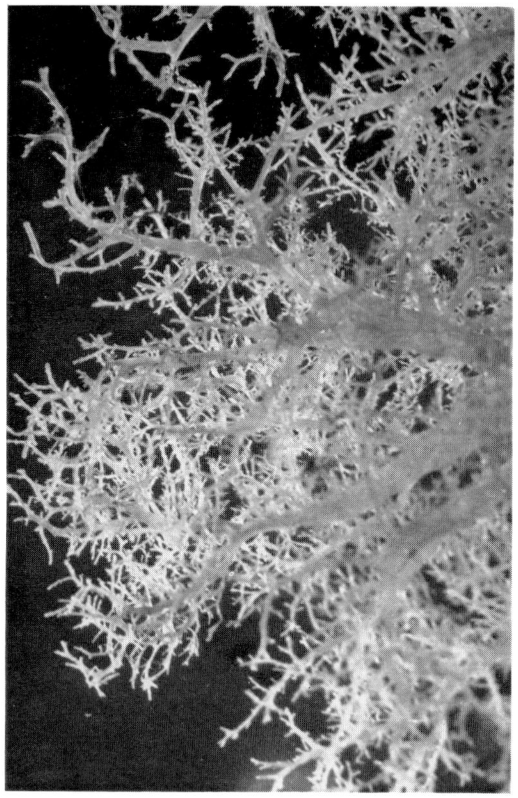

Fig. 129 Branches of the pulmonary vein (resin cast).

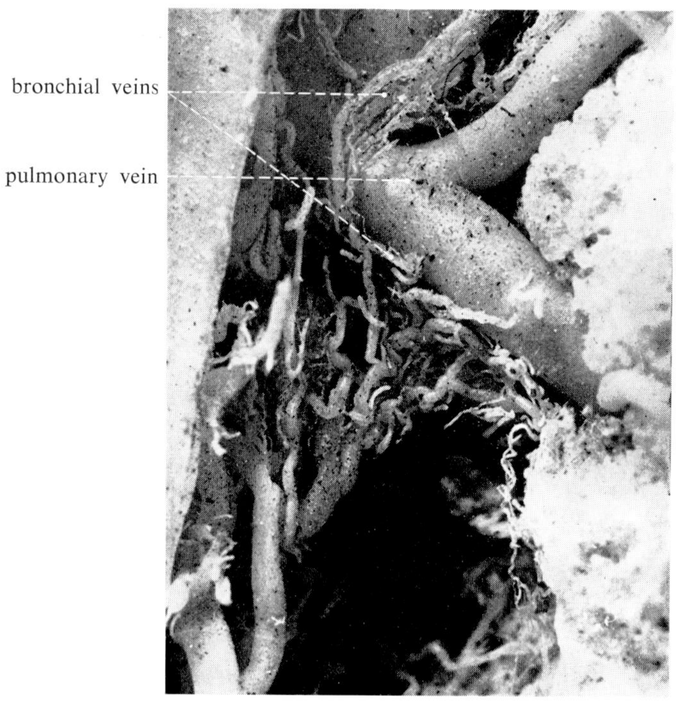

Fig. 130 Pulmonary vein and bronchial veins (resin cast).

Fig. 130 shows a long deep intrapulmonary bronchial vein in relationship with the wall of the pulmonary vein.

Fig. 131 demonstrates an anastomosis of a long deep bronchial vein and a branch of a superficial bronchial vein. As can be seen, numerous anastomoses exist between such intrapulmonary bronchial veins.

Deep Short Bronchial Veins: The short branches show the finest and most extensive distribution of all the intrapulmonary bronchial veins.

Fig. 132 is a resin casting to show the short branches of the deep bronchial vein in the region where segmental bronchi are formed.

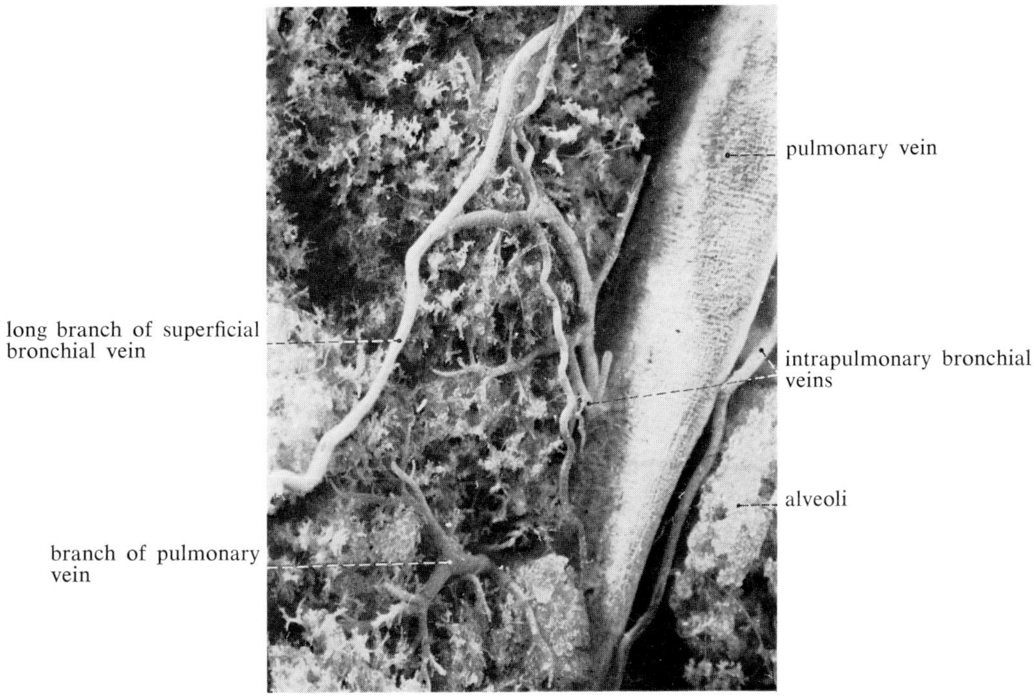

Fig. 131 Pulmonary vein and bronchial veins (resin cast).

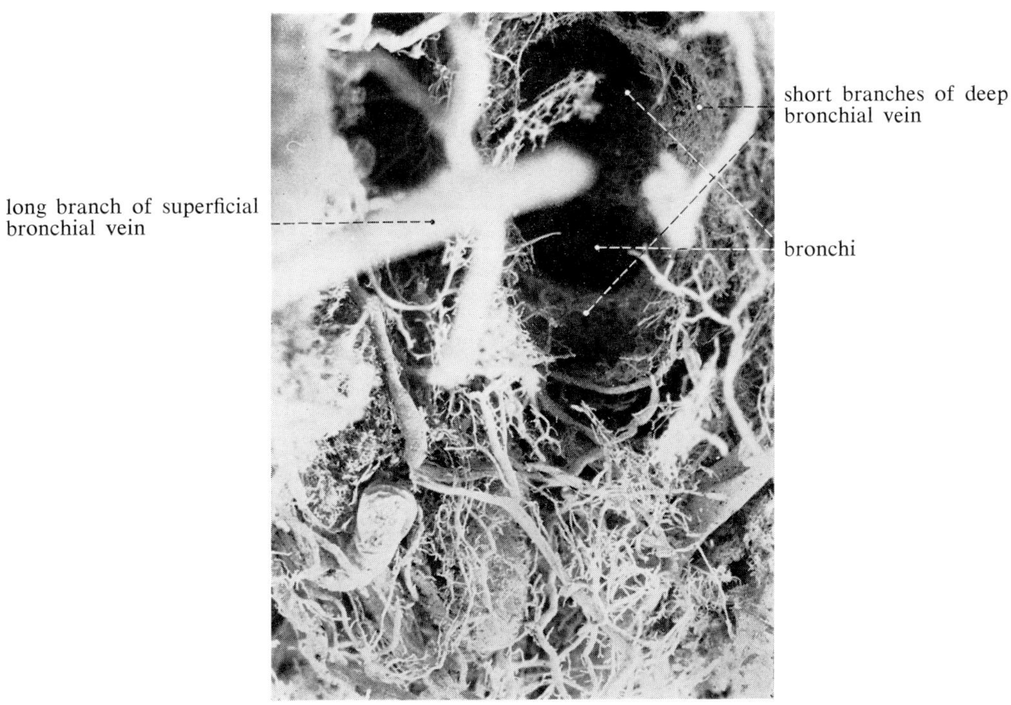

Fig. 132 Bronchial veins (resin cast).

In general, short branches of the deep bronchial vein show dense distribution. Each vessel distributes in quite narrow regions, but each has abundant anastomoses which resemble a venous sinus. From such morphological relationships, the short branches of the deep bronchial veins are considered to be functionally equivalent to venous sinuses; they participate actively in regulation of the pulmonary circulation.

The following is a summary of the above studies:

Intrapulmonary bronchial veins are classified as either the superficial or deep veins, and are further subdivided into long and short branches.

The superficial intrapulmonary bronchial veins drain mainly the pulmonary pleura; their long branches run along the mediastinal surface of the pulmonary pleura with lengthy courses along the interlobar fissures or along subpleural branches of the pulmonary veins. Morphologically these bronchial veins have a striking resemblance to the bronchial arteries.

In the region of the hilum these vessels anastomose with the long branches of the deep intrapulmonary bronchial veins and join the pulmonary veins of the region.

Extensively distributed to the surface of the pleura, the short branches form anastomoses with branches of the subpleural pulmonary veins.

The long branches of the deep bronchial veins drain the walls of the bronchi, and pulmonary arteries and veins to join the pulmonary vein in the vicinity of the hilum.

Short branches of the deep bronchial vein anastomose with neighboring branches of the pulmonary vein in many places. Although each branch distributes in limited regions, abundant anastomoses are found which resemble venous sinuses.

Unlike the pulmonary artery and vein, the bronchial vein is almost the same size in its central and peripheral portions. Its direction and pattern are not so regular as those of the pulmonary artery and vein.

The bronchial vein of the pulmonary arterial wall has fine anastomoses with the bronchial vein of the bronchial wall. The pulmonary venous wall does not form so fine anastomoses as those of the bronchial wall, excepting in the region of the hilum.

As a rule the bronchial arteries and veins run parallel, as shown in Fig. 133.

As shown in Fig. 134, irregular polygonal capillary networks are observed between the bronchial arteries and the bronchial veins.

The diameter and the arrangement of the capillaries stemming from the bronchial artery and the capillaries originating in the pulmonary artery are completely different.

In the normal lung, communication between the bronchial artery and vein is made only by capillary beds, as shown in Fig. 135.

As with other peripheral systemic veins, valves are observed in extrapulmonary bronchial veins, but the intrapulmonary bronchial veins are devoid of valves, as is also the case for pulmonary veins.

The fact that the intrapulmonary bronchial veins are devoid of valves at first gives the impression that one may be dealing with a branch of the pulmonary vein, but when the distribution, arrangement, and

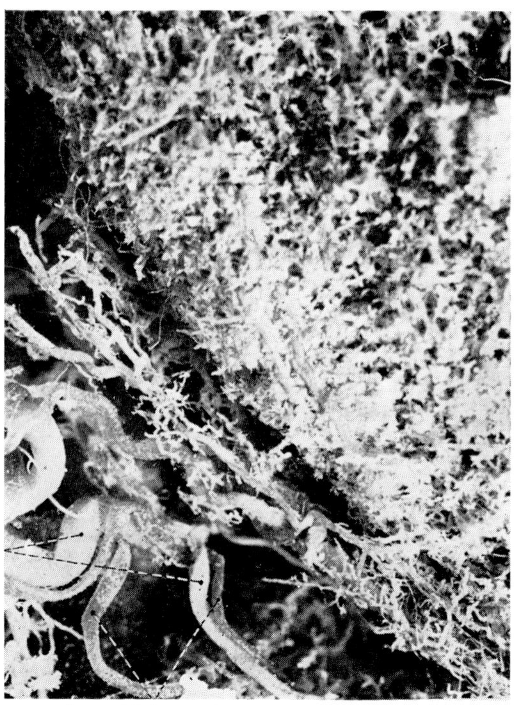

Fig. 133 Bronchial arteries and veins (resin cast).

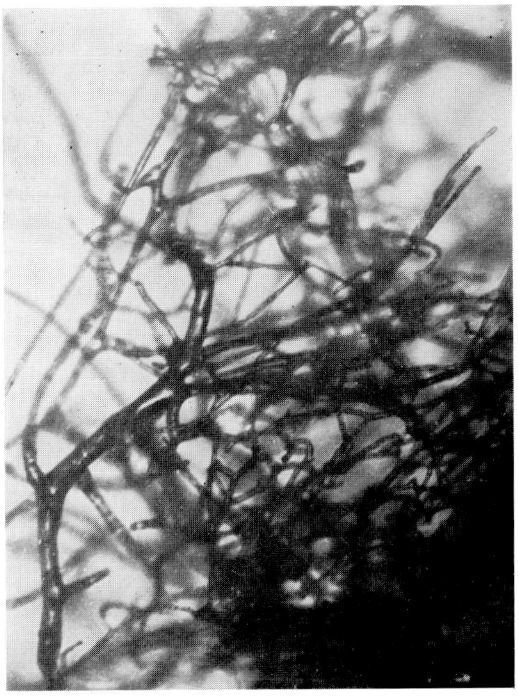

Fig. 134 Capillary nets of the bronchial vascular system (resin cast).

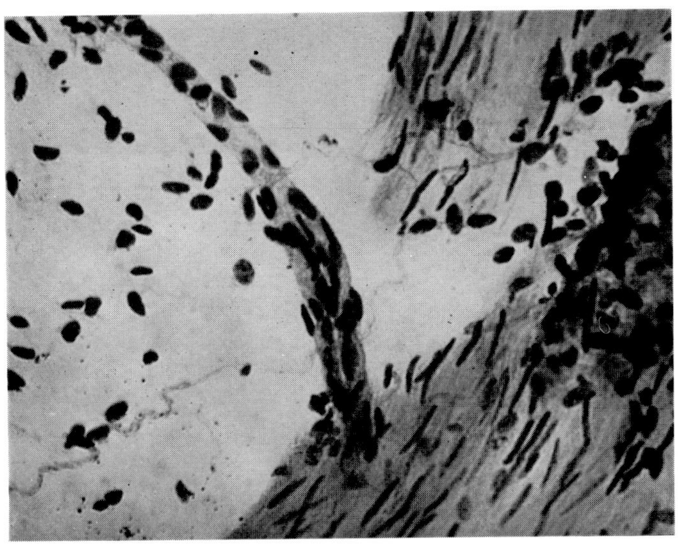

Fig. 135 Capillary of the bronchial vascular system (Bielschowsky's method modified by SUZUKI).

relation with the bronchial artery are taken into consideration, it is possible to distinguish between bronchial and pulmonary veins.

III. RELATIONSHIP BETWEEN PULMONARY AND BRONCHIAL VASCULAR SYSTEMS

The elucidation of the relationship between the pulmonary and the systemic circulations is significant, both for anatomical studies and for the clarification of various problems, *e.g.*, surgical collapse therapy, chemotherapy, pathology of emphysema, bronchiectasis, hematogenous metastases of intrapulmonary or extrapulmonary primary malignant tumors, etc. Studies of physiology and pathophysiology of the pulmonary circulation also depend on this relationship.

A. In Normal Lung

As to the interrelation of the pulmonary and bronchial vascular systems, studies carried out by OMOCHI (1937), MILLER (1947), VERLOOP (1948), LIEBOW, HALES and LINDSKOG (1949), NAGAISHI and M.

YAMASHITA (1950–1957), HAYEK (1953), AOKI (1954), NAKAMURA, TAKIZAWA and KATORI (1955, 1957) and others have opened questions involving a diversity of opinion.

The authors, Nagaishi and M. Yamashita, studied this problem in detail, using human lung (normal lung, accidental death), freshly resected specimens, or lungs of dogs.

The methods of study used by the authors were as follows:

1) The irrigation of saline solution containing dyes into the bronchial artery.

2) Investigation of resin castings prepared by insufflating three colored acrylic resins via the pulmonary artery, pulmonary vein and the bronchial artery.

3) Histological investigations on sections prepared by injecting gelatin solution containing dyes of different colors into these blood vessels.

4) Investigation of sections, of 5–10 mm thickness, made from specimens, cleared with oliganum oil.

Three dimensional and microscopic observations were made on resin castings.

The following is the result of studies carried out by the present authors (NAGAISHI and M. YAMASHITA).

These studies were first carried out by the above authors in 1950–1957, and were later elaborated by U. TAKAHASHI (1959), and by H. YAMAMOTO and M. ITO (1970) of the authors' group.

The capillary networks of the intrapulmonary bronchial artery origin are connected to the alveolar capillary networks of pulmonary artery origin by a few capillary rami communicates; but most of the capillary networks of the intrapulmonary bronchial artery form anastomoses, and then are connected to the pulmonary vein, in the so-called postcapillary region, via the intrapulmonary bronchial veins.

Such findings as the capillary networks of the intrapulmonary bronchial artery and those of the pulmonary artery being one above the other, or having a direct and close anastomoses between them, have not been observed in the normal lung.

Central to the terminal bronchioles, the capillaries of the bronchial artery also form anastomoses with the pulmonary vein via the intrapulmonary bronchial vein. However, in this region, infrequently direct arterio-arterial shunts are observed between the branches of the bronchial and pulmonary arteries. In addition to these anastomoses many vasa vasorum of bronchial artery origin are observed on the wall of the pulmonary artery.

In the region between the pulmonary artery branch and the bronchial artery branch, where arterio-arterial shunts exist, HAYEK (1940) observed a specific structure which is called "Sperrarterien", on the vascular wall of the region corresponding to the former.

"Sperrarterien" indicate that arteries whose longitudinal muscular layers are seen between the intima, and the annular muscular layer of the tunica media of the arterial wall; and by the remarkable development of the longitudinal muscular layer sometimes the vascular lumen is said to be narrowed or sometimes closed.

"Sperrarterien" are said to be observed in other organs of the body such as the liver, thyroid gland, suprarenal body, testicles, etc., but existence of this on the bronchial artery branch was reported for the first time by KULL (1925) and FEYRTER (1927).

Of the arterio-arterial shunts between the pulmonary artery branch and the intrapulmonary bronchial artery branch, HAYEK (1940) and MIZUGUCHI (1952) said that the "Sperrarterien" were observed in the region corresponding to the former, whereas KULL (1915), FEYRTER (1927), WATZKA (1936), MERKEL (1940), VERLOOP (1948), LAPP (1951), MEESEN (1951) and T. NAKAMURA, et al. (1955–1958) said that it was observed in the region corresponding to the latter.

Especially T. NAKAMURA, TAKIZAWA and KATORI (1958) made a detailed description of the "Sperrarterien" in their book "Studies on the Bronchial Vascular System".

According to them, the external diameter of the "Bronchiale Sperrarterien" is about 100 μ and the branch of the pulmonary artery which joins it is not a muscular artery but is an elastic type artery. They also observed the "Sperrarterien" not only on small bronchi with internal diameters of less than 1.2–1.3 mm, which still have cartilages, but on some parts of the mediastinal pleura. The "Sperrarterien" are said to have been observed in the human lung but not in the lung of dog.

The book by T. NAKAMURA, et al. describes the bronchial vascular system morphologically and physiologically; this book is a fine one in making their relationship clear.

In 1950–1957 the present authors histologically did not prove the existence of "Sperrarterien"; since then U. TAKAHASHI (1959) of the author's group, confirmed, although infrequently, its existence in human lung. However, the physiological and pathological significance of the "Sperrarterien" remains still in question.

LAPP (1951) was of the opinion that "Bronchiale Sperrarterien" had a physiological significance, but T. NAKAMURA, et al. (1955–1958) supposed that it did not, except in those case where a remarkable change in the pressure in either the pulmonary or the bronchial artery, occurs when the mixture of the blood stream of both arteries may be caused by the existence of the "Sperrarterien".

The present authors investigated not only the significance of "Sperrarterien" patho-physiologically on human adults, but considered that an investigation from the standpoint of the physiological regulation of the blood circulation in the fetus may be necessary. This is from the viewpoint that "Sperrarterien" belong in the same category with the Botallo's duct or ovoid fenestra. However, the authors at present hold no datum to support the above standpoint.

Toward a better understanding on these points, the authors' (M. YAMASHITA and NAGAISHI (1954)) studies will be described in the following as to the relationship between the pulmonary and bronchial vascular systems, after ligation of pulmonary blood vessels (using dogs and other experimental animals), and in the course of certain pulmonary diseases.

B. After Ligation of Pulmonary Blood Vessels

1. Ligation of Pulmonary Artery

Ligation of the pulmonary artery results in dilation of the bronchial artery.

When perfusion was made through a bronchial artery after the ligation of a pulmonary artery, most of the blood in the lobe was forced out. When Berlin blue was perfused through the bronchial artery after ligation of the pulmonary artery, a large amount of dye was found in the lung, as compared with controls. After ligation of a pulmonary artery, numerous bronchial arterial branches were observed to run toward the periphery from the hilum.

Enlargement and dilatation of the bronchial artery after ligation of the pulmonary artery correlated with time lapse, changes being greatest three months or more after the ligation.

Moreover, precapillary anastomoses were seen between the pulmonary and bronchial vascular systems in addition to the usual postcapillary anastomoses found in normal lungs.

These anastomoses between the pulmonary and bronchial arteries were mainly observed in the periphery of pulmonary lobes after ligation of a pulmonary artery. Similar findings have been reported by BLOOMER, HARRISON, LINDSKOG and LIEBOW (1949), by COCKETT and VASS (1951), and by ELLIS and GRINDLAY (1951). However, the authors hesitate to completely confirm the observation of Bloomer that if a shunt is formed by such anastomoses, dilation of the bronchial artery occurs, with the result that the vascular bed is enlarged, producing an increase in the volume of blood flow to the lung.

In any case, the ligation of the pulmonary artery produces enlargement and dilatation of the bronchial artery, resulting in the increase of precapillary anastomoses and the development of various abnormal flow routes.

2. Ligation of Pulmonary Vein

Total ligation of the pulmonary vein of one side usually results in death.

When the lives of experimental animals are prolonged for more than 3 months under this condition a proliferation and dilatation of intrapulmonary bronchial veins can be observed, evident shunts being formed between these and the pulmonary veins.

If the occlusion of the pulmonary vein continues, the blood flow from the pulmonary artery will take abnormal pathways, *e.g.* to the caval system.

3. Ligation of Bronchial Artery

If the bronchial artery is ligated, pathological changes occur in the lung; the degree of change depends on the region of vascular ligation.

For instance if a bronchial artery to a lower lobe is ligated immediately proximal to the lobar bronchus, no significant change is seen in the related lobe, but if all the bronchial arteries of the side are ligated, prominent changes are observed. In the former case, anastomoses of the bronchial artery with small branches distributing to the mediastinum or diaphragm and with branches of other bronchial arteries extending to other lobes may have prevented the changes.

These experimental results are similar to those of ELLIS, et al. (1951), in their studies on the upper lobe.

When ligations are performed on all bronchial arteries of one side, most animals will die of pneumonia within one week.

Surviving animals may exhibit ulceration, thrombosis, or submucous bleeding at the roots of lobar bronchi or of the main bronchus, on the side of the ligations.

These ulcers are found only in the bronchi of large diameter, *i.e.*, in the roots of the main stem or lobar bronchi. This phenomenon may be due to a scarcity of anastomoses in the central portion of the hilum, as contrasted with a richness of anastomosis in peripheral portions.

4. Ligation of Pulmonary and Bronchial Arteries

If ligations are made at the root of the lobar branches of the pulmonary artery, and also at that portion of the lobar branches of the bronchial artery immediately before it reaches the lobar bronchus, the blood flow of the pulmonary arteries will be blocked completely, making irrigation from the right ventricle impossible. However, if the irrigation is made from the root of the aorta the fluid flows into the lobes in which the pulmonary artery has been ligated. If the irrigation is continued, the blood in the lobe flows from the pulmonary vein.

Severe fibrous changes, bronchiectasis, and marked over-development of new blood vessels were observed in lobes of animals in which the above-mentioned procedures were tried, and in which survival occurred.

Fig. 136 shows the conditions of both arteries three months after ligation. It is quite interesting to see the extent of bronchiectasis.

Fig. 137 demonstrates roentogenographically the marked development of newly developed blood vessels.

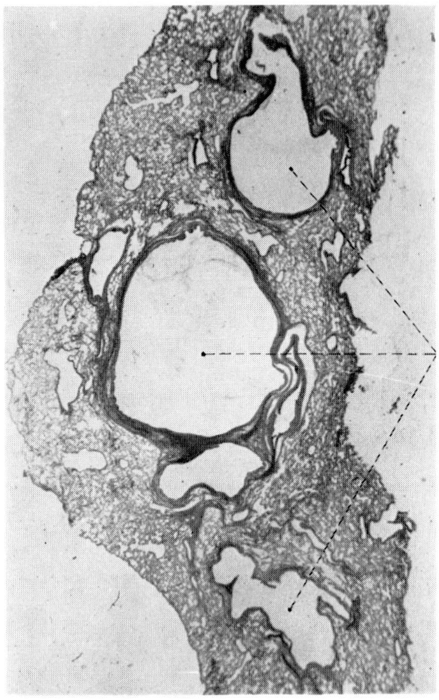

Fig. 136 Experimental bronchiectasis of the dog (three monthus after the ligation of both pulmonary artery and bronchial artery).

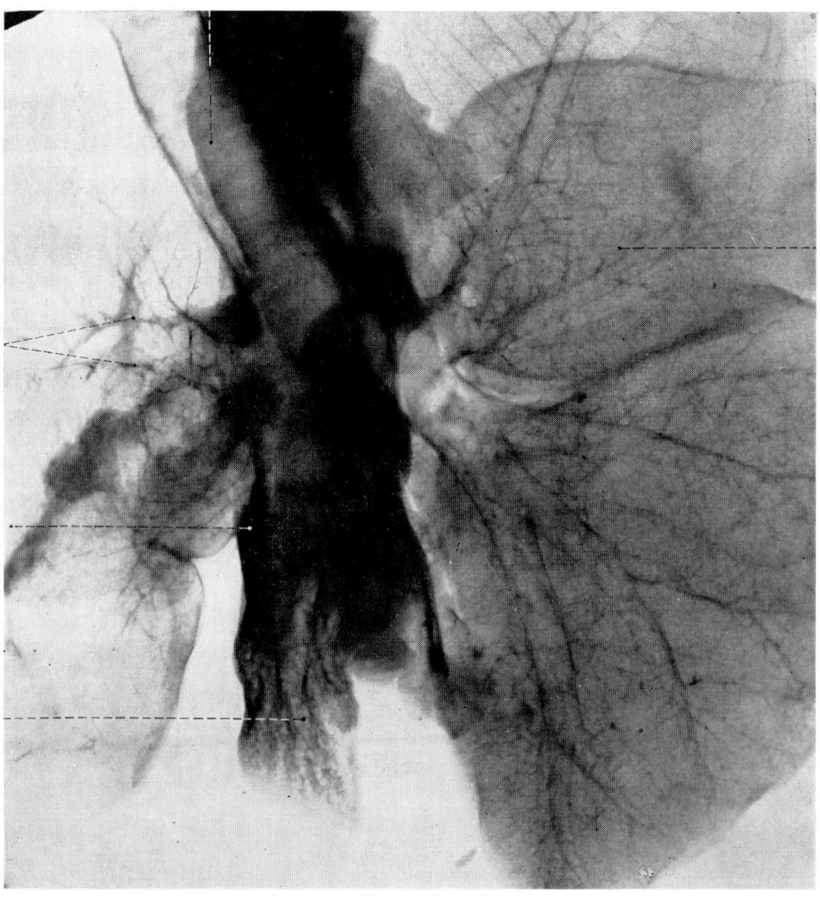

Fig. 137 Proliferated bronchial arteries in the experimental bronchiectasis (three months after the ligation of both right lower lobe artery and bronchial artery).

These new blood vessels develop from branches of small arteries to the diaphragm or mediastinum, and from bronchial arteries supplying other lobes. However, the lobes in which the pulmonary and bronchial arteries have been ligated become atelectatic and gas exchange is not performed.

C. Relationship between Pulmonary and Bronchial Vascular Systems in Certain Lung Diseases.

1. Pulmonary Tuberculosis

Pathological changes in the pulmonary artery and vein in the tuberculous lung have been studied at length, but studies on the bronchial artery and vein have been relatively few.

CALMETTE (1923) and LAUFMAN (1929) claimed that the aneurysmic changes seen in the tuberculous lung involved the bronchial artery. WRIGHT (1938) stated that the abundant supply of arterial blood through the bronchial artery promoted the hyperplasia of the collagenous fibers in the tuberculous lung.

Regarding the bronchial artery in the tuberculous lung, detailed studies have been carried out by WOOD and MILLER (1938), N. NAGASAWA, M. YAMASHITA and NAGAISHI, et al. (1950–1955), CUDKOWITZ (1951), AOKI (1954), MATSUO (1954) and T. NAKAMURA (1954). These studies noted proliferation of branches of the bronchial arteries in the region of tuberculous foci.

The relation between the pulmonary and the bronchial vascular systems in the tuberculous lung is somewhat different from that of the normal lung. In the tuberculous lung, depending on the nature of the focus in individual cases, the extent of bronchiectasis, emphysema, atelectasis, or pleural adhesion, the relation between the pulmonary and the bronchial vascular systems may present a diversity of aspects.

Predominant changes seen in and around the tuberculous foci include obstruction and new growth of blood vessels.

Obstruction is mainly found in the pulmonary vascular system of the region, new growth mainly involves the bronchial vascular system. Often obstructions of the blood vessels are caused by mechanisms such as diffuse infiltration in the adventitia, or by the perivasculitis accompanying caseous changes; these cause hypertrophy of the intima, producing vascular obstruction.

As indicated by BOYD (1950), these pathological changes are frequently observed in the pulmonary artery immediately before or adjacent to the tuberculous foci.

In the bronchial artery similar changes are seen in regions adjacent to caseous foci.

Development of obstruction in the pulmonary artery precedes new growth of the bronchial artery and vein in the tuberculous lung.

However, in the cases in which long-term chemotherapy has been carried out, the new growth of the blood vessels arising from the bronchial artery frequently extends into the infectious foci and these presumably participates in the absorption or excretion of the caseous substance, and also in the healing of the tuberculous foci.

Once obstruction occurs in the pulmonary artery, resulting in the transformation or disappearance of the alveolar capillary networks, a new growth of blood vessels derived from the bronchial artery arises in vessels corresponding to the former alveolar capillary networks; these join the pulmonary vein, by-passing the bronchial vein.

Figs. 138–140 demonstrate the appearance of fine blood vessels related to tuberculous foci. They show a complicated appearance, differing from the normal.

New growth of blood vessels (arising from the bronchial artery) is often observed in regions surrounding cavities.

Fig. 141 is a schema indicating the relationship of the pulmonary and the bronchial vascular systems to the tuberculous cavity and its surrounding regions, in cases in which no chemotherapeutic agent was used.

Unlike new growth of the bronchial artery in the cavity wall there is little new growth of it in the capsulated caseous foci.

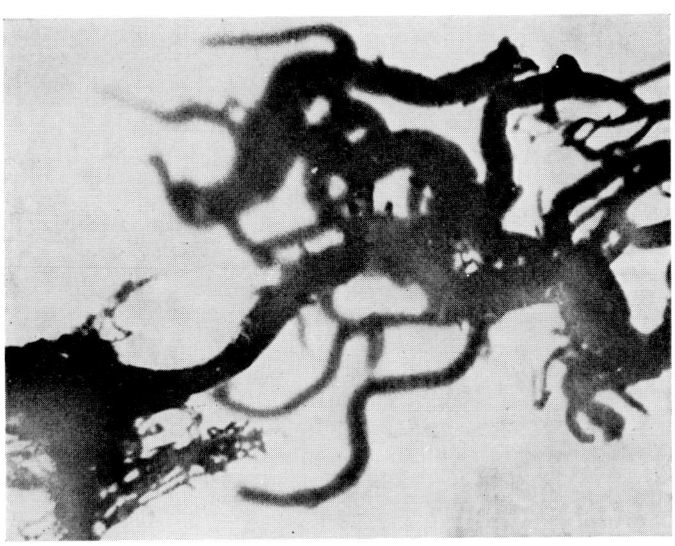

Fig. 138 Proliferated vessels in the neighborhood of the tuberculosis focus (resin cast).

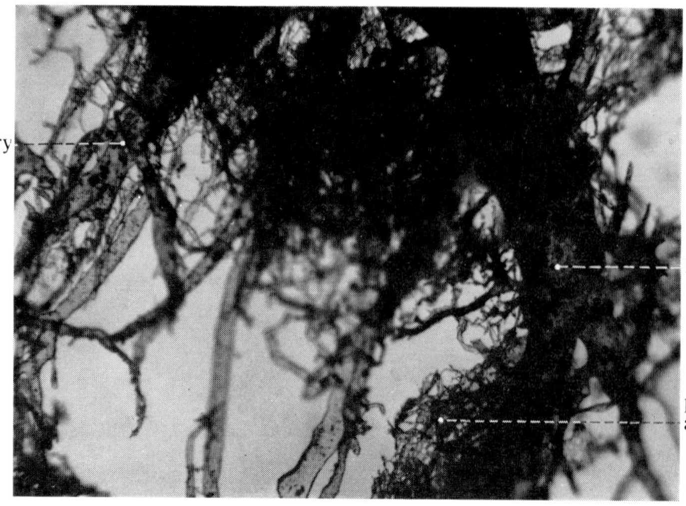

Fig. 139 Proliferated capillaries of the bronchial artery (resin cast).

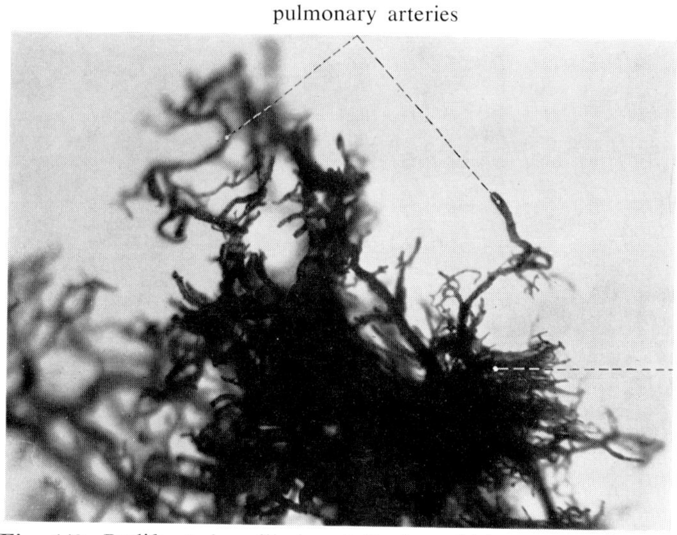

Fig. 140 Proliferated capillaries of the bronchial artery (resin cast).

New growth of the bronchial artery is observed predominantly in the regions surrounding encapsulated foci. In particular, when long-term chemotherapy was performed (using principally INH, and its derivatives), newly grown vessels frequently intruded into the caseous foci, or into the wall of cavity thereof.

2. Bronchiectasis

Regarding the relationship between the pulmonary vascular system and the bronchial vascular system in normal lung and in bronchiectasis, investigations were made in detail, by Liebow, et al. (1949) and by Cockett, et al. (1951).

A marked proliferation of the bronchial vessels was observed in the case of bronchiectasis, in which the bronchial artery bends and winds, is dilated and hypertrophied.

The newly developed vessels, arising from branches of the bronchial artery, anastomose with the pulmonary vascular system via precapillary, capillary or postcapillary networks.

3. Pulmonary Emphysema

In emphysema, generally, the caliber of the alveolar capillary networks is smaller. Frequently the normal structure of the capillary networks has disappeared and somewhat enlarged branches of bronchial vessels are observed to occupy those areas.

The newly developed blood vessels stemming from the bronchial artery form prominent anastomoses with the pulmonary artery in the region of the precapillary networks.

If a chronic inflammation is seen in the emphysematous lung, not only is the respiratory area diminished, but the capillary networks of the pulmonary vascular system disappear, and are replaced by the blood vessels of the bronchial vascular system, resulting in a functionally unfavorable condition.

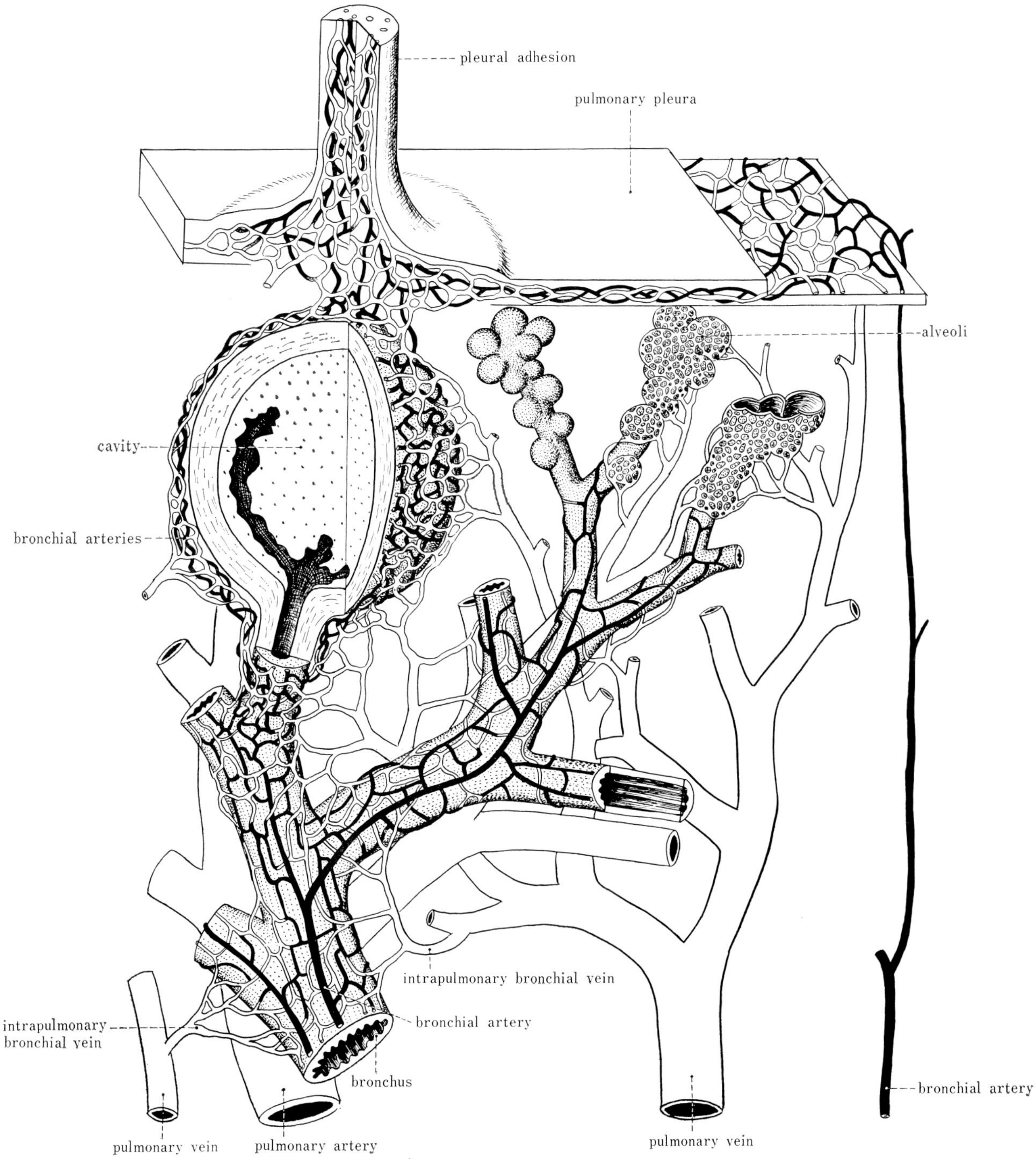

Fig. 141 Relationship between pulmonary and bronchial vascular systems in the surrounding part of tuberculous cavity.

4. Pulmonary Atelectatasis

The following is the result of an investigation by the authors (1952) (using resin castings) on the relationship between the pulmonary and the bronchial vascular systems in atelectatic areas after pneumothorax.

In the atelectatic area, the pulmonary arteries and veins are gathered together in the shape of a closed umbrella, with arrangement in layers, in parallel with the main axis of each lobe.

The pulmonary vessels are greatly diminished in caliber, and in those portions where complete atelectasis has existed for a long time the alveolar capillary networks are found to disappear. Meanwhile, as stated by Aoki (1949), an evident proliferation of branches of the bronchial artery is observed.

These newly grown blood vessels stemming from the bronchial artery, together with the branches of small mediastinal arteries in sisterly relationship with the bronchial artery proceed into the lung from the hilum, bending, winding and forming rich anastomoses with the pulmonary system.

So it is that in abnormal conditions, as a rule, stenosis of the blood vessels of the pulmonary vascular system is generally related to a proliferation and dilatation of vessels of the bronchial vascular system.

Chapter III. Lymphatic System

The lymphatic system of the lung is, in principle, the same as that of other organs. However, since the lung is an organ which is prone to be affected by external factors, hence its lymphatic system is possibly more significant as a part of the defense mechanisms of the organism.

It is a well known fact that the lymphatic system is closely involved in the genesis and development of pulmonary tuberculosis, and in the metastasis of lung cancer.

The character of the lymphatic system is complicated by the fact that although it participates in the defense mechanism of the organism, it also takes part in the development of disease process.

This is a most important point to bear in mind in making observations on the dynamic nature of the pulmonary lymphatic system.

In elucidating the structure of the pulmonary lymphatic system from a physiological point of view, its character as a dynamic reation system must be the starting point.

In this connection, the authors (NAGAISHI and OKADA, 1952–1969) carried out morphologic and functional studies on the pulmonary lymphatic system. However, for present purposes, descriptions were mainly concentrated on the anatomical and histological relationships within the system.

In our previously published book on the lung, the lymphatic system was described in two parts: the lymph vascular system, and the lymphoid tissues located in the region of the lymph vessels. The authors intend also to describe the extravascular fluid pathway system of KIHARA, "Das extravasculäre Saftbahnensystem", in the following.

In a broad sense, the lymphatic system is a part of the circulatory system and, particularly in relation to the lungs or pleura, is also involved in the manifestations of pulmonary anthracosis, and in absorption of various substances through the bronchial wall or the parietal pleura.

It is also useful to understand the relationship between circulating body fluids and the lymphoid tissues.

I. ABSORPTION FROM RESPIRATORY SYSTEM

As is well known, the lung is an organ whose functions include removal of oxygen from the air inhaled into the respiratory system, and release of carbon dioxide from the blood into alveolar space.

In short, the lung is an organ which regulates external respiration, participating in gas exchange. It also participates in the absorption of fluid and solid particles entering the respiratory system.

This absorptive capacity is an important pulmonary function which cannot be overlooked as, for example, in the resolution of pulmonary edema or in bacterial infections.

Substances entering the respiratory system, depending on their nature and on particular circumstances, will be absorbed into the capillaries through the alveolar wall, or absorbed into the lymph vessels from the epithelial spaces of the respiratory system.

The latter route belongs to HIHARA's "the extravascular fluid pathway system".

A. Brief History

An absorbing function for normal lung was mentioned by BERNARD, et al. as early as 1857.

In the latter half of the nineteenth century, it was proved that blood corpuscles or charcoal powders entering the respiratory system were carried into the lung tissues and hilar lymph nodes (KNAUFF, 1867; NOTHNAGEL, 1877; RUPPER, 1878; and ARNOLD, 1888).

Later, studies on the route of absorption of these substances were pursued in animal experiments.

For instance, charcoal powder (SOYKA, 1878; LUBENEAU, 1907; TOMITA, 1918), silica powder (v. INS, 1878; CHARLETON, 1924; GROSS, 1927), or blood corpuscles (PERL and LIPMAN, 1870; SOMMERBRODT, 1872; FLEINER, 1888), were studied after inhalation. These substances were absorbed lymphatogenously and reached the hilar lymph nodes. The routes of absorption are gradually being clarified.

The time required for these substances to appear in the blood stream or hilar lymph nodes was also studied by the above researchers. Further, the time required for these substances to disappear completely from the respiratory system was studied by YOSHIDA (1926).

Many researchers were also studying the varieties of substances which could be absorbed from the respiratory system, such as: absorption of water (Colin, 1873; Peiper, 1884), low molecular weight compounds (Sehrwald, 1886 Laqueur, et al., 1919, 1921), dyes (Heubner, 1920; Hirakawa, 1925), various proteins (Besredka, 1920; Suzuki, 1922; Jones, 1924; Fox, 1936; Drinker, et al., 1937), and bacteria (Sewell, 1918; Hirakawa, 1925; Umeda, 1929; Schultz, et al., 1938).

Although there were differences in quantity or velocity of absorption according to the size of the particles, all of the above-mentioned substances were definitely shown to be absorbed through the respiratory system.

Moreover, it became evident that there were two routes of absorption, the one into blood capillaries through the alveolar wall, the other proceeding lymphatogenously via the epithelium of the tracheobronchial wall. Determinations of route of absorption depended, among other factors, on the size of particles (Umeda, 1929; Drinker, et al., 1941).

Nishikawa (1940, 1941) examined histologically the route of movement of inhaled charcoal powder from the tracheobronchial wall to the lymph vessels, his studies revealed that absorption of the charcoal powder occurred at certain specific points.

Later, T. Kihara (1956) showed this route to be a part of the extravascular fluid pathway system of the lung.

Coworkers of Drinker (1945, 1947) and of Courtice (1946) made quantitative measurements of pulmonary lymph flow. Their methods involved obtaining lymph directly from the right lymphatic trunk and determining the absorbing ability of the lung quantitatively by measuring the increase or decrease in volume, or by change in composition. The validity of the method stemmed from the observation that in the dog lung most lymph drains into the right lymphatic trunk.

However, these methods involved technical difficulties in the procedure of obtaining lymph samples.

Sagawa, T. Yokoyama, and Iwata (1955), of the author's group, devised a new procedure for this purpose. In this method, each of the veins connecting with the right venous angle are ligated, and a small vinyl tube is inserted into the isolated sac-like segment of the vein formed as a result of the ligation; the lymph is thus obtained indirectly from the right lymphatic trunk.

This method is especially convenient because it does not require thoracotomy, and is especially useful in the experimental study of mechanisms of the pulmonary edema formation.

Furthermore, other methods were also developed to follow the absorption of insufflated radioisotope labeled substances (Qualls, et al., 1953), and for determination of lymphatogenous absorption or for application of radioactive colloidal substances in the radiotherapy of lung cancer (Taplin, et al., 1951; Bahn, et al., 1953; Bryant, et al., 1953; Berg, et al., 1953; Meneely, 1953).

Similar studies were made by Sagawa and Okada (1957) of the author's group; they applied several of these methods.

B. Substances Absorbed

1. Water and Crystalloids

Experiments performed by Colin (1873) in the horse and, by Peiper (1884) in the dog and rabbit, proved that water was easily absorbed into the normal lung.

In particular, Colin carried out an experiment in which 21 liters of water were insufflated slowly into the trachea of a horse in three and half hours time, and without noticeable bad effect.

Rapid absorption of solutions of inorganic salts, such as sodium chloride or iodide, or potassium ferrocyanide was also demonstrated by Sehrwald (1886), Winternitz, et al. (1920), and Umeda (1929).

2. Dyes

Slavjansky (1869), Küttner (1875), Hirakawa (1925), and Umeda (1929) carried out investigations on the absorption of various dyes, and showed that phenolphthalein, gentian violet, methylene blue, trypan blue, or orange G were absorbed through the respiratory tract.

Hirakawa (1925) performed experiments with rabbits using various kinds of dyes to investigate the permeability of the wall of the respiratory system; he reported that basic dyes pass through the wall of the respiratory system easily, whereas acid dyes which were lipoid soluble were more freely diffusible.

Also found to influence the absorption of dyes were the quantity, concentration and degree of lipoid solubility; however, detailed investigation of these parameters has not yet been made. Hirakawa (1925) reported that the diffusibility of dyes did not differ in experiments in which alcohol was used in place of water as solvent.

3. Albumin

Besredka (1920) showed that horse serum and albumen were absorbed by the respiratory system, in experiments with guinea pig.

Levaditi (1922), D'Aunoy (1922), Jones (1924), and Suzuki (1932) also stated that albumin was absorbed through the respiratory tract, and that animals could be sensitized by insufflating antigen via the tracheobronchial route.

Jones showed that animals were sensitized by insufflating cattle serum or horse serum into the respiratory system, but since the repetition of insufflation of the antigen did not cause anaphylactic shock, and since the increase of antibodies in the blood was quite slow, it was apparent that these antigens were absorbed slowly and in quite small quantities.

Drinker, et al. (1937) noted that horse serum, hemoglobin or albumin insufflated into the respiratory system appeared first in serum and then in lymph, and that the absorbed quantities were quite small, in accord with the observations of Jones.

4. Solid Particles

Absorption of charcoal powder or dust into the human lung was verified in a number of animal experiments. In addition to charcoal powder, silica powder, blood corpuscles, and carmine (UMEDA, 1929), calcium carbonate (FUJIMOTO, 1925; UMEDA, 1929), nickel silicate (DRINKER, et al., 1947); cinnabar (SCHOTTELIUS, 1878; SHESTOPAL, 1879; KAWAHARA, 1924), and radioactive colloidal gold (BRYANT, et al., 1953), were found to be absorbed through the respiratory system. These observations were repeatedly confirmed in animal experiments.

These solid corpuscles were shown to be absorbed lymphatogenously, and are thus favored in experiments to detect routes of absorption, and especially to determine routes to regional lymph nodes.

However, in the absorption of corpuscles by the respiratory system, there are certain limits to the size of particles. Thus, GILLIAN, et al. (1938) stated that the maximum size of corpuscles was 2 μ in an experiment in the snake, and DRINKER, et al. (1947) stated that particles of pyrex glass of 4 μ dia. were not absorbed in the dog lung.

5. Bacteria

As to bacteria, staphylococcus (SEWELL, 1918), tubercle bacillus (SAKAMOTO, 1916; UMEDA, 1929), hay bacillus, bacillus pyocyaneus and chromobacterium prodigiosum (UMEDA, 1929), pneumococcus (SCHULZ, et al., 1938), and whooping cough bacillus (OTANI, et al., 1943) were shown to be absorbed by the respiratory system, based on documented experimental findings.

Thus, UMEDA (1929) reported that he could prove that the tubercle bacilli (and other bacteria) which he had insufflated into the respiratory system of the rabbit or dog were found in the hilar lymph nodes or in the pleural cavity, depending on the case; however, no detailed description was available as to the route to the latter.

The sizes of the bacteria absorbed from the respiratory system were generally in the range of about 0.5 μ–3 μ. Although the nature of the bacteria differed, they were absorbed evenly from the respiratory system in the normal lung.

6. Oily Substances

Absorption of oily substances was investigated in detail using radiopaque contrast media.

SICARD, et al. (1922) stated that lipiodol insufflated into the respiratory system could be rapidly absorbed; however, according to ARCHIBALD, et al. (1927), and UMEDA (1929), absorption was quite slow, and the disappearance of lipiodol from some radiograms was mostly due to expectoration from the respiratory tract.

UMEDA verified histologically the process whereby lipiodol broke into droplets and was absorbed by the phagocytes, but the quantity involved was said to be very small.

In contrast to lipiodol, dionosil (X-ray contrast medium) disappears from the respiratory system in a short time. This is presumed due to the rapidity of absorption as well as to expectoration; variation in the rate of absorption of these substances may be due to physico-chemical differences.

C. Mechanism of Absorption

1. Route

The route of absorption by the respiratory tract differs according to the nature of the substances involved and particularly according to the size and physical state of the particles.

Those of small molecular size will be absorbed into the capillaries (as well as into the lymph vessels) through the alveolar wall.

Those of larger particulate size will not be absorbed directly into the blood vessels, but will enter lymph vessels.

According to UMEDA (1929), insufflation of sodium iodide solution into the respiratory system will yield iodide in the blood within one minute.

Therefore, it is evident that ionic substances (such as I^- and Na^+), will be rapidly absorbed into the blood, penetrating the alveolar wall almost instantly, in a manner similar to the diffusion of gas molecules.

These findings were confirmed by QUALLS, et al. (1953), and by IWASE, N. NAGASAWA, M. YAMASHITA and NAGAISHI (1959), as shown in Fig. 142.

As described by the above investigators, when the size of the particle is extremely small it will be absorbed into lymph vessels, but absorption into blood vessels will be faster than into the lymph vessels, and the quantity absorbed into the blood vessels will be far larger.

Thus, according to HAGIHARA (1951), the particles of the pigment insufflated into the respiratory system of the resected toad lung were found first in the blood vessel, 30 minutes later, and then in the lymph vessels.

Albumin is also absorbed into blood and lymph vessels, and appears in the blood in a short time (DRINKER, et al., 1937). The route of absorption is considered to be similar to that of the other above-mentioned substances.

On the other hand, particles of about the same size as charcoal powder will not be absorbed directly into the blood, but are absorbed lymphatogenously. BORCHARDT(1929) proved this by animal experiment.

It is also evident from the results of autopsies performed by BEITZKE (1925) that absorbed charcoal powder or dust will not move into the blood vessels.

NISHIKAWA (1941) stated that the route of lymphatogenous absorption of charcoal powder to be as follows: 1) In the passages lined by ciliated epithelium, particularly as shown in Fig. 143, charcoal powder penetrates freely and moves into the lymph tissues; 2) in the passages lined by cuboidal or squamous epithelium the powder penetrates the tissue of the wall of the respiratory system either freely or in the phagocytosed condition. Most of the particles move into the lymph capillaries, and adhere to the lymph tissues, or will be carried into regional lymph nodes. Absorption will be faster for smaller sized charcoal powders.

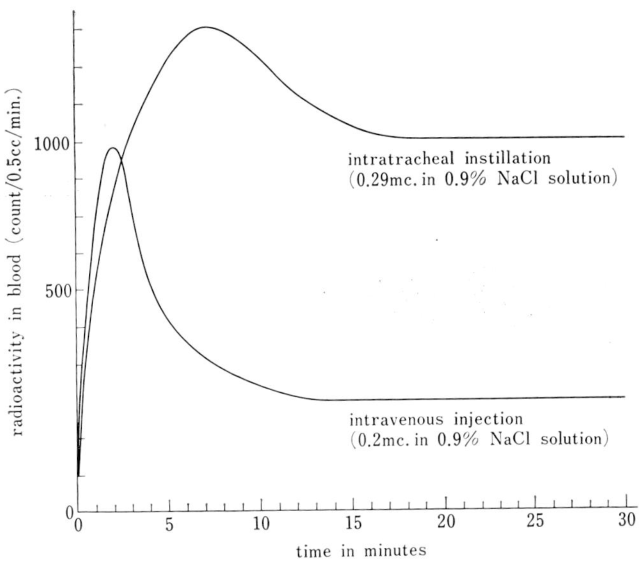

Fig. 142 Concentration of radioactive substance in the blood after intrabronchial instillation.

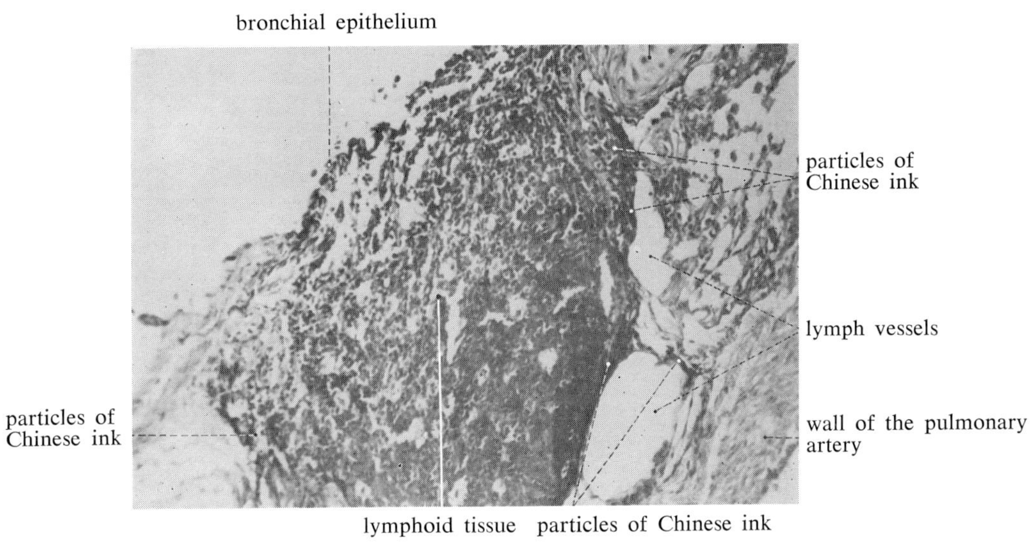

Fig. 143 Absorption of Chinese ink through the bronchial lymphoid tissue.

As to bacteria NISHIKAWA's report is the most detailed. However, according to studies by OTANI and TAKAWA (1943), the route of absorption is considered to be similar to that for charcoal powder.

In summary, the route of absorption of substances from the respiratory system differs depending on the size of the particles. Fig. 144 is a schema showing three routes of absorption, *i.e.*, hematogenous, lymphatogenous, and by phagocytosis.

2. Velocity and Rate

The gas exchange in the alveole is a result of diffusion, a physical phenomenon. Since Na^+, I^-, and PO_4^{---}, etc. are quite rapidly absorbed into the blood, diffusion is also thought to play the principal role in these cases.

The blood capillary pressure in the human lung is said to be within the range of 8–10 mm Hg (SASAMOTO, 1952; TASAKA, 1953; SAGAWA, et al., 1955); osmotic pressure of the blood is said to be in the range of 32–38 cm H_2O (ITO, et al., 1929; KYLIN, 1931).

Various solutions insufflated into the respiratory system are considered to be absorbed immediately into blood vessels.

This is also evident from the results of experiments by QUALLS, et al. (1953), who stated that when I^{131} or Na^{24} were insufflated into the respiratory system (in the form of NaI or NaCl), radioactivity was instantly detected in the blood. They also stated that the distilled water was more easily absorbed than was physiological saline solution.

As to the velocity of the absorption into lymph vessels, NOTHNAGEL (1877) stated that erythrocytes in the respiratory passages moved into the lung tissue after 3–5 minutes; and UMEDA (1929) said that Orange G instilled into the respiratory system was found in bronchial lymph nodes within 15 minutes.

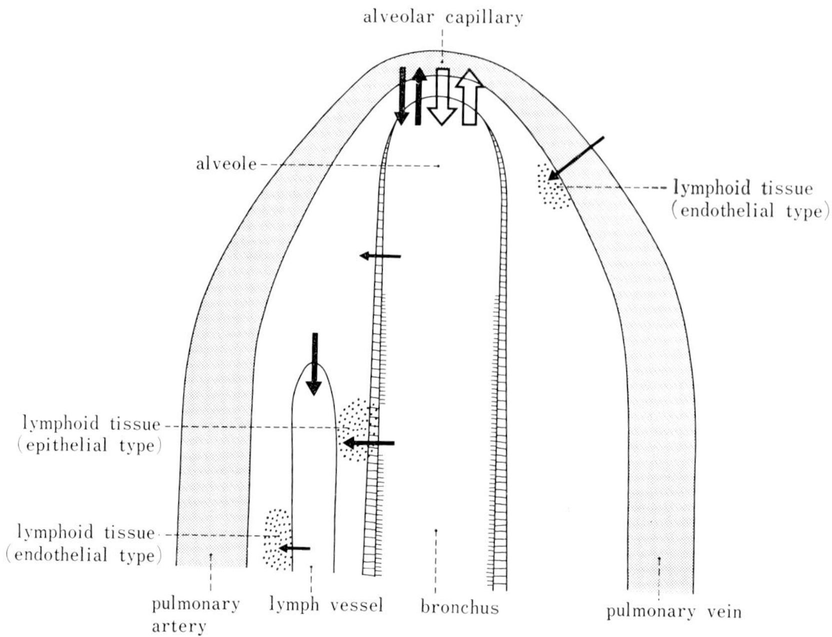

Fig. 144 Absorption of various substances in the bronchoalveolar system.

DRINKER (1945) showed that EVANS blue dye (T-1824) instilled into the respiratory system appeared in the right lymphatic trunk in 20–30 minutes.

Y. SENDA (1958), of the author's group, proved that particles of India ink instilled into the respiratory system appeared in hilar lymph nodes within 15 minutes.

IWASE (1959), of the author's group, used P^{32} as a tracer, and examined the velocity of absorption of various kind of solutions or antibiotics from the respiratory system, obtaining the following results:

1) The absorption of a solution will start immediately after insufflation;

2) The rate of absorption of a solution will vary depending on its concentration. As shown in Fig. 145, a solution of high concentration is slower in absorption;

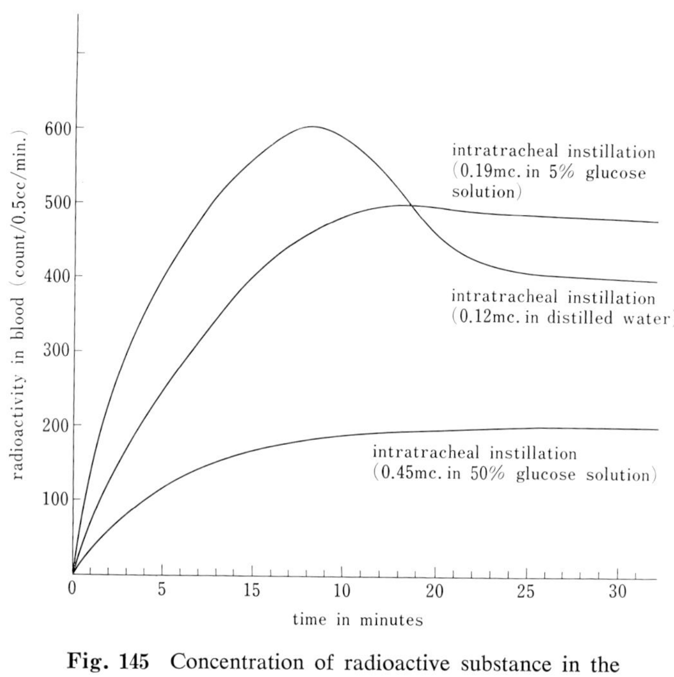

Fig. 145 Concentration of radioactive substance in the blood after intratracheal instillation.

3) The rate of absorption of the solution will also fluctuate according to the solute. In general, the absorption of larger particles will be slower. Changes in pH will have some influence, but excepting instances of actual damage to tissues, the influence is relatively small;

4) The absorption of solutions occurs predominantly in the alveolar region;
5) Addition of certain agents, such as pilocarpine or adrenalin, will somewhat delay the absorption;
6) Interruption of the vagus nerves will not affect the absorption of solutions in most instances;
7) For antituberculous agents, such as streptomycin and PAS or INH, absorption is in inverse proportion to the molecular weight;
8) Insufflation of antituberculous agents into the respiratory system yields high concentrations in the blood. By this method enhanced local effects can also be expected.

As mentioned, absorption from the respiratory system into lymph vessels or blood vessels is generally rapid. Whether the fluctuation in the velocity of the absorption varies by kinds of substances is as yet unknown, but many researchers have verified that the rate of absorption is decreased in inverse proportion to the size of particle.

Iwase (1959), of the author's group, made observations on the microautoradiograms of sections of the resected lung of rabbit which had been insufflated intrabronchially with IHMS (isonicotinyl hydrazide methanesulfonate (Na-salt) labeled with isotope C^{14}.

IHMS labeled with C^{14} was found to localize in large quantities in the regions of caseous tuberculous foci.

Following the example of Iwase (1959), N. Nagasawa, M. Yamashita, Iwase and Nagaishi (1960) using the Métras' catheter performed intracavitary insufflation of chemotherapeutic agents in patients with pulmonary tuberculosis or lung abscess, obtaining useful results.

II. PULMONARY LYMPH VESSELS

The lymph vessels form a closed circulatory system lined continuously by endothelium.

According to size, they are called lymph capillaries, lymph vessels (in narrow sense), and collecting lymph vessels.

The lymph passes through the endothelium of the lymph capillaries, but the capillaries do not communicate directly with the connective tissue spaces, nor do they have direct communication with the pleural cavity, through stomata.

The lymph capillaries consist of single layers of endothelium; the small lymph vessels consist of single layers of endothelium and thin fibro-elastic tissues.

Collecting lymph vessels have smooth muscles in the wall, the fibers of which run longitudinally or obliquely.

The lymph is carried from the capillaries of the most peripheral regions to the collecting lymph vessels by the lymph vessels (in the narrow sense).

As described earlier, body fluids are absorbed into the lymph vessels of the periphery, but some of the lymph is released into surrounding tissues on the way to central regions. This is a distinguishing trait of the lymphatic system. Therefore, the caliber of central lymph vessels is not always large; in some regions the caliber of the vessels in peripheral regions is found to be larger.

Fig. 146 shows a schema of the lymph vessels of the lung of the cow.

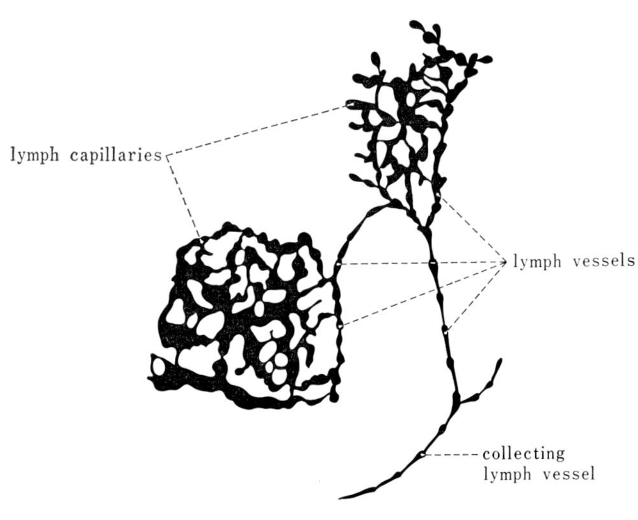

Fig. 146 Schema of the lymph vessel.

The lymph capillaries form complicated networks, showing both sac-like expanded portions and extremely small portions.

The diameter of the vessel varies according to the region. At quite short intervals it suddenly becomes narrow or expands.

The lymph originating in the lymph capillary networks is carried into small vessels of a rosary-like appearance. Valves are observed in these rosary-like vessels. In more central regions the valves in collecting lymph vessels are less frequent.

The pulmonary lymph vessels are considered to be significant from the clinical standpoint, since they participate in the development of tumor, inflammation, and fluid derangements.

In the instance of pulmonary edema, the fluid that leaked into the lung tissues or into the alveolar spaces will be absorbed by the alveolar capillary net or lymph capillary when the edema vanishes; some researchers such as WATANABE (1955), on the contrary, say that the congestion of the fluid inside lymph vessels may actually promote the development of pulmonary edema.

As is well known, when the primary infection of pulmonary tuberculosis takes place, changes arising in the intrapulmonary primary focus extend lymphatogenously to the hilar lymph node.

RICH (1951) stated that in the tuberculous lung small foci are found along the lymph route between the intrapulmonary foci and regional hilar lymph nodes; and AMANO (1947) reported that one manifestation of late dissemination of pulmonary tuberculosis was a lymphangitis.

All through the various stages of pulmonary tuberculosis there are possibilities of lymphatogenous extension of the disease process.

AMANO (1947) further stated that allergic reactions will cause obstructive or thrombotic lymphangitis which will alter the development of inflammation. However, this is mainly the case in individuals who are already sensitized.

In cases of malignant tumor, lymph vessels are not able to prevent the development of tumor; rather they appear to serve as routes for spread, or for metastasis.

The pulmonary lymph vessels have an important role in the development of various chest diseases. On the other hand, they serve also to mediate the healing process as seen, for example, in the recovery stages of pneumonia or pulmonary edema.

In order to have a thorough understanding of the origin and development of lung diseases, the data obtained from studies of lymph vessels of the lung are indispensable.

A. Outline of Structure

The lymph vessels of the lung, as well as those of other organs, originate in capillary networks, which consist of a single layer of endothelium.

The subpleural lymph vessels are called "superficial lymph vessels" and others are called "deep lymph vessels".

Those related to subpleural, interlobular and pulmonary veins are considered to belong to the same system. NAGAISHI and OKADA (1958) refer to these collectively as "interstitial-venous" or "interstitial lymph vessels".

The lymph vessels surrounding parts of the bronchi and the pulmonary artery are considered to belong to a system other than that designated "interstitial"; NAGAISHI and OKADA refer to these as "broncho-arterial lymph vessels" or, in short, as "parenchymal lymph vessels".

The subpleural lymph vessels are observed in the deepest layer of the subpleural connective tissue. The lung is literally surrounded by these dense lymph vessel networks.

The interlobular lymph vessels are located near the central regions of the interlobular connective tissue; here they form fine networks, as do the subpleural vessels.

Lymph vessels occurring in the adventitia of the pulmonary vein also form fine networks, surrounding continuously the circumference of relatively large branches of the pulmonary vein.

The lymph vessels related to the larger cartilaginous bronchi are distributed in the submucosa and adventitia; however, in the small non-cartilaginous bronchi lymph vessels are supplied only in the submucous layer. Thus the large bronchi are surrounded by two layers of networks and the smaller ones by a single layer or network.

The lymph vessels of the submucosa and the adventitia anastomose through lymph vessels running in spaces in the cartilages; hence, the lymph of the submucosa moves into the vessels of the adventitia.

The lymph vessels related to the pulmonary artery form fine networks in the adventitia. In many instances these lymph vessels are far larger than those of other intrapulmonary regions; in some cases it looks as if the pulmonary artery appears as if floating in a lymph space. HAYEK (1960) termed this the "periarterielle Lymphräume" (periarterial lymph space), and stated that it played the role of a buffer zone to protect the pulmonary artery from the influence of respiratory movements.

The interstitial lymph vessels are located along the pulmonary veins, but their distribution is limited to the area surrounding relatively large branches of the pulmonary vein.

The parenchymal lymph vessels related to the pulmonary artery distribute more in peripheral portions than those related to the bronchus. But even the former does not distribute more in peripheral portion where the terminal bronchiole change to the respiratory bronchiole; lymph vessels are not observed in regions further peripheral. In other words, the alveolar wall is devoid of the lymph vessels. Interchange of the body fluid in regions peripheral to the respiratory bronchiole are considered to be made through the clefts in the tissues.

Lymph from the lymph capillary networks of the outermost peripheral region moves into the lymph vessels proper and then flows further into the collecting lymph vessels of the central portion.

Observation of the pulmonary lymph vessels from the above viewpoint may be summarized in the following.

Most of the lymph originating in the subpleural lymph capillary networks is carried to the hilum by the subpleural collecting lymph vessels, some being carried by the collecting lymph vessels accompanying the pulmonary vein.

The lymph originating in the capillary networks of the pulmonary vein is carried by the collecting vessels accompanying the pulmonary vein, to the hilum.

The lymph originating in the capillary networks of the bronchi and the pulmonary artery is carried to the hilum by the collecting lymph vessels accompanying the pulmonary artery.

B. Brief History

RUDBECK (1653) first observed the lymph vessels of the lung. His observation was made on the pulmonary pleura of the dog.

And in the posthumus manuscript "Opera Omnia" of WILLIS (1673), a fine picture of the superficial lymph vessels of calf lung is shown.

About 100 years later, with the studies of MASCAGNI (1781) and CRUIKSHANK (1790), general knowledge of the morphology of the lymph vessels became somewhat more widespread. In particular, they mentioned that the superficial lymph and deep lymph vessels distribute in the lung, and those vessels intercommunicate.

More evident progress in the study of lymph vessels has occurred since the middle of the 19th century. WYWODZOFF (1866) reported on the lymph vessels of dog and horse; his report was one of the first to detail the anatomy of the lymphatic system of the lung.

According to WYWODZOFF, deep lymph vessels arise in the alveolar wall and distribute to the vascular or bronchial walls, communicating with each other; superficial lymph vessels, unlike the deep vessels, are devoid of valves and originate in the pleura, join the deep vessels, and run along the veins.

SIKORSKY (1970), and SAPPY, et al. (1874, 1888), also reported their studies.

SIKORSKY's statement that lymph capillaries originate in the alveolar wall or in relation to bronchial epithelium, and KLEIN's (1875), that the lymph vessels of the pulmonary pleura communicate with the pleural cavity through stomata, became the focus of dispute in later years.

From the end of the 19th century to the beginning of the 20th century, however, the greatest contribution to the study of the lymph vessels of the lung was made by MILLER.

In his paper published in 1896, MILLER divided the lymph vessels of the lung into four groups according to their distribution, *i.e.* subpleural, peribronchial, periarterial and perivenous. The subpleural lymph vessels were said to anastomose with other deep lymph vessels in the region of the hilum.

Later, in 1919, more detailed studies on the lymph vessels of the lung were reported by MILLER, a summary of which was reprinted in his monograph "The Lung" (1947).

MILLER's work on the structure of the lymph vessels of the lung must have been epoch-making in those years, although some of his findings did not escape criticism in later years.

His observations can be summarized as follows: In the normal lung, lymph flows toward the hilum in both superficial lymph vessels and deep lymph vessels.

Those vessels accompanying the bronchi form fine networks on the bronchial wall. The networks are two-layered in the case of the large bronchi (having cartilage in their walls); however, small bronchi (lacking cartilages) have only a single layer of vessels. Lymph capillaries were not observed in the regions peripheral to alveolar ducts.

The lymph vessels along the pulmonary artery also form networks; these anastomose in many places with vessels accompanying the bronchi, and are particularly frequent in the region of bifurcation of the bronchi.

The lymph vessels along the pulmonary veins arise from three regions, *i.e.* alveolar ducts, bronchial walls, and pulmonary pleura. They are observed to be most abundant about the interlobular veins and connective tissues.

The superficial lymph vessels, such as subpleural lymph vessels, form fine networks, bearing many valves. This contrasts with the paucity of valves in the interlobular lymph vessels. In regions close to the surface of the lung, the valves of the lymph vessels, connecting the subpleural and deep vessels, open toward the pleural side. In other words, the usual direction of lymph flow from the pulmonary pleura and the lung is toward the hilum.

MILLER's studies on the direction of lymph flow from the pulmonary pleura were cited by many researchers (JOSSIFOW, 1930; DRINKER and YOFFEY, 1941; GRAY, 1948; MAXIMOW and BLOOM, 1952), and for some time his summary was considered to be authoritative.

This is the history of the study of the lymph vessels of the pulmonary pleura and the lung. However, in later years, studies have continued on the drainage pathways of regional vessels.

For example, MOST (1908) injected dye solution subpleurally in 10 still-born infants and showed that lymph from the upper part of the lung runs to both right and left tracheobronchial lymph nodes, whereas that of the lower part of the lungs runs into lymph nodes of the bifurcation. Efferent lymph vessels stemming from the lymph nodes exhibited anastomoses between the right and left sides.

FRANKE (1912) also reported on subpleural injection of dye solutions in still-born infants. Part of the lymph of the lung was found to drain directly into lymph nodes behind the pancreas by way of lymph vessels in the pulmonary ligament, without passing to the hilum of the lung.

ROUVIÈRE (1938) elaborated on the description of the lymphatic regions of the lungs in his famous work "Anatomie des lymphatiques de l'homme". Based on the observations of 200 autopsy specimens, he classified three lymphatic regions, upper, middle, and lower, and right and left respectively.

There are many reports about the lymph vessels of the lung of various mammals, but many of them were based on simple descriptions of two or three animals. The reports of BAUM (1909, 1912, 1918, 1926), however, gave detailed observations.

BAUM published a series of books about the lymphatic system of several domestic animals, including detailed descriptions of the lymph vessels of the lung. His works are of significance in the history of studies of lymph vessels.

About the same time, FLINT (1906), CUNNINGHAM (1916), KAMPMEIER (1928), and HARVEY and ZIMMERMAN (1935) investigated the origin of the lymph vessels of the lung, using embryos of pig and man. These investigators made a number of reports on the origin of the lymph vessels of the lung and on the development of lymph vessels at various embryonal and fetal ages.

OTTAVIANI (1938) reported in detail on morphological changes in the lymph vessels of the lung during development in the fetus.

SIMER (1952), and TOBIN, et al. (1954) reported on their anatomical studies of the lymph vessels of the lung; the former presented evidences against the Miller's concept of lymph flow from the pulmonary pleura; the latter reported that the alveolar wall did have lymph vessels, contrary to the general knowledge of that time. However, their interpretations were not generally accepted.

Of the books published in these years, "Die menschliche Lunge" (1953) by HAYEK was of excellent quality. The following is a summary of his observations.

The lymph vessels of the lung are observed to accompany the connective tissues, with origin in the tissues surrounding the branches of the pulmonary artery. These are also connected with the peribronchial networks, which have valves in the more central vessels. Since the lymph vessels appear to be encircling the branches of the pulmonary artery, HAYEK termed these "Lymphräume" (lymph spaces), and he regarded them as a kind of mechanical buffer zone. This view point must be considered to have a certain validity.

"Le Poumon" by POLICARD (1955) is also famous as a monograph, but as to the lymph vessels it mainly refers to the works of other investigators.

These are the major studies which have been made in Europe and in the U.S.A.

In Japan, also many such investigations have been carried out from the beginning of the twenty century.

KIHARA (1924) injected dye solutions directly into pulmonary lymph vessels. He classified the deep lymph vessels into three systems, *i.e.* those accompanying pulmonary artery, pulmonary vein and bronchi. He also noted the existence of valves in the deep lymph vessels. In contrast to MILLER's observations, KIHARA reported lymph vessels running from the pulmonary pleura to the deep portions of the lung.

TORII (1931) investigated the efferent lymph vessels of the human fetus and new-born, and of young dogs. SHIMAZAKI (1931) carried out detailed investigations on the efferent lymph vessels of the human lung. According to SHIMAZAKI there is an efferent route that runs into the retroperitoneal lymph nodes through the esophageal and caval openings. This is in addition to the general route which runs into the lymph nodes of the hilum.

SHIDA (1932) injected dye solution into the thoracic cavity of rabbits and cats, investigating the movement of the dyes to the regional lymph nodes. His investigations revealed that the regional nodes of the lung and of the thoracic cavity are evidently separate, and there is little or no communication between the vessels of the lung and those of the thoracic cavity.

With the purpose of clarifying the existence of the lymph vessels on the alveolar wall, KUTSUNA (1935) injected dye solution into dog lung using the intrapulmonary injection method; he reported the presence of lymph vessels in the alveolar wall.

MORI (1940) performed thoractomies on cattle, horses and pigs and investigated by injecting dye solution directly into the bronchial wall. According to MORI some of the lymph vessels of the lung are of subpleural, and others are of bronchial origin. Those accompanying the blood vessels are lymph vessels arising from the bronchial wall; lymph vessels arising in the subpleural regions and those that go into the subpleural regions from the interior of the lung are quite different, with completely separate routes of drainage.

The authors (NAGAISHI and OKADA, 1955) have made several investigations on the lymph vessels of the lung of several mammals and man, and have issued detailed reports on their morphological findings.

Their studies are in three categories: 1) the regions of distribution of the lymph vessels of the lung (particularly, whether the alveolar wall has lymph vessels), 2) the relationship between the subpleural and deep lymph vessels (particularly, whether they anastomose, and if they do, in which direction does the lymph run in the anastomoses), and 3) the lymphatic regions of the lung.

The authors (NAGAISHI and OKADA) intend to describe these points in detail.

Supplement: Methods of Investigation

To assist in the understanding of cited studies or interpretation of illustration provided, several methods used in the study of lymph vessels of the lung will be described.

1) Injection Methods

The contents of the pulmonary lymph vessels are transparent and therefore, in order to make observations, it is necessary to visualize the vessels by some method, *e.g.*, by injection of dye solution into the lymph vessels.

Since the relatively central lymph vessels have many valves and retrograde injection is difficult, injections are generally made from the periphery.

The puncture method, using a fine injection needle, is commonly used. One method involves injection directly (blindly) into the tissue; the other involves insertion of the needle directly into the lymph vessels, followed by injection of the material.

In our early studies, quicksilver was used as an injection material; more recently, various dyes have been used with facility.

As MAGNUS (1922) reported, sometimes a small amount of air or hydrogen peroxide is purposefully injected into the lymph vessels as a procedure preparatory to injection, thus expanding the lumen and making it more convenient for the injection of material. In general, such a preparatory procedure is considered to be unnecessary. The injection of hydrogen peroxide, for example, may produce bubbles in the surrounding tissues, and often damages the specimen.

a) Dye Injection Methods

The injection of dye solutions is the most commonly used method for the investigation of lymph vessels. By this method one can determine the macroscopic route of lymph flow and the vessels can also be pursued histologically.

The dyes for injection must not be too coarse, and at the same time not so fine as to easily penetrate vessels or stain surrounding tissues.

In this sense, suspensions of India ink or Berlin blue are favored. Methylene blue is not suitable because it stains the surrounding tissues.

The mixture of GEROTA (1896) involves combining ethyl ether with turpentine oil, and adding various dyes. This method is convenient since the viscosity of the injection mass can be altered by varying the mixing ratio.

b) X-ray Contrast Media Injection Method

MENKES (1932) and SHDANOW (1932) tried the injection of X-ray contrast media (using lipiodol instead of turpentine oil) in GEROTA's method.

OKADA and NAGAISHI (1959) mixed ether or benzene with the X-ray contrast media to give an appropriate fluidity, and added to this suspensions of red lead, white lead or Berlin blue, which have desirable characteristics as dyes and contrast media.

This method is very convenient for roentgenographical study of the pulmonary lymph vessels, and also for histological examination.

Fig. 147 is a roentogenogram of lymph vessels of the human lung.

c) Injection with Silver Nitrate Solution

Injection of silver nitrate solution is used to stain the outline of the endothelial cells of the lymph vessels.

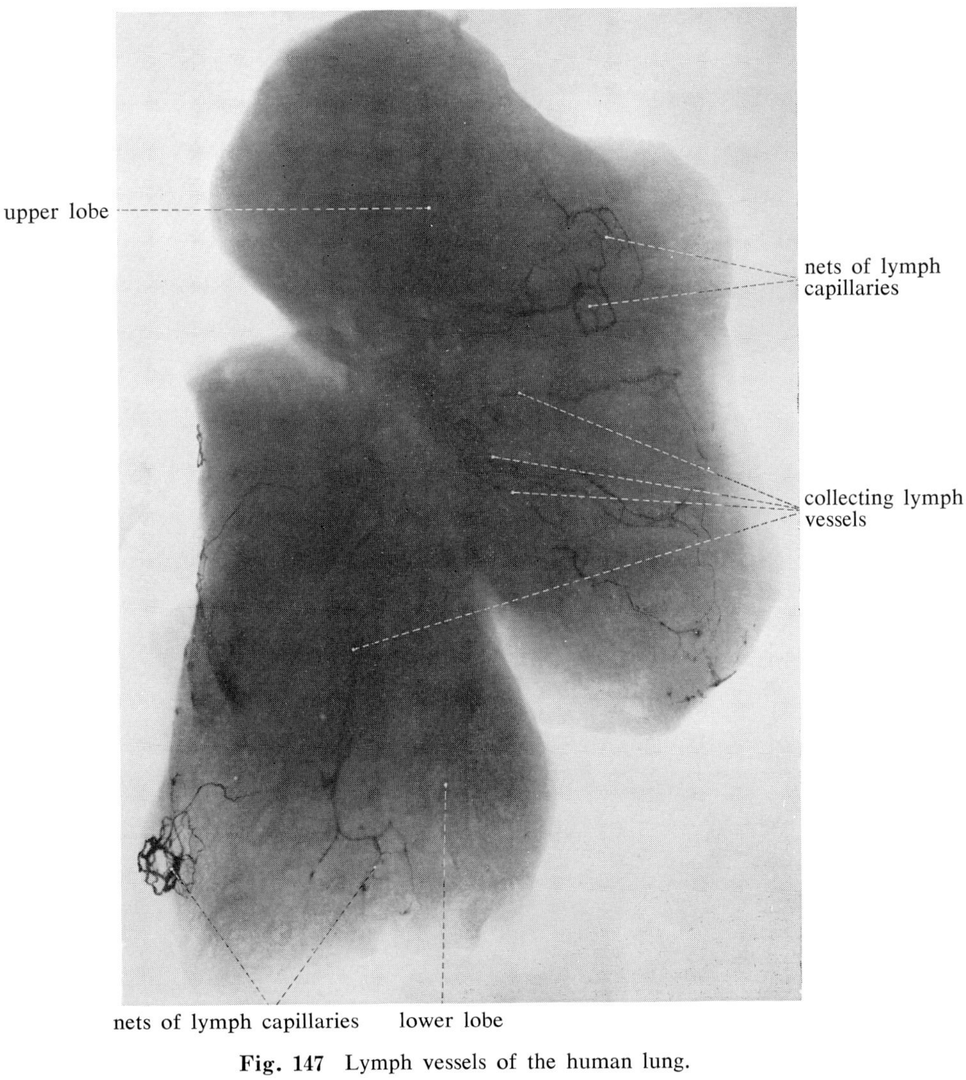

Fig. 147 Lymph vessels of the human lung.

The authors inject silver nitrate solution (0.25%) into the lymph vessels, expose the specimens to sunshine, and then make observations. Fig. 148 is an example of the appearance of the intercellular cement-substance of the lymph vessels, as seen by microscopic examination.

This method is suitable for the observation of stripped and flattened specimens of pleura but is not adequate to permit the macroscopic study of lymph vessels.

d) Injection with Acrylic Resin

The authors have adapted a method similar to that explained in Chapter I. When injecting methylmethacrylate into the lymph vessels it is also essential to inject blood vessels and bronchi in order to prevent the collapse of the resin casting.

This method was used by TOBIN (1954).

Fig. 149 shows an example of resin casting of the subpleural lymph networks of the dog lung.

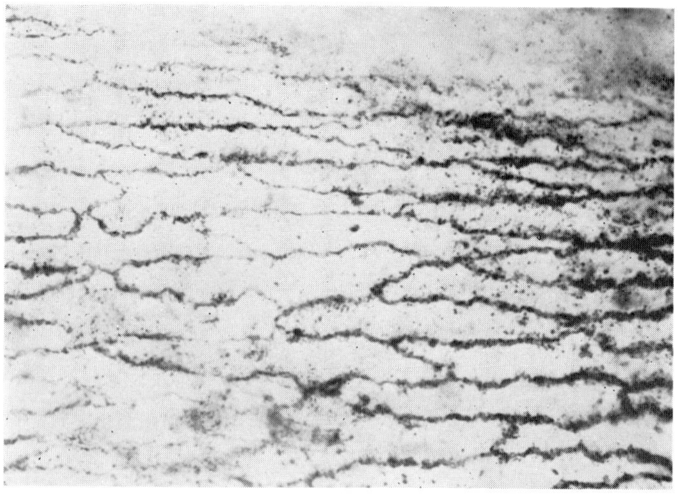

Fig. 148 Intercellular cement-substance of the pulmonary lymph vessel (by silver nitrate injection).

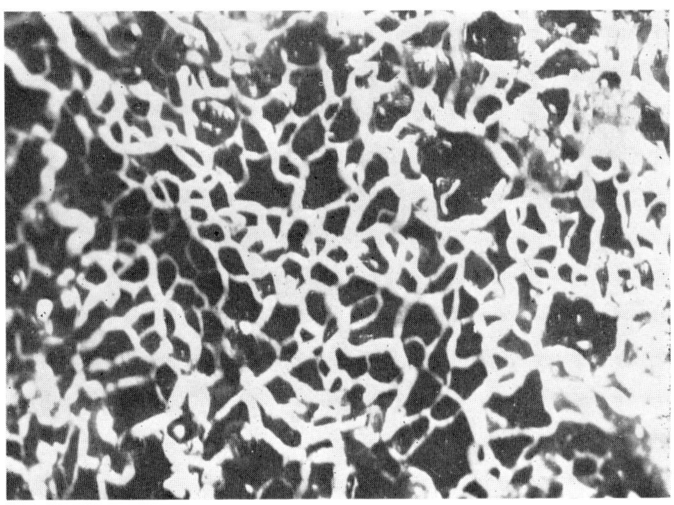

Fig. 149 Lymph vessel net of the pleura (resin cast, dog).

2) Studies of Routes of Absorption *in vivo*

The injection or insufflation of dyes or fine corpuscles into the respiratory passages or into lung tissues of living animals is done for the purpose of pursuing the routes of absorption and lymphatogenous transportation.

This method is indispensable in the investigation of pathways of lymph flow and for the designation of regional lymph nodes.

3) Histological Methods

Histological observation of lymph vessels without previous injection of dyes is somewhat difficult. The authors' method is to observe the lymph vessels by hematoxylin-eosin staining of sections of tissues, after first detecting the distribution and morphology of the lymph vessels by injecting of dye solution.

Fig. 150 shows an example of lymph vessels in the intersegmental connective tissues of an infant.

It is not always easy to distinguish between lymph and blood vessels. Even if a lymph vessel cannot be positively identified histologically it is impossible to say that lymph vessels are completely lacking; therefore, one must be conservative in making reference to lymph vessels.

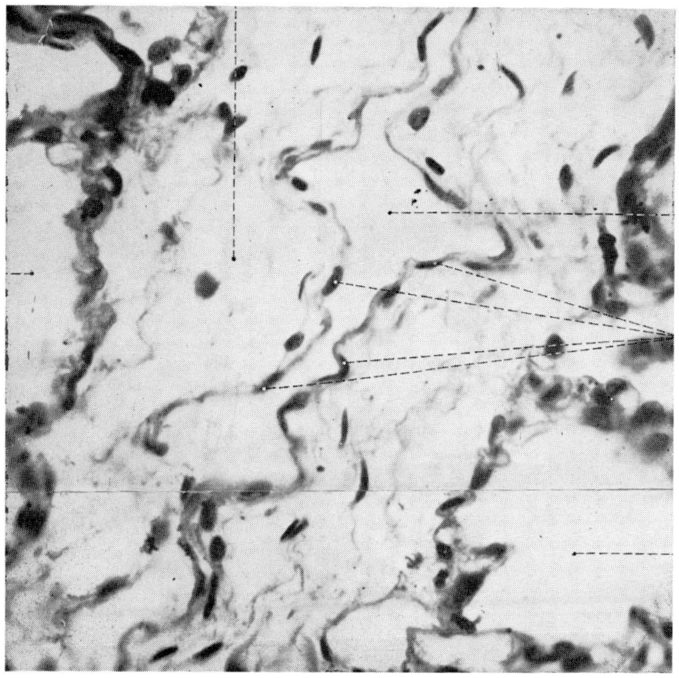

Fig. 150 Lymph vessel of the intersegmental connective tissue (infant).

However, when a vessel with a typical valve is found inside the lung, it can definitely be identified as a lymph vessel.

In a cleared specimen of the pulmonary pleura, lymph vessels may frequently be stained by silver impregnation, but for most investigations of the lymph vessels hematoxylin-eosin staining is generally recommended.

The authors use other specific staining methods when particularly required.

C. Origin and Development

1. Centrifugal and Centripetal Theories

There are symmetrical and unsymmetrical portions in the lymphatic system.

Those belonging to the former are lymph sacs in the cervical, subclavicular and retroiliac regions; those of the latter are retroperitoneal lymph sacs or cisterna chyli (cistern of Pecquet).

The thoracic duct is derived from cervical and retroperitoneal lymph sacs, and the peripheral lymph vessels are said to originate in all of the above-mentioned lymph sacs (Lewis, 1905; Sabin, 1913).

Since the end of 19th century there have been two theories about the mode of development of lymph vessels.

One is the centripetal theory of Budge (1880), and of Huntington and McClure (1910); the other is the centrifugal theory of Ranvier (1897), and of Sabin (1909).

The centripetal is based on the idea that the lymph vessels develop by fusion of lymph spaces in tissue interstices; the centrifugal holds that lymph vessels develop by differentiation of venous endothelium.

Regarding the lymph vessels of the lung, there are two similar theories.

Cunningham (1916) was definitely on the side of the centrifugal theory, whereas Kampmeier (1928) supported the centripetal theory.

As in the study of Heuer (1909) on the intestine, Cunningham made retrograde injections of dye solution into the lymph vessels of the lung at early stages of embryonal life. It was found that along with the stage of development of the embryonal lung, the regional distribution of the lymph vessels increased proportionately. These results were considered to support the centrifugal theory.

Kampmeier (1928), without injecting dye solutions, observed the existence of discontinuous tissue spaces, lined by endothelium, in the peripheral portion of the lung; he regarded these as lymph vessels. Similar secluded canals were observed by Harry and Zimmerman (1935).

One must note that investigators such as Cunningham and Ottaviani, who adopted the injection method, were inclined to support the centrifugal theory. This cannot be considered as merely coincidental; interpretations were affected by the method of study.

Whether Cunningham overlooked such tissue lymph spaces (being preoccupied by the lymph vessels which were injected with dye solution), or whether the secluded lymph spaces designated by Kampmeier were in fact in communication with central lymph vessels, is as yet uncertain.

As Sabin said, quoting from Ludwig, "Method is everything". Further investigation may be necessary to the solution of this vexing problem.

However, since the lymph vessels are formed as one continuous canal system, and whether or not the lymph vessels in regions are formed by budding of endothelium or by fusion of clefts in the tissues, there is no divergence of opinion that the development of the major lymph vessels of the lung is centrifugal.

2. Origin and Development during Embryonic and Early Fetal Life

Regarding the origin of the lymph vessel of the lungs of mammals, relatively detailed investigations have been carried out by KAMPMEIER (1928), HARVEY and ZIMMERMAN (1935), OTTAVIANI (1938), and AKIYAMA (1952) on human lungs, and by FLINT (1906), and CUNNINGHAM (1916) on pigs.

The lymph vessels in the lung of the fetal pig develop, according to FLINT and CUNNINGHAM, from the thoracic duct, right lymphatic trunk and the retroperitoneal lymph sac.

When the body length of the fetus is about 2.5–3 cm, vessels extend from the thoracic duct along the trachea; the plexus of lymph vessels extends from the ventral side of the trachea to the region of the tracheal bifurcation.

The lymph vessels arising from the right lymphatic trunk join the above, and from the plexus of the lymph vessels of the hilum thus formed, lymph vessels penetrate into the lung.

In addition to these lymph vessels from the upper part, other lymph vessels arising from the retroperitoneal lymph sac ascend posterior to the diaphragm, to form a plexus of lymph vessels inside the lower lobe. These lymph vessels anastomose with vessels to the upper part, in the fetus of about 4 cm body length.

The lymph vessels of the lung of the pig can roughly be divided into two groups according to their locus of development, i.e. accompanying the veins or connective tissues, or accompanying the bronchi or arteries.

The former develop very rapidly and reach the pleural surface in a short time; the latter are slower in development but finally reach the periphery, surrounding the bronchial tree (CUNNINGHAM, 1916).

The formation of the lymph vessels of the lung of the fetal pig is almost completed when the body length is about 6 cm.

The lymph vessels of the lung develop from the plexus of the lymph vessels in the region of the hilum, in both human and pig fetal lung.

According to KAMPMEIER (1928), the plexus of lymph vessels around the hilum of the human fetus is said to connect directly with the thoracic duct in the upper portion, and in the portion lower than the hilum is said to descend in the pulmonary ligament and form anastomoses with the plexus of lymph vessels around the esophagus. He said that in the 2.2 months embryo, the lymph vessels move from the hilum into the lung along the bronchus, artery and vein. By 2.5 months, development is said to be noted in all regions of the lung. Similar findings have been ascertained in studies by the authors' group.

Then, at 3.5 months of age, the lymph vessels extending to the peripheral portions along the bronchus, artery, and vein, further extend to the subpleural regions, and the lymph vessels of the diaphragmatic surface of the pulmonary pleura are found to bear valves.

HARVEY and ZIMMERMAN (1935) stated that in the fetus of 11.2 cm crown-ramp height the endothelium of the lymph vessels showed valve-like structures. Function of valves was found to occur when the fetal height reached 32.5 cm. This conclusion was based on histological findings.

This was also shown by the results of the authors' experiments wherein the injection of dye solution into the fetal lymph vessels from any region, dispersed the solution widely in the lymph vessels, indicating incompetence of the valvular system.

As explained above, for the human fetus, the lymph vessels of the lung can be observed in the early period of the embryonal life in the region surrounding the bronchus, artery and vein, and in the subpleural, interlobular and intersegmental regions. The time of such development is said to be almost in accord with the time of completion of formation of the pulmonary lobule.

In such early period of the embryonal life, when a dye solution is injected into the subpleural lymph vessels, the solution will be found to distribute in most of the vessels of the pulmonary lobe. Histological observation of these specimens reveals the existence of many large lymph vessels in the lung tissues.

The lymph vessels are particularly abundant in the subpleural and interlobular connective tissues, around large bronchi and in the regions surrounding the blood vessels. Particularly in the interlobular connective tissues the vessels are found to be large in number and caliber. Therefore, in the fetus, each pulmonary lobule, as shown in Fig. 151, is replete with lymphatic networks which separate it from adjacent lobules.

3. Further Development during Fetal Life

The distribution of the lymph vessels of the lung in later fetal life does not differ significantly from conditions extant during embryonal life, as shown in Fig. 152.

According to the authors' investigations, lymph vessels were observed to develop in the regions surrounding the bronchi in fetuses up to the age of seven months. The vessels were seen in the adventitia of the bronchi and distributed about the bronchial cartilages. At these stages, lymph vessels were not observed in the submucous layer of the bronchi. However, in the bronchial submucous layers of the new-born or still-born baby well developed lymph vessels were observed. Accordingly, the lymph vessels of the mucous membrane of the bronchi were considered to develop in the last stages of fetal life.

There have been no reports describing in detail the development of submucous lymph vessels of the bronchus in either the embryonal or fetal stages in the human lung but, considering the above results and also the mentioned finding in the pig (FLINT, 1906), the submucous lymph vessels of the bronchus can be regarded as the last of the lymph vessels to develop in the lung.

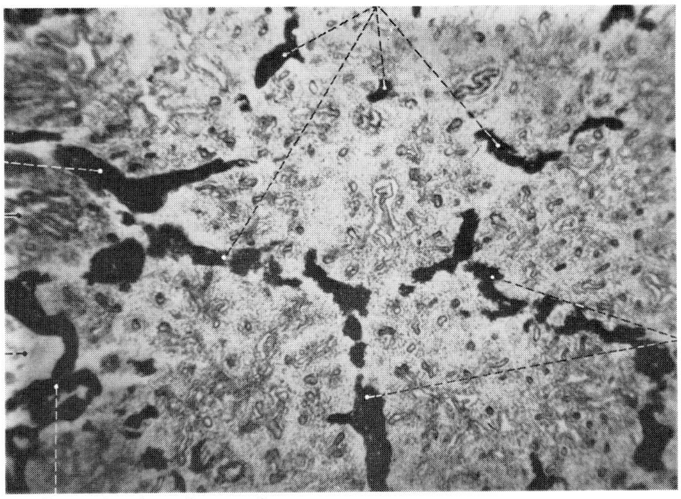

Fig. 151 Interlobular lymph vessels in the lung of the human embryo.

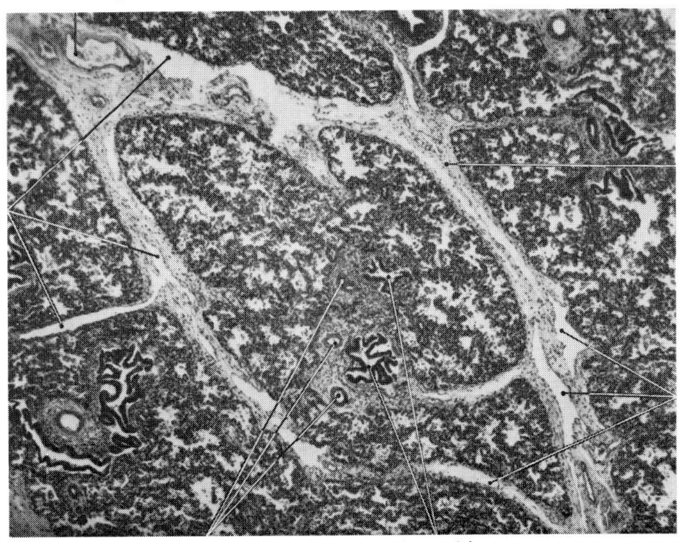

Fig. 152 Interlobular connective tissue in the lung of the human embryo.

The subpleural lymph vessels can be observed on the surface of the lung after the injection of dye solution. In particular, OTTAVIANI (1938) made detailed observations on the subpleural lymph vessels in the embryo and fetus, concentrating especially on the phenomenon of "Verdichtung" in the later period of fetal life.

The lymph vessels form widespread networks in the early period of embryonal life; in the later part of embryonal life, mediastinal, diaphragmatic and interlobar subpleural networks become more prominent than those of other regions.

This distinction gradually becomes less and vanishes after birth; at the age of one year the differences between the lymph vessels in the regions of "Verdichtung" and other regions is less evident.

The phenomenon of "Verdichtung" is caused by the flow of a large amount of lymph into the lymph vessels of a certain region; this can be observed in interlobular and subpleural lymph vessels, and in lymph vessels running to the hilum. These, as a whole, can be considered to have the function of collecting vessels.

According to the authors' studies, a dye solution injected subpleurally into the fetal lung flows to the hilum by a relatively short route.

The subpleural lymph vessels seem to play the role of collecting vessels.

As mentioned earlier, when a dye solution is injected subpleurally into the fetal lung the dye disperses diffusely in the lymph vessels of the pulmonary lobe. It is supposed from this fact that, in the fetal lung, the flow of lymph is not subject to valvular competence.

However, after 7 months of fetal age, when dye solution is injected into the S^{1+2} of the left lung, the injected solution may spread as far as S^3, although not to the lingular segment. This doubtless indicates that at the later period of fetal life valves develop, become competent, and lymph flow then takes a certain direction, becoming fixed gradually as the valves develop and become competent.

D. Morphology

Lymph vessels can be followed from periphery to central regions by injecting dye solution into the subpleural lymph vessels or into lymph vessels surrounding the bronchi.

In the lymph capillary networks, as shown in Fig. 153, both cyst-like expanded and extremely small vessels are intermingled forming complicated networks, and the diameter of the vessels show substantial irregularities.

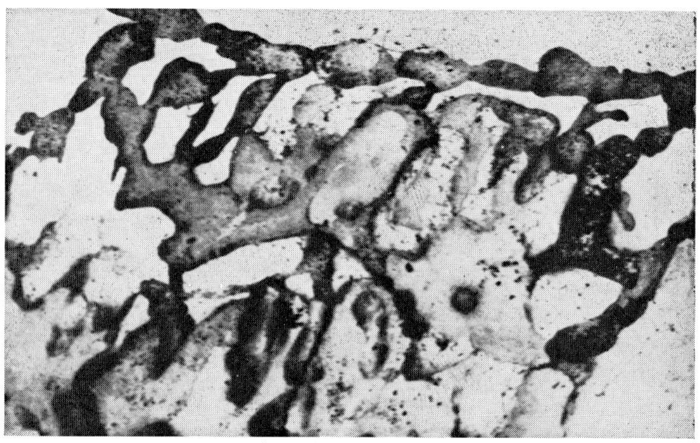

Fig. 153 Pleural lymph vessel of the cattle.

The lymph from the capillary networks first moves into small tubular vessels which have a rosary-like appearance. The tubular portion is short, with valves in the narrow part. These are the vessels in which the most dense accumulations of valves are found.

In regions more central, the valves are observed to be less frequent. These vessels are called collecting lymph vessels.

The above is a general account of the lymph vessels of the lung of cattle; in the human lung the pattern of movement from the lymph capillary to the collecting lymph vessels is not as evident as in cattle.

In the dog lung, as shown in Fig. 154, the lymph vessels of the lung are tubular as a whole and the differentiation of the vessels is not as evident as in cattle.

The lymph vessels are lined by endothelium; as they leave the organs as efferent vessels smooth muscle and elastic fibers are seen to develop in the walls (KIHARA, 1954).

MILLER (1937) stated that the intima, media and advantitia of lymph vessels are more differentiated in the central regions; MORIKAWA (1943) obtained similar results on histological investigation.

The lymph capillaries of the human lung consist only of an endothelial layer. Staining of intercellular cement substance (by silver nitrate) shows the outline of endothelial cells, as shown above in Fig. 148. The capillaries have somewhat larger endothelial cells as compared with those of blood capillaries.

MORIKAWA (1943) reported observation of the connective tissue fibers running around the endothelium in some smaller lymph vessels, but it is relatively rare that such layers can be clearly distinguished from those of the surrounding connective tissues.

In the vessels central to the lymph capillaries smooth muscle fibers may be noted, as shown in Fig. 155.

Some of the muscle fibers run in longitudinal directions, as shown in Fig. 156.

The smooth muscle shown by BALTISBERGER (1921) to be present in the pleura was considered by MILLER (1937) to be smooth muscle belonging to subpleural and collecting lymph vessels.

MORIKAWA (1943) made histological studies of the larger lymph vessels (internal dia 0.3–0.9 mm) in the region of the hilum, and of efferent vessels from the broncho-pulmonary lymph nodes; he reported

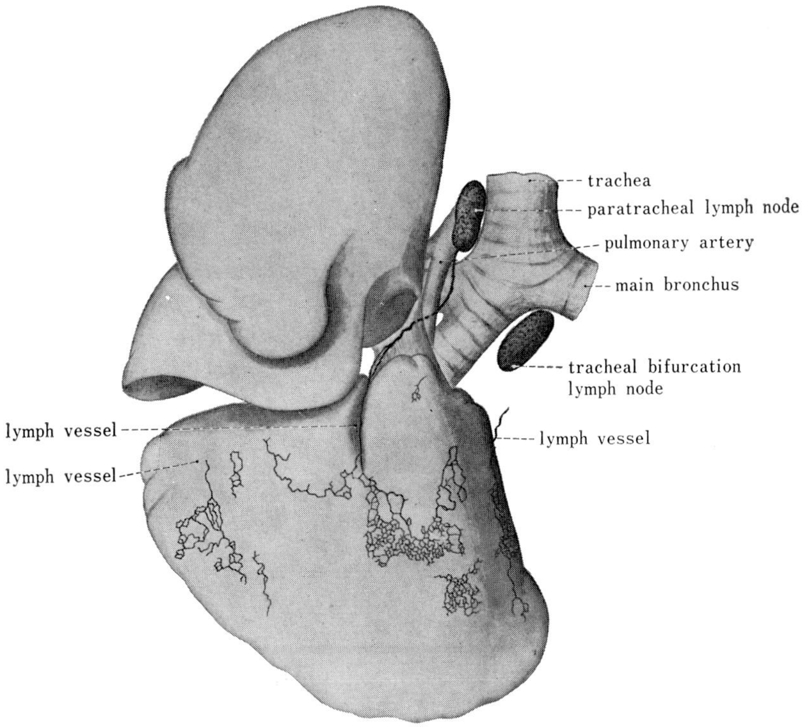

Fig. 154 Pleural lymph vessel (dog).

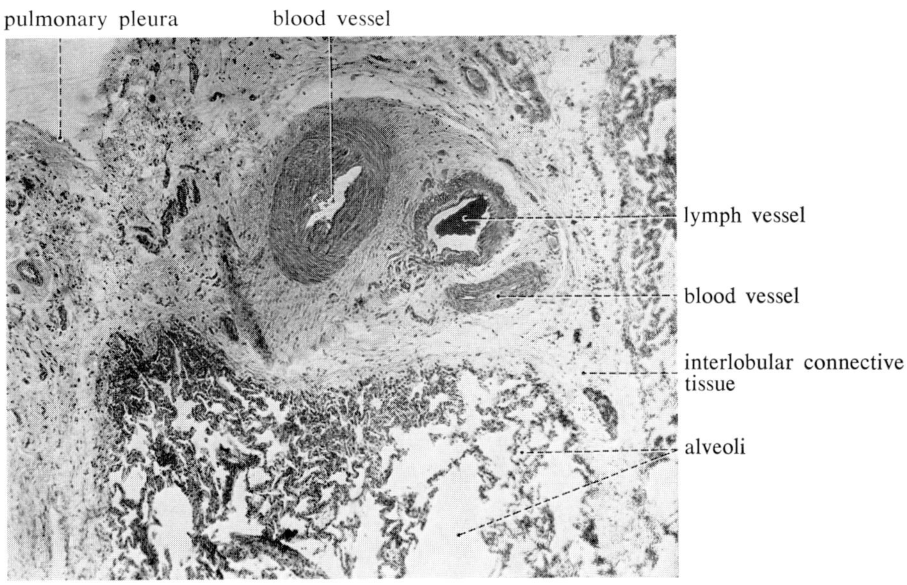

Fig. 155 Lymph vessel with muscle fibers (cattle lung).

the observation of an obvious muscular layer in vessels in the region of the hilum. Unlike those in the periphery, the muscular layer encircled vessels and ran in longitudinal and annular directions in the media.

The adventitia, *i.e.* the capsule of connective tissue, was not well developed in any portion of the lymph vessels of the lung. The observation of formed capsules which could be differentiated from surrounding connective tissue was quite rare.

Varying according to the animal, the histological structure of lymph vessels of the lung shows some differences. For example, in cattle, as compared with the human, muscular layers are found to develop in a relatively more peripheral position as shown in Figs. 156 and 157.

Judging from the above histological findings, the movement of lymph in the peripheral regions of the lung is supposed to be mainly passive. It is also for this reason that congestion of lymph in peripheral vessels may occur. On the contrary the muscular layers in the walls of central vessels are presumed to promote a smooth movement of lymph.

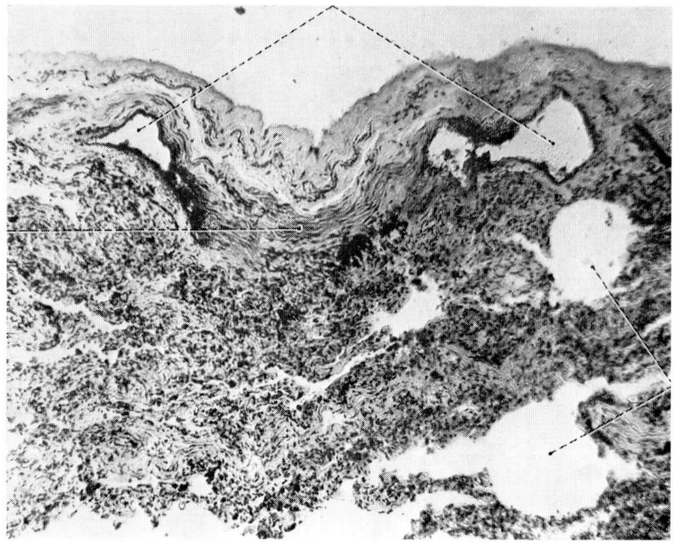

Fig. 156 Muscle fibers of the subpleural lymph vessel.

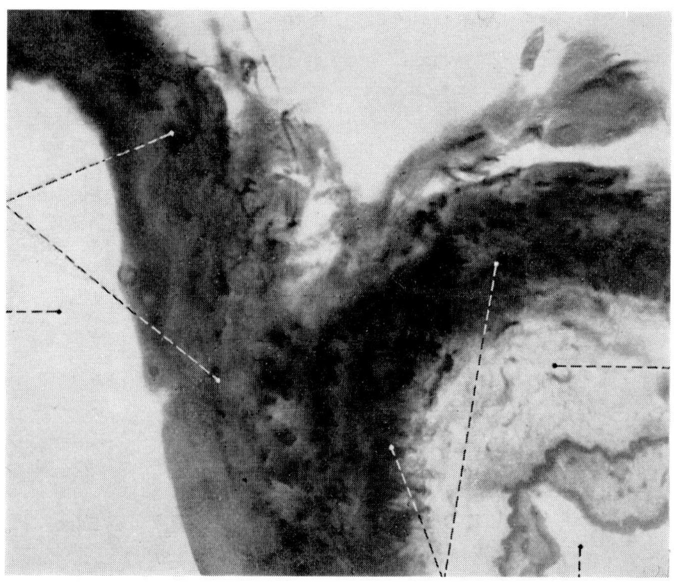

Fig. 157 Elastic fibers in the wall of the lymph vessel.

Valves of the lymph vessels are considered to be formed by folds of endothelium which have projected into the vascular lumen. In the earliest stage of development these folds cannot be considered to function as valves (HARVEY and ZIMMERMAN, 1935).

Fig. 158 shows an example of a completed valve.

According to KAMPMEIER (1928), subpleural lymph vessels in the region of the hilum are the first to exhibit valves.

MILLER (1937) and MORI (1940) stated that the valves of lymph vessels were usually bilobate and occasionally unilobate; we have observed the same.

MILLER (1937) counted numbers of valves in serial sections from various regions of the lung. MORI (1940) investigated the distribution of valves in the lymph vessels of the lungs of cattle, horses and pigs; he reported that in the lymph vessels accompanying pulmonary arteries, pulmonary veins and bronchi, the valves were found to be most numerous in vessels of dia >0.5 mm. The frequency of valves decreased in the more central regions.

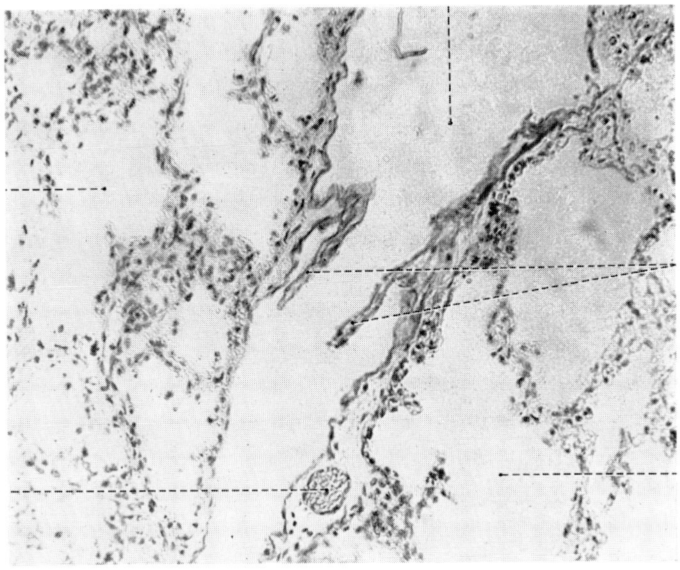

Fig. 158 Valve of the pulmonary lymph vessel.

E. Classification and Distribution

MASCAGNI (1787) and CRUIKSHANK (1790) divided the lymph vessels of the lung into the superficial, distributing in the pulmonary pleura, and the deep lymph vessels, distributing in the intrapulmonary tissues.

Later, MILLER and many other researchers classified the lymph vessels of the lung according to their regional distribution. More recently, they have been classified, as shown in Table 6.

Table 6 Classification of the pulmonary lymph vessel.

A. superficial lymph vessel
 subpleural lymph vessel

B. deep lymph vessel
 1) lymph vessel in the interlobular connective tissue
 2) lymph vessel related to the pulmonary veins
 3) lymph vessel related to the bronchi
  a) lymph vessel in the submucous layer
  b) lymph vessel in the adventitia
 4) lymph vessel related to the pulmonary arteries

The lymph flowing through these lymph vessels was observed to follow a certain pathway. MORI (1940) ascertained this pattern of flow in cattle, horses and pigs.

The authors (NAGAISHI and OKADA, 1958) have made investigations in detail, mainly on the lymph flow in human lung, and also in dog and cattle lungs. In the description of these studies the authors adopted the generally used classification, as shown above in Table 6.

1. Subpleural Lymph Vessels

The lymph vessels of the pulmonary pleura are called superficial, pleural, or subserous, however, the authors consider it to be appropriate to call them the subpleural vessels, as histological observations show the lymph vessels distribute in the subpleural interstitial layers rather than in the pleura itself.

a. In Dog Lung

When the normal surface of the dog lung is illuminated and observed obliquely, transparent subpleural lymph vessel networks can be observed, in many instances.

Especially suitable for observation is the costal surface of the lower lobe; the puncture and injection of dye solution can easily be performed in vessels of this portion.

Although the subpleural tissue of the dog is relatively thin, it is well developed, as shown in Fig. 159, and lymph vessel networks are quite apparent.

The lymph vessel networks in the dog lung differ from those of man or cattle in showing relatively uniform networks, as shown in Fig. 160.

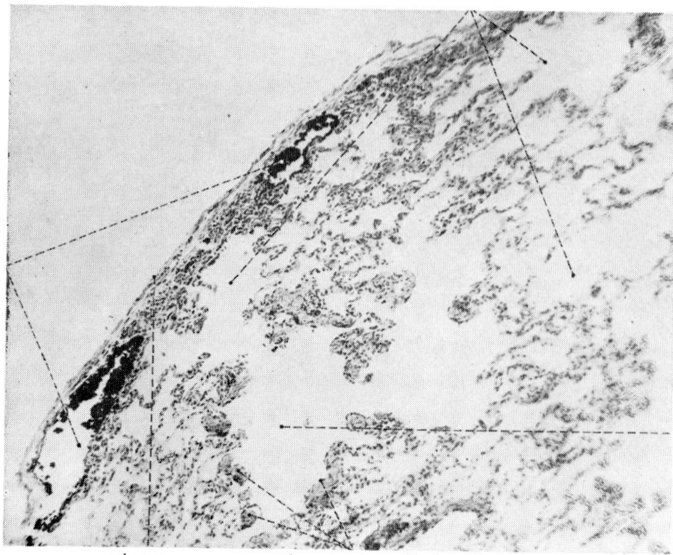

Fig. 159 Subpleural lymph vessel (dog).

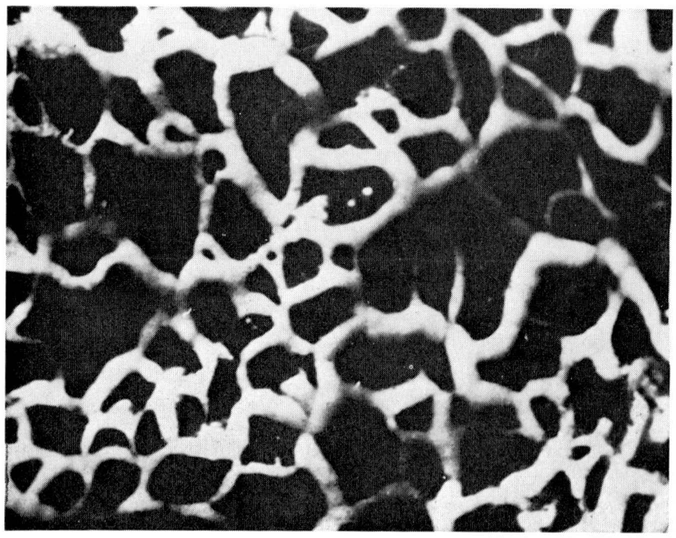

Fig. 160 Subpleural lymph vessel (resin cast, dog).

The differentiation of lymph vessels (in the narrow sense) and of collecting lymph vessels is somewhat difficult in the dog, their sizes being almost the same.

Several subpleural collecting lymph vessels are observed on each pulmonary lobe. The vessels run along the interlobar fissures, forming a part of the collecting vessels related to the pulmonary vein in the region of the hilum, as shown above in Fig. 154.

As noted, the subpleural lymph vessels of the dog lung run mainly on the surface of the lung toward the hilum, but some of them, as mentioned by BAUM (1918), dip into the lung and return to the subpleural layer, and some run further into the deep portion of the lung, as mentioned by MATHIS, et al. (1932). In such cases, lymph flows from the subpleural lymph vessel networks into the collecting lymph vessels of the deep portion of the lung, and reaches the hilum running along the blood vessels.

According to the authors' investigation, retrograde flow of dye toward the perivascular lymph vessel networks was not observed when the dyes had once entered the collecting lymph vessels related to the blood vessels.

Table 7 is a summary of investigations on the subpleural lymph vessels of the dog.

According to the authors' experiments, only small amounts of dye solution could injected into the subpleural lymph vessels of the dog, even though the injection needle was inserted exactly into the lymph vessels. Injection of larger quantities was impossible even if the pressure of injection was increased.

Table 7 Lymph-flow of the subpleural lymph vessel in the dog lung.

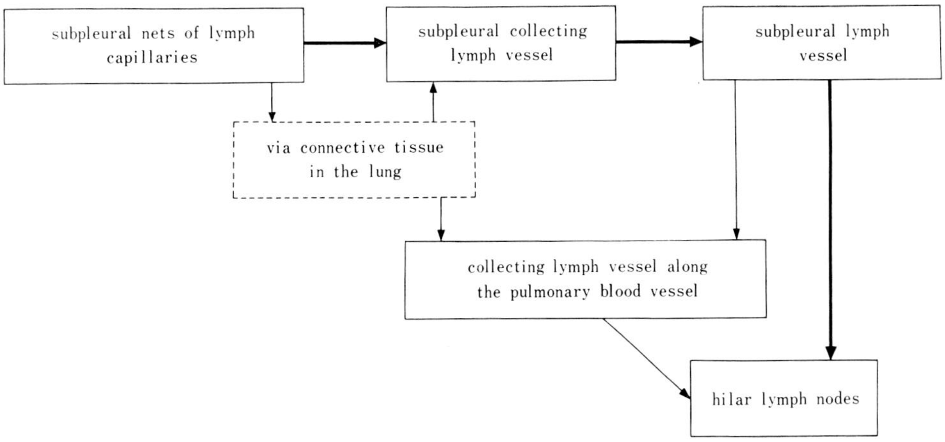

In these cases, there was no evidence of the spreading of dyes into other lymph vessels on the pleural surface. It was therefore assumed that these vessels were probably solitary, and without communication with other lymph vessels.

These findings were often seen in the lung of the dog, but not in the lung of man or cattle.

It is not yet known how such closed or restricted lymph vessels develop; they may be residual to solitary lymph spaces developed in the periphery of the lung in embryonal or fetal life.

b. In Cattle Lung

Subpleural lymph vessels of cattle are also observed in the subpleural interstitial layers, as shown in Fig. 161. The injection of dye solution is easier here than in the dog since the lymph vessel network is dense and many portions are dilated, as if cystic.

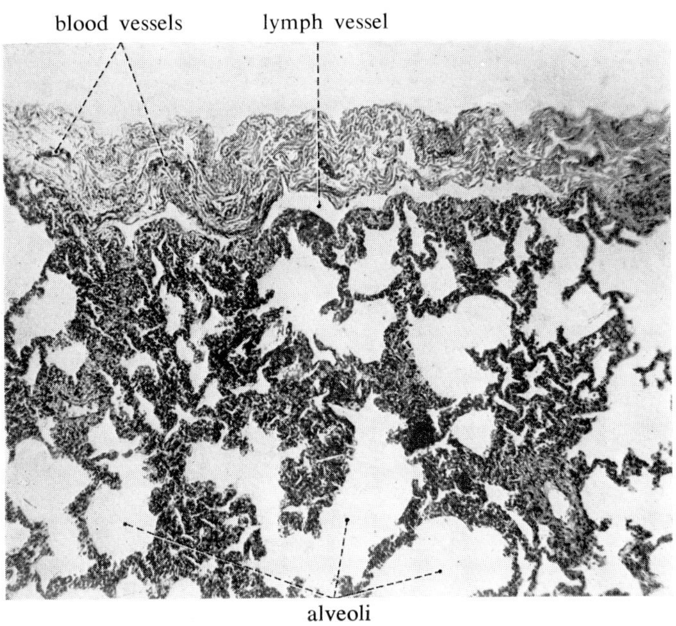

Fig. 161 Subpleural lymph vessels of the cattle.

Subpleural lymph vessels of cattle are not valved, as shown in Fig. 162. The diameter of the vessels differs, varying from large and sac-like to thread-like vessels. These resemble a rosary, and interconnect.

The lymph flowing out from the capillary networks moves into vessels which run nearly parallel along the borders of the lobules.

The lymph vessels in cattle are better developed than in the dog. Vessels containing valves appear to be constricted and can be readily differentiated from lymph capillaries.

Thus, a dye solution injected into a subpleural lymph capillary spreads into the capillary network and then moves into the collecting lymph vessels. Flow does not occur in a retrograde fashion, nor into neighboring lobules.

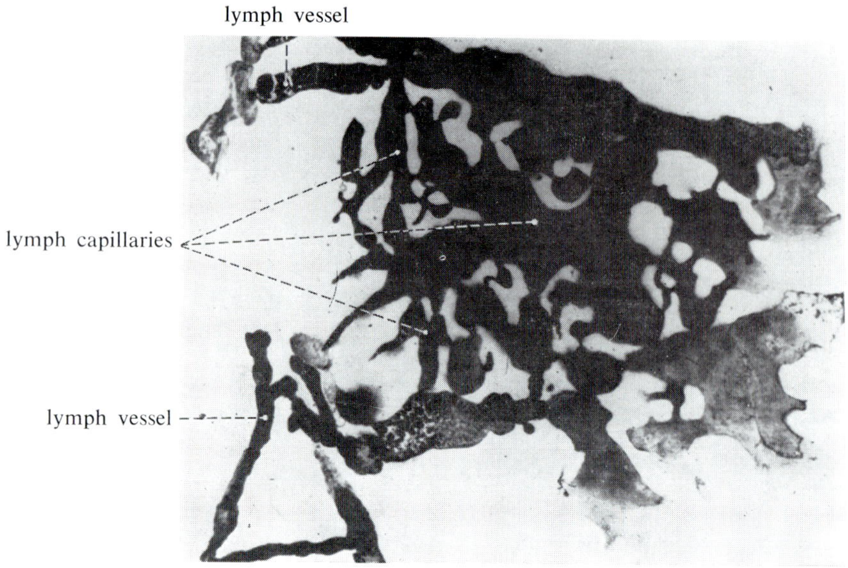

Fig. 162 Subpleural lymph vessel of the cattle.

The lymph from a group of lobules (several, up to ten) flows into a collecting lymph vessel, then further to the hilum via regional lymph vessels of the surrounding portion of the lobule. Some of the collecting lymph vessels of cattle reach the hilum in a bundle of two or three vessels, but most of them run along pulmonary veins, or along the margin of a pulmonary lobe, immediately under the pleura, and without forming anastomoses. In this region, several collecting lymph vessels run parallel, presenting a different aspect as compared to those of dog or man.

Fig. 163 is a schema of subpleural lymph vessels of cattle.

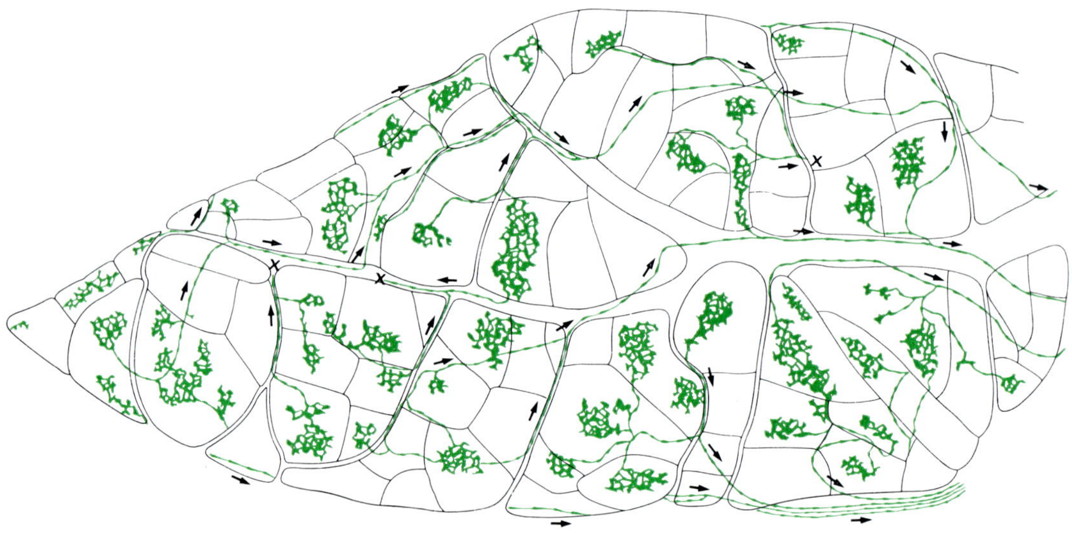

Fig. 163 Lymph-flow in the subpleural lymph vessel of the cattle.

As is seen from the above, the collecting lymph vessels usually are immediately beneath the pleura, but in not a few instances, after once entering the interlobular connective tissue, the vessels reappear in other portions of pleural surface, as stated by Baum (1912), or directly extend to the hilum along the pulmonary artery, pulmonary vein or bronchus.

The subpleural collecting lymph vessels include vessels arising from the bronchial wall, as will be described later. As stated by Mori (1940), these are an entirely different set of collecting lymph vessels, shown by the fact that a dye solution injected into the subpleural lymph capillary network will not move into such collecting lymph vessels.

c. In Human Lung

According to Kampmeier (1928), and Harvey and Zimmerman (1935), spaces in the subpleural connective tissue, which are similar to lymph vessels, are said to be observed in the embryo of 2.5–3.0 months of age.

The time of development of the subpleural lymph vessels is different from those in the hilum and is somewhat later, according to OTTAVIANI (1938); the embryonic height is about 70 mm or, according to KAMPMEIER (1928), about 85 mm in height, which corresponds to about 3.5 months of embryological age.

The subpleural lymph vessels of a fetus of about 70 mm in height are found to form extremely rough and simple networks; in the fetus of about 90 mm in height small lymph vessels develop among the rough networks and the networks are more finely divided.

In the fetus of more than 90 cm in height, *i.e.* in the fifth months of fetal age, as shown in Fig. 164, differentiation of the subpleural lymph vessels takes place, showing the outline of the lobules; the lymph vessels divide the surface of the lobule into further fine networks and the arrangement of the lymph vessels is almost completed.

Fig. 165 presents an example of the histological finding in a lymph vessel at this stage.

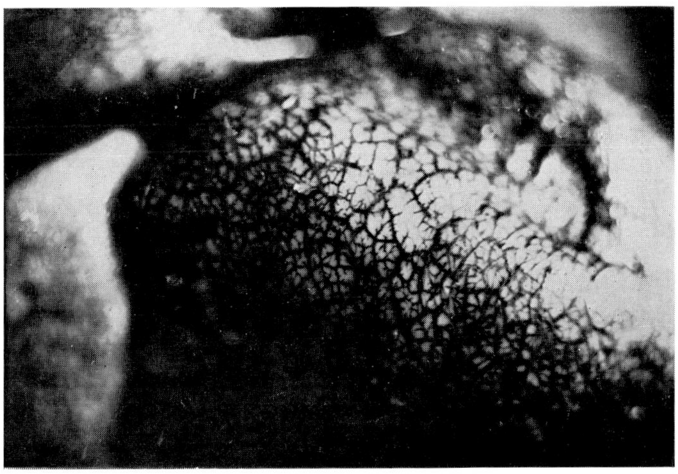

Fig. 164 Subpleural lymph vessel of the human embryo.

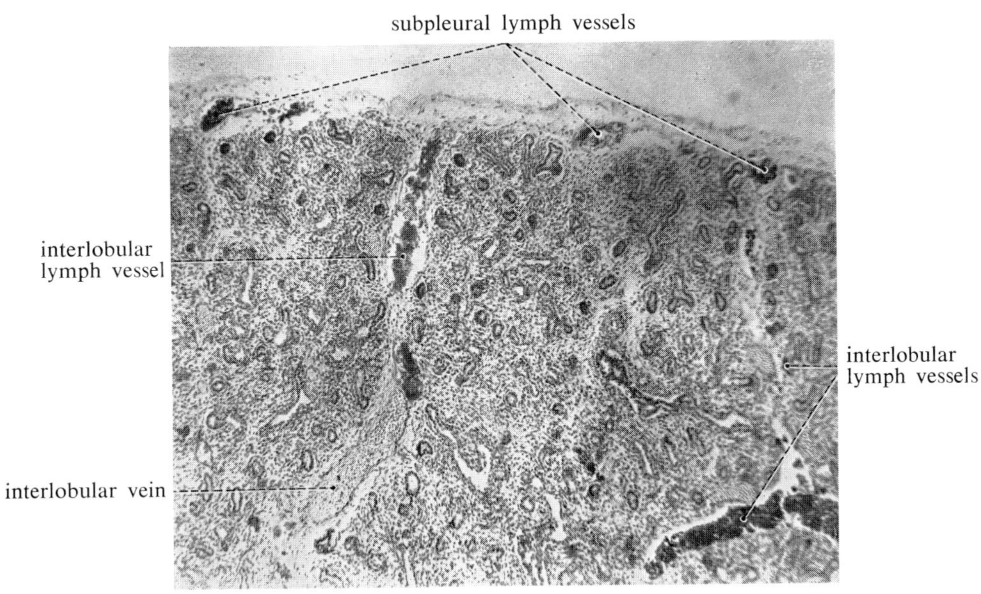

Fig. 165 Subpleural and interlobular lymph vessels of the fetal lung.

Around the same time, the aforementioned phenomenon of "Verdichtung" (OTTAVIANI) takes place, to be observed more markedly in the later periods of fetal life.

For example, in the fetus of 17 cm height, the lymph vessels in the region of the hilum are observed to become particularly enlarged and with dense distribution.

Then, at the height of about 19 cm, the subpleural lymph vessels of the base and fissures start to show similar morphological changes.

In the later part of fetal life, generally, no notable change is observed, other than the phenomenon of "Verdichtung". The subpleural lymph vessels at this stage are morphologically the same as in the new-born, as shown in Fig. 166.

Fig. 167 is an example of the histological appearance of the subpleural lymph vessels in a new-born.

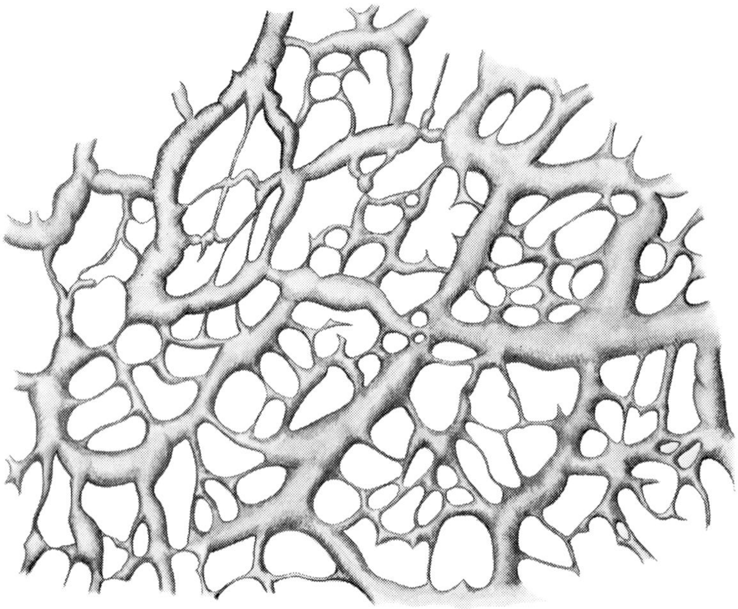

Fig. 166 Subpleural lymph vessel of the human embryo (sketch).

pleural surface subpleural lymph vessels

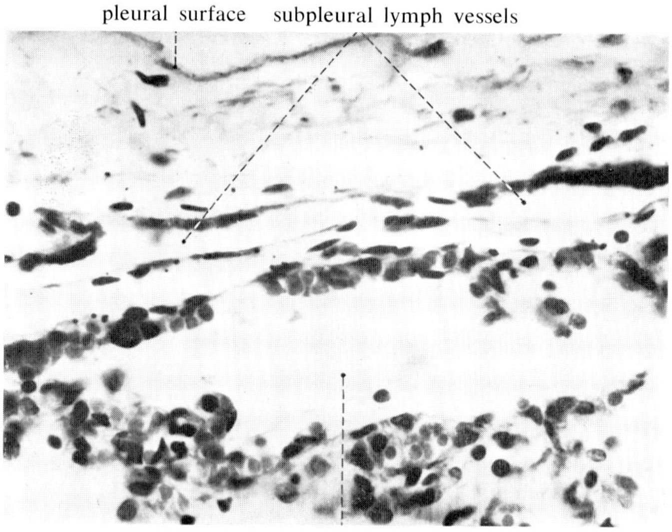

alveole

Fig. 167 Subpleural lymph vessel of the human new-born lung.

In the lungs of either child or adult the subpleural lymph vessels are observed macroscopically as transparent canals. On the diaphragmatic margin of the lower lobe they can be observed most readily, but in general macroscopic observation without injection of dye solution is difficult.

When dye solution is injected into the fetal or new-born lung, the solution will spread easily into a wide area, as described earlier, and exchange of lymph flow is seen within the networks. In the adult lung, however, the injected solution does not spread widely but flows into the networks of smaller areas,

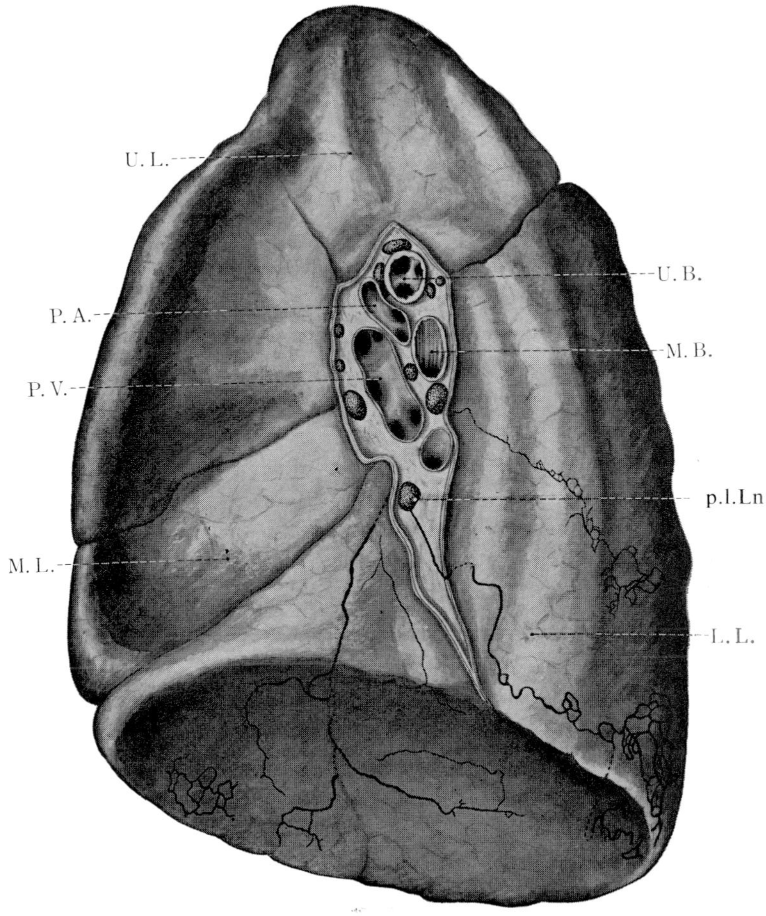

Fig. 168 a Lymph vessel of the human right lung.
U.L.: upper lobe, P.A.: pulmonary artery, P.V.: pulmonary vein, M.L.: middle lobe, M.B.: main bronchus, p.l.L.n.: pulmonary ligament lymph node, L.L.: lower lobe, U.L.: upper lobe bronchus.

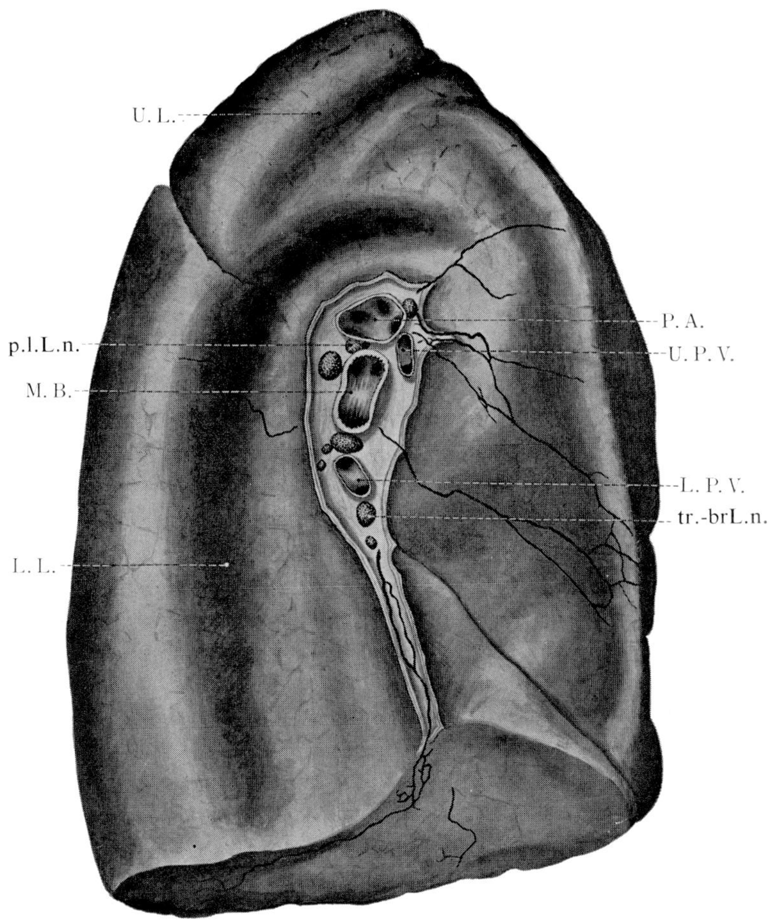

Fig. 168 b Lymph vessel of the human left lung.
U.L.: upper lobe, tr.-br.Ln.: tracheo-bronchial lymph node, M.B.: main bronchus, L.L.: lower lobe, P.A.: pulmonary artery, U.P.V.: upper pulmonary vein, L.P.V.: lower pulmonary vein, p.l.Ln.: pulmonary ligament lymph node.

as shown in Fig. 168(a), (b), and then runs immediately into the collecting lymph vessel, via the lymph vessels in the narrow sense. In the lymph vessels of adults, valves are well developed and therefore the injected solution flows in a directed manner.

In the adult, as shown in Figs. 169–171, the form of lymph vessel networks is midway as compared with those of the dog and cattle.

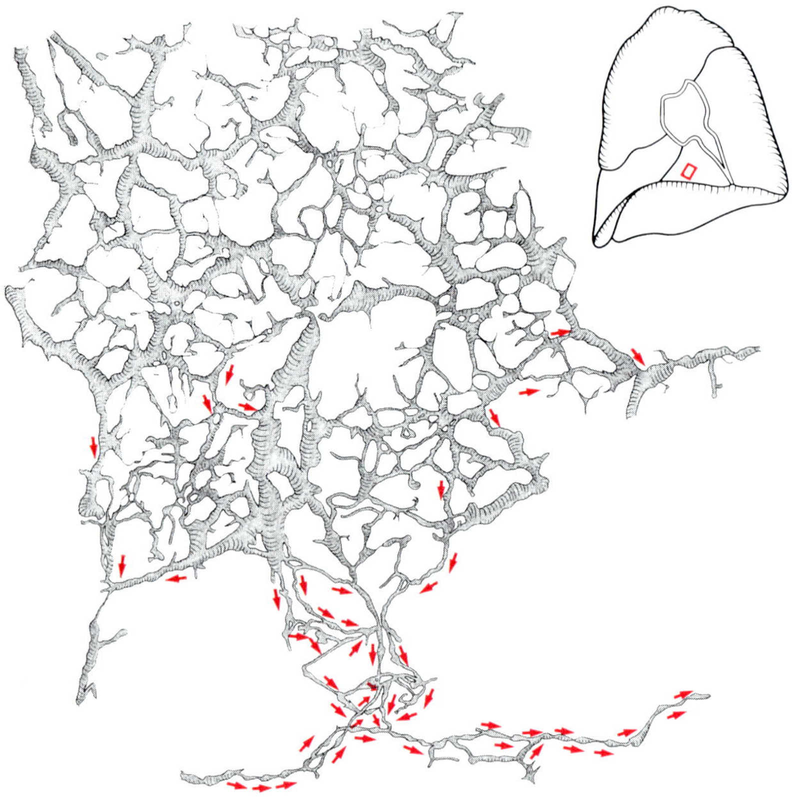

Fig. 169 Subpleural lymph vessel of an adult human lung.

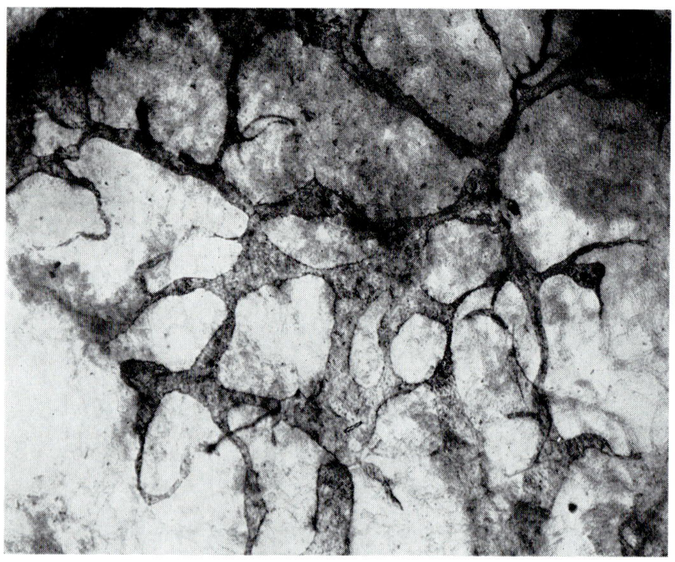

Fig. 170 Subpleural lymph vessels (Chinese ink instillated specimen, human adult).

The collecting lymph vessels joining the subpleural lymph vessels are observed to be most abundant on the mediastinal surface of the pulmonary pleura, *i.e.* in the region where "Verdichtung" is observed, and not as well developed on the costal surfaces.

The collecting lymph vessels of the human lung run in solitary fashion, mainly along the intersegmental or interlobular regions where abundant connective tissue is observed. Observation of several collecting

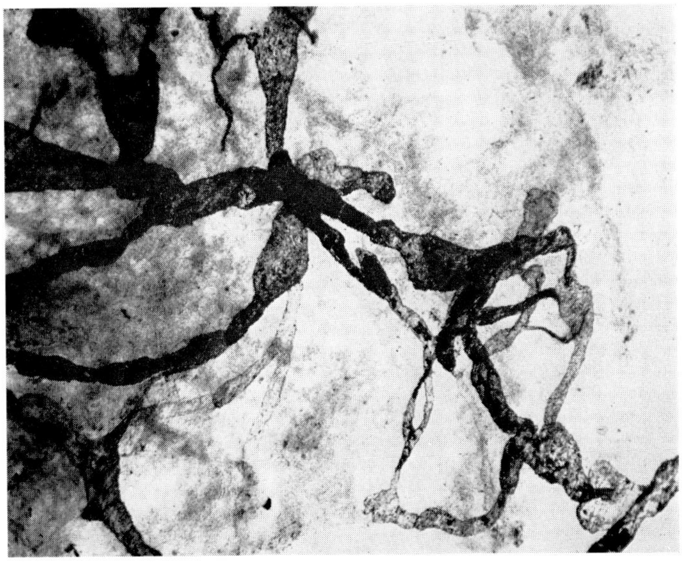

Fig. 171 Subpleural lymph vessels and collecting lymph vessels (Chinese ink instillated specimen, human adult).

lymph vessels running parallel along the margin of the lobe, as in cattle, is not often observed.

Figs. 172 and 173 are examples of histological findings in subpleural lymph vessels of adult and infant, respectively.

Passage of lymph from the subpleural to the intrapulmonary lymph vessels is seen in adults as well as in the fetus or new-born: however, in the latter, the lymph flows freely in all directions, whereas in the former, the lymph flow is fixed in certain directions.

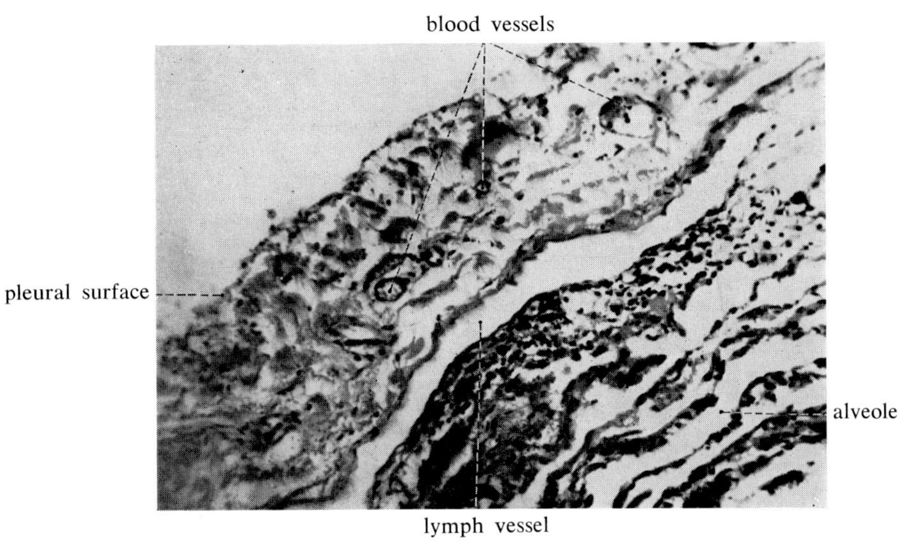

Fig. 172 Subpleural lymph vessel of the human lung.

Fig. 174(a) and (b) are radiographic illustrations (using soft X-ray apparatus) obtained after injection of X-ray contrast media into the subpleural lymph vessels in the lung of an adult (deceased). In this specimen, free communication is found between the subpleural lymph vessels and those of the interlobular connective tissue.

In adults free communication between these vessels is observed only in specific regions; for example, at the diaphragmatic margin of the lower lobe. This finding is in accordance with the findings of Kampmeier (1928) and Miller (1947).

Fig. 175 shows the lymph pathways from the subpleural tissues to the connective tissues surrounding the bronchus or pulmonary artery.

Fig. 176 shows the lymph pathway from the subpleural tissues to the connective tissues surrounding the bronchus.

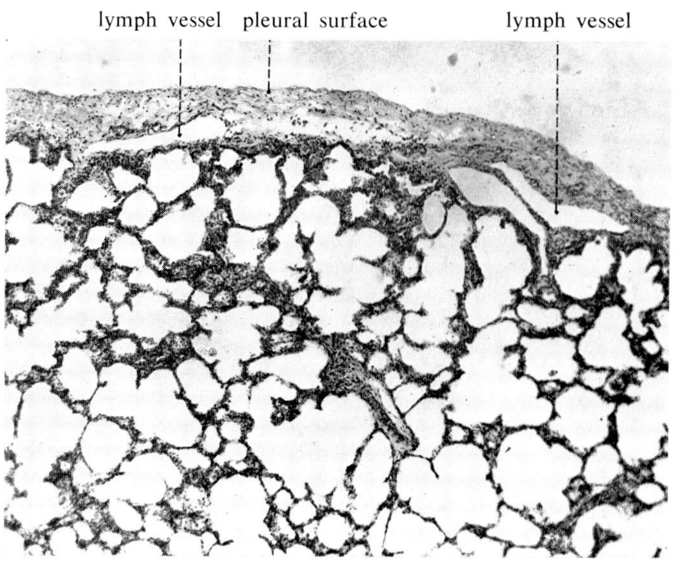

Fig. 173 Subpleural lymph vessel of the human lung.

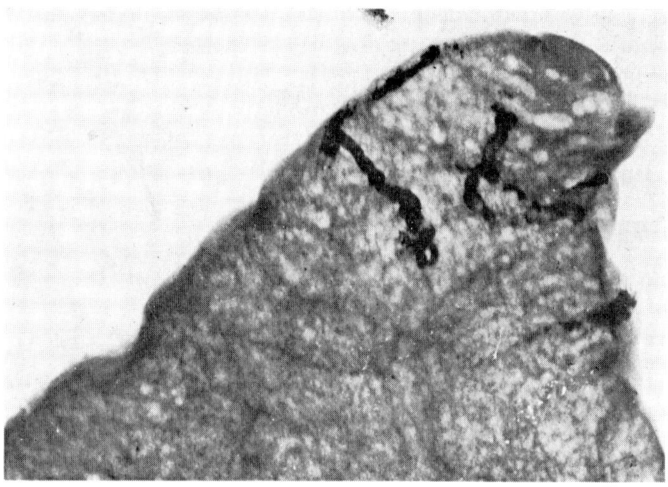

a

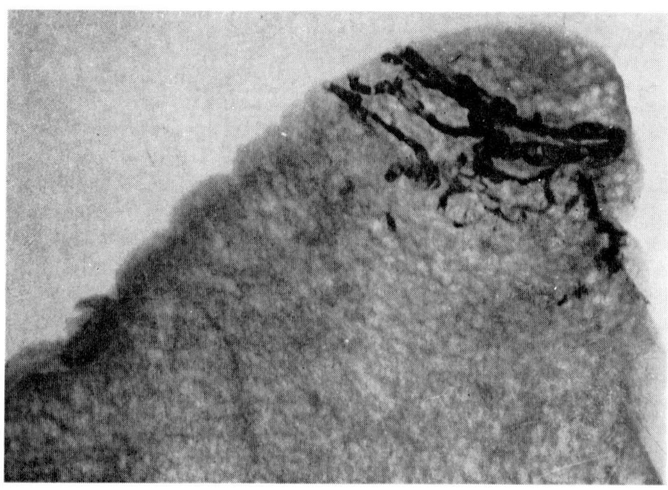

b

Fig. 174 a, b Roentgenogram showing anastomoses between the subpleural lymph vessel and the interlobular lymph vessel.

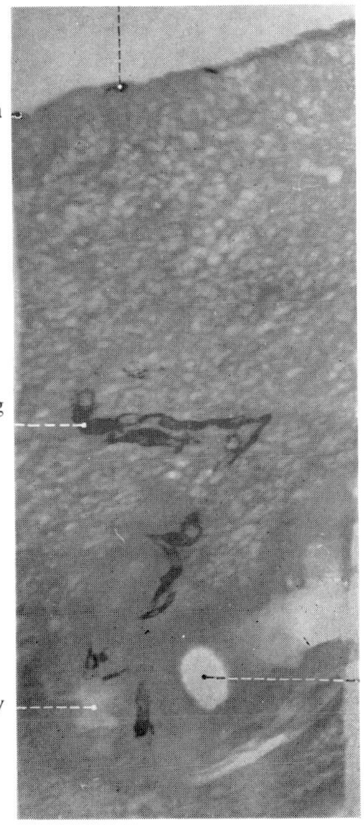

Fig. 175 Subpleural and deep lymph vessels of the human lung (roentgenogram with contrast medium).

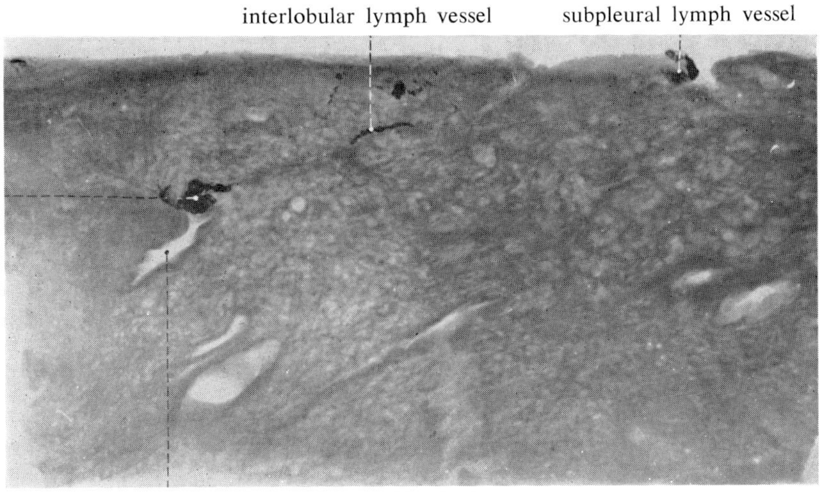

Fig. 176 Subpleural and deep lymph vessels of the humans lung (roentgenogram with contrast medium).

The lymph of the subpleural tissues runs, as is well known, toward the hilum along the surface of the lung, but in the adult there definitely exists an additional pathway which runs from the subpleural tissue to the intrapulmonary tissue (FRANKE, 1912; KIHARA, 1924; SHIMAZAKI, 1931 and SIMER, 1952), it is appropriate to say that the subpleural vessels run toward the hilum, joining the deep lymph vessels.

From the results of the authors' investigations, opinions about the relation of the subpleural lymph vessel of adults and the deep lymph vessel of the lung can be restated as follows. The observations of MASCAGNI (1787) and CRUIKSHANK (1790) that free communications exist between both lymphatic systems seem not to necessarily be correct; statements by MILLER (1896) and KAMPMEIER (1928) that free communications can be observed in specific regions to be valid.

However, the view of MILLER that a connection between the subpleural and intrapulmonary deep lymph vessels does not exist should be corrected.

That the lymph of the subpleural tissues flows mainly into the hilum through vessels along the surface of the lung, but that some runs to the pulmonary vein or tissues surrounding the bronchus by way of the interlobular tissues, may be considered an appropriate view.

Table 8 is a schematic presentation of arrangement of the subpleural lymph vessels of human adult.

Table 8 Subpleural lymph-flow in the human adult lung.

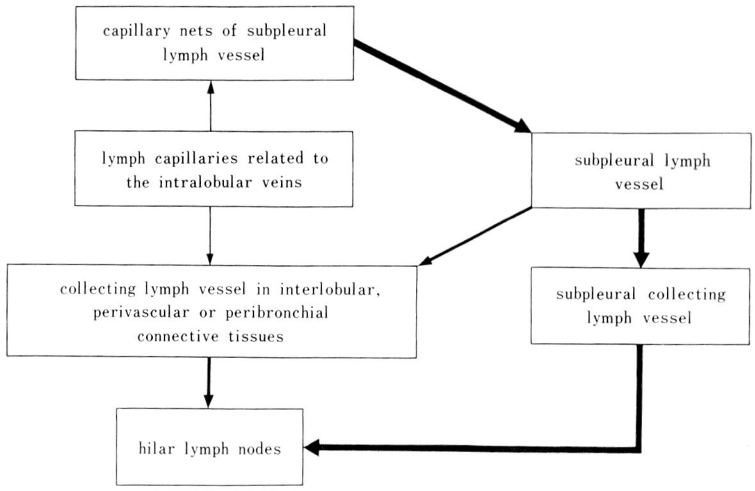

2. Lymph Vessels in Interlobular Connective Tissue

OTTAVIANI (1938) stated that in the human fetus of about 12 cm in height the arrangement of lymph vessels around each pulmonary lobule became distinct and additional to those lymph vessels related to blood vessels. AKIYAMA (1952) reported that, at 14–16 weeks of fetalage and again at the 23rd week, lymph vessels surrounding the pulmonary lobule develop markedly.

The lymph networks of the interlobular connective tissue of man show a regular arrangement after 4–5 months of fetal age, as shown in Fig. 177.

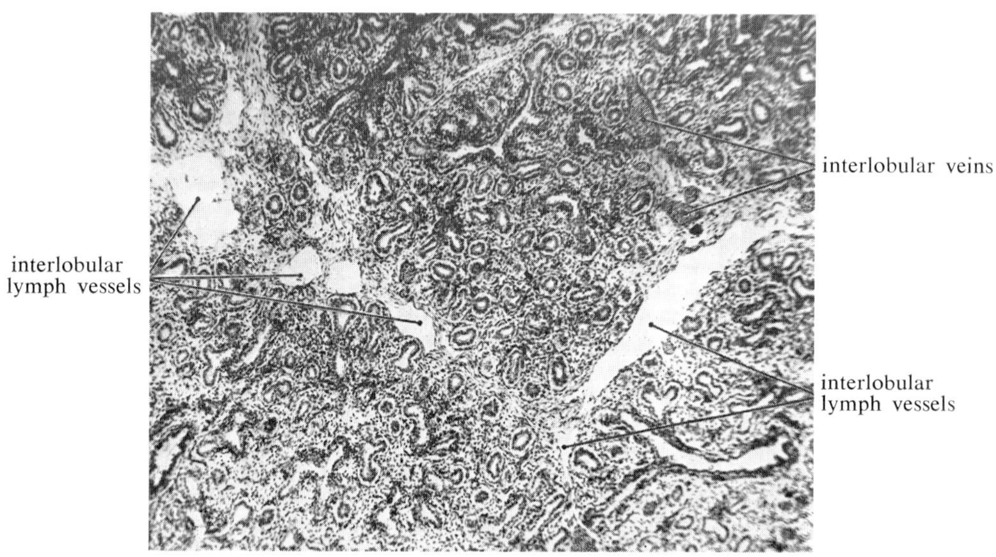

Fig. 177 Interlobular lymph vessels of the human embryo.

Fig. 178 shows an example of the histological findings of interlobar and interlobular lymph vessels near the hilum, in a fetus of a later stage than the above.

MILLER (1947) stated that in the dog lung the interlobular connective tissue is lacking, and that the lymph vessels related to pulmonary veins are observed in place of those of the interlobular connective tissue, as in other animals. In cattle, or example the interlobular connective tissue is well developed.

In this interlobular connective tissue of cattle two routes are observed: one reaches the hilum via the

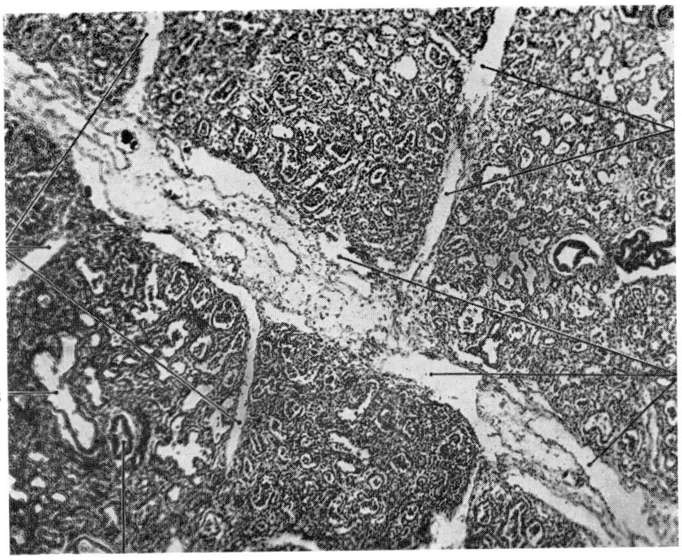

Fig. 178 Interlobar and interlobular lymph vessels of the human fetus near the hilum.

collecting vessel of the subpleural lymph vessel, and the other reaches the hilum via the lymph vessel networks of the bronchial wall; however, proper lymph vessels are not observed in the interlobular connective tissue.

Contrary to this, in the interlobular tissue of the human lung no such marked development of lymph vessel networks is observed.

Figs. 179 and 180 illustrate the histological appearances of intersegmental and interlobular lymph vessels of new-born and adult.

CUNNINGHAM (1916) made observations on the lung of the pig and reported that the interlobular and subpleural lymph vessels are differentiated embryologically from those lymph vessels that are related to the pulmonary vein.

In interlobular connective tissues, in addition to the proper interlobular or collecting lymph vessels, lymph vessels related to the pulmonary vein and collecting vessels for the subpleural lymph vessels are also observed, as shown in Figs. 181 and 182.

The proper lymph vessel of the interlobular connective tissue is capillary in type and forms networks similar to the subpleural lymph capillary networks, as shown in Fig. 183.

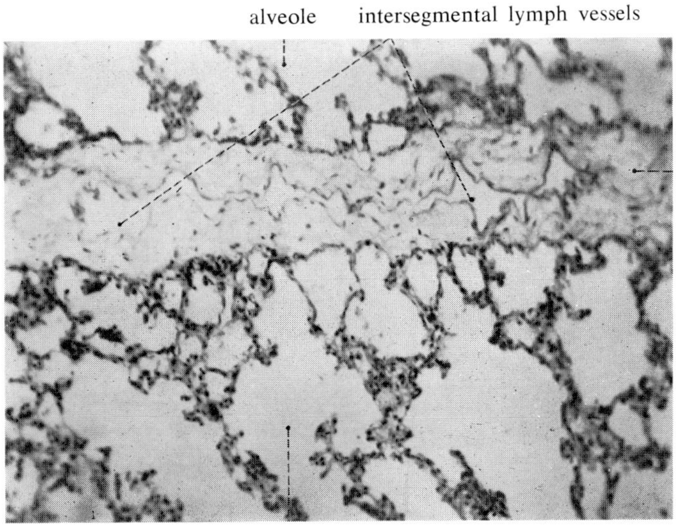

Fig. 179 Lymph vessel of the intersegmental connective tissue.

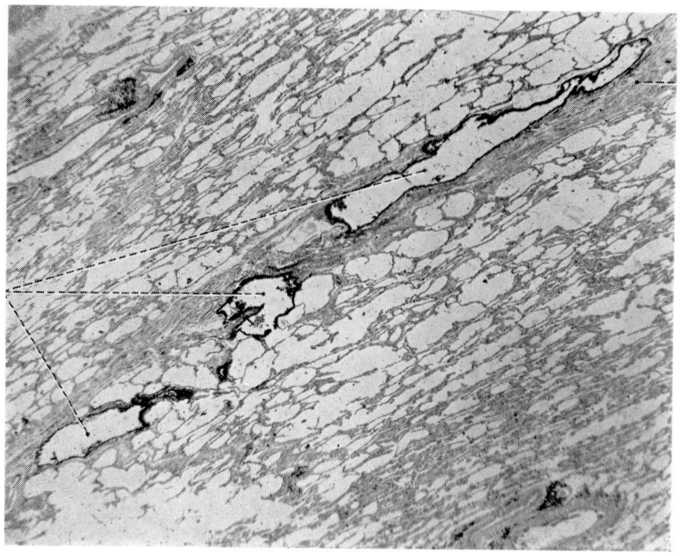

Fig. 180 Lymph vessels of the interlobular connective tissue.

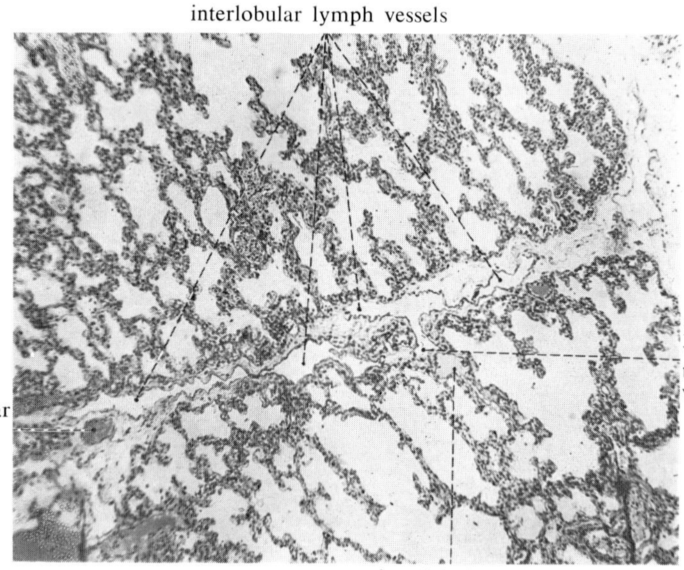

Fig. 181 Interlobular and intralobular lymph vessels.

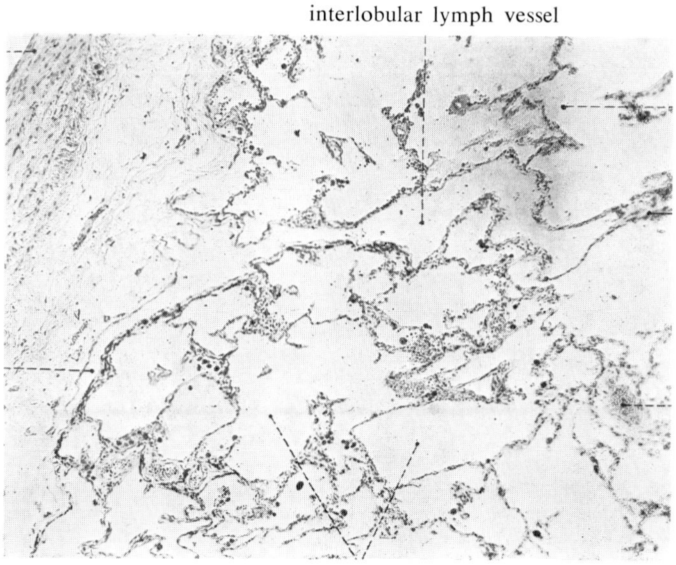

Fig. 182 Interlobular and periarterial lymph vessels.

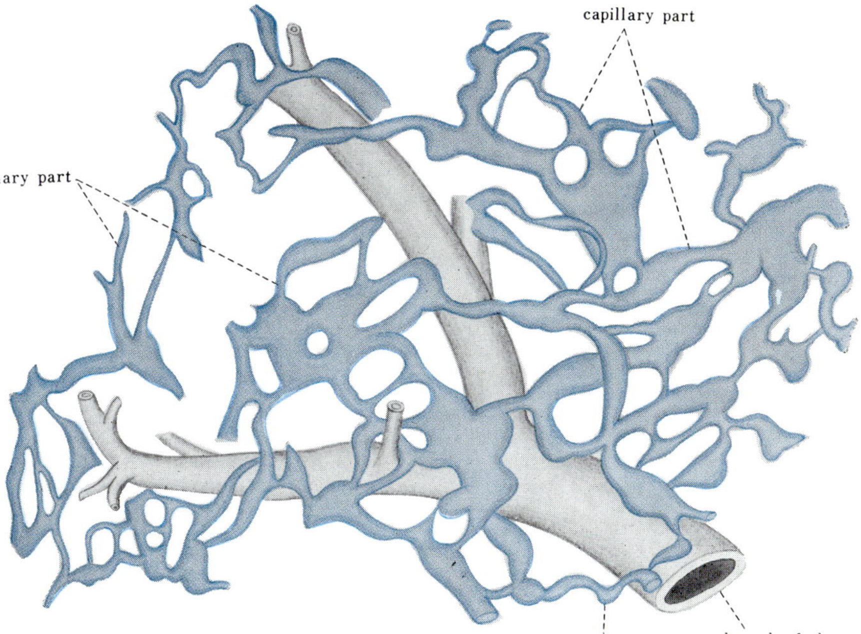

Fig. 183 Lymph vessels and pulmonary veins in the interlobular connective tissue.

In fetus and new-born the dye injected specimen shows the formation of lymph vessel network, anastomosing with the subpleural lymph vessel networks in many places. In the adult, free anastomoses are not observed except in particular regions.

Thus, the subpleural lymph of adults flows into collecting lymph vessels without causing retrograde flows; lymph, however, does not flow into the interlobular lymph capillary networks.

The interlobular pulmonary veins are accompanied by lymph vessels which are considered, from their form and arrangements, to play the role of collecting vessel for the interlobular lymph vessels. Lymph vessels accompanying large veins show the same typical shape as collecting vessels.

As explained above, in cattle, some of the collecting lymph vessels arising from the bronchial wall reach the subpleural tissues via the interlobular tissue, but in man, the existence of these collecting lymph vessels remains undemonstrated.

As will be explained later, the relationship between lymph vessels of the bronchial wall and of the region surrounding the pulmonary artery in man is more intimate; consequently, lymph flows into peribronchial or collecting lymph vessels related to the bronchus and pulmonary artery. The existence of collecting lymph vessels from bronchus to interlobular tissue can not definitely be considered to exist.

Tables 9 and 10 are schemas of lymph flow in the interlobular connective tissues of man and cattle.

3. Lymph Vessels related to Pulmonary Vein

As shown in Figs. 184 and 185, branches of intralobular veins accompany lymph vessels in many instances. Part of these are adjacent to alveolar walls. Tobin (1954) stated that the alveolar wall itself contains lymph vessels. He may have misunderstood the above findings.

The pulmonary vein is extremely small in its intralobular portions, but is relatively large in its interlobular portions; the accompanying lymph vessels also become larger, as shown in Figs. 186 and 187. Further, when veins become larger, the accompanying lymph vessel networks will also increase in number, as shown in Fig. 188.

The lymph vessels related to the pulmonary vein as shown in Fig. 189, have anastomoses in many portions with the surrounding interlobular lymph vessels.

In addition to the intralobular lymph vessels which have a general route toward the intralobular tissues, some are found to run toward the subpleural tissues.

On examining these vessels, one notes that they run to the pulmonary pleura from the intrapulmonary regions. In the normal human lung these are the only lymph vessels which proceed toward the subpleural tissue from the intrapulmonary lymph vessels.

Miller (1947) stated that the lymph vessels lying immediately beneath the pleura do not flow into the

Table 9 Lymph-flow in the interlobular lymph vessel and in the lymph vessel related to the pulmonary vein of the human lung.

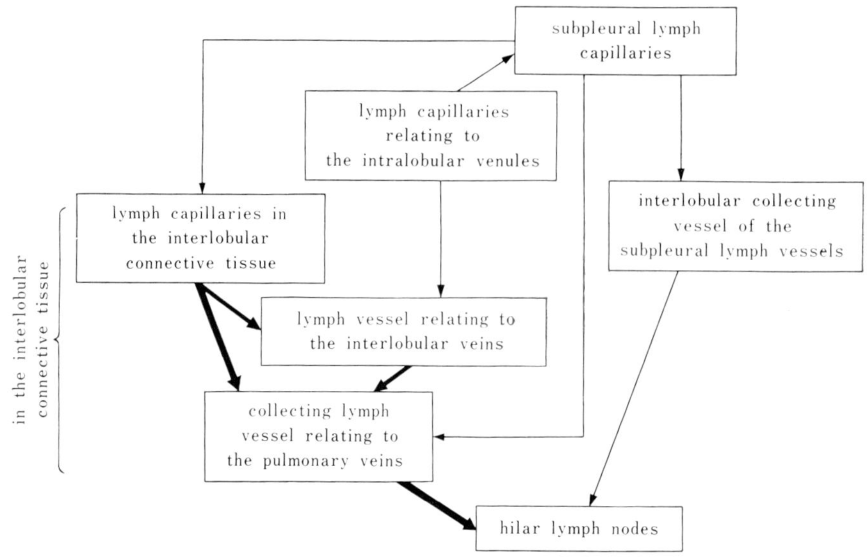

Table 10 Lymph-flow in the interlobular lymph vessel of the cattle lung.

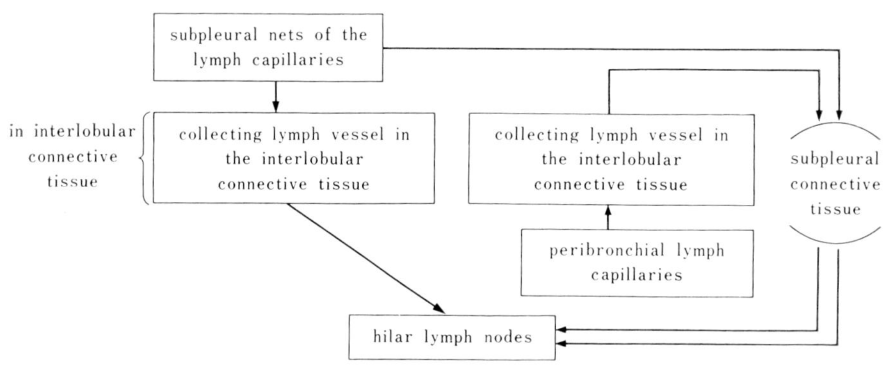

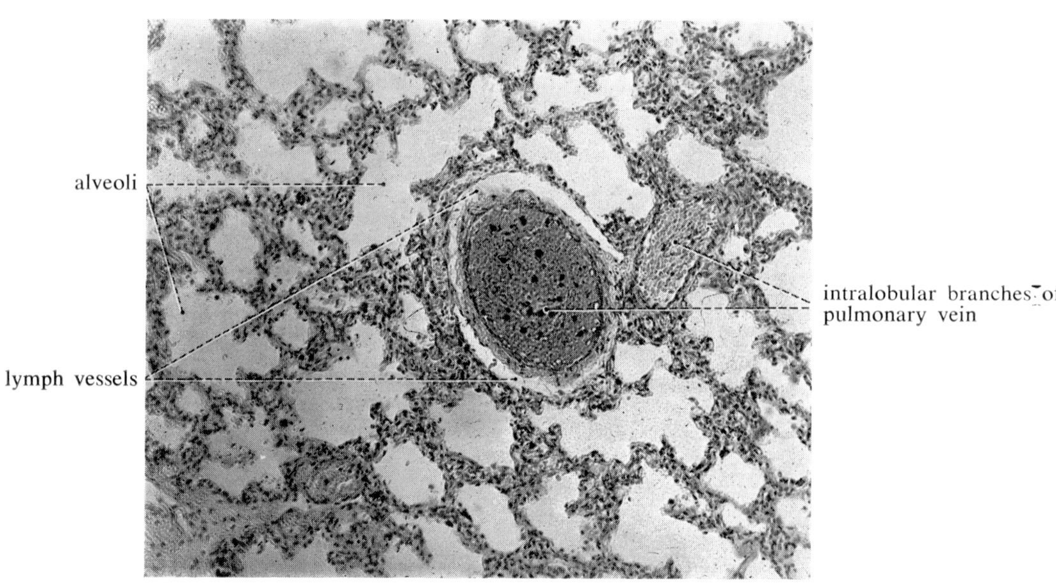

Fig. 184 Lymph vessels related to the pulmonary vein.

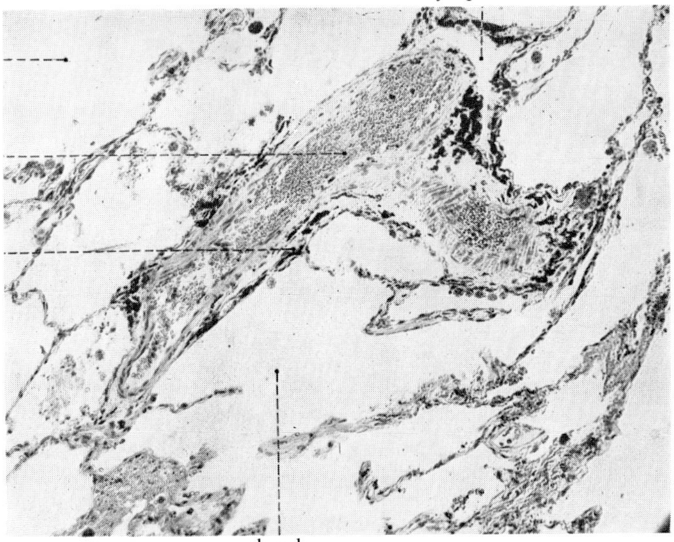

Fig. 185 Lymph vessel related to the pulmonary vein.

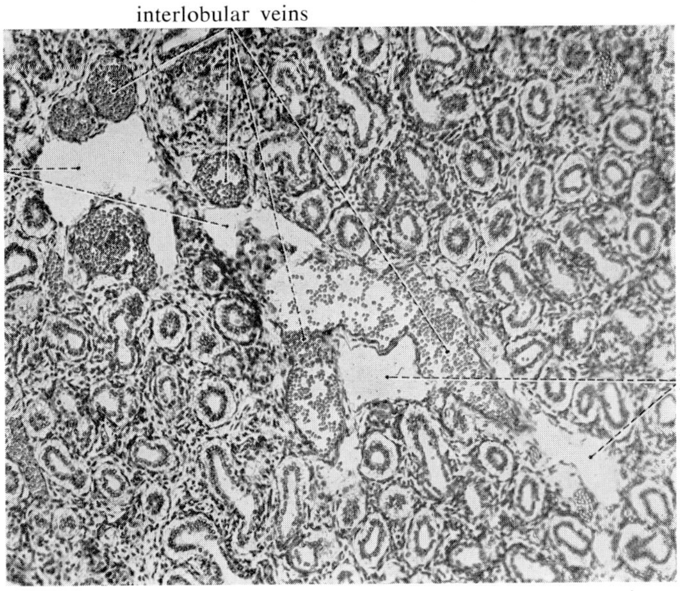

Fig. 186 Lymph vessels related to the interlobular vein in the embryo lung.

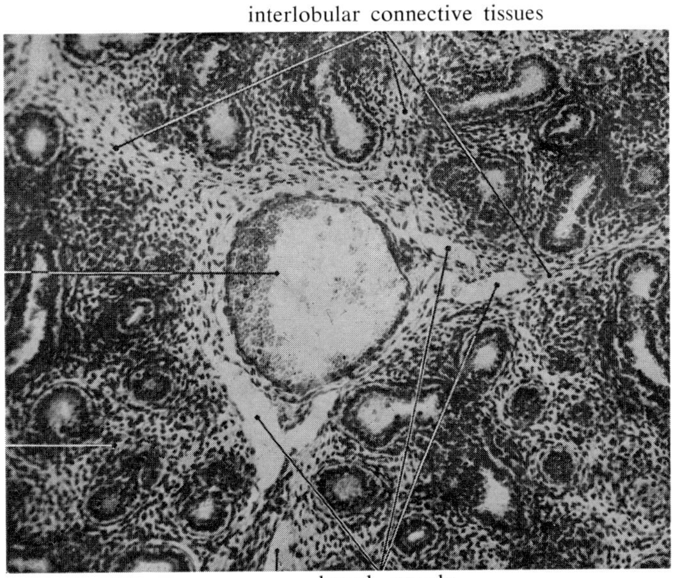

Fig. 187 Lymph vessels related to the interlobular vein.

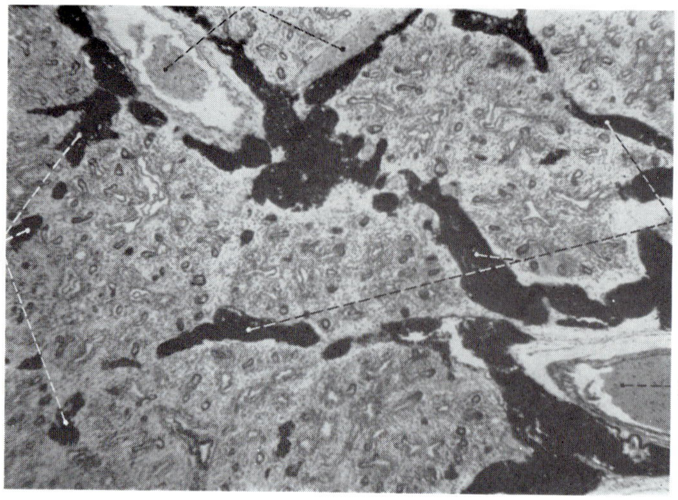

Fig. 188 Lymph vessels related to the interlobular vein.

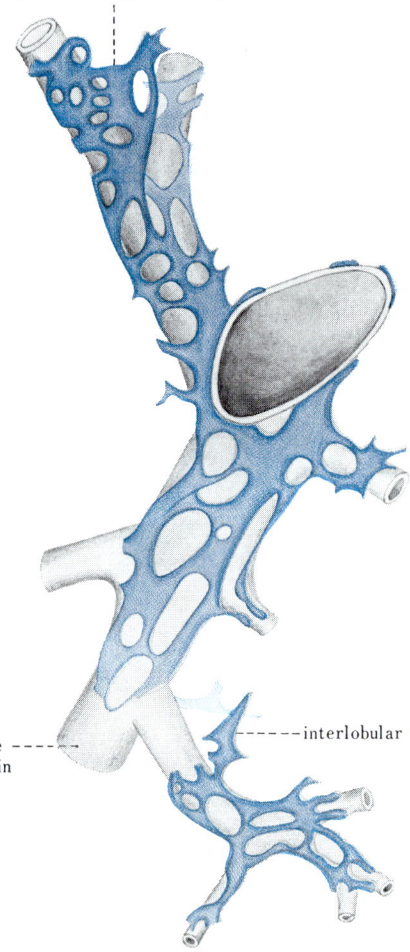

Fig. 189 Lymph vessel nets related to the pulmonary vein.

deep portion of the lung but join into the subpleural lymph vessels. This statement seems to have been made upon observation of the above lymph vessels.

It is well known that anthracosis is observed in the subpleural tissues of the human lung, but this charcoal powder deposition is too great in amount to have arisen only from the alveolar walls immediately under the pleura. It is appropriate to consider that it was carried from the depths of the lung tissue via the above-mentioned route. The deposition of charcoal powder in the subpleural tissues strongly suggests that it is carried lymphatogenously.

Table 11 is a schema showing the lymph vessels related to the pulmonary vein.

Table 11 Lymph-flow in the lymph vessels related to the branches of the pulmonary vein.

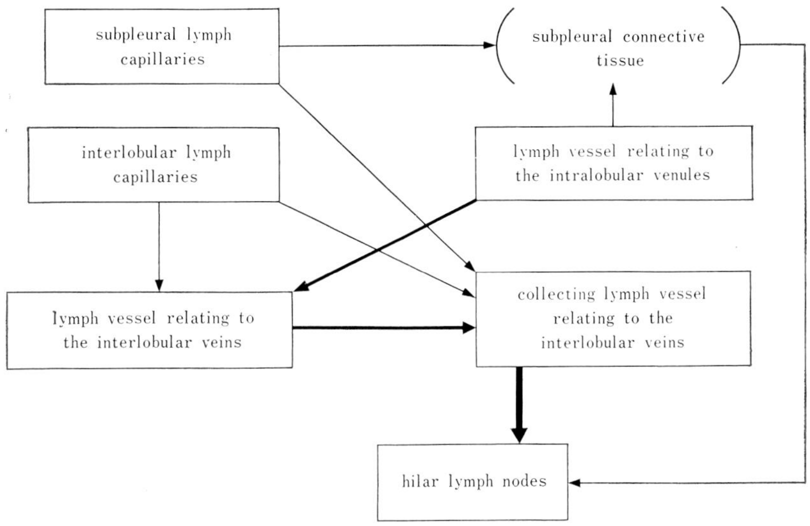

4. Lymph Vessels related to Bronchus

As shown in Figs. 190 and 191, lymph vessel networks of the bronchus of the human lung are observed in the adventitia and submucosa.

The former shown in Fig. 192 develops early in fetal life; the latter arises in later stages. The submucosal vessels are considered to be the last to develop.

Thus, the bronchi of adults are surrounded by the lymph vessels of submucous and adventitial origin.

The submucosal lymph vessels are situated between the muscular layer of mucous membrane and bronchial cartilage, as shown in Fig. 193. The submucosal vessels are of the capillary type, being extremely small, they form networks, and are devoid of valves.

Compared to the submucosal vessels, the vessels of the adventitia are larger, and form finer networks as shown in Fig. 194.

Between the above lymphatic networks many anastomoses are observed. The submucosal lymph flows into the adventitial vessels through these networks.

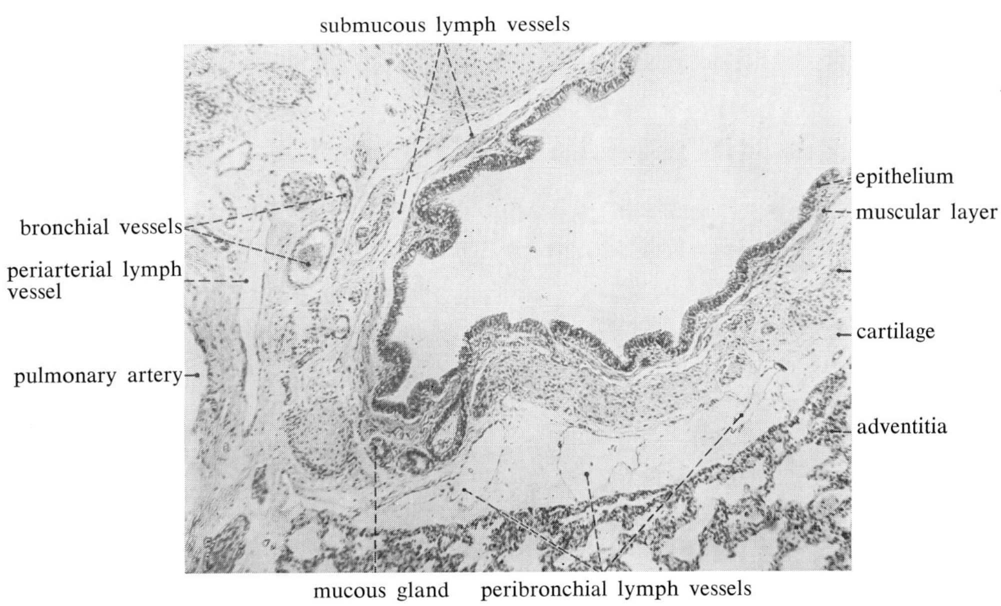

Fig. 190 Lymph vessels related to the bronchus.

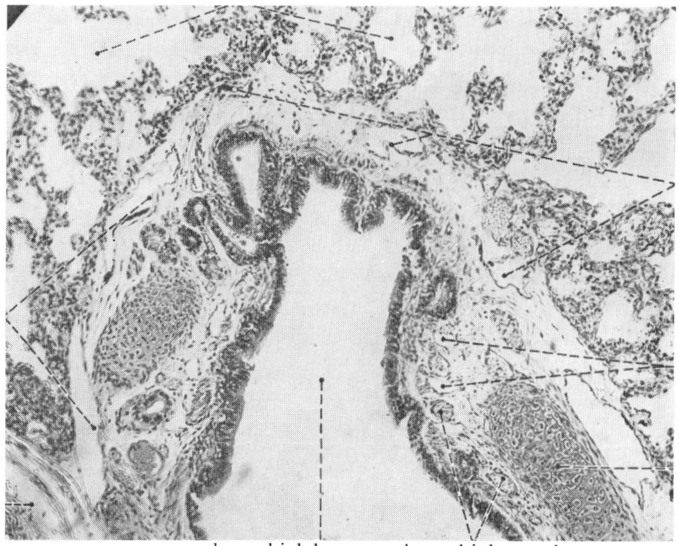

Fig. 191 Lymph vessels related to the bronchus.

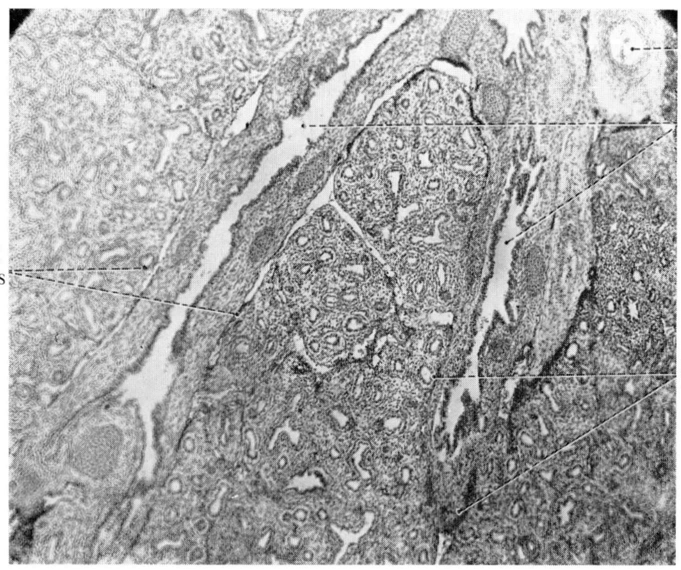

Fig. 192 Lymph vessels related to the bronchus in the human lung.

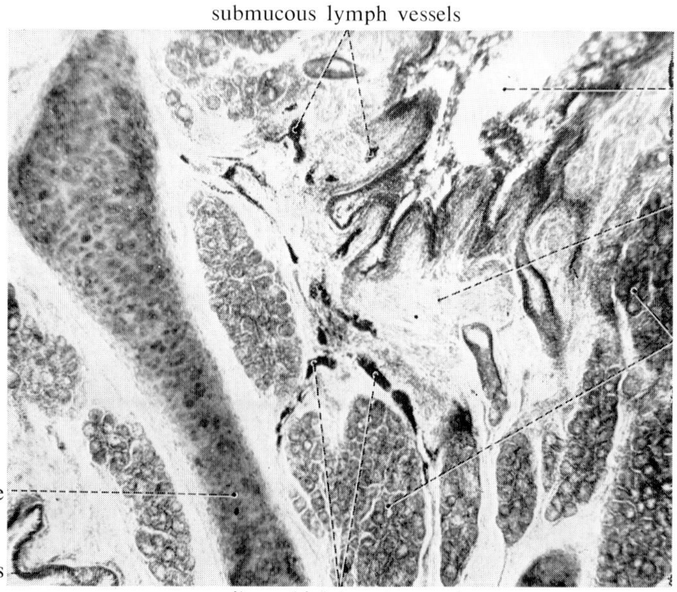

Fig. 193 Lymph vessels related to the bronchus.

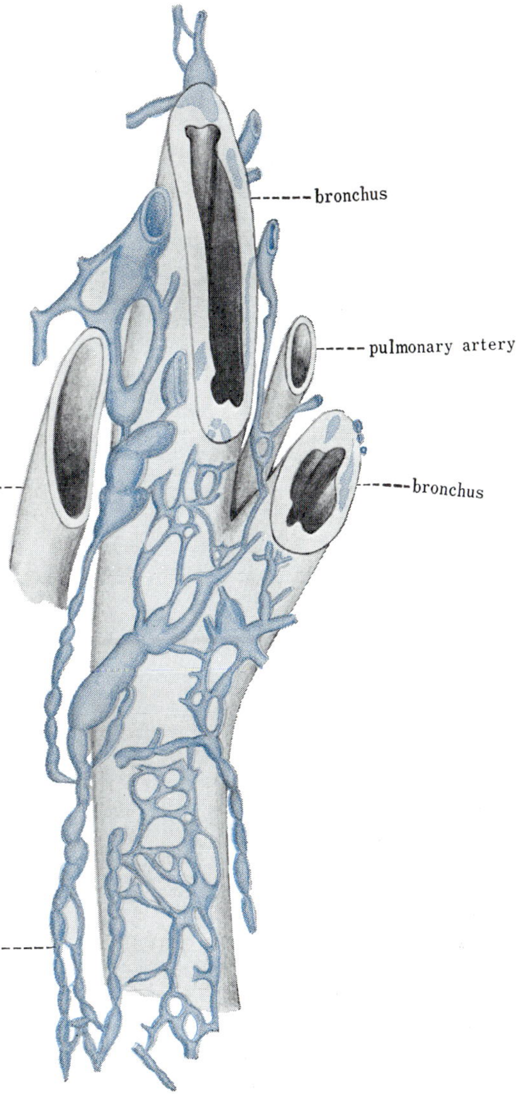

Fig. 194 Lymph vessel nets related to the bronchus (human lung).

The adventitial lymph vessels pass into one of several collecting vessels found in the connective tissue surrounding the bronchus or pulmonary artery; however, since many anastomoses are found between the lymph vessels of the adventitia and periarterial tissues, part of the lymph originating in the bronchial wall can be considered to penetrate first into the periarterial lymph vessels and then to flow into collecting lymph vessels.

Figs. 195 and 196 show histological findings of the lymph vessels related to the bronchus and pulmonary artery of the human new-born.

Fig. 197 illustrates similar findings of the guinea pig lymph vessels.

As shown in Fig. 198, the lymphatic networks of bronchi (which have cartilages in the wall) are arranged in two layers. The networks are found in a single layer in peripheral regions where the arrangement of the cartilages is loose, as shown in Fig. 199(a) and (b), and in the outermost peripheral regions, where cartilages are lacking, the lymph vessel networks are also sparse, as shown in Fig. 199(c), (d), (e), (f).

Various opinions are reported as to how lymph vessels are related to the bronchi in the most peripheral regions.

For example, WYWODZOFF (1866), SIKORSKY (1870) and KUTSUNA (1935) reported that lymph vessels of the bronchial wall extend to the most peripheral region, *i.e.*, to the alveolar wall. Later, TOBIN (1954) reported the same opinion.

Although KUTSUNA (1935) described diagrammatically the existence of lymph vessels in the alveolar wall of dog, the histological investigations by the authors (NAGAISHI and OKADA, 1958) revealed that lymph vessels could not be found in the alveolar wall of dog. Nor could electron microscopic observa-

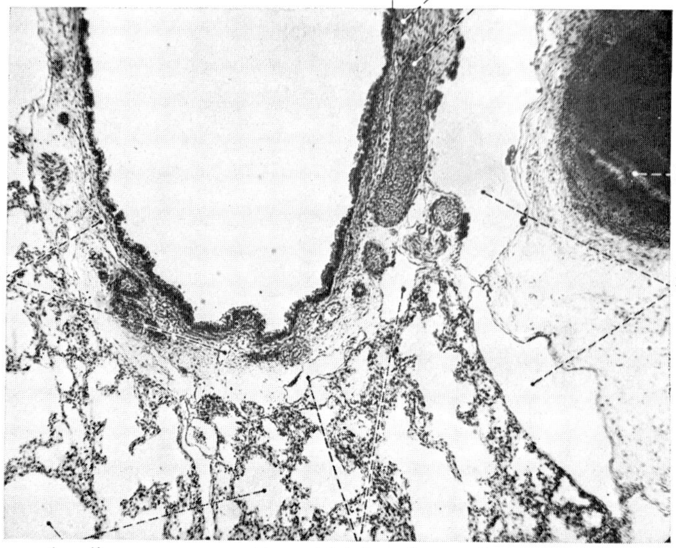

Fig. 195 Lymph vessel related to the bronchus and the pulmonary artery (human new-born).

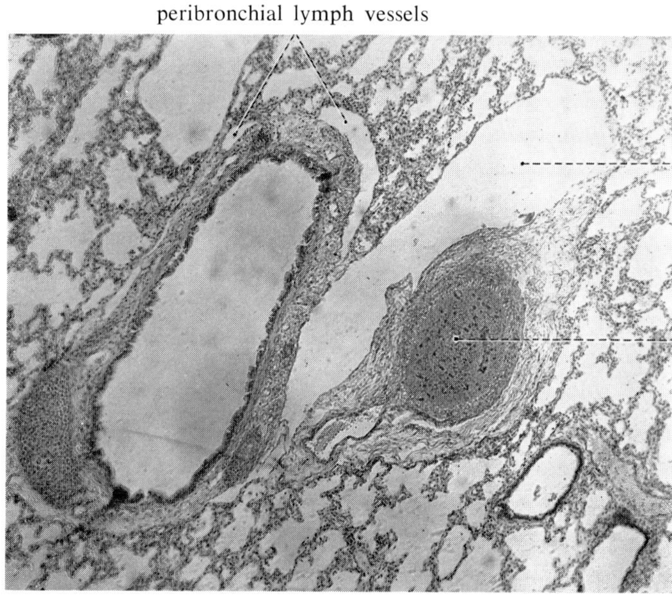

Fig. 196 Lymph vessels related to the pulmonary artery (human new-born).

tions of the human lung disclose the vessels in the alveolar wall which could be considered to be lymph vessels.

TOBIN (1954) stated, as mentioned earlier, that lymph vessels do not exist in all the alveolar walls, but that some, related to small blood vessels, were found adjacent to the alveolar wall.

The question is then, in what region can lymph vessels related to the bronchus be clearly observed? MILLER (1947) gave a definite answer to this question.

He stated clearly that lymph vessels can be observed only up to the peripheral end of the alveolar duct.

However, according to the authors' investigations on the human lung, lymph vessels extended only as far peripherally as the region between the terminal and respiratory bronchioles.

Fig. 200 (a)–(d), shows that it is perhaps better to regard the lymph vessels in this region as accompanying the adjoining pulmonary artery rather than the bronchus.

MORI (1940) carried out investigations by injecting dye solution into the lymph vessels of the bron-

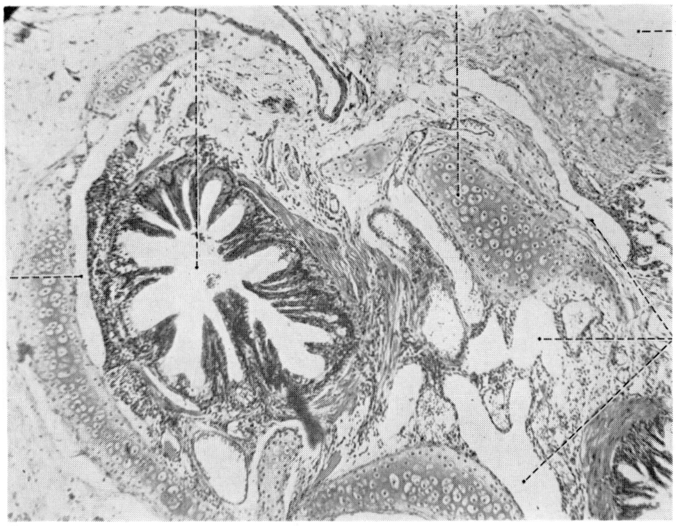

Fig. 197 Lymph vessels related to the bronchus (guinea pig).

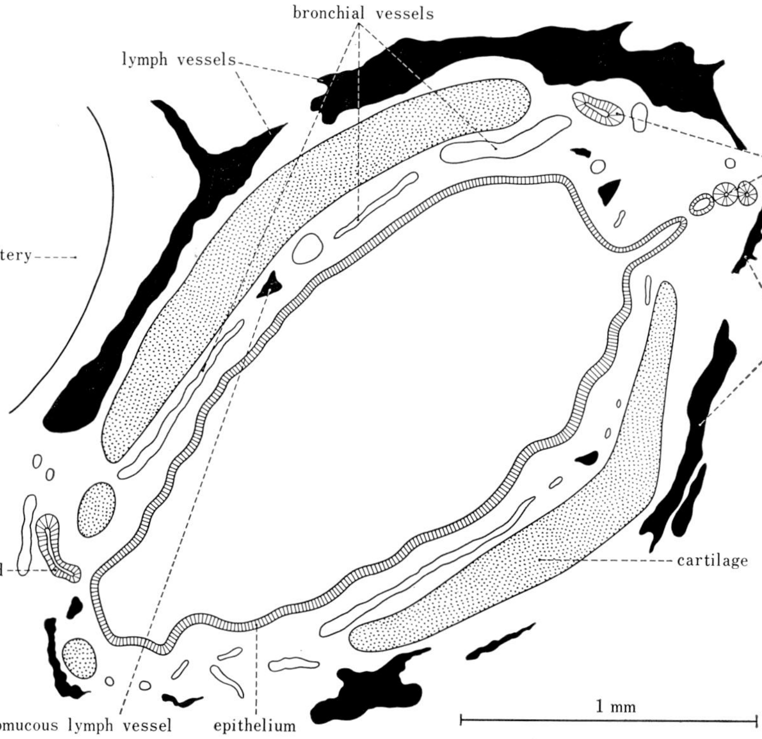

Fig. 198 Lymph vessels related to the bronchus.

chial wall of cattle, horse and pig, and claimed that he found three routes in the collecting lymph vessels in this region, *i.e.*, one arising from the bronchial wall, and proceeding toward the tissues surrounding the pulmonary artery, one which proceeds toward the tissue surrounding the pulmonary vein, and one proceeding toward the subpleural tissue via the interlobular tissues.

The authors (NAGAISHI and OKADA) confirmed MORI's experiments on the cattle lung.

As shown in Fig. 201, it is obvious that vessels from the peripheral lung frequently reach the subpleural tissue via the interlobular tissues, those from the central portions run directly toward the hilum along the bronchus, and others run along the pulmonary vein toward the subpleural tissues.

Thus in the cattle lung, unlike human lung, collecting vessels from the bronchial walls run along the pulmonary vein or interlobular tissue to the subpleural tissue.

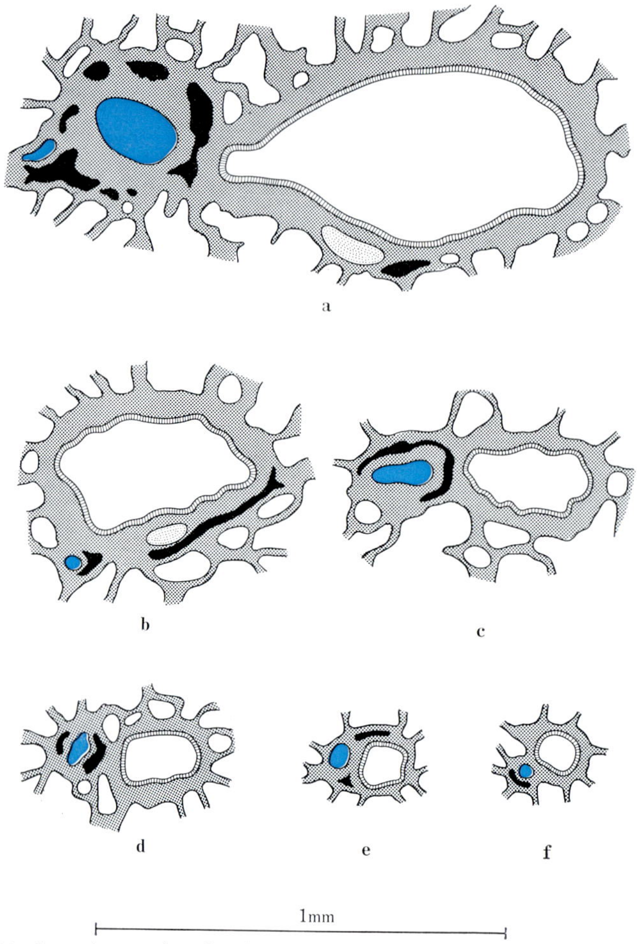

Fig. 199 Lymph vessels related to the pulmonary artery and the bronchus.

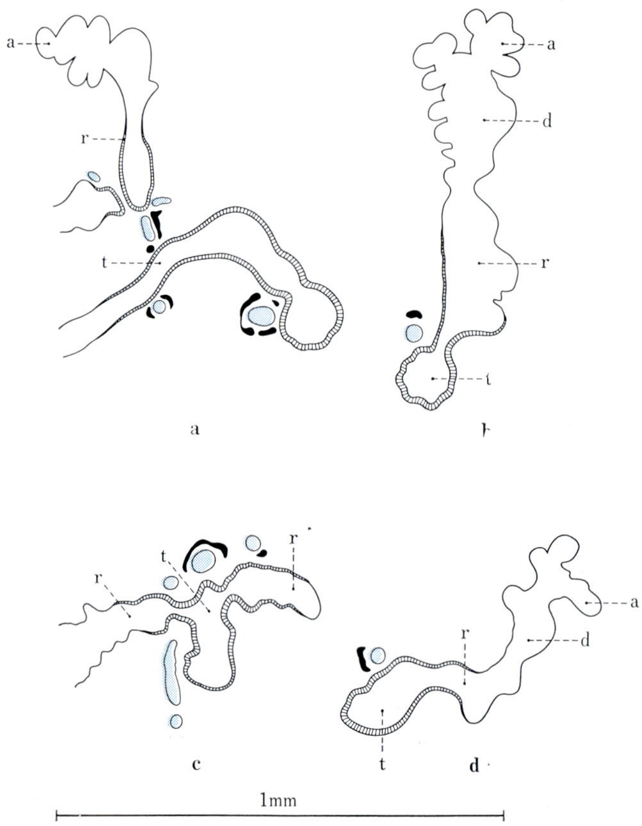

Fig. 200 Lymph vessel related to the bronchiole.
t: terminal bronchiole, r: respiratory bronchiole
d: alveolar duct, a: alveolar sac

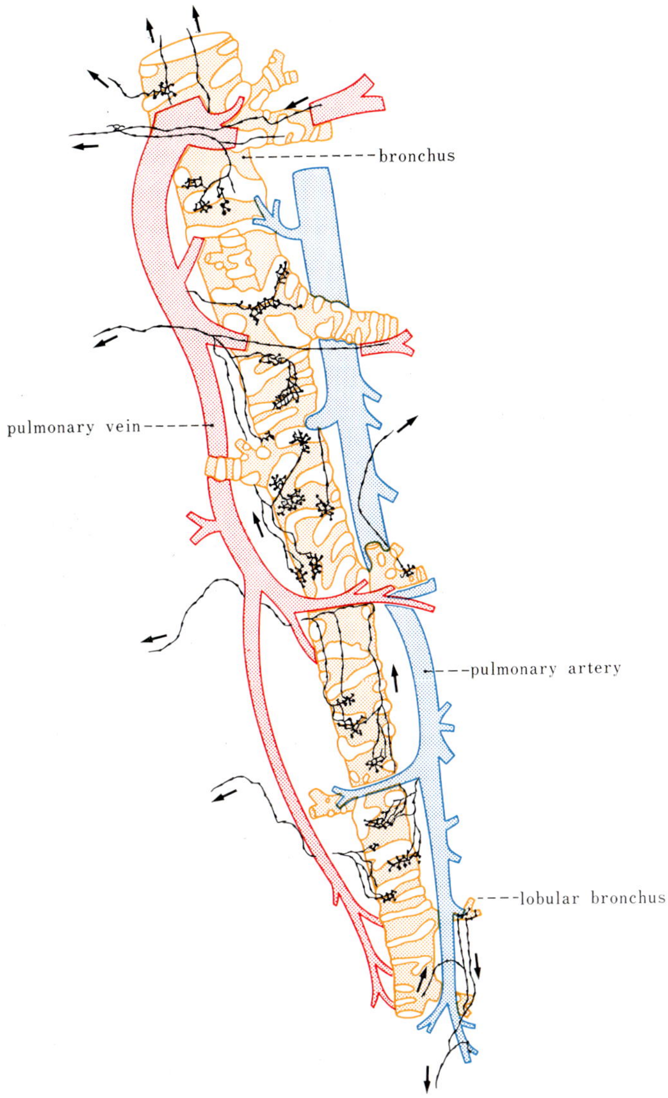

Fig. 201 Lymph vessel related to the bronchus (cattle lung).

Table 12 Peribronchial and periarterial lymph flows.

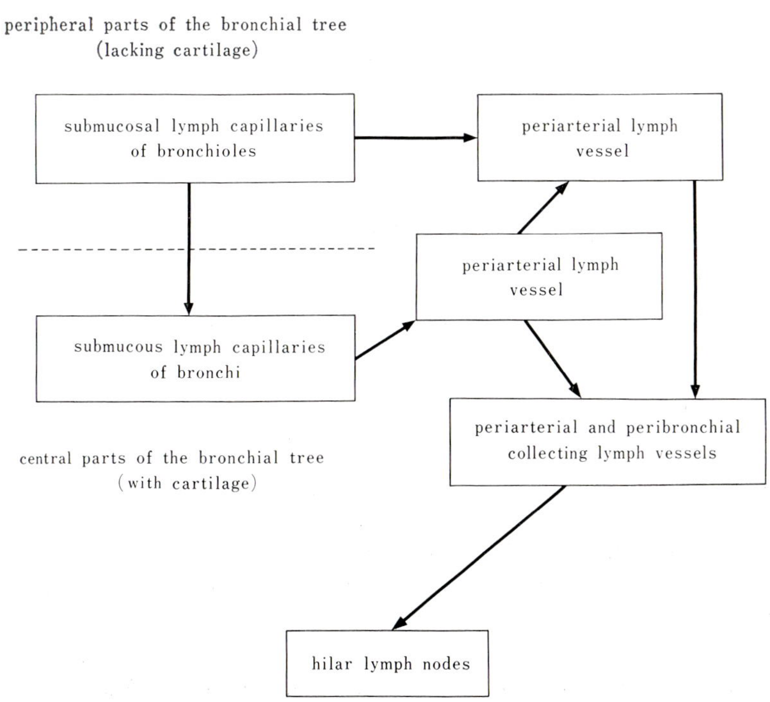

Table 12 is a schema showing the route of flow in the lymph vessels related to the pumlonary artery and in the vessels related to the bronchus in the human lung.

5. Lymph Vessels related to Pulmonary Artery

In regions close to the central portion of the pulmonary artery the lymph vessel networks show marked development in the immediate area, giving the impression that the pulmonary artery is floating in a large lymph space, as shown in Figs. 202, 203, and 204.

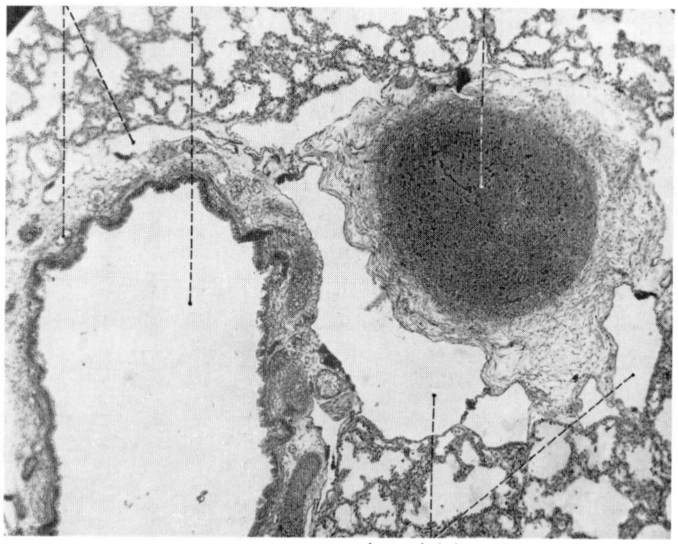

Fig. 202 Lymph vessel realted to the pulmonary artery.

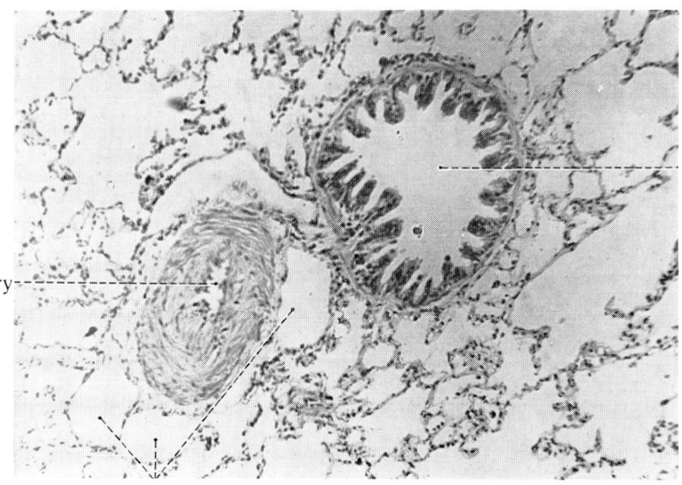

Fig. 203 Lymph vessel related to the pulmonary artery.

HAYEK (1953) designated the lymph vessels of the tissues surrounding the pulmonary artery as "periarterialle Lymphräume", and stated that this specialization acts as a buffer zone, protecting the pulmonary artery against outside influences, such as those resulting from respiratory movements.

In peripheral regions, as shown in Fig. 205, the bronchus and the pulmonary artery are surrounded by a single layer of lymph vessel networks, which anastomose with each other.

Figs. 206 and 207 present histological findings of the lymph vessels related to the pulmonary artery in fetal life. As will be seen, the lymph vessels surrounding the pulmonary artery are better developed than those surrounding the bronchus, even in fetal life.

As noted above, the lymph vessels related to the pulmonary artery are observed to run to the outermost peripheral regions, as compared with those related to the bronchi. According to the investigations

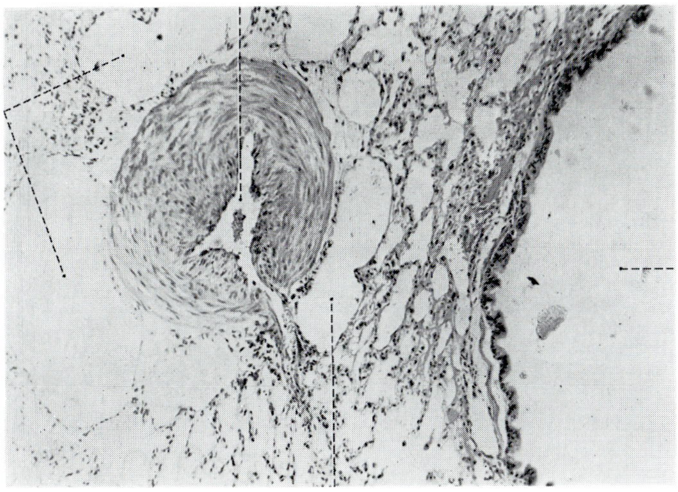

Fig. 204 Lymph vessel related to the pulmonary artery (rabbit lung).

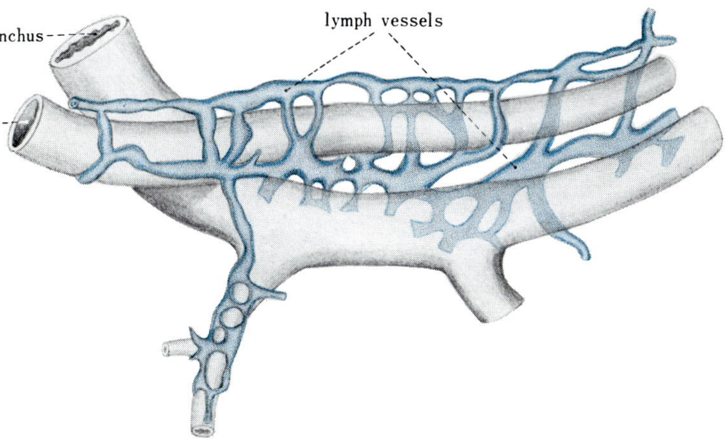

Fig. 205 Lymph vessel nets related to the bronchus and the pulmonary artery (human lung).

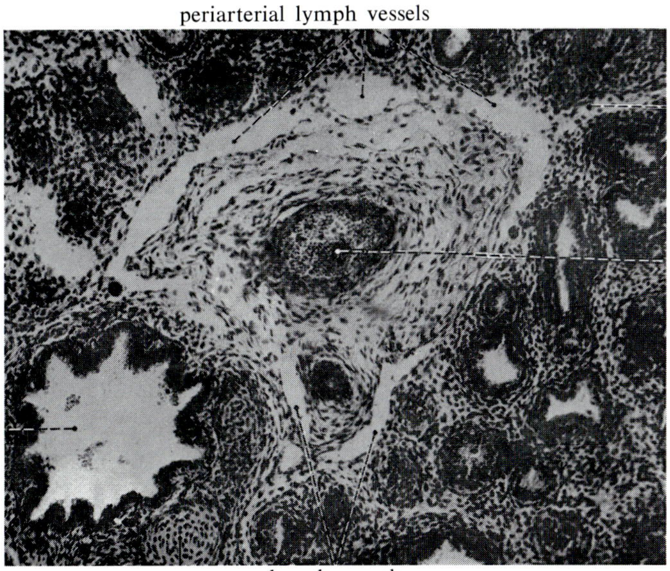

Fig. 206 Periarterial lymph vessel in the lung of the human embryo.

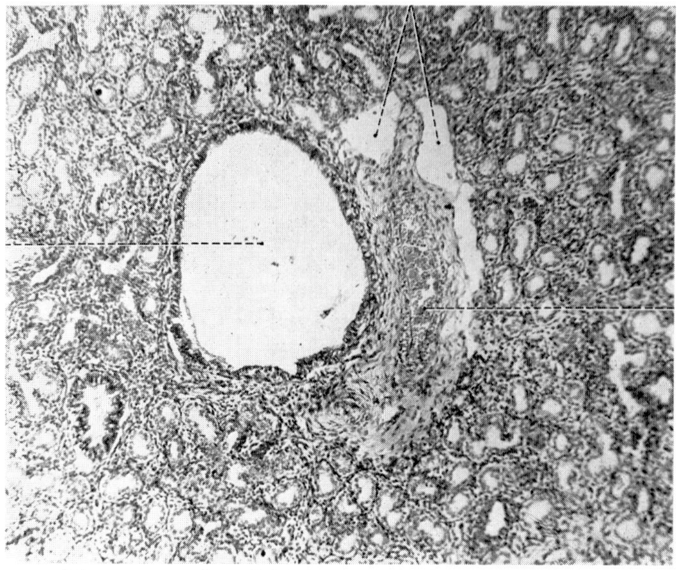

Fig. 207 Periarterial lymph vessel in the lung of the human embryo.

carried out by the authors, the former principally, are observed to extend as far as the region of the terminal bronchioles. Depending on the specimen, they sometimes extend to the respiratory bronchiole, as shown in Fig. 208.

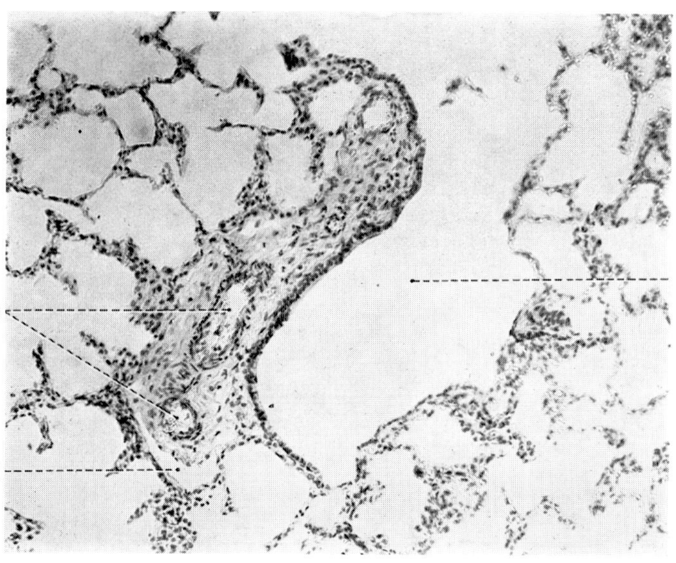

Fig. 208 Lymph vessel related to the small branch of the pulmonary artery.

6. Classification of Pulmonary Lymph Vessels according to Lymph Flow

In general, lymph vessels are well developed in regions with abundant connective tissues.

As shown in Fig. 209, this relation holds in the case of the lung, and lymph vessels are observed to have developed markedly in the regions with abundant connective tissues, such as the subpleural and interlobular tissues, and surrounding the pulmonary artery and vein, and about the bronchus.

The connective tissues in these regions can also be divided into those in the mesenchyma (*i.e.*, subpleural, interlobular, and surrounding the pulmonary vein), and those in the parenchyma of the lung (*i.e.*, surrounding the bronchus and the pulmonary artery).

The lymph vessels in these regions are also considered, from the direction of their lymph flow, to belong to different systems.

For this reason, the authors (NAGAISHI and OKADA) have classified the lymph vessels of the lung as

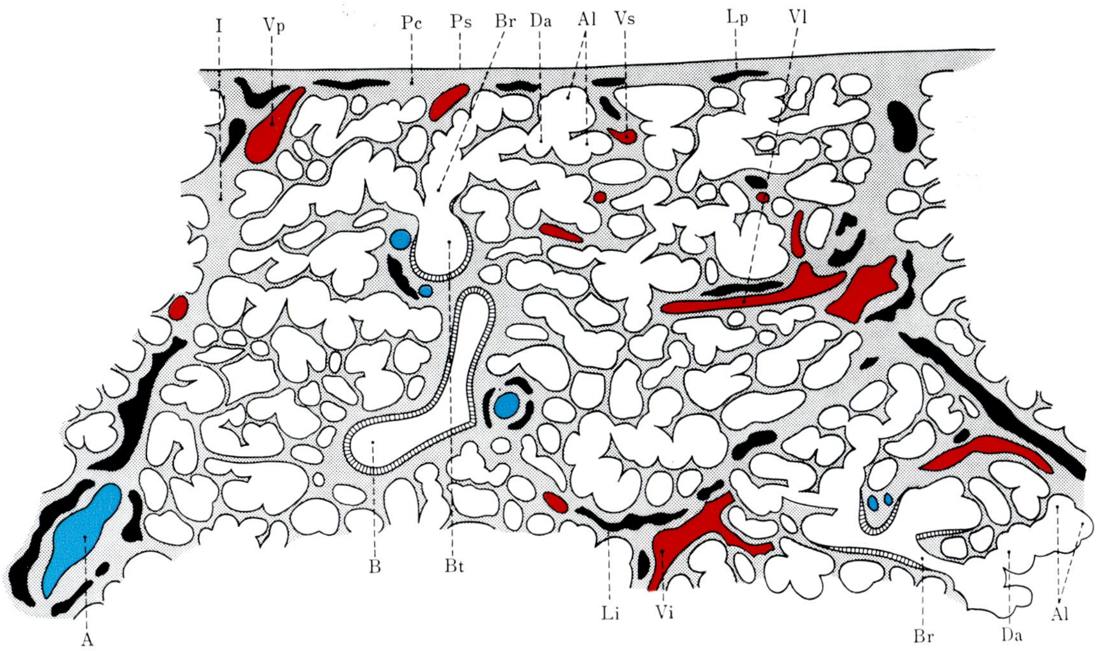

Fig. 209 Distribution of lymph vessel in the pulmonary lobule.

I: interlobular connective tissue, Vp: interlobular vein, Pc: subpleural connective tissue, Ps: pleura, Br: respiratory bronchus, Al: alveole, Da: Alveolar cuct, Lp; subpleural lymph vessel, Vs: intralobular vein emptying into the subpleural vein, Vl: intralobular vein, A: pulmonary artery, B; bronchus, Bt: terminal bronchus, Li: interlobular lymph vessel, Br: bronchus, Da: alveolar duct

broncho-arterial and interstitial-venous; in simplified terms these are called "parenchymal" and "interstitial" lymph vessels.

Table 13 shows a classification of the lymph vessels of the lung. In Fig. 210 distribution of the lymph vessels is shown in a three-dimensional schema.

Table 13 Pulmonary lymph vessel.

- interstitial-venous lymph vessel (interstitial lymph vessel)
  - subpleural lymph vessel
  - lymph vessel in the interlobular connective tissue
  - lymph vessel related to the pulmonary vein
- bronchio-arterial lymph vessel (parenchymal lymph vessel)
  - lymph vessel related to the bronchus
    - submucous lymph vessel
    - lymph vessel in the bronchial adventitia
  - lymph vessel related to the pulmonary artery

F. Lymphatic Region of Lung

To which lymph nodes will the lymph, originating in the intrapulmonary tissues, flow? The question of the specificity of direction of lymph flow is closely related to the direction of spread of such diseases as pulmonary tuberculosis and lung cancer, etc.

SHIDA (1932) examined the rabbit and cat lungs and stated that the regional lymph nodes included the aortic, innominate vein angle, paratracheal, and tracheobronchial lymph nodes. The lymph of the lung predominantly flows into these lymph nodes, whereas lymph from extra-pulmonary regions of the thoracic cavity flows independently into other lymph nodes.

However, the lymph of the lung does not flow only into the above lymph nodes.

As stated by BAUM (1926), in cattle, horse, pig or dog, some efferent lymph vessels are found to run toward abdominal lymph nodes.

This can readily be appreciated from the fact that the lymph vessels of the lung arise embryologically from the retroperitoneal lymph sac, and not only from the thoracic and right lymphatic trunk.

It is quite interesting that similar findings are observed for the human lung, as will be explained later.

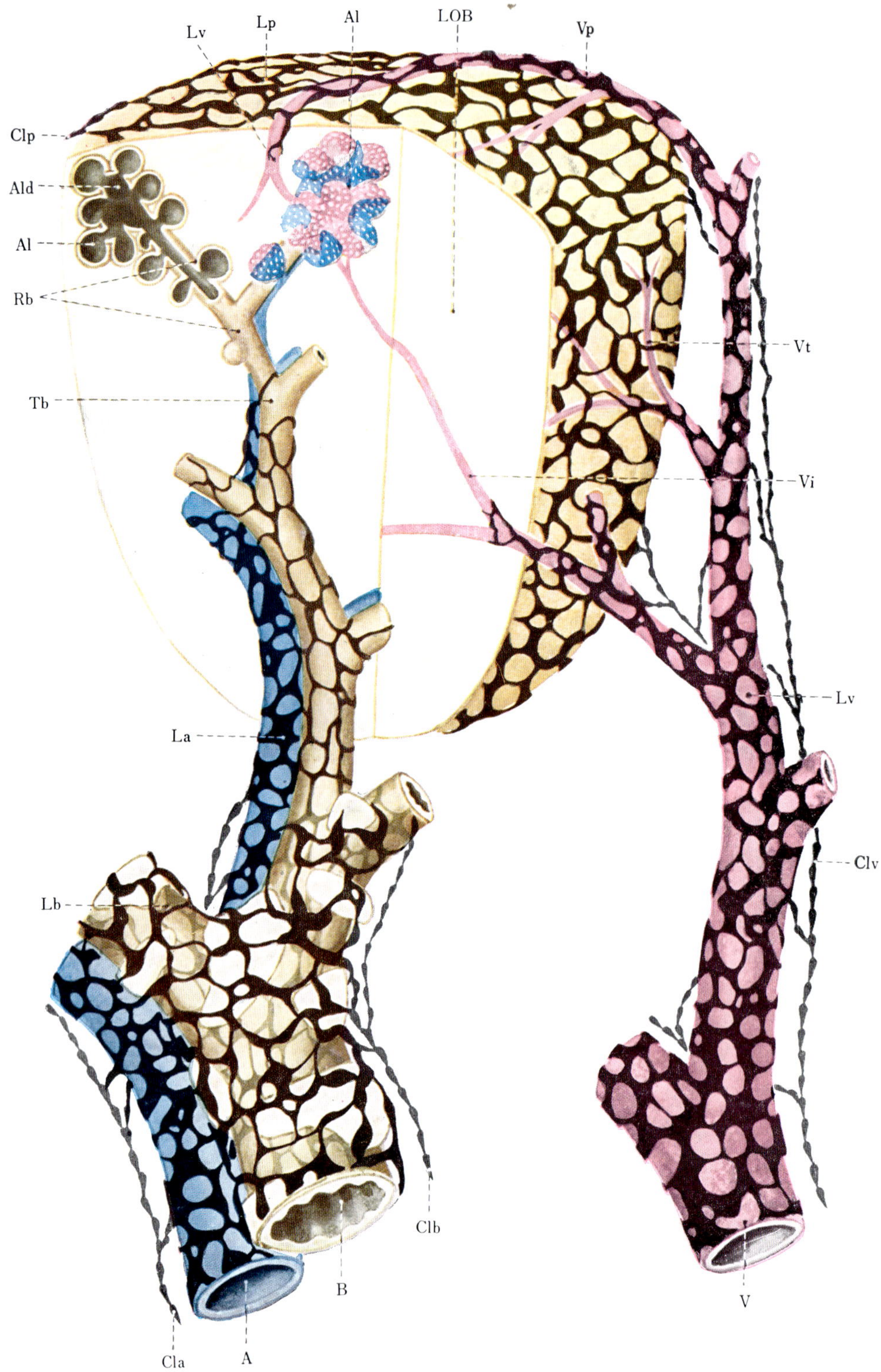

Fig. 210 Distribution of the pulmonary lymph vessels.
A: pulmonary artery, Al: alveole, Ald: alveolar duct, B: bronchus, Rb: respiratory bronchiole, Tb: terminal bronchiole, Cla: collecting lymph vessel related to the pulmonary artery, CLb: collecting lymph vessel related to the bronchus, Clp: subpleural collecting lymph vessel, Clv: collecting lymph vessel related to the pulmonary vein, La: periarterial lymph vessel, Lb: peribronchial lymph vessel, LOB: lobule, Lp: subpleural lymph vessel, Lv: perivenous lymph vessel, V: pulmonary vein, Vi: intralobular branches of the pulmonary vein, Vp: subpleural branches of the pulmonary vein, Vt: interlobular branches of the pulmonary vein.

As to the lymphatic drainage areas of the human lung, various investigations will be described in the following brief history.

Of these investigations, the studies of OKA (1929) on the role of the hilar lymph nodes in the primary complex of tuberculosis, and those of SHIMAZAKI (1931) and ROUVIÈRE (1932) using dye injection methods, are highly valued.

Based on abundant clinical experience and pathological data, H. OKA (1929) schematized the hilar lymph nodes as shown in Table 14; and ROUVIÈRE concisely reported on the lymphatic regions of the lung, based on 200 autopsies.

Table 14 Efferent lymph flows from lungs and their regional lymph nodes (OKA, H. 1929).

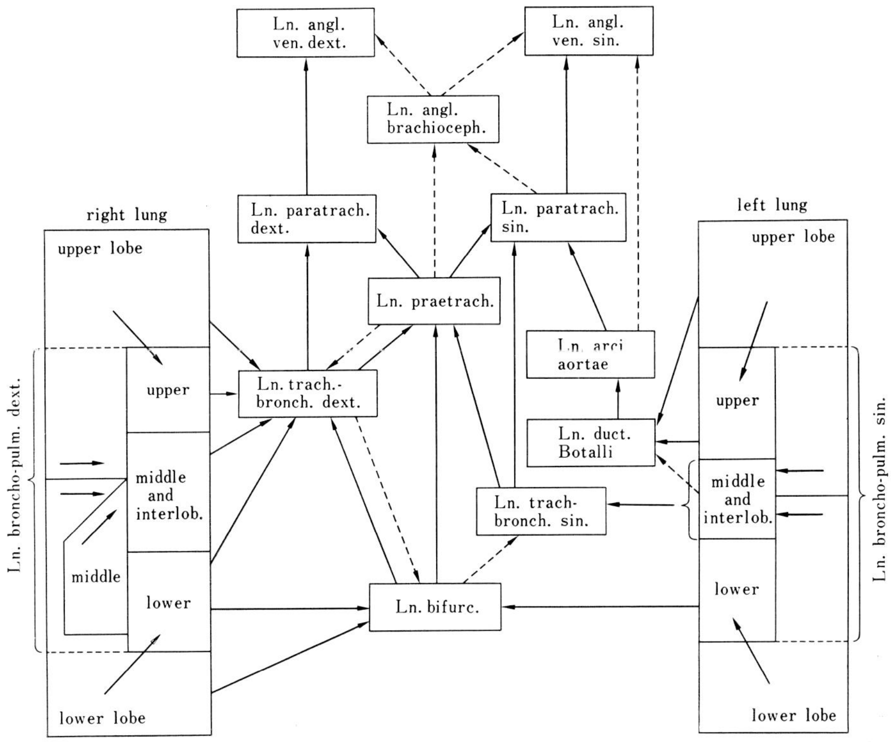

However, as to the exact details, all investigations were not of the same opinion. Particularly as to the description of the lymphatic regions, each investigator described these in his own way. Descriptions of the borders of each region frequently contain certain degrees of obscurity.

One reason is that in the lymphatic system the injection of dye solution from the center to the periphery is impossible; another is that many variations exist in the patterns of lymph vessels.

The author will here describe the lymphatic regions of the lobes of the lung based on the above studies and on his group's investigations. Although fundamental principles are stressed, it must be kept in mind that there are many variations in the lymphatic drainage system.

1. Right Lung

a. Upper Lobe

SHIMAZAKI (1931) investigated the lymphatic drainage patterns of the right upper lobe. The lymph from the mediastinal surface of the lung flows into the right paratracheal and venous angle nodes via the right tracheobronchial node; the lymph from the pleural surface flows to the tracheal bifurcation node or to the right paratracheal node; the lymph from the posterosuperior region of the interlobar surface of the right upper lobe flows to the bifurcation node via the right bronchopulmonary lymph node; the lymph from the anteroinferior region of the interlobar surface of the right upper lobe flows to the tracheobronchial node via the upper part of the right bronchopulmonary node, and lymph from the deep portion of the lung takes the same route as that from the interlobar surface.

ROUVIÈRE (1932) divided the lymphatic region of the right upper lobe broadly into the anteroinferior and posterolateral portions, and stated that the lymph coming from the former flows into the right paratracheal lymph node and from the latter into the right paratracheal or bifurcation lymph nodes. OKA (1929) stated that the lymph of the right upper lobe flows into the right tracheobronchial node either directly or via the bronchopulmonary node and then runs to the right paratracheal node.

As will be seen from the above, only one part of the lymph which originates in the right upper lobe flows to the tracheal bifurcation node.

b. Middle Lobe

OKA (1929) stated that the lymph of the middle lobe does not flow to the tracheal bifurcation node, but SHIMAZAKI (1931) claimed that middle lobe lymph runs to the right paratracheal node via the bronchopulmonary node, or via the right tracheobronchial or tracheal bifurcation lymph node.

Thus, their views are in accord on the point that the middle lobe lymph finally flows to the right paratracheal node.

c. Lower Lobe

SHIMAZAKI (1931) stated that the lymph from the diaphragmatic and costal surfaces flows into the tracheal bifurcation node, and the lymph of the interlobar surface and deep portion flows to the tracheal bifurcation lymph node or to the right tracheobronchial node.

His results almost coincide with those of OKA and ROUVIÈRE.

It seems certain that much of the lymph flows into the tracheal bifurcation node; however, FRANKE (1912) and SHIMAZAKI (1931) stated that in addition to the lymph drainage to the hilar node, some was observed to descend in the pulmonary ligament from the diaphragmatic surface of the lower lobe and to flow into the node in the region of the inferior vena caval opening.

FRANKE (1912) attributed certain abdominal symptoms in pneumonia to the above-mentioned lymphatic route.

A part from its clinical significance, the observation of such a lymphatic route is quite interesting from both the embryological and the comparative anatomical points of view.

Besides the above, some lymph from the lower lobe flows into the node of the pulmonary ligament.

2. Left Lung

a. Upper Lobe

The observation that most of the lymph of the upper part of the left lobe runs into the left paratracheal lymph node (via the node of Botallo's ligament) and to the aortic arch node has been verified by several investigators.

SHIMAZAKI (1931) stated that the lymph from the anteroinferior portion of the mediastinal surface, from the costal and interlobar surfaces, and from the deep portions of the lung, flows to the left tracheobronchial or to the tracheal bifurcation node. ROUVIÈRE (1932) also stated that a part of the lymph of the inferior portion of the upper lobe runs to the left paratracheal node, and some flows to the tracheal bifurcation lymph node.

OKA (1929) did not mention the route from the left upper lobe to the tracheal bifurcation lymph node; however, he stated that the lymph of the inferior portion of the upper lobe runs mainly to the right tracheobronchial lymph node.

In short, most of the lymph of the upper part of the left upper lobe flows into the left paratracheal node via the above-mentioned routes, and that from the lower part run into the left tracheobronchial node, excepting that which runs into the tracheal bifurcation node.

b. Lower Lobe

Lymph from the left lower lobe runs primarily to the tracheal bifurcation node.

From the lower lobe there is also a route running to the lymph node of the pulmonary ligament.

SHIMAZAKI (1931) stated that the lymph from the interlobar surface of the lower lobe, from the upper part of the costal surfaces, and from a small portion of the deep portion of the lung may occasionally run to the left tracheobronchial node.

G. Lymph Flow from Parietal Pleura and Diaphragm

The lymph vessels of the parietal pleura form fine networks in the subpleural region and flow into the collecting vessels of the intercostal spaces. These collecting vessels number one or two for each space.

The lymph flow from the parietal pleura flows in different directions, according to the region of origin.

The lymph originating in the regions anterior to the anterior axillary line flows anteriorly, and via the anterior intercostal lymph nodes, the internal mammary nodes and substernal nodes into the venous angle.

The lymph originating in the region posterior to the anterior axillary line flows posteriorly, and via the posterior intercostal and prevertebral lymph nodes, into the thoracic duct and then into the venous angle.

However, the lymph flow from the first and the second intercostal spaces usually runs into the supraclavicular nodes.

The lymph flow originating in the diaphragm runs in different directions according to the region of origin.

The lymph originating in the anterior region of the diaphragm flows anteriorly via the anterior diaphragmatic nodes, which are located on the anterior edge of the diaphragm; the flow then runs to the internal mammary vessels which run along the edges of the posterior wall of the sternum, or via the sternal lymph vessels, where it flows into the venous angle of the same side, as shown in Fig. 211 (a).

The lymph originating in the posterior region of the diaphragm takes a different course from the above. In many instances the vessels perforate the muscle, or pass through the esophageal or aortic openings, and run to the retroperitoneal nodes or to the lymph nodes situated along the lesser curvature of the stomach or the pancreas, as shown in Fig. 211 (b).

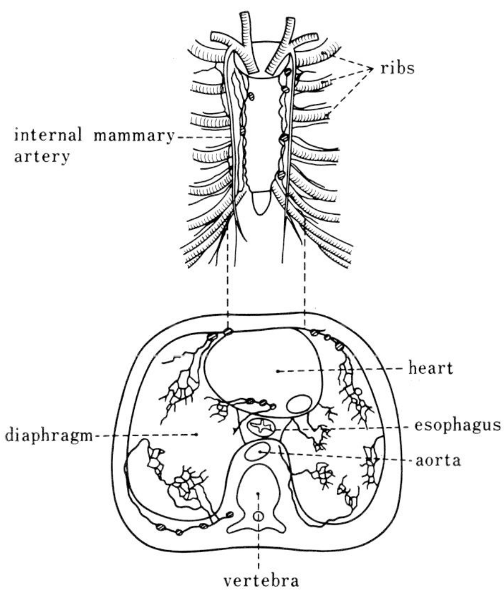

Fig. 211 a Lymph-flow from the anterior portion of the diaphragm.

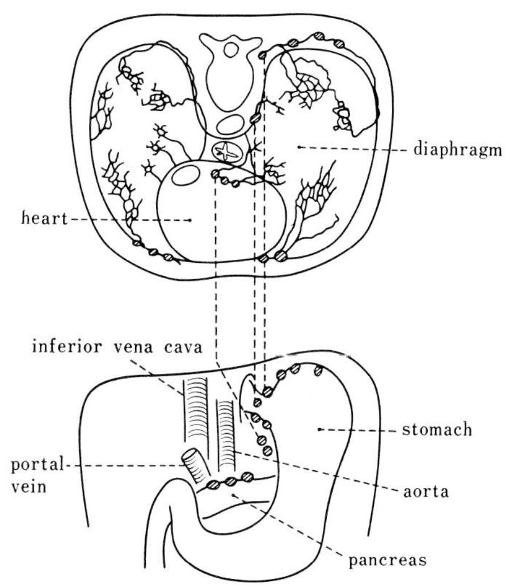

Fig. 211 b Lymph-flow from the posterior portion of the diaphragm.

Some of the lymph flows medially along the posterior border of the diaphragm and enters the thoracic duct via prevertebral lymph nodes.

In view of the above, it is not unexpected that a tumor in the neighborhood of the diaphragm may have either a thoracic or an abdominal metastatic extension.

H. Routes of Efferent Lymph Flow

The efferent lymph flow runs via the regional bronchopulmonary nodes of the respective pulmonary lobes to the nodes of the trancheal bifurcation, or to the right and left tracheobronchial lymph nodes. The route from these lymph nodes to the right and left venous angles runs in two ways, as shown in Fig. 212. One route ascends along the bronchus and via the paratracheal lymph node, running to the venous angle. NAGAISHI and OKADA called it the paratracheal route.

The right paratracheal route arises from the right tracheobronchial or tracheal bifurcation lymph nodes, and, passing through the right paratracheal lymph node and deep cervical nodes, runs into the right venous angle. The left paratracheal route arises from the left tracheobronchial or the tracheal bifurcation lymph nodes and reaches the left venous angle via the left paratracheal lymph node and the deep cervical lymph node.

Another route does not pass through the paratracheal lymph nodes. Slight differences are observed in the right and the left of this route.

The right route arises from the bifurcation or the right tracheobronchial lymph nodes, and, passing the innominate vein angle nodes, reaches the venous angle. This is called the innominate vein angle route. The left arises from the tracheobronchial node (or Botallo's node), and passing through the aortic arch lymph nodes, reaches the left venous angle. This is called the aortic arch route.

Observation of the efferent lymph flow in each pulmonary lobe reveals that, as shown in Fig. 213, the lymph from the right upper lobe flows to the tracheobronchial lymph nodes or to the upper part of the tracheal bifurcation nodes via the bronchopulmonary nodes at the root of the upper lobe bronchus; taking the right paratracheal route the flow is then to the right venous angle.

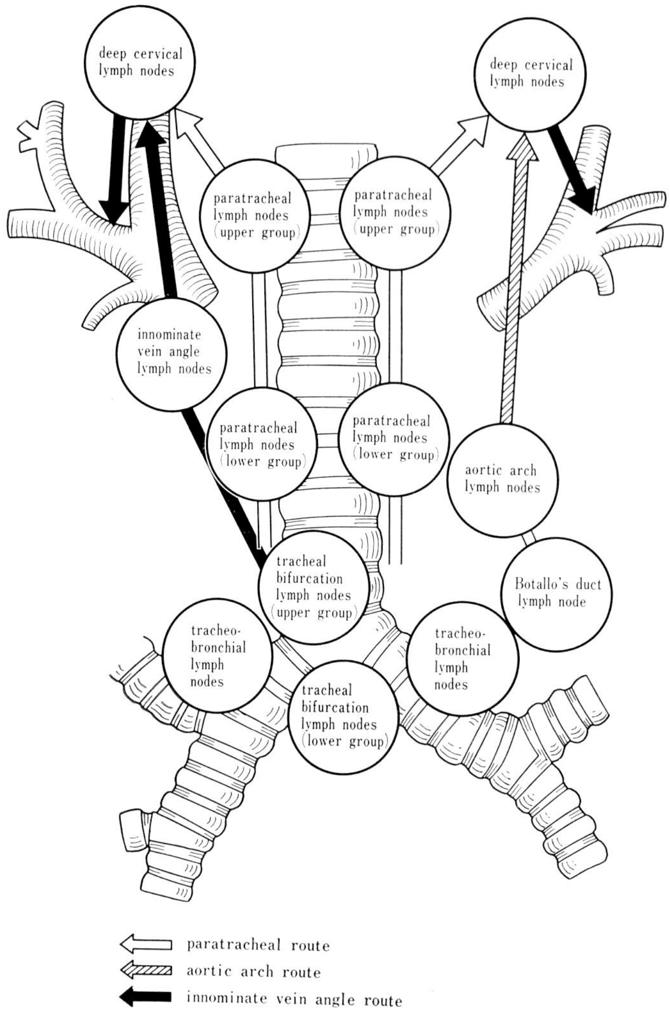

Fig. 212 Efferent lymph flow of the lung.

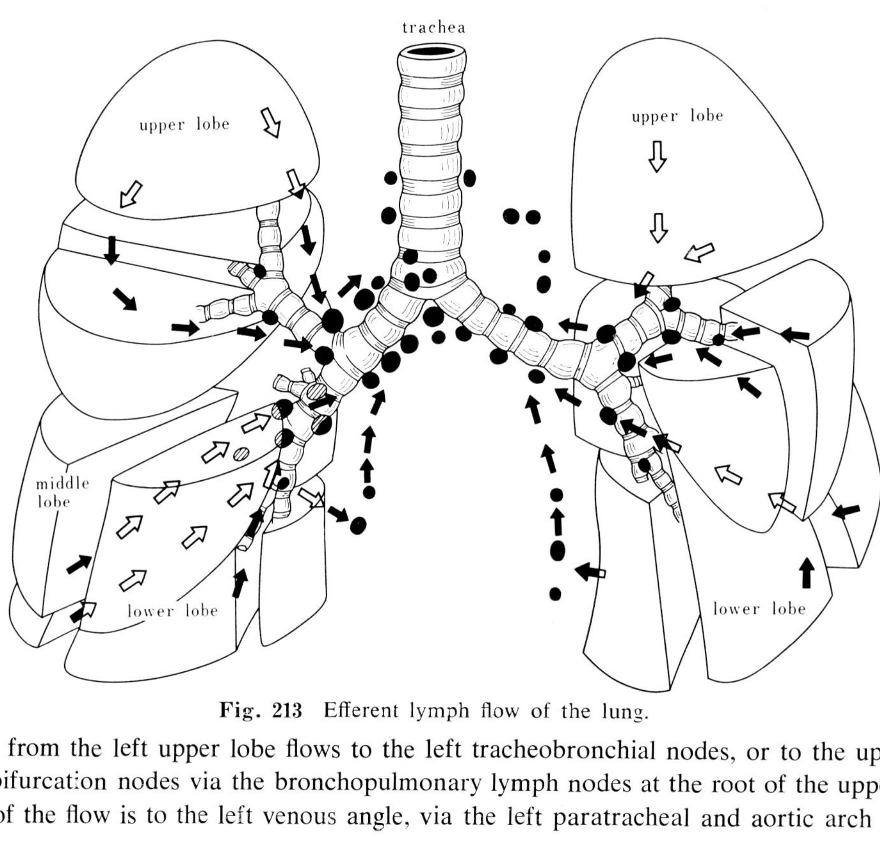

Fig. 213 Efferent lymph flow of the lung.

The lymph from the left upper lobe flows to the left tracheobronchial nodes, or to the upper group of the tracheal bifurcation nodes via the bronchopulmonary lymph nodes at the root of the upper lobe bronchus. Most of the flow is to the left venous angle, via the left paratracheal and aortic arch routes.

However, the lymph from the left upper lobe flows not only to the venous angle of the same side but to the venous angle of the opposite side via the tracheal bifurcation lymph node.

The lymph from the right middle lobe, through the bronchopulmonary nodes at the root of the middle lobe bronchus, flows to the lower group of the tracheal bifurcation nodes. Lymph flow from the middle lobe may flow not only into the venous angle of the same side but also into that of the opposite side.

The lymph from the right and left lower lobes passes through the bronchopulmonary nodes at the root of the lower lobe bronchus or the pulmonary ligament lymph nodes, and flows into the lymph nodes of the tracheal bifurcation. This lymph may flow to the venous angle of the opposite as well as to the same side.

When performing lung cancer surgery, removal of the lymph nodes must be made systematically, considering the mentioned routes for the efferent lymph flow of the lung.

The lymphatogenous spread of lung cancer usually takes place in the regional lymph nodes of the lobe in which the primary focus is located; it rarely takes place in the nodes of other routes, at least, in the case of relatively early tumor growth.

For this reason, the author will describe the minimal extent of removal of lymph nodes, in the case of lung cancer surgery:

Removal of the regional bronchopulmonary node of the lobe in which the primary foci is located, is indicated, but also, when the primary focus is found in the right upper lobe, removal of also of the paratracheal and the innominate vein angle route of the same side. When the primary foci is in the left upper lobe, the paratracheal and aortic arch route of the same side should be removed, systematically and in the direction of the venous angle. At the same time, the regional lymph nodes of the middle lobe and lower lobe in the vicinity of the root of the upper lobe and the tracheal bifurcation lymph nodes must be removed.

When the primary focus is in the middle lobe, or in the right or left lower lobe, the regional bronchopulmonary lymph nodes in that region and also the pulmonary ligament lymph nodes and the tracheal bifurcation lymph nodes must also be removed.

In the event that cancer infiltration has extended to the thoracic wall, and yet presenting an indication for surgery, when the infiltration is found in the region anterior to the mid-axillary line the thoracic wall must be removed in the anterior direction, and when it is found posterior to the mid-axillary line the thoracic wall must be sufficiently removed in the posterior direction.

Lung cancer surgery and the removal of lymph nodes are performed according to indications; however, when nodectomy is required, the lymphatic system must be removed extensively according to the conditions but avoiding the clearing of unnecessary portions. This is what the authors (NAGAISHI and OKADA) wish to emphasize.

Because lung cancer is a disease which is frequently found in people in their 5th or 6th decades, one must be cautious not to proceed too extensively when operating.

III. LYMPHOID TISSUE OF LUNG

In general, lymphoid tissue consists of interstitial reticular tissue and lymphocytic free cells. It is widely dispersed in various parts of the human body in the shape of lymph nodes, lymph nodules or lymph infiltrations.

Many researchers have investigated the function of these lymphoid tissues. Lymphoid tissues contribute to production of lymphocytes and to protective mechanisms of the organism.

When we consider that the lung is an organ consistently exposed to irritation from the external environment it is not unexpected that abundant lymph tissues will be found within the confines of that organ.

Following the pathological investigations of CORNET (1907) and GHON (1912) on the changes in hilar lymph nodes at the time of primary infection by pulmonary tuberculosis, RANKE (1916) reported his theory on the stadia of tuberculosis, and the conception of the primary complex was established. Regarding the role of the hilar lymph node in pulmonary tuberculosis as being mainly of pathological importance, early investigations were not carried out with an immediate concern for anatomical relationships.

A number of studies have been done on the hilar lymph nodes but, up to the present, not many studies have been reported, excepting these of KIHARA, HORII, et al. (1954), and the author's group, on the lymph nodules or the lymph infiltrations so widely distributed in the peripheral portions of the lung.

A. Outline of Structure of Pulmonary Lymphoid Tissue

Lymphoid tissues consist of interstitial reticular tissues and free lymphocytes, which are distributed in the lung as well as in the hilum. In principle, all these tissues are related to the lymphatic vascular system.

The pulmonary lymphoid tissue includes the hilar nodes, lymphoid tissues related to the bronchi and to the pulmonary blood vessels, subpleural lymphoid tissues, and lymphoid tissues in the interlobular connective tissue.

From its structure, the lymphoid tissue can also be divided into lymph infiltrations, nodules, or nodes.

The lymph infiltrations and nodules are predominately distributed in the periphery of the lung, usually adjacent to lymph capillaries, venules, or bronchial wall.

Nodes are seldom found in the periphery of the lung; rather they are mainly adjacent to the collecting vessels of the hilum, and are generically termed the hilar lymph nodes.

Most of the lymphoid tissues distributed in regions peripheral to the bronchopulmonary nodes are in the form of nodules or lymph infiltrations, mainly located in the bifurcations of the bronchi. The amount of such tissues differs according to age or condition.

The lymphoid tissues in the periphery have a function similar to that of the hilar lymph nodes, *i.e.* producing lymphocytes or isolating foreign bodies or bacteria. This tissue also plays a very important role as a part of the extravascular fluid pathway system of KIHARA.

The greater part of the bronchial lining is formed by ciliated epithelium; solid corpuscles or bacteria are not absorbed from this portion. However, in that part of the bronchial wall in which epithelial type lymphoid tissues occur, the infiltration of lymphocytes affects the subepithelial or the epithelial layer, solid corpuscles or bacteria being absorbed from this portion and carried into the lymph vessels. The epithelial lining in these regions becomes cuboidal and devoid of cilia. The epithelial type lymphoid tissues, such as those found on the wall of the bronchus in the periphery, form a part of the pulmonary extravascular fluid pathway system.

B. Brief History

The history of studies of the hilar lymph nodes and of the intrapulmonary lymphoid tissues will be later described in some detail but here only in outline.

BURDON-SANDERSON (1870) pointed out the existence of diffuse lymphoid masses located in the connective tissues between the bronchi and neighboring pulmonary arterial branches in the lung of the guinea pig.

FRANKENHAÜSER (1879) noted the presence of lymphoid cells with clear borders in the bronchial wall of the rat, cat and deer; however, in the human lung, these cells were observed around the excretory ducts of the mucous glands of bronchi (dia. >8 mm).

The above studies, demonstrated the existence of lymphoid tissues in the bronchial wall or in tissues surrounding the bronchi in various mammals.

KLEIN (1875) stated that the lymph nodules accompanying the bronchus of rabbit or guinea pig extended to the tunica propria of the mucous membrane.

TURNER (1877) claimed that in the human lung, unlike those of the rabbit or guinea pig, lymph nodule were always observed to be external to the muscular layers.

STÖHR and KÖLLIKER (1881), and TOLDT (1888) also reported finding lymphoid tissue along the bronchus. The above finding of KLEIN was not confirmed by them.

ARNOLD (1880) indicated that lymphoid tissues were found on the pulmonary pleura and in regions surrounding blood vessels, not only in mammals but also in the normal human lung. Thus, he regarded lymphoid tissue as one of the normal components of the lung.

The existence of lymphoid tissue in the subpleural tissue was also confirmed by LÜDERS (1892), and the views of HELLER and SCHRÖTTER (1897), and also of ARNOLD (1880) regarding the intrapulmonary lymphoid tissues were recognized and cited by many investigators.

OPPEL (1905) studied various kinds of vertebrates (from monotremata to human beings) and concluded that lymphoid tissues were a part of the normal structure of the lung; with this study, the existence of intrapulmonary lymphoid tissue became widely known.

Of the intrapulmonary lymphoid tissues, those accompanying the bronchus are particularly noteworthy; however, investigators have held differing opinions as to whether or not these are found only in extramuscular layers of mucous membrane.

Although EBNER (1899) stated that the lymphoid tissues of the bronchus of the human lung are found mainly in the region of the tracheal bifurcation, he found that some of them reach the layer of the mucous membrane after penetrating the muscular layers; MERKEL (1902), however, submitted a negative opinion.

MILLER made a collective statement in his book "The Lung" (1947) on the distribution of the intrapulmonary lymphoid tissues. His viewpoint was not very different from that of ARNOLD. As to the lymphoid tissues related to the bronchus, he joined ARNOLD in stating that he was unable to observe that the lymphoid tissues penetrated the muscular layer to reach the layers of the mucous membrane.

His opinion was that the lymphoid tissues were related to the bronchus and blood vessels as a component of normal lung; those lying on the pulmonary pleura were principally related to the pulmonary veins. According to his opinion, the intrapulmonary lymphoid tissues proliferated upon stimulation by anthracotic deposits.

HAYEK (1945, 1953) reported that lymphoid tissues were found in regions surrounding the bronchi and blood vessels, and also on the pulmonary pleura. He said that lymph infiltrations were observed adjacent to the blind end of the diverticulum of the bronchus; he termed this apparatus the "Lymphoepitheliales Organ". His view about the lymphoid tissue of the bronchial wall is notable for its uniqueness.

Considering the opinions of ASCHOFF (1926), WASSERMANN (1933) and POLICARD (1950, 1955), HAYEK divided the intrapulmonary lymphatic tissues into five constituents: the lymph vessels, adipose tissues, dust cells of mesothelial origin, lymphoid tissues containing dusts, and lymphoid tissues not containing dusts. He stated that each lymphoid tissues is composed of a combination of some of these five constituents.

In Japan, detailed investigations on the pulmonary lymphoid tissues were made by KIHARA and HORII and their followers (1924–1956).

For example, NISHIKAWA (1940, 1941) insufflated charcoal powder into the respiratory system of rabbits and examined the route of absorption; the absorption of the charcoal powder occurred only in that part of the tracheobronchial mucous membrane covered by ciliated epithelium.

His classification of the intrapulmonary lymphoid tissue followed numerous subsequent investigations.

OTANI and ARISHIGE, et al. (1952), and BOKU (1954) made observations on the development and distribution of the pulmonary lymphoid tissues, using materials from the fetus and the mature rabbit; BOKU and HASEGAWA, et al. (1949) made similar observations on the human lung.

These studies were reported collectively by KIHARA (1954). This report is possibly the most detailed available which deals specifically with the development and distribution of pulmonary lymphoid tissue.

C. Development

Table 15 shows the results of studies made by OTANI and ARISHIGE (1952), and by BOKU (1954), on the development of intrapulmonary lymphoid tissues of the rabbit.

Table 15 Development of lymphoid tissue in rabbit lung (OTANI, T. and ARISHIGE, Y., 1952; BOKU, S., 1954).

BOKU (righ whole lung or upper lobe)				OTANI & ARISHIGE (right lower lobe)			
animals	peri-lymphatic	peri-bronchial	peri-vascular	animals	peri-bronchial	peri-vascular	sub-pleural
28 D fetus (whole)	0	0	0				
2 D (whole)	0	0	0				
7 D (upper)	1	0	0	1 W	16	0	0
14 D (upper)	1	19	1	2 〃	18	0	1
				3 〃	18	0	0
				1 M	27	3	1
				2 〃	55	7	1
				3 〃	62	13	2
				4 〃	56	10	1
				5 〃	84	12	1
				6 〃	90	18	2
				adult	91	14	3

According to these studies intrapulmonary lymphoid tissue was not observed in fetal life, but after birth could be found in the region of the hilum. With aging it begins to appear in the lung parenchyma, and in the course of development the amount of the lymphoid tissue increases until a certain stage.

Judging from the pattern of development, the lymphoid tissue which appears in the wall of lymph vessels can be considered to be the precursor of a lymph node. The lymphoid tissues on the bronchial wall or venous wall do not develop into nodes, but remain in the form of nodules or infiltration.

With the purpose of determining the exact time of development of intrapulmonary lymphoid tissue, OTANI and ARISHIGE, et al. (1952) made investigations in the rabbit. Their calculations were as follows:

$$\frac{\text{number of lymph infiltrations}}{\text{number of bifurcation of bronchi}} \times 100$$

They made comparative studies on changes in this ratio at various stages in development.

The percentage of lymphoid tissues gradually increase after birth, reaching in the 4th month, almost the same percentage (about 30%) as for the mature rabbit.

STEINERT (1928), HARVEY and ZIMMERMAN (1935) and KIHARA, et al. (1954) stated that the lymphoid tissue of the human lung is observed from the 3rd month of embryonal age.

These lymphoid tissues emerge from the region of the tracheal bifurcation along the right and left main bronchi, and later develop into hilar nodes.

In the beginning, small lymph infiltrations are observed in regions where lymph vessels are found to be most dense, as shown in Fig. 214.

In the latter stages of fetal life, as shown in Figs. 215 and 216, the nodes are observed as masses of tissue along the vessels, projecting like a peninsula into the vessel lumen. By this time the border of the lymph infiltration becomes defined, showing that it is evidently the site or origin of the lymph node.

Judging from these processes of development the close relation between the nodes and vessels becomes quite evident.

The lymph space surrounding the germinal center of the lymph node, as shown in Figs. 217 and 218, will develop into the marginal sinus of the lymph node.

At a later period of the fetal life secondary nodules and reticulum bridges in the marginal sinus will develop in these germinal centers, as shown in Fig. 219.

Table 16 Development of lymphoid tissue in the human lung (Boku, S., 1952; Hase, H., 1945).

	materials	lymph nodes	lymphoid tissues
Boku, S. (1952)	4 M. fetus	8 { hilar .... 1; subpleural ...... 1; deep .... 1 }	0
	6 M. fetus	7 { hilar .... 5; deep .... 1; peribronchial ... 1 }	4 { peribronchial ... 2; subpleural ...... 2 }
	9 M. fetus	15 { hilar ....13; subpleural ...... 1; deep .... 1 }	62 { peribronchial ...55; perivascular .... 7 }
Hase, H. (1945)	7.5 M. child	24	
	9 M. child	22	
	16 M. child	20	
	18 M. child	21	

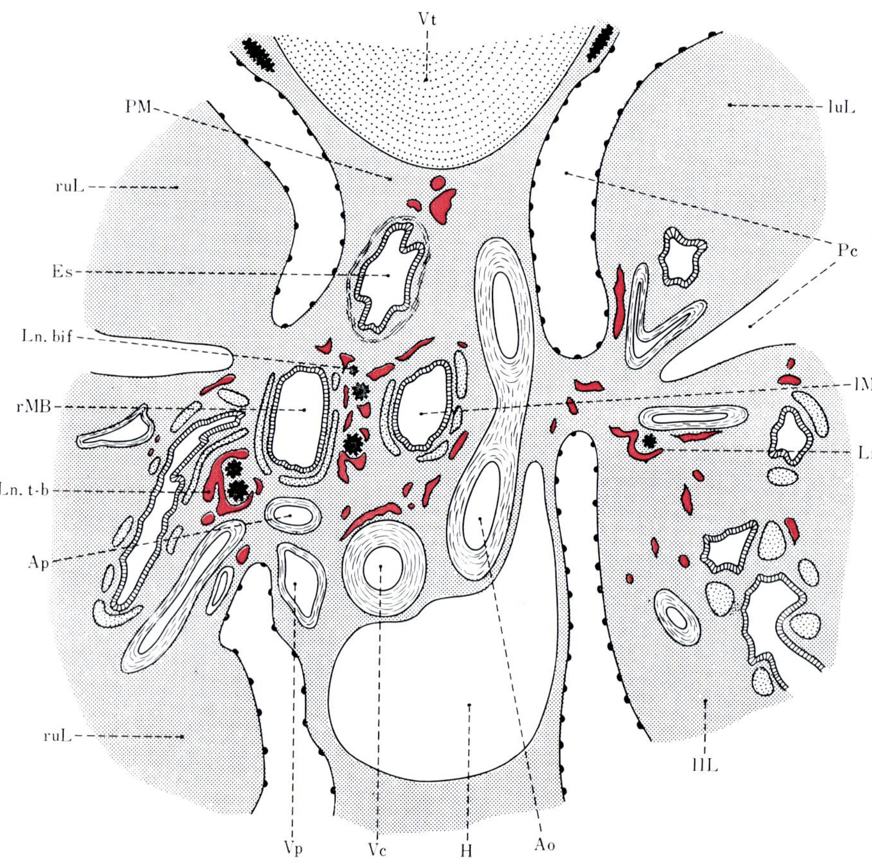

Fig. 214 Development of the hilar lymphoid tissue (human fetus, 4M.).

Vt: vertebra, PM: post. mediastrium, ruL: right upper lobe, Es: esophagus, Ln.bif: bifurcation lymph nodes, rMB: right main bronchus, Ln.t-b: tracheo-bronchial lymph nodes, Ap: pulmonary artery, ruL: right lower lobe, luL: left upper lobe, Pc: pleural cavity, lMB: left main bronchus, Ln.b-p: bronchopulmonary lymph nodes, Vp: pulmonary vein, Vc: vena cava, H: heart, Ao: aorta, llL: left lower lobe

According to the observation by Boku (1954), lymph infiltrations in the human lung are found far later than lymph nodes.

As shown in Table 16, these infiltrations are said to develop about the sixth month of fetal age.

This, then, raises the question as to whether the lymphoid tissue of the human lung increase steadily in amount with aging.

Miller (1937, 1947) concluded that in the human lung, since the lymphoid tissue would increase in proportion to the extent of anthracosis, there would be a close relationship between the development of lymphoid tissues and irritation.

On the basis of an experimental study on the development of animals in a germ free environment, Miyakawa (1954) stated that the development of lymphoid tissue was the result of exogenous irritation. However, from the comparative anatomical and ontogenical points of view, Kihara (1954) stated that the development of

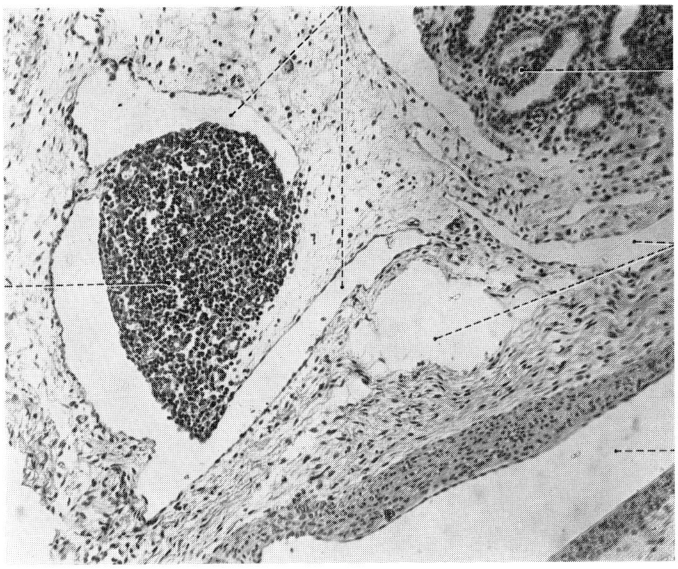

Fig. 215 Origin of the hilar lymph node (in fetus).

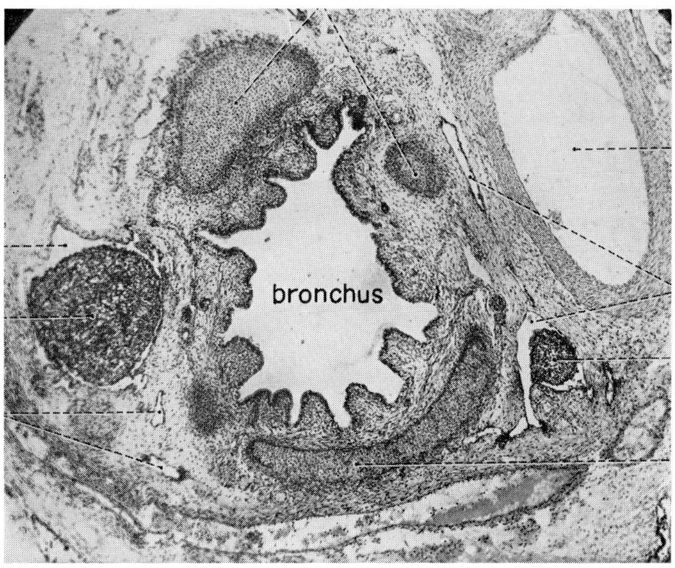

Fig. 216 Origin of the hilar lymph node (in fetus).

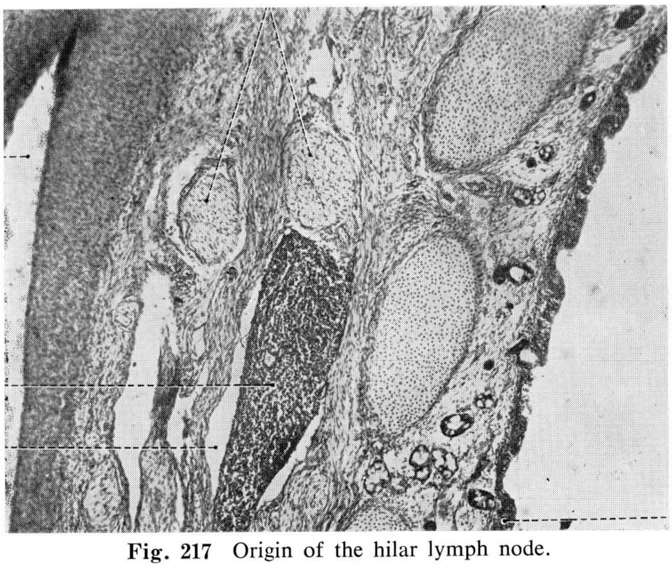

Fig. 217 Origin of the hilar lymph node.

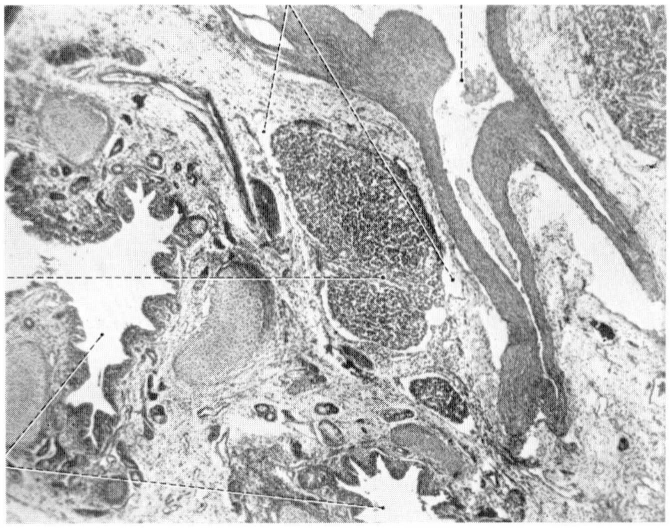

Fig. 218 Origin of the hilar lymph node.

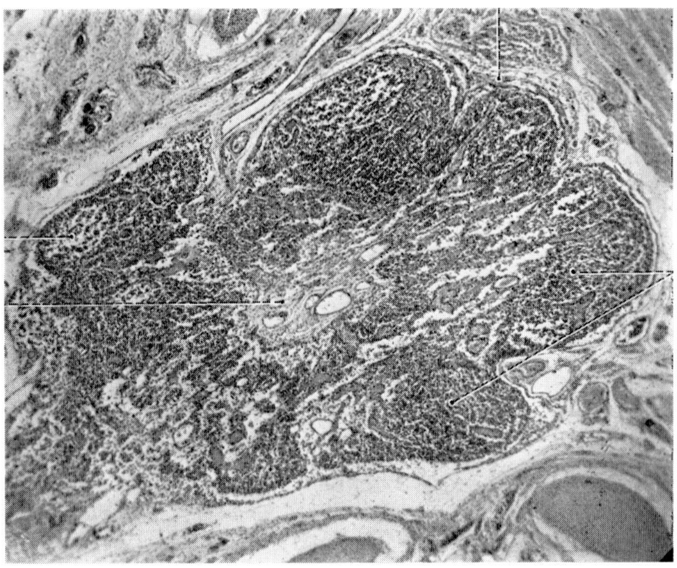

Fig. 219 Hilar lymph node of new-born child.

lymphoid tissue was not incidental; rather there was a potential for development which was independent of external stimuli.

From the results of investigations made by OTANI and ARISHIGE, et al. (1952) and by KIHARA (1954), it is presumed that in the human lung the lymphoid tissue develops to an uncertain extent, and that the degree of development is influenced by external or exogenous stimuli.

In general, lymphoid tissues are considered to increase up to a certain age, and to decrease thereafter, but as in the study of OGO (1935), the cases were investigated too few to warrant an exact conclusion.

D. Morphology and Classification

1. Morphology of Lymphoid Tissue of Lung

Morphologically, the lymphoid tissue is a kind of reticular tissue. The free cells are mainly lymphocytes and are distributed in the form of lymph nodes, nodules and lymph infiltration.

Many lymphoid tissues are observed in the lung as well as in other parts of the body. No particular specialization is observed in the lung.

Lymph node: In many instances, the nodes are large enough for macroscopical observation, with obvious capsule and trabecula. The most common type in the lung is the so-called hilar lymph node. Fig. 220 is an example of the histological structure of such a node.

Lymph nodule: The lymph nodule has a structure similar to that of a primary nodule in a lymph

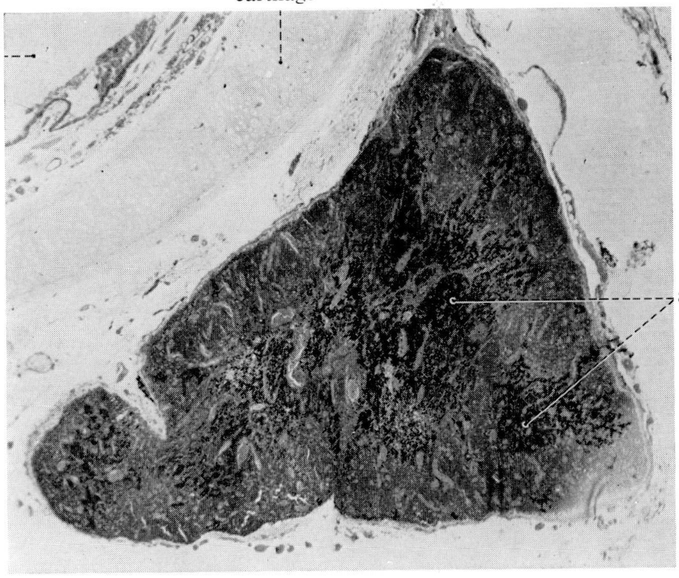

Fig. 220 Hilar lymph node.

node. The nodule lacks obvious capsule or trabecula, and the relation with the lymph vessel is not as close as is that of the node. Some lymph nodules have secondary nodules, i.e. germinal centers (FLEMMING) or "Reaktionscentrum" (HELLMAN).

In the lung nodules are frequently observed along the large bronchi, occasionally they are observed in the periphery.

Lymph infiltration: Lymph infiltrations are a type of lymphoid tissue which is observed to be diffusively and widely distributed even in relatively peripheral regions of the lung, as will be described later.

The above three types of lymphoid tissues are sometimes difficultly distinguishable, one from another. In what follows, however, they are classified according to the above criteria.

2. Classification

The pulmonary lymphoid tissue is, in general, classified into lymph node, lymph nodule and lymph infiltration, according to morphological characteristics. KIHARA (1954) reported on a different but systematic classification according to the relationship of the lymphoid tissues to the circulatory system.

The classification by KIHARA was made from the embryological and comparative anatomical point of view and is interesting, but its use requires detailed microscopic investigation in order to distinguish accurately whether a particular lymphoid tissue belongs to lymph or blood vessels. Since it is troublesome in most studies to make such serial sections, we prefer the customary and more practical classification according to distribution and gross morphology.

Thus, we classify the lymphoid tissues of the lung as hilar nodes, lymphoid tissues related to bronchi and pulmonary blood vessels, subpleural lymphoid tissues, and interlobular lymphoid tissues.

a. Hilar Nodes

Definition:

Opinions vary as to the nodes to be included in the hilar group.

ENGEL (1926) divided the bronchial lymph nodes into hilar and extrahilar nodes, defining the former as those generally called bronchopulmonary; tracheobronchial nodes, tracheal bifurcation nodes, aortic arch nodes and Botallo's ligament nodes were included in the latter. OKA (1929) designated bronchopulmonary nodes as belongings to the hilar lymph node group.

Therefore, in a narrow sense, hilar lymph node may be taken to mean bronchopulmonary lymph node, although the term "hilar lymph node" is generally also used by clinicians to include the extrahilar nodes.

In order to comply with clinical usage, the hilar lymph node group is interpreted to include the bronchopulmonary lymph nodes and the neighboring two or three lymph nodes.

Topography and Classification of Hilar Lymph Nodes:

Topographic relationships and classifications of hilar lymph nodes have been reported in some detail.

SUKIENNIKOW (1903), BARTELS (1909), ENGEL (1926), STEINERT (1928), JOSSIFOW (1930), SHIMAZAKI (1931), TORII (1931), SHIDA (1932), ROUVIÈRE (1938), from a purely anatomical standpoint, and GHON and POTOTSCHNIG (1919), OKA (1929), KITA (1953), SCHWARZ (1953) and YAMAGATA (1954), from patho-anatomical or clinical standpoints have all made topographic-anatomical studies on the hilar lymph nodes.

In this book, the authors use the following classifications: bronchopulmonary nodes, right and left tracheobronchial nodes, aortic arch nodes, Botallo's ligament node, pretracheal nodes, tracheal bifurcation nodes, right and left paratracheal nodes, and innominate vein angle nodes.

i. Bronchopulmonary Lymph Nodes

Fig. 221 shows the distribution of bronchopulmonary nodes in the human lung.

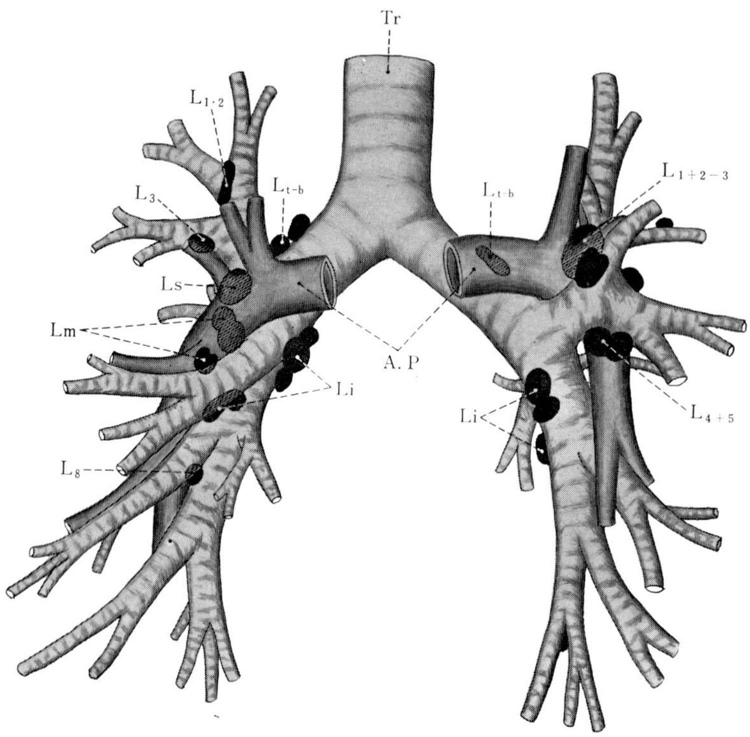

Fig. 221 Bronchopulmonary lymph nodes of the human lung. Tracheobronchial and bronchopulmonary lymph nodes (human lung, ventral view)
A.P.: pulmonary artery, Tr: trachea, Lt-b: Abbrevations of bronchopulmonary lymph nodes are proposed by the authors.

These are the nodes in the region where right and left upper lobe bronchi diverge from the main bronchi, as well as those lymph nodes distributed peripherally along the bronchi.

These lymph nodes correspond to the hilar lymph node group as described by ENGEL (1950), but some are located too peripheral to the hilum to be called hilar lymph nodes.

The pulmonary lymph nodes mentioned by BAUM (1929) correspond to the bronchopulmonary lymph nodes.

The authors consider, as stated also by SUKIENNIHOW (1903), and BARTELS (1909), that it is appropriate to use the term "pulmonary lymph node" exclusively for those lymph nodes which are observed indeterminately in the peripheral portion of the lung.

SUKIENNIKOW (1903) stated that the bronchopulmonary lymph nodes are located along the bronchial system, particularly its bifurcating portions, but ENGEL (1926) and OKA (1927), stated that the bronchopulmonary lymph nodes are located along the pulmonary artery and not along the bronchial system. STEINERT (1928) claimed that since the dividing bronchi and pulmonary artery and vein are so very close to each other, it is difficult to judge to which system the hilar lymph nodes belong.

As can be seen in Fig. 222, the hilar lymph nodes are observed in regions other than the bifurcation of the bronchi, although there may be differences in numbers. This was also pointed out by ROUVIÈRE (1932) and by KITA (1953).

The authors consider that since lymph nodes essentially belong to the lymphatic system, and not to the bronchial or blood vascular system, it is meaningless to argue as to whether or not the lymph nodes belong to either of the latter.

However, in order to clarify the topographic-anatomical relation of the bronchopulmonary nodes, it is convenient to regard them as related to the bronchi. Therefore, the lymph nodes will be described in connection with the bronchial system.

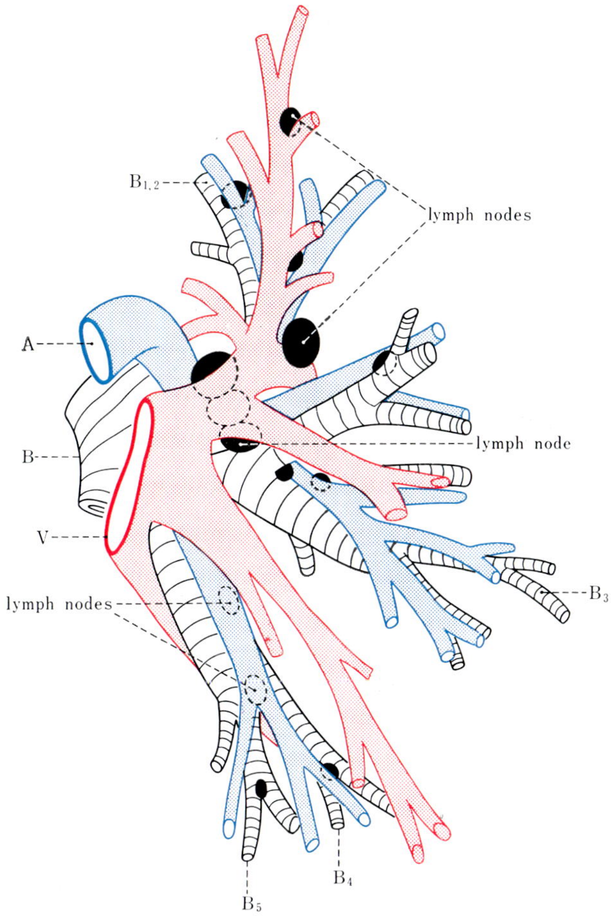

Fig. 222 Bronchopulmonary lymph nodes founded in a left upper lobe (human adult).
red: pulmonary vein, blue: pulmonary artery, black: lymph nodes

SUKIENNIKOW (1903) classified the bronchopulmonary lymph nodes in relation to the brnochial system. As shown in Fig. 223, he termed those in the first bronchial bifurcation as "Lgll. bronchopulmonales I Ordnung" and those of the second bifurcation as "Lgll. bronchopulmonales II Ordnung". This classification was adopted partially by BARTELS (1909), by H. OKA (1929).

In the papers reported in 1926, ENGEL classified the bronchopulmonary lymph nodes as follows:
1) "Lgll. hilares ant. dext."
2) "Lgll. hilares post. dext."
3) "Lgll. hilares ant. sin."
4) "Lgll. hilares post. sin."

In his book published in 1950, ENGEL classified the right and left hilar lymph nodes into "postero-laterale Drüsen" and "medio-anteriore Drüsen".

STEINERT (1928) made a similar classification into "hintere Hiluslymphknoten" and "vordere Hiluslymphknoten".

There are thus two classifications for the bronchopulmonary lymph nodes, one by bronchial bifurcation order and the other by positional relation to the hilum; practically, both classifications are used.

For instance, SUKIENNIKOW used the term "Lgll. bronchopulmonary ventr. I Ordnung od. II Ordnung". Although the term "dorsal" was not used in his classification, the term "ventral" was adopted; therefore, his classification is supposed to have been made by considering the dorsoventral positional relation to the hilum. Series of lymph nodes, "Verbindungskette", so-called by him, evidently correspond to the "Lgll. hilares post. oder interlobares" of ENGEL; therefore the classification by SUKIENNIKOW was not made according to the order of bronchial bifurcation.

Evidently the classification and nomenclature of bronchopulmonary lymph node is in a complicated state, and should be clarified.

H. OKA (1929) suggested that the bronchopulmonary lymph nodes would be better described by adding the words right or left pulmonary, anterior and posterior, superior and inferior, interlobar, and in order of bronchial branching, etc.

His method is convenient in pinpointing the exact location of each lymph node, but it is too complicated. A more concise new classification is needed. YAMAGATA's system of abbreviations (1954) for hilar lymph nodes was concise and convenient for clinical use (made by considering roentgenological observations), but it is easily confused with other classifications.

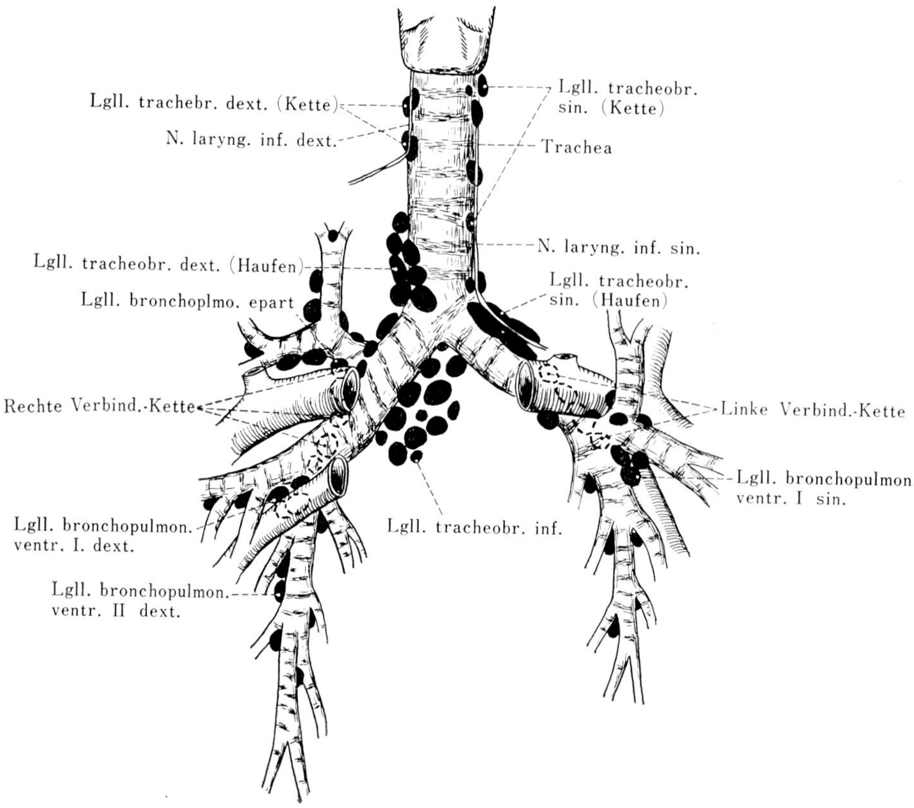

Fig. 223 Broncho-pulmonary lymph nodes (SUKIENNIKOW, W. 1903).

Supplement:

Authors' (NAGAISHI and OKADA) Nomenclature for the Bronchopulmonary Lymph Nodes:

This nomenclature of the hilar lymph nodes is based on the sequence of bronchial branching. In this way the position of lymph nodes can be described simply and accurately.

The bronchopulmonary lymph nodes are all represented by the letter "L" or "LL" (plural).

The positional relationship of each node is designated by adding the abbreviation or number of the corresponding bronchus. The abbreviation or number is to be put under the right side of the "L".

For the abbreviation of the bronchi, "s" (superior) "m" (middle) and "i" (inferior) are used; as for the number of the bronchi, the nomenclature of the bronchial branching is used.

For the lymph nodes in regions where the bronchus divides, the abbreviation or numbers of the two bronchi may be used.

For example, the lymph node at the root of the upper lobe bronchus is shown as L_s, that in the root of B^6 as L_6, that in the division between B^4 and B^5 as $L_{4 \cdot 5}$, and that in the region where B^{1a} and B^{1b} divide as $L_{1a \cdot b}$.

When right and left are required, "r" or "l" is put before the "L". Anterior and posterior designations can also be shown by a combination of these marks, *i.e.*, L_a, and L_p.

Since the bronchi and lymph nodes can hardly be considered as lines or dots, the exact positional relationship of all lymph nodes can obviously not be shown by the above nomenclature; however, this method has an advantage in allowing for the description of bronchopulmonary lymph nodes up to the bifurcation of subsegmental bronchi.

Right Bronchopulmonary Lymph Nodes

Figs. 224 and 225 are schema showing right bronchopulmonary lymph nodes. Representative among them are L_s, L_m, L_i and L_6.

L_s, *i.e.* the lymph nodes at the root of the upper lobe bronchus, are arranged as if they surround the bronchus. Particularly, they are observed in great numbers in the region between the upper lobe bronchus and A^{1+3}, or between the upper lobe bronchus and the right trunk of the pulmonary artery.

SUKIENNIKOW (1903), BARTELS (1909) and SCHWARTZ (1950) designated the latter group as "Lgll. bronchopulm. eparterialle"; they were also called "right superior bronchopulmonary lymph nodes", by SHIMAZAKI (1931), but from the viewpoint of relation with the bronchus these lymph nodes are located under the root of the upper lobe bronchus, and should be considered as belonging to L_s.

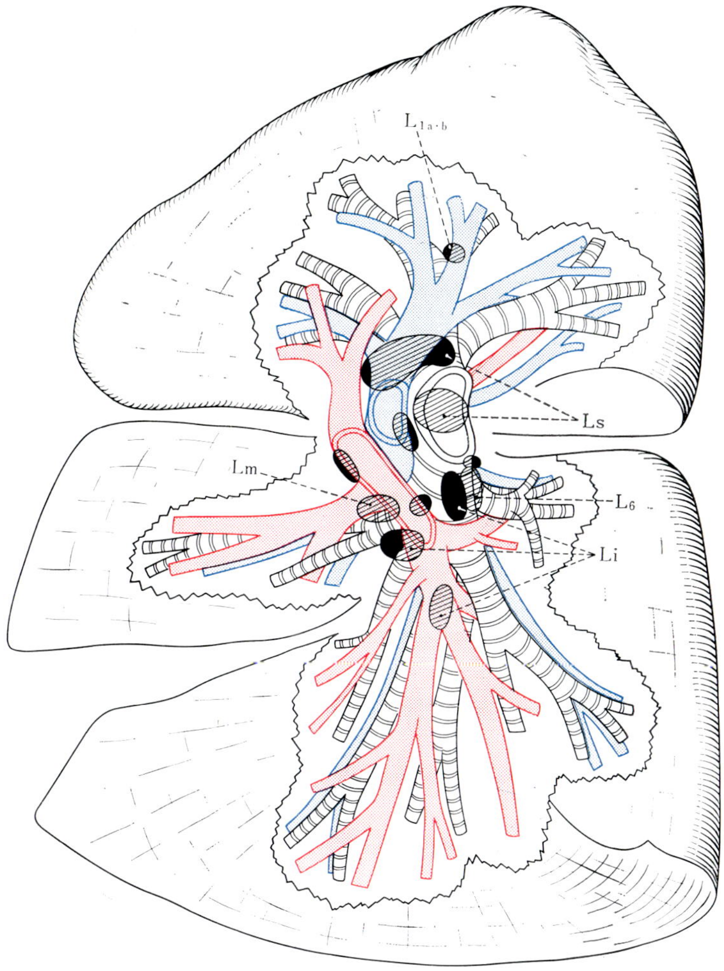

Fig. 224 Hilar lymph nodes (human right lung).
red: pulmonary vein, blue: pulmonary artery,
black: lymph nodes and nodules

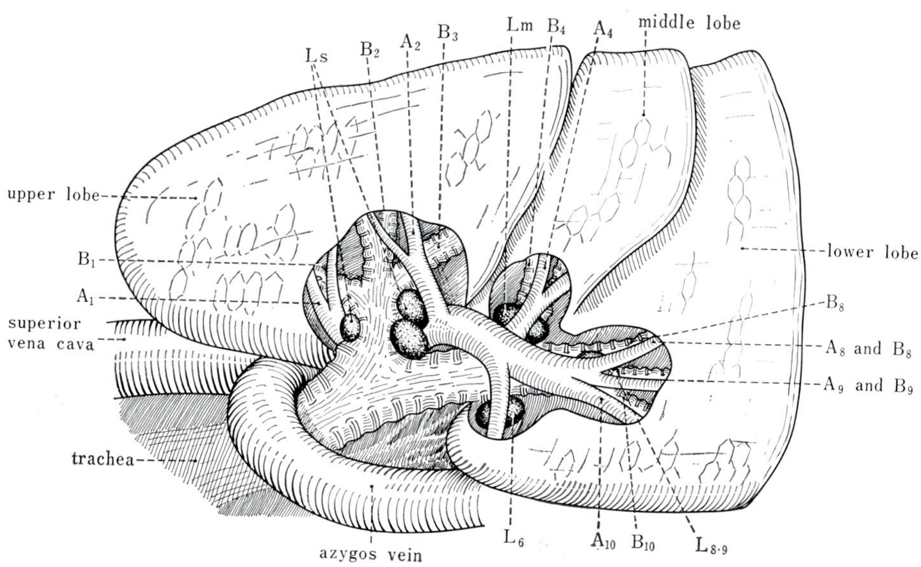

Fig. 225 Bronchopulmonary lymph nodes (human right lung).

The "Verbindungskette" (Sukiennikow, 1903; Ghon and Pototschnig, 1919), and parts of the hilar lymph nodes (Engel, 1950), also belong to L_s.

The major right bronchopulmonary lymph node is L_s, but along the right upper lobe bronchus or in the regions where B^1, B^2 and B^3 divide, rather large lymph nodes are observed in almost all instances. The regions of bifurcation of the three segmental bronchi are close to one another, so the nodes may be indicated as $L_{1\cdot2\cdot3}$.

L_m, the lymph nodes at the root of the middle lobe bronchus, are almost as well developed as L_s; in many cases, $L_{4\cdot5}$ are observed to be rather large nodes.

Nodes at the root of the middle lobe bronchus are located between the middle lobe artery and bronchus. SCHWARTZ (1953) termed these the infra-arterial nodes, and SHIMAZAKI (1931) referred to the right inferior bronchopulmonary nodes.

Nodes at the root of the middle lobe bronchus were called by SUKIENNIKOW "Lgll. bronchopulm. ventr. I Ordnung", abbreviated as $LL_{m\cdot i}$.

Thus, at the root of the middle lobe bronchus, the nodes are well developed; when they enlarge and press upon the middle lobe bronchus the pressure may cause atelectasis, resulting in the so-called middle lobe syndrome.

L_i, *i.e.* the lymph nodes at the root of the lower lobe bronchus, are not observed to be a definite group, differing from L_s or L_m. The nodes are scattered in regions from $L_{m\cdot i}$ to the region of bifurcation of the segmental bronchi of the basal segment.

Rather than to indicate these lymph nodes as L_i it would be more appropriate to consider them as belonging to the bronchi of basal segments. Among these nodes $L_{8\cdot9}$ are observed frequently to be relatively large. L_6 is also well developed.

Left Bronchopulmonary Lymph Nodes

Figs. 226 and 227 are schema to show the left bronchopulmonary lymph nodes. L_s, L_{4+5}, $L_{s\cdot i}$ and L_i are respresentative nodes.

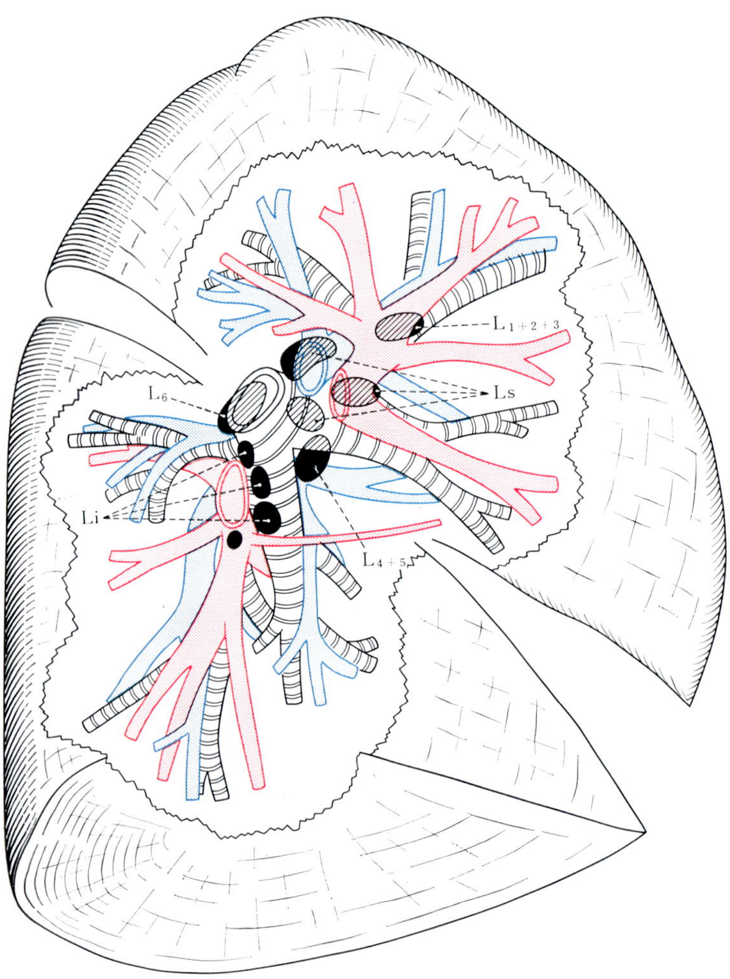

Fig. 226 Bronchopulmonary lymph nodes (human left lung).

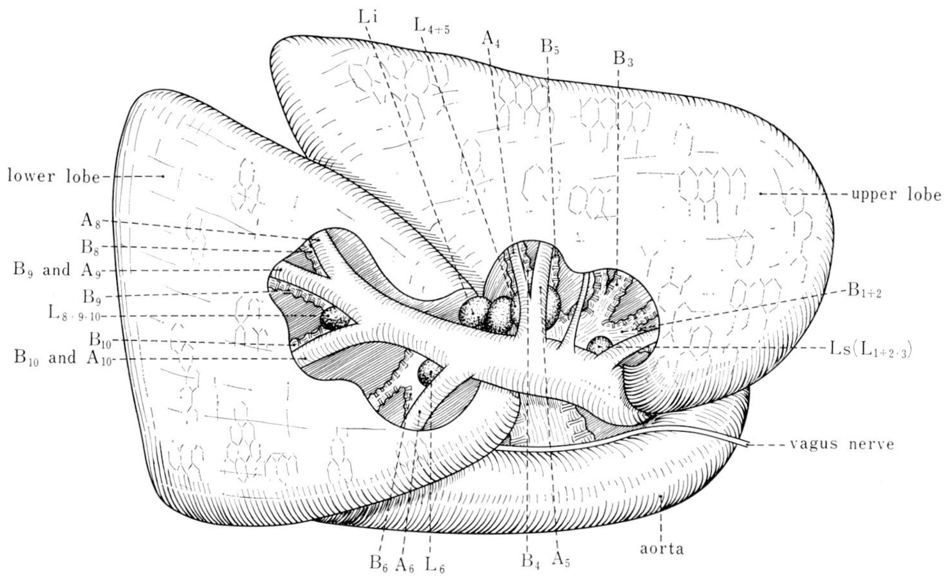

Fig. 227 Bronchopulmonary lymph nodes (human left lung).

LL_s, the lymph nodes at the root of the upper lobe bronchus, are frequently observed between the pulmonary artery or vein and the upper lobe bronchus. The circumference of the root of the upper lobe bronchus is literally surrounded by nodes.

As a result, the left upper lobe has a tendency to atelectasis, secondary to pressure occlusion by nodes.

This is also the reason why the left upper lobe, next to the right upper lobe, was a predilected region of the formerly common "Epituberkulose".

In the left upper lobe, segmental bronchi divide in relatively short distances, and because the lymph nodes in the surrounding region are relatively large, the peripheral part of L_s sometimes shifts into $L_{1\cdot 2\cdot 3}$ and $L_{4\cdot 5}$. These are all independent lymph node groups, each of relatively large size.

The "Lgll. bronchopulm. ventr. I Ordnung, sin." mentioned by SHKIENNIKOW (1930) indicates the group lying under L_s. These can be abbreviated as $L_{s\cdot 1}$, but primarily the group belongs to the upper lobe.

L_2, *i.e.* the lymph nodes at the root of the lower lobe bronchus, are not observed to form a definite group as in the right lung; but L_6 is found to be rather large in size. L_{7-10} are observed to be scattered in the regions around the branches of the basal segmental bronchi, more on the peripheral side than L_6, and are of various sizes.

ii. Pulmonary Ligament Lymph Nodes

Fig. 228 is a schema showing the pulmonary ligament lymph nodes.

Inferior to the trunk of the inferior pulmonary vein, nodes are observed to exist in the pulmonary ligament. Their numbers vary from 1 to 5 respectively, being 2 in many instances.

The nodes in this region receive the lymph partly from the basal segments of the lower lobe. From the point of lymph flow, these are considered to be bronchopulmonary nodes.

iii. Tracheobronchial Lymph Nodes

As shown in Fig. 229, the lymph nodes in this region are the group which are seen about the lower part of trachea, tracheal bifurcation and origins of the right and left main bronchi. Their numbers are 3 or 4 on each side.

The right tracheobronchial lymph nodes merge with the paratracheal nodes in the central portion, and with L_s in the peripheral; the boundary can sometimes be inadequately distinguished.

For instance, the "Lgll. tracheobronch. dext. Haufen" of SUKIENNIKOW (1903) shows definitely the tracheobronchial nodes; however, those in the upper part can be considered as paratracheal, in view of their positions.

The left tracheobronchial lymph nodes are distributed from the left side of the lower part of the trachea to that portion where the left trunk of the pulmonary artery crosses the left main bronchus.

These are called by various names, *e.g.*, "Lgl. hilares post. suprema (ENGEL)", "Lgl. epibronchialis sin. (ENGEL)", "linke obere tracheobronchiale Lymphknoten (GHON, POTOTSCHNIG)", left epibronchial lymph node (SHIMAZAKI), or epitracheal lymph node.

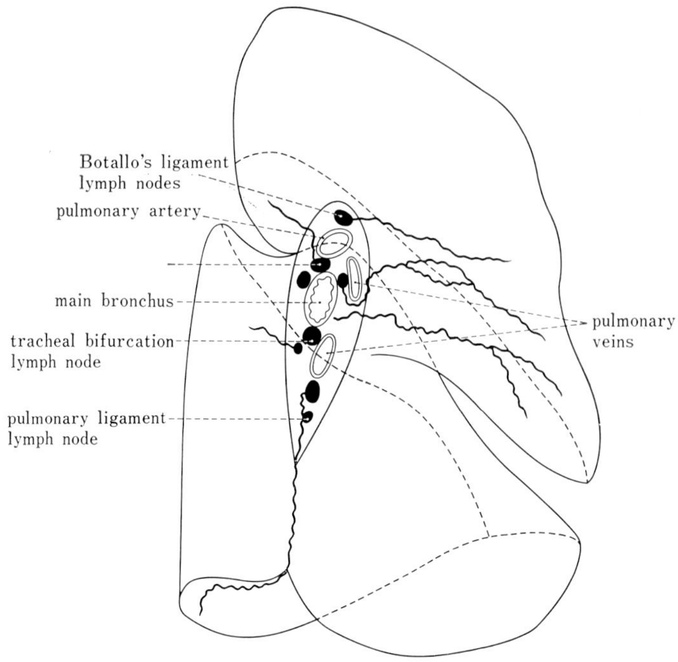

Fig. 228 Hilar lymph nodes (left lung).

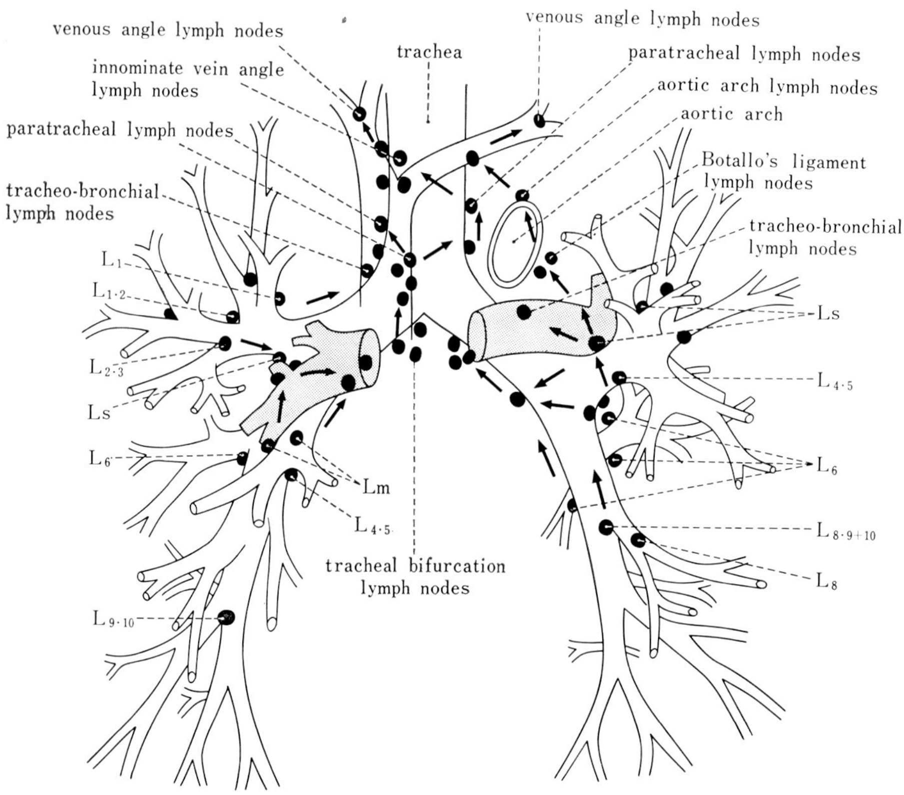

Fig. 229 Distribution of the hilar lymph nodes.

As claimed by OKA (1929) Botallo's ligament and aortic arch nodes should be included in the tracheobronchial lymph nodes. However, in this book, the nodes of Botallo's ligament and of the aortic arch will be described separately.

iv. Botallo's Ligament Lymph Nodes

Fig. 229 shows that these nodes, usually one or two in number, are located on the left side of the ligament (or duct).

Since these nodes receive lymph from the lung, there is a tendency to anthracosis. When performing thoracotomy these nodes, together with the aortic arch nodes, are often observed through the mediastinal pleura and are blackish in color.

v. Aortic Arch Lymph Nodes

As was shown in Fig. 229, the aortic arch nodes are a group of nodes in the region surrounding the aortic arch. They are usually 5–7 in number. Sometimes more than 10 of them are observed; however, not all of these receive lymph from the intrapulmonary vessels.

SHIMAZAKI (1931) included in the category of the aortic arch nodes all those in the area at the upper border of the Botallo's duct (ligament).

vi. Tracheal Bifurcation Lymph Nodes

As shown in Figs. 223 and 229 the bifurcation nodes extend from immediately under the tracheal bifurcation to the inferior aspect of the proximal portion of the main bronchi of both sides, and frequently are three in number.

These nodes are called "Lgll. tracheobronch. inf. (SUKIENNIKOW), or "Untere tracheobronchiale Lymphknoten (GHON and POTOTSCHNIG)".

vii. Pretracheal Lymph Nodes

Fig. 229 shows the pretracheal nodes as located anterior to the lower part of the trachea, *i.e.* in the adipose tissue on the posterior aspect of the bifurcation of the pulmonary artery. Their numbers are usually two or three.

viii. Innominate Vein Angle Lymph Nodes

The innominate vein angle nodes are found where the bilateral innominate veins unite to form the superior vena cava. There may be as many as a dozen of these nodes.

ix. Paratracheal Lymph Nodes

As shown in Figs. 223 and 229, the paratracheal lymph nodes are distributed along the sides of the trachea, and are usually 5–6 in number on each side.

SUKIENNIKOW (1903) designated these as "Lgll. tracheobronch. dext. et sin. Kette".

Those on the right side join the upper part of the right tracheobronchial lymph nodes.

Those on the left side are distributed in the area on the right side of the aortic arch, superior to the left side of the tracheal bifurcation.

Since these nodes are adjacent to the anterior wall of the esophagus, tuberculous foci may rarely perforate the esophageal wall.

Hilar Lymph Nodes in Mammals:

The distribution of hilar nodes in mammals is almost the same as in the human lung. Lymph nodes can thus be designated according to classifications used for the human lung.

Differing from the human lung, however, anthracosis is rarely observed in the hilar nodes of mammals; this is probably due to the difference in span of life or in environment. For similar reasons, anthracosis is also rarely observed in youths or young girls.

Strictly speaking, certain histological differences are found as between the lymph nodes of various animals, as stated by HORII (1954). The development of bronchopulmonary lymph nodes is extremely poor in most mammals, excepting man.

For example, in the rabbit, the extent of development of bronchopulmonary and tracheobronchial nodes is rather unimpressive. The number of tracheobronchial lymph nodes is observed to increase in higher animals. However, according to KIHARA and TESHIMA, et al. (1935), bronchopulmonary lymph nodes are observed very rarely even in higher animals or primates, and lymph nodes are not observed in any great number in regions peripheral to lobar bronchi, differing in this respect from the situation in the human lung.

Fig. 230 shows the hilar nodes of a dog. In the region peripheral to the tracheobronchial nodes, nodes are hardly observed.

X-ray Examination of Hilar Lymph Nodes

In the normal lung, the hilar lymph nodes cannot ordinarily be defined radiologically. When the nodes enlarge beyond a certain size or when calcification occurs, their location can be disclosed.

In order to find exactly which lymph node is shown in the X-ray picture, dorsoventral or lateral bronchography, and post-bronchographic tomography may be utilized, in addition to routine radiography. However, approximate positional relationships of hilar nodes can be found by routine radiography.

The pulmonary image is schematized in Fig. 231 (a), (b).

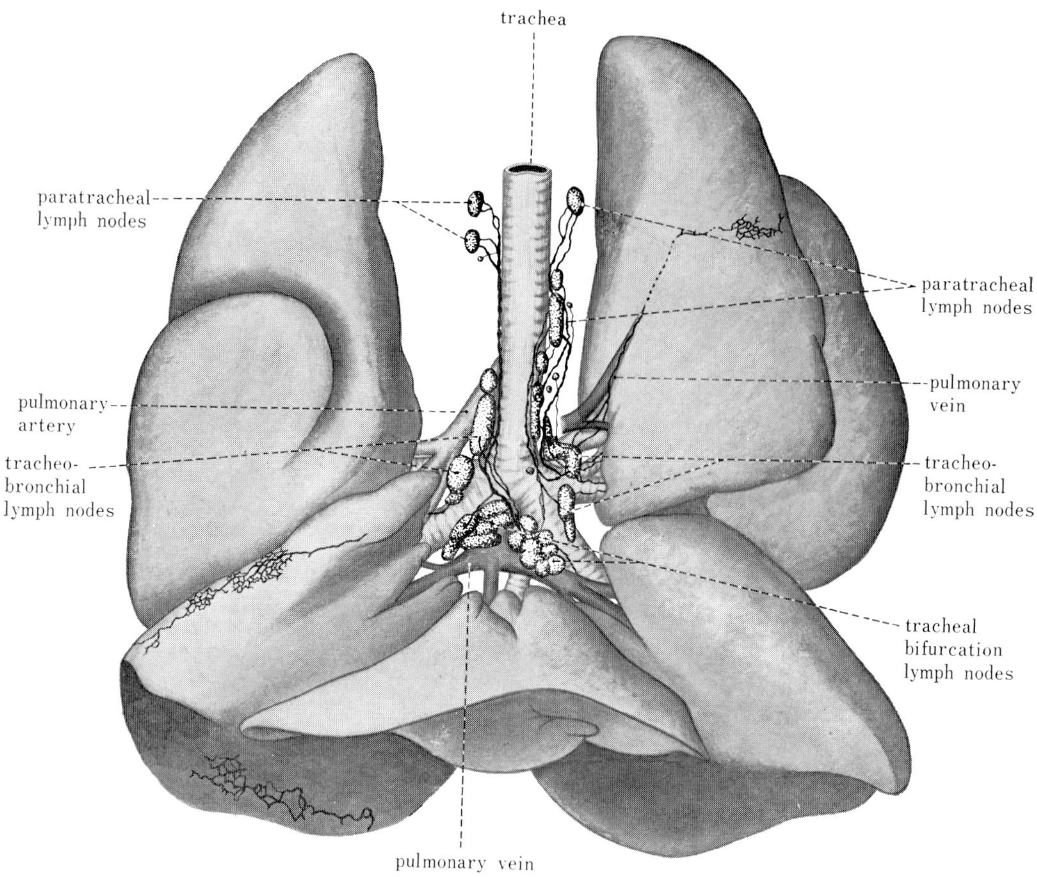

Fig. 230 Hilar lymph node (dog lung).

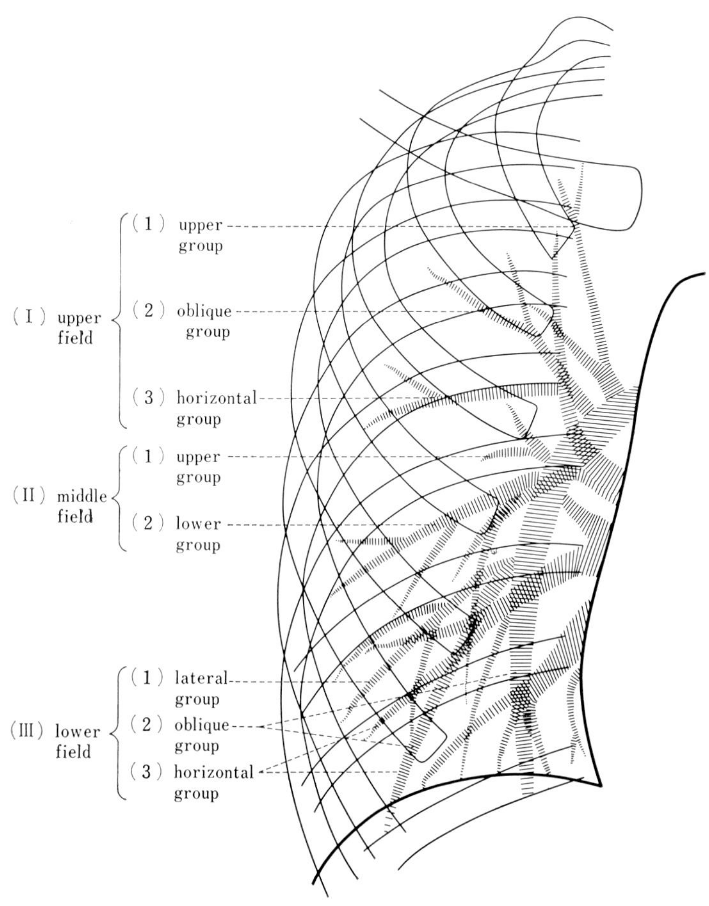

Fig. 231 a Pulmonary artery of the right lung.

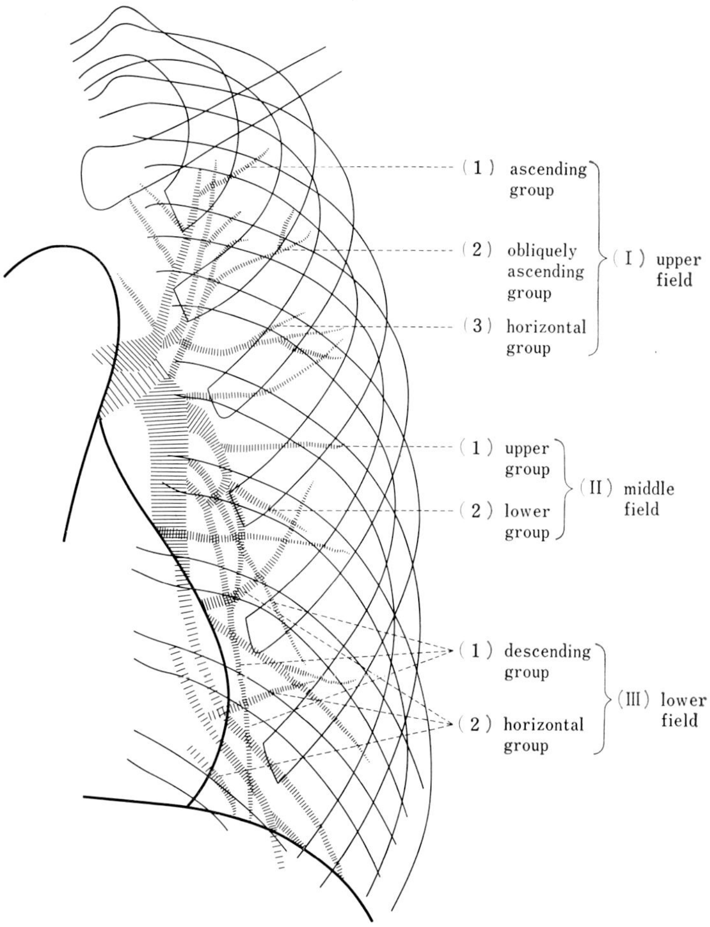

Fig. 231 b Pulmonary artery of left lung.

Fig. 232 shows the pulmonary image and the location of each hilar lymph node.

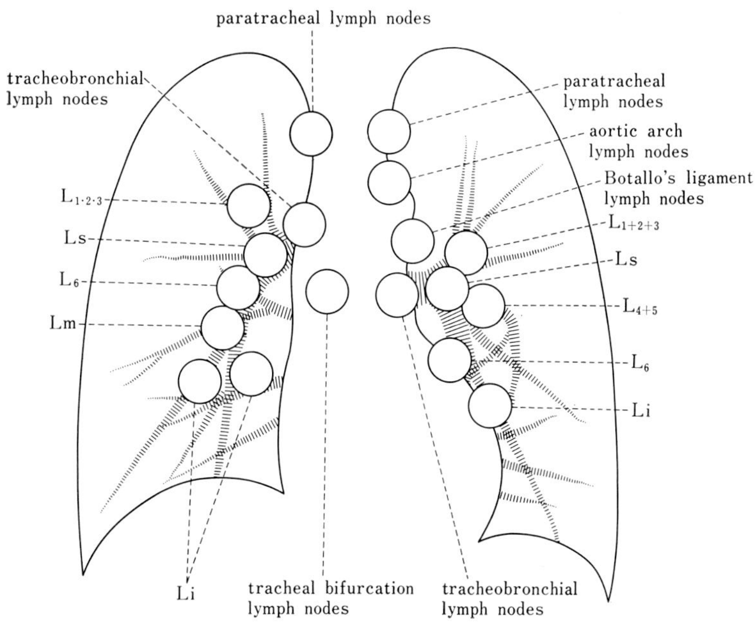

Fig. 232 Pulmonary pattern and hilar lymph nodes.

b. Lymphoid Tissue related to Bronchi

The lymphoid tissues are observed also in the regions surrounding the bronchi.

In the human lung, in the 5th or 6th order bifurcation of the bronchi, the lymphoid tissues are observed in the majority of instances; however, in regions more peripheral, it is rare to detect obvious lymphoid tissues.

The lymphoid tissues belonging to the bronchial wall are classified into the following three types in man, cattle, rabbit, and guinea pig:

1) epithelial type
2) tunica propria type
3) adventitial type

The lymphoid tissue related to the bronchus was investigated by BURDEN-SANDERSON (1870), studying the guinea pig. Thereafter some researchers stated that lymphoid tissues were observed in the region surrounding the bronchi in some kinds of mammals but not in man (ARNOLD, 1880); FRANKENHÄUSER (1879) stated that noticeable lymphoid tissues were not found in the region surrounding the bronchi of man.

With the lapse of time, such investigators as KÖLLIKER (1854), TURNER (1877), TOLDT (1888), v. EBNER (1899), OPPEL (1905), and MILLER (1947) were inclined to recognize the existence of lymphoid tissues about the bronchus of man as well as in other mammals; presently, lymphoid tissues are regarded to exist in the region surrounding the bronchi of normal human lungs.

On the other hand, regarding the distribution of lymphoid tissues on the tracheobronchial wall, there have been many opinions, *e.g.*, lymphoid tissues were observed only in the adventitia but not in the mucous layer (TURNER, 1877; MILLER, 1911); in some kind of animals, lymphoid tissues were not observed in the mucous layer (ARNOLD, 1880; STÖHR and KÖLLIKER, 1881); or the distribution differed according to the region. In the large bronchi (with cartilages) they were observed in the adventitia, but in small bronchi (lacking cartilages) they were distributed in the mucous layers, etc.

Presently, it is considered that lymphoid tissues are observed in the adventitia and mucous layers of the bronchi; in some instances, lymph infiltration is said to have reached even to the subepithelial layer.

Of the animals which are commonly used for experiments, lymph infiltrations related to the bronchi have been observed abundantly in rabbits and guinea pigs, whereas in the dog fewer observations have been reported.

NISHIKAWA (1941) counted the number of lymph infiltrations in the lung of rabbit and reported that 89 were observed on the bronchial walls.

EBNER (1899) and STEINERT (1928) reported that many lymphoid tissues were observed in the bifurcating portion of the bronchi; OTANI and ARISHIGE (1952) stated that in the rabbit 99% of lymphoid tissues were located in the region of the bifurcating bronchi.

As was described earlier, lymphoid tissues were rarely observed in regions distal to 5th–6th order bifurcating bronchi, in human lung.

According to NISHIKAWA (1940), lymph infiltrations were observed frequently at the level of terminal bronchioles, and could also be found in the second order respiratory bronchioles in the lung of rabbit. MILLER (1947) also reported on observations in the cat lung, stating that lymphoid tissues were noted in the region surrounding the respiratory bronchioles.

According to investigation by the authors, as shown in Fig. 233, in cattle lymph infiltrations were observed many times on the wall of terminal bronchioles, whereas in the dog it was quite rare that lymph infiltrations were observed on the bronchial wall.

As to the relation between the tracheobronchial wall and lymphoid tissues, NISHIKAWA (1940, 1941) classified three types:

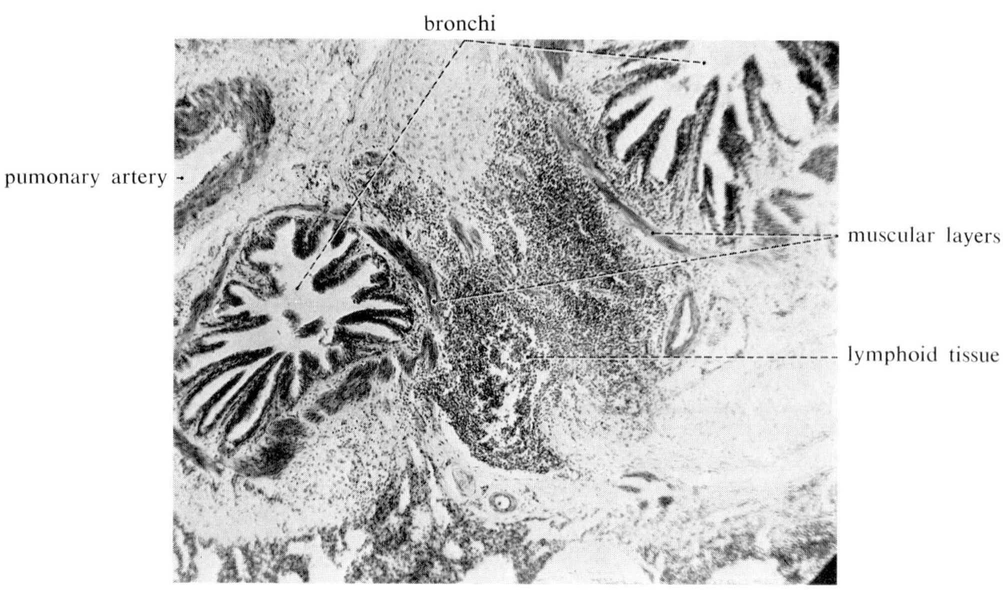

Fig. 233 Lymphoid tissue of the bronchial bifurcation.

Epithelial type: In the regions where lymphoid tissues exist in the subepithelial layer the mucous membrane lacks folds, as shown in Fig. 234, and epithelial cells are cuboidal or low columnar in shape.

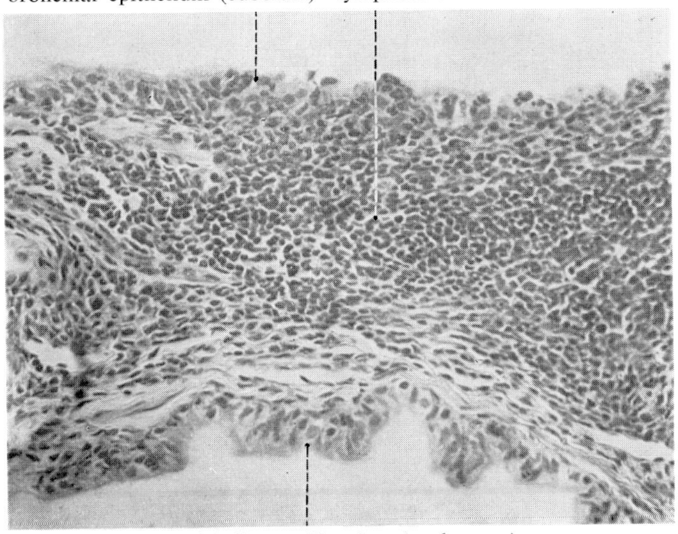

Fig. 234 Lymphoid tissue (epithelial type).

Tunica propria type: Lymphoid tissue of this type is distributed from adventitia to tunica propria, as shown in Figs. 235 and 236 (the muscular layer is torn in the section).

Adventitial type: Lymphoid tissue of this type is shown in Fig. 237.

The authors have also made investigations on the lymphoid tissues related to the bronchus of guinea pig, cattle and man, and have confirmed that they belong to one of the three types of NISHIKAWA (1940).

According to BOKU (1954) the ratio of these types is highest in the tunica propria type, less in epithelial or adventitial types.

The epithelial type lymphoid tissue definitely relates to the epithelium. As shown in Fig. 238, the mucous membrane of the bronchial epithelium in this region has a specific shape, unlike that of other regions.

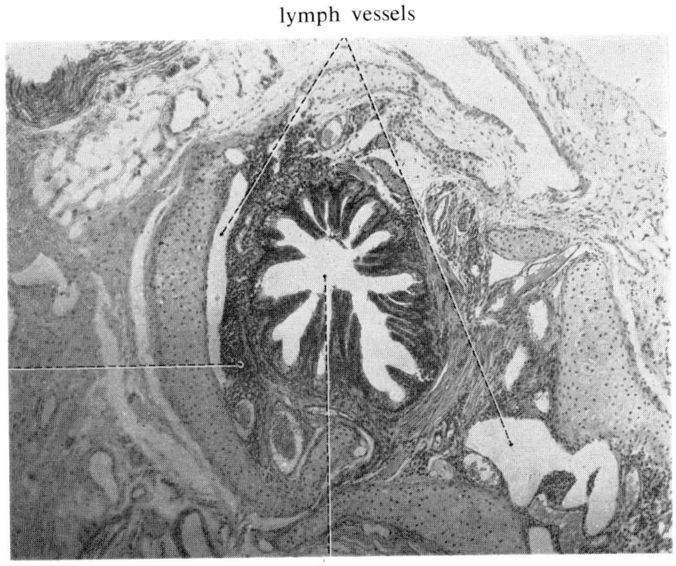

Fig. 235 Lymphoid tissue (tunica propria type).

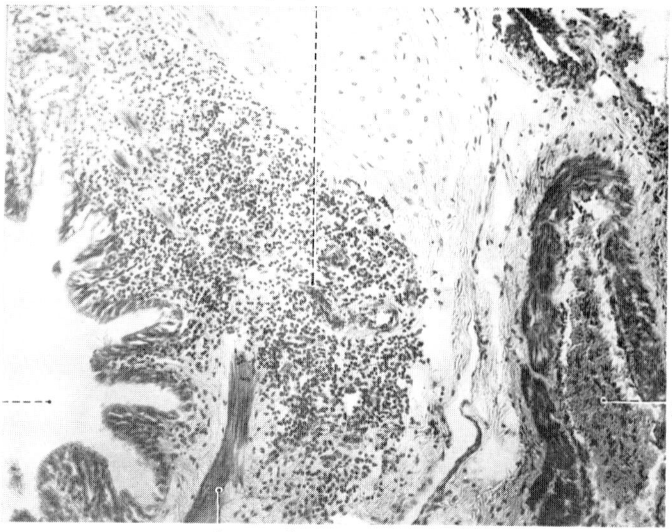

Fig. 236 Lymphoid tissue (tunica propria type).

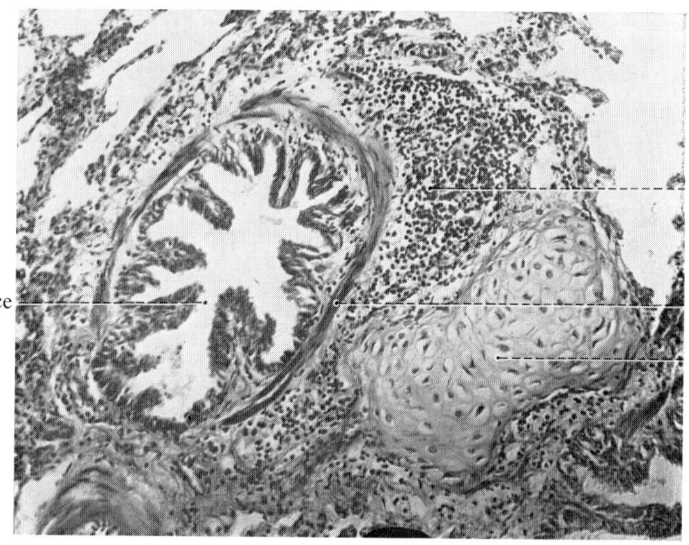

Fig. 237 Lymphoid tissue (adventitial type).

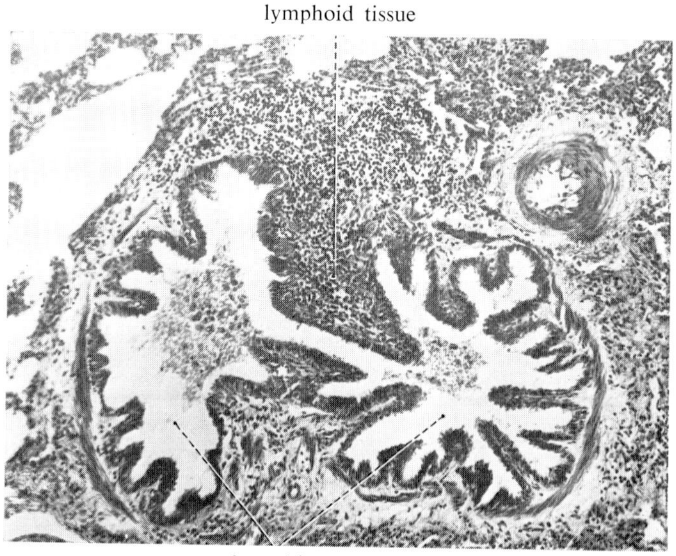

Fig. 238 Lymphoid tissue (epithelial type).

Kölliker (1854) stated that some of the lymphoid tissue found on the lymph vessels frequently surrounded gland vesicles or ducts in the bronchial mucous membrane; Hayek (1953) stated that many "Schleimhaut-divertikel" were found in the bronchi, and that a close relationship was observed between the "Schleimhaut-divertikel" and lymphoid tissues or lymph vessels.

The relationship resembles to that of the epithelial type of lymphoid tissue described by (Nishikawa, 1940 and 1941). Hayek (1953) called this specific apparatus the lympho-epithelial organ or pulmonary tonsil; the present authors have not as yet confirmed this.

The tunica propria and adventitial types of lymphoid tissues are histologically always adjacent to lymph vessels.

This relation is observed, as shown in Fig. 235, to be particularly evident in the region surrounding the bronchus of the guinea pig or rabbit, in which development of lymphoid tissue and lymph vessels is remarkable. Some are not only adjacent to the lymph vessel on one side, but also may appear to sit astride two lymph vessels, in bridge-like form.

c. Lymphoid Tissue related to Pulmonary Blood Vessels

Lymph infiltrations or lymph nodules are found along the pulmonary artery and vein, and in the regions of division of branches and tributaries.

The tissues are found mostly along the pulmonary vein, and fewer along the pulmonary artery, but not found along the bronchial artery and vein. The number of lymphoid tissues related to the pulmonary blood vessels is less than that of for the bronchi.

Arnold (1888), Miller (1896), and Guieysse-Pellissier (1920) reported that the lymphoid tissues are found with the pulmonary blood vessels. In particular, Miller emphasized that lymphoid tissues were observed frequently in the bifurcating portions of the pulmonary veins.

According to Nishikawa (1940, 1941), about 10% of the intrapulmonary lymphoid tissues in the rabbit lung is observed along vessel walls, of which 86% was found along the branches of the pulmonary vein, the residual 14% along the branches of the pulmonary artery. No lymphoid tissue was found in relationship to the bronchial artery and vein.

The lymphoid tissues were observed to be limited to the ramifying portions of the pulmonary artery or vein.

Lymphoid tissues are also observed along the walls of the pulmonary artery and vein of the human lung, but fewer than along the bronchial wall. According to Boku (1954), lymphoid tissues were observed in 12–21% of the ramifying portions of the pulmonary artery, and in 6–7% of the corresponding regions of the pulmonary vein. Accordingly, the percentage of the lymphoid tissues along the pulmonary blood vessels is far lower than for the bronchi, where lymphoid tissues were observed in half of the ramifying portions up to 5th or 6th order bifurcations.

Histologically, the lymphoid tissue related to the pulmonary artery was observed in the adventitia and did not reach the endothelium. For instance, Nishikawa (1940, 1941) and Otani and Arishige (1952) reported that their histological investigations on the lymphoid tissue related to the pulmonary artery of the rabbit revealed all of the lymphoid tissues to be of the adventitial type.

As mentioned earlier, the pulmonary artery is accompanied by an abundance of lymph vessels, and lymphoid tissues are always found adjacent to the arteries, as shown in Fig. 239.

The lymphoid tissue related to the pulmonary veins is of the endothelial as well as the adventitial type. Nishikawa (1940, 1941) and Otani and Arishige (1952) reported the ratio of the amount of the former to the latter to be about 4:1 in the rabbit.

As for the pulmonary vein, the adventitial type of lymphoid tissue is found in the lymph vessels in regions surrounding the pulmonary veins, whereas the endothelial type is characteristic of the pulmonary vein itself, as shown in Fig. 240.

As mentioned previously, lymphoid tissue is observed on the walls of venules and it is often found between the alveoli. The result is that it is sometimes interpreted as belonging to the walls of the peripheral bronchi. Therefore, when lymphoid tissue is found among the alveolar region, the relationship to the pulmonary vein must be ascertained.

d. Subpleural Lymphoid Tissues

Although the quantity is small, lymphoid tissue is observed in the subpleural regions.

The observation of lymphoid tissue in the subpleural region was reported by Kölliker (1854), Arnold (1880), Lüders (1892) Heller and v. Schrötter (1897).

Some researchers (Guieysse-Pellisier, 1920) denied its existence, but later Schaffer (1933) and Stöhr (1951) took an affirmative attitude and described it in the text books.

Today it is generally accepted that lymphoid tissues occur in subpleural regions.

However, since there have been very few observations of subpleural lymphoid tissues, some investigators doubt that it can always be found in normal lungs. Miller (1937) claimed that lymphoid tissue could not be found in the normal lung, and that its development took place only under abnormal conditions. Nishikawa (1940, 1941) and Otani and Agishige (1952), however, reported on the observation of lymphoid tissues in the normal subpleural region in rabbits.

Nishikawa (1940) stated that in the mature rabbit the subpleural lymphoid tissue amounted to 1% of the lymphoid tissues of the lung. Otani and Arishige (1952) reported that they could constantly find subpleural

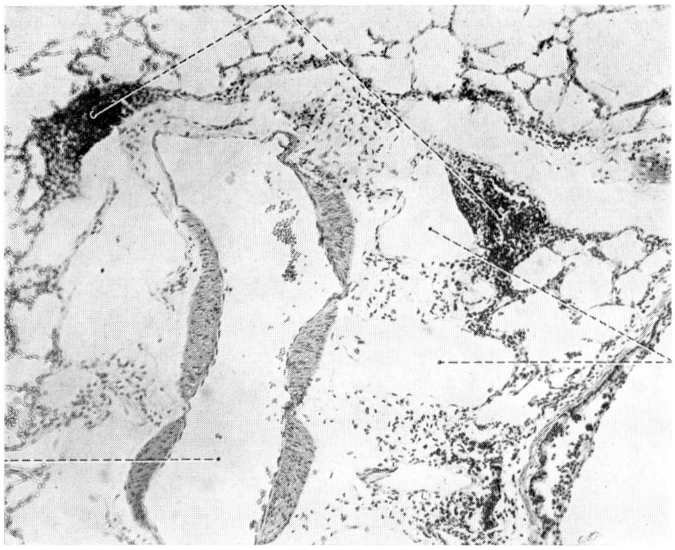

Fig. 239 Lymphoid tissue related to the lymph vessel.

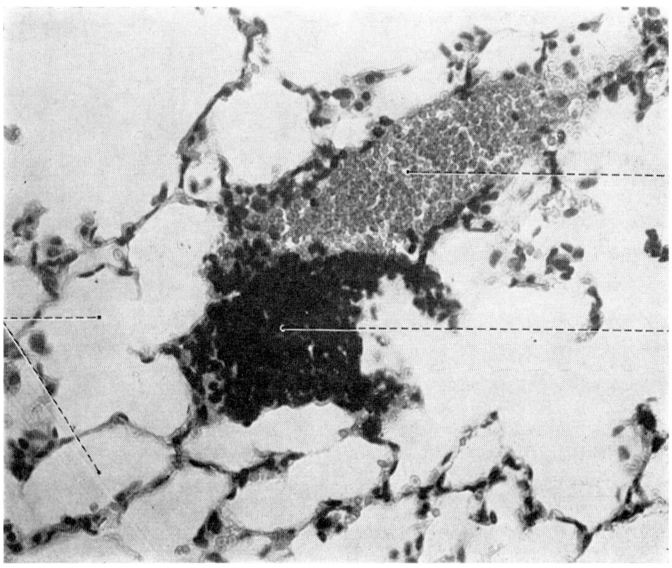

Fig. 240 Lymphoid tissue related to the pulmonary vein.

lymphoid tissues in the rabbit examined in various stages from 2 weeks after birth to maturity.

OGO (1935) stated that only in the case of a 6 year-old child, many lymphoid tissues were observed in the subpleural region (130 in the right lung and 112 in the left lung), but he did not find the same conditions in adults 52 or 59 years of age, or in an infant 3 months in age.

When the surface of the pulmonary pleura is observed carefully during thoracotomy, circumscribed anthracosis can frequently be found. The authors consider that it is not so rare to find lymphoid tissue in the subpleural region of human lung.

Subpleural lymphoid tissue is also observed in the transitional region between interlobular and subpleural connective tissues.

Lymph nodules are found in the interstitial layer of the pulmonary pleura, but not in the submesothelial layer of the pleura. The subpleural lymphoid tissue is considered to belong to lymph vessel or blood vessel, but this has not yet been definitely determined.

e. Lymphoid Tissues in Interlobular Connective Tissue

KÖLLIKER (1854), ARNOLD (1880) and OGO (1935) reported the observation of lymphoid tissue in interlobular connective tissues.

The authors have not confirmed this yet with human lung, but experienced one case in cattle lung.

MILLER (1937) said that he found lymphoid tissue in the interlobular connective tissue, in addition to that related to the pulmonary vein. He interpreted this to be the result of anthracosis or some other irritation; however, the authors consider lymphoid tissue in the interlobular tissue to be physiological, since the interlobular connective tissues have the same character as the subpleural connective tissues.

It is premature to say that these lymphoid tissues belong to either lymph vessels or to pulmonary veins.

E. Function of Lymphoid Tissue of Lung

In order to understand the structure of the lymphoid tissue of the lung as a whole, and aslo in order to assist in understanding the relationship of lymphoid tissues to lymph vessels, the function of the lymphoid tissue will now be discussed.

1. Lymphoid Tissue and Extravascular Fluid Pathway System (Kihara)

The extravascular fluid pathway system refers to reticular or spongy clefts in tissues which consist of specific argyrophilic fibers of connective tissue.

Kihara (1950) reported the finding of such fluid pathway, and designated it the extravascular fluid pathway system.

He published this finding in his book "Das Extravaskuläre Saftbahnensystem" (1950, 1956).

The extravascular fluid pathway system is widely distributed in various portions of the body.

Kihara classified the system into pre-lymphovascular fluid pathway ("Prälymphovaskuläre Saftbahnen"); para-lymphovascular fluid pathway ("Paralymphovaskuläre Saftbahnen") and para-venule fluid pathway ("Paravenule Saftbahnen").

Pre-lymphovascular fluid pathway: This is a route leading from tissues to lymph vessels.

The macula cribriformis of the parietal pleura is representative; it will be further described in Chapter VI (Pulmonary Pleura).

Nishikawa (1940) investigated the route of absorption by insufflating charcoal powder into the respiratory system of rabbits. The inhaled charcoal powder was absorbed only from regions where epithelial type lymphoid tissue was found. The epithelial type lymphoid tissue observed in the walls of the respiratory passages is in the pre-lymphovascular fluid pathways.

Para-lymphovascular fluid pathway: This is a pathway accompanying the efferent lymph vessel.

It indicates the route by which lymph leaks out of lymph vessels into the tissues, and is later reabsorbed into lymph vessels or venules.

Teshima (1935) reported that this pathway was found in the chest, along with the internal mammary lymph vessel.

The peribronchial and the adventitial type lymphoid tissues related to the pulmonary artery and vein have a close relation to lymph vessels; the lymph is presumed to go in and out through the clefts of the reticular tissues. Accordingly, such lymphoid tissue can be considered to form a station in the para-lymphovascular fluid pathway in the lung.

Para-venule Fluid Pathway: This pathway is observed along the venule. Its main function is to act as an absorption route, but leakage may also occur.

Nishikawa (1940) made an investigation of this pathway by injecting India ink into veins of the rabbit. According to his investigation, leakage of India ink was seen only in portions where the intima type lymphoid tissue was observed, that is to say in the walls of pulmonary veins. Thus the endothelial type lymphoid tissue related to the pulmonary vein was considered to belong to the para-venule fluid pathway.

Krause (1926) stated that when tubercle bacilli were injected intravenously in rabbits, the first foci emerged in lymphoid tissues; the injected bacilli were localized in the lung in a manner similar to that of India ink particles.

The extravascular fluid pathway system is undoubtedly a very important component of the circulatory system. Further studies on this point are necessary.

2. Production of Lymphocytes by Pulmonary Lymphoid Tissues

Production of lymphocytes by hilar lymph nodes can easily be inferred from the results of many experiments on other lymph nodes.

By quantitative investigations, Horii and Tamaki,et al. (1951) revealed that the total amount of the intrapulmonary lymphoid tissues is not inconsiderable; they judged these lymphoid tissues to have the capability of producing lymphocytes.

They compared numbers of lymphocytes, and numbers of mitochondria in lymphocytes. The unit number of lymphocytes in pulmonary arterial blood was 1,850, and the average number of mitochondria was 5.9. They reported the number of lymphocytes in the pulmonary venous blood to be far greater, namely, 4,610, and the number of mitochondria as 6.7.

Although samples were not large they made similar studies on lymphocytes in bronchial arteries and veins, and found that here there was not so much fluctuation. From the results of these investigations, they concluded that a considerable number of lymphocytes were produced by intrapulmonary lymphoid tissues, and that these lymphocytes moved into the systemic circulation through the pulmonary vein.

Horii and Tamaki, et al. (1951) tried to decrease the number of lymphocytes in the peripheral blood of rabbits by X-ray irradiation; they counted the number of lymphocytes in the pulmonary artery and vein during the irradiation and stated that the decrease of lymphocytes in the peripheral circulation was caused by the folmulation of lymphocytes in the lung.

Kihara (1954) observed reticular fiber networks, similar to those of the extravascular fluid pathway system, in the tissues surrounding the pulmonary artery. He observed that the lymphocytes degenerated by X-ray irridation accumulated in these regions. On the basis of these studies, Horii and Tamaki, et al. (1951) stated that the lung has the important function of regulating and adjusting the lymphocyte levels in the blood.

3. Pulmonary Lymphoid Tissue in Defensive Processes

The lymphoid tissue contributes to defense mechanisms as well as to the production of lymphocytes.

Foreign bodies may reach the lymphatic system of the lung by the tracheobronchial or hematogenous routes.

The author will describe these routes.

i. Foreign Bodies or Bacteria in Respiratory System

Whenever foreign bodies or bacteria in the respiratory system are taken into the lymphatic system of the lung, the aforementioned epithelial type lymphoid tissues and the extravascular fluid pathway system (Kihara) will play important roles.

Otani and Takawa (1943) made experimental studies on the role of lymphoid tissue during infection by whooping cough bacilli and revealed that infection will be less evident in individuals whose lymphoid tissues are well developed.

From their results it can be understood that the epithelial type lymphoid tissue contributes to the defense process.

However, results of experiments on insufflation of India ink made by Y. Senda, (1958) of the author's group, showed that the particles of India ink passed through lymphoid tissues, and moved rapidly into the surrounding lymph vessels. Therefore there is a possibility that exogenous bacteria may also move into lymph vessels without being filtrated by lymphoid tissues.

Particularly, tubercle bacilli said to elicit tissue reactions only in the beginning of infection may take the same route as the particles of India ink. This was confirmed for hay bacilli, pyocyaneus bacilli and tubercle bacilli, by the experiments of Umeda (1929).

Nishikawa (1940) stated that pulmonary lymphoid tissue was mainly distributed in the region of bifurcations of bronchi, structures most easily affected by exogenous injuries. Nishikawa considered this to be significant, from the point of the defense process of the organism; however, according to our own investigations the defense ability of the lymphoid tissue should not be overestimated.

In addition to the above, foreign bodies or bacteria which infiltrate into the respiratory system may take other routes to enter lymph vessels, *e.g.*, via the connective tissue from that portion of the bronchial wall which is covered by cuboidal or squamous epithelium.

Whichever the route may be, bacteria taken into the lung tissue from the respiratory system will not be disposed of completely before reaching lymph vessels.

Bacteria once taken into the lymph vessels will be carried to the hilum by lymph flow; however, in the human lung, enroute to the hilar lymph node, the lymph nodes and tissues which participate in the filtration of lymph are very few; it is relatively rare that foreign bodies or bacteria are stopped before reaching the hilar nodes.

In the instance of primary tuberculosis in which immunity is not established, even though primary foci and foci in the hilar lymph nodes are established it is rare to observe other foci along the lymph route connecting them.

On the other hand, in guinea pig or rabbit lungs, the endothelial type lymphoid tissue of the extravascular fluid pathway system (Kihara) is found very often to have developed on the wall of lymph vessel in relatively peripheral regions. According to the experiments of Y. Senda (1958), who studied insufflation of India ink into the respiratory system, this type of lymphoid tissue was observed to function as part of the paralymphovascular fluid pathway in releasing particles of India ink into lymph vessels.

From the results of his experiment of the lymph to conclude that foreign bodies or bacteria in the peripheral portion of the lymph vessel may also be partially stopped by endothelial type lymphoid tissue before reaching the hilar lymph nodes.

In the human lung the development of lymphoid tissue in the peripheral portion is poor, but highly developed lymph nodes are found in the hilum. Foreign bodies or bacteria which enter the lymph are disposed of mainly in the nodes of this latter region.

The lymph coming from the afferent lymph vessel flows into the central sinus from the marginal sinus of the lymph node, is filtrated through the node, and then enters the efferent lymph vessel.

When this is considered from the point of the mechanism of filtration of charcoal powder, anthracosis is first found only in the central sinus, as shown in Fig. 241, and later begins to appear in the intermediate sinus or marginal sinus.

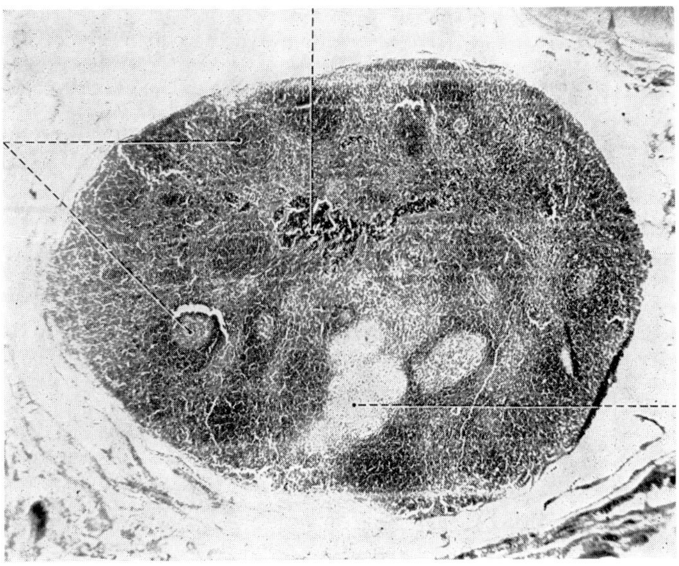

Fig. 241 Hilar lymph node with tuberculous lesion.

Similarly, when bacteria enter the node lymphatogenously they frequently localize in the central sinus. In other words, when the foci are found in this portion they can be considered to be lymphatogenous in origin.

When lymph nodes encompass many foreign bodies their reactivity may be decreased as a result of sclerosing processes; their ability to dispose of foreign bodies may also be decreased.

As can be seen from the above, lymph nodes have a function in the defensive processes; however, this role may be less significant if certain limits are exceeded; in fact, nodes may then degenerate partially or totally.

Fig. 242 shows a lymph node specimen from a 61 year-old man.

A portion of the lymph node covered by capsule looks like adipose tissue; lymphoid tissue containing secondary nodules is observed only in the remaining portion. It is particularly interesting to note that a cancer metastasis is found in this degenerated lymph node. The metastasis is observed only in the region where considerable lymphoid tissue remains.

ii. Foreign Bodies and Bacteria in Blood Vessels

When India ink is injected intravenously, particles of ink appear in the lymphoid tissue of the lung in a relatively short time.

This finding is the same for the subendothelial lymphoid tissue of the pulmonary vein, as well as for the lymphoid tissues of other regions.

Particles of India ink move directly from blood vessels into the lymphatic system, in the region of the lymphoid tissues. Such a direct relation of the blood vascular system to the lymphatic system is found only in the lymphoid tissues.

The mechanism whereby foreign bodies or bacteria move into lymphoid tissues from the blood vascular system has been under investigation for a long time; two points of view regarding this matter are roughly the following:

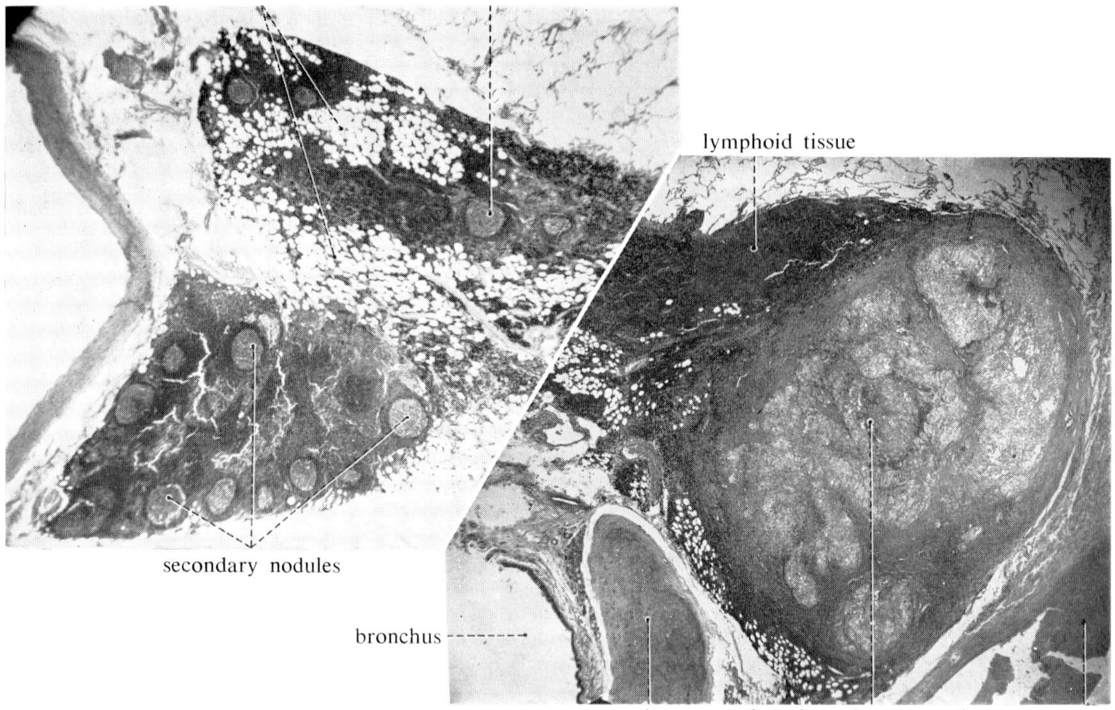

Fig. 242 Lung cancer metastasis founded in the hilar lymph node (61 year-old male).

One view is that various substances move into the lymphoid tissue from those parts of the venules in which the endothelium is highly cuboidal in shape (ZIMMERMAN, 1923; TEI, 1937).

The other view is that the arteriole forms a glomus in the secondary nodule of lymphatic tissue, and that various substances enter the lymphoid tissues from this arrangement (OGO, 1934).

Thus, according to either view, the direct movement of substances from the blood vascular system into the lymphatic system is probably performed chiefly through the lymphoid tissues. Pathologically the most interesting observations relate to hematogenous dissemination of tubercle bacilli.

KRAUSS (1926) reported that when tubercle bacilli were injected in the vein of the rabbit particularly evident foci were formed in the intrapulmonary lymphoid tissue. From this report it can also be considered that bacteria in the blood enter the lymphatic system in the region of the lymphoid tissues.

As will be seen from the above discussion, lymphoid tissues are observed in many places in the lung. Exogenous foreign bodies or bacteria may be disposed in these tissues, but, they may not be disposed of by filtration through only one lymph node.

However, since many lymph nodes lie in the hilum of the human lung, and endothelial type lymphoid tissues are observed in peripheral regions, the release of foreign bodies or bacteria into the vascular system may be stopped by filtration through lymphoid tissues.

Fig. 243 is a schema of the pulmonary lymphoid tissues.

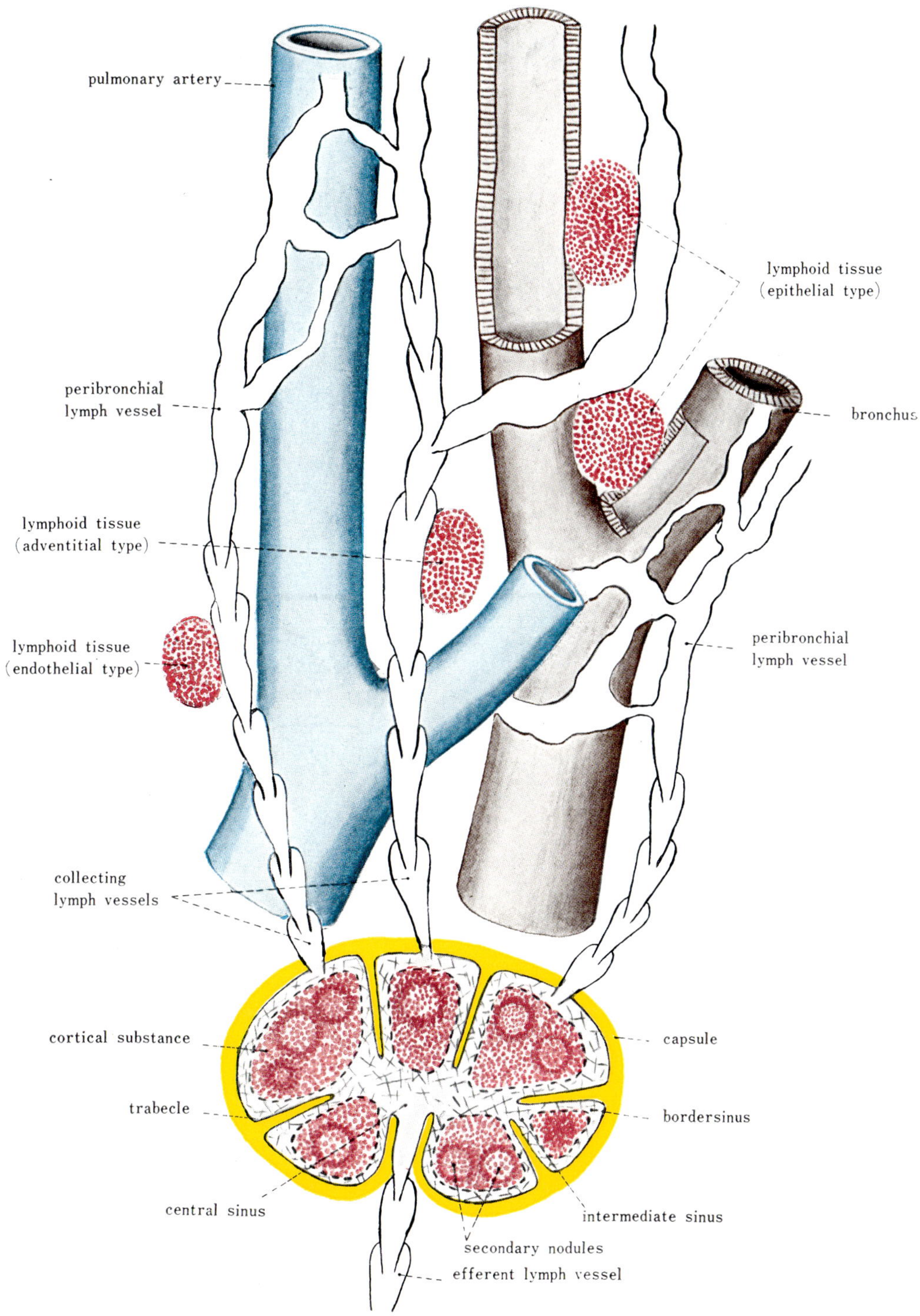

Fig. 243 Distribution of the lymphoid tissues in the lung.

Chapter IV. Nervous System

It has been well known since the beginning of 20th century that the lung is an organ which is innervated by the vegetative nervous system.

In general the lung is considered as a respiratory apparatus which inflates or collapses passively upon movement of the thorax and diaphragm, but it must not be forgotten that it is also an organ which has an automaticity of its own under the influence of the vegetative nervous system.

The neuromuscular and the neurovascular systems represent the anatomical basis of the automaticity of the lung.

In this chapter the systematic description is based on studies performed by the authors (NAGAISHI and INABA), of the anatomical and histological structures of the above system, as well as of the various reflexes.

I. OUTLINE OF INNERVATION OF LUNG

The lung is innervated by branches of the sympathetic, vagus and phrenic nerves. On the anterior and posterior surfaces of the hilum branches of these nerves form the pulmonary nerve plexuses.

The nerve fibers arising from these plexuses are distributed along bronchi and blood vessels.

Nerve fibers different from the above are found to distribute on the pulmonary pleura, forming fine networks. These nerve fibers originate also in the anterior and posterior pulmonary plexuses of the hlium.

The vegetative nerve fibers which run along the bronchi form bundles in the region of the bronchial cartilages, and are distributed in the lung, relayed by many ganglion cells along their way. Most of these are multipolar ganglion cells.

The postganglionic nerve fibers, arising from the ganglion cells which are observed along the bronchi, distribute in the lung, giving out many branches. However, ganglion cells are not observed along the branches of the pulmonary artery except in the region of the root of the artery.

The nerve fibers distributing in the lung can be classified as of two types, from functional and histological standpoints.

One, afferent nerve fibers, belong to the visceral sensory nervous system, and the other, efferent nerve fibers, belong to the vegetative nervous system.

The nerve endings of the visceral afferent system are composed of large myelinated nerve fibers, originating in free nerve endings.

These sensory nerve endings are distributed in the bronchi, blood vessels, parenchyma, and pleura.

The nerve endings observed in the pulmonary parenchyma are presumed to participate in the respiratory self-regulatory (HERING-BREUER) reflex.

These reflexes belong to the bronchial system, and are considered to participate in the regulation of the rhythm and depth of respiration. The cough reflex is also one of the reflexes arising in the tracheobronchial system.

The sensory nerve endings which are located in the pulmonary artery and vein are presumed to participate in the regulation of blood pressure in the systemic and pulmonary circulations.

The reflexes arising from the pulmonary vascular system are those of the pulmonary artery blood pressure regulating reflex, *i.e.* "Lungenentlastungs Reflex", the Bainbridge reflex.

In the muco-muscular layer of the bronchi, sensory nerve endings showing specific histological findings are observed. These endings are considered to participate in the vago-vagal reflex.

Besides the above, there is a pleuropulmonary reflex.

The efferent nerve fibers of the lung include the sympathetic and parasympathetic. The preganglionic fibers of the above system are myelinated; the postganglionic are non-myelinated.

The vegetative nerve endings, in the form of extremely fine nerve fibrils, are distributed in the bronchi, pulmonary parenchyma, pulmonary blood vessels, pulmonary muscle, and pulmonary pleura.

Among these the vasomotor nerves have a unique distribution.

In general, vasomotor nerves to the pulmonary artery and vein are exceedingly sparse, as compared with the distribution to bronchial arteries and veins; moreover, the vasomotor nerves of the vein are fewer than those of the artery.

The postganglionic fibers of the sympathetic nerves are not observed in alveolar capillaries or arterioles of less than 100 μ (inside dia.). This observation was confirmed by KAI and SAGAWA (1969) of the author's group using rapid freezing and Falck-Hillarp's fluorescent methods.

The vegetative nerve fibers distributing in the bronchi form networks of extremely fine nerve fibers in the tunica propria, submucous tissue and smooth muscle of the bronchial wall.

These vegetative nerve fibers are considered to participate in the contraction and dilation of the bronchus.

As it will be understood from the above, the nervous system of the lung distributes in all the tissues of the lung, including muscular and vascular systems, and participates in the secretion of the mucus and serous fluid of the bronchial walls, as well as in the neurovascular and neuromuscular regulations of pulmonary functions.

Table 17 shows the structure and the functional role of the nervous system in the lung.

Table 17 Structure and Function of the Nervous System of the Lung.

1) Afferent Nerve Fibers (Visceral Sensory Nervous System):
  a) Those distributed in the bronchial system
    i) Intracutaneous nerve; Regulates the cough reflex.
    ii) Sensory nerve ending in the tunica propria of the mucous membrane and submucous tissue: Regulates the cough reflex.
    iii) Sensory nerve ending in the bronchial branch and intrapulmonary smooth muscle: Relays the sense of air hunger (such as in an attack of bronchial asthma).
    iv) Sensory nerve ending in the alveolar duct peripheral from the respiratory bronchiole and interalveolar interstice: Participates in the pulmonary vagus nerve reflex (Hering-Breuer's reflex) and forms the centripetal pathway.
    v) Specific sensory nerve ending in the muco-muscular layer of the bronchus: Decreases the blood pressure or causes cardiac arrest reflectively.
  b) Those distributed in the vascular system
    i) Sensory nerve ending in the wall of the pulmonary artery: Participates in the pulmonary artery stem reflex (TAKINO).
    ii) Sensory nerve ending in the wall of the pulmonary vein: Participates in the reflex similar to Bainbridge's reflex.
    iii) Sensory nerve ending in the wall of the bronchial artery and vein: Regulates the sense of pain of the blood vessel.
  c) Those distributed in the pulmonary pleura
    Sensory nerve ending in the pulmonary pleura: Participates in the pulmonary vagus nerve reflex (Hering-Breuer's reflex) and respiratory reflex

2) Efferent Nerve Fibers (Vegetative Nervous System):
  a) Those distributed in the bronchial system
    i) Those in the bronchial mucous gland and serous gland: Participate in the bronchial mucous and fluid serection.
    ii) Those in the bronchial submucous tissue: Regulate the innervation of the connective tissue cell of the submucous tissue and tunica propria of the mucous membrane.
    iii) Those in the bronchial smooth muscle: Participate in the contraction and relaxation of the bronchial smooth muscle and pulmonary muscle.
    iv) Those in the pulmonary parenchyma: Participate in the contraction, dilatation and permeability of the alveolar capillary.
  b) Those distributed in the vascular system
    i) Vasomotric nerve of the pulmonary artery: Regulates the contraction and dilation of the pulmonary artery.
    ii) Vasomotoric nerve of the pulmonary vein: Regulates the contraction and dilation of the pulmonary vein.
    iii) Vasomotoric nerve of the bronchial artery and vein: Regulates the contraction and dilation of the bronchial artery and vein.
  c) Those distributed in the pulmonary pleura
    Those in the mesothelium of the pulmonary pleura and blood vessels: Participate in the permeability of the mesothelium of the pulmonary pleura and regulate the contraction and dilation of the capillary of pulmonary pleura.

Supplement: Staining Methods and Materials

The authors (NAGAISHI and INABA) used mainly Bielschowsky's method as modified by SUZUKI (1952), so-called Sugamo myelin sheath staining method (combined methods of KULSCHITZKY and PALQ), and FALCK-HILLARP's fluorescent method (1962).

When necessary, hematoxylin-eosin staining, or VAN GIESON's elastic fiber staining method was adopted.

CAJAL's method, GOLGI's method, methylene blue staining, BIELSCHOWSKY's method, and their modified methods were generally used for the staining of the nerve tissues; in the author's experiences, BIELSCHOWSKY's method as modified by SUZUKI was found to be the most simple in procedure and gave the best staining results.

Materials for investigation were obtained from fresh human or dog lungs. As regards the human lung, the normal portion of a freshly resected lobe was used. The tissue was fixed in 20% neutral formalin immediately after resection and was kept for two or three months. Thereafter, according to purpose, it was prepared by frozen section, paraffin section or celloidin section, etc. and by various staining methods.

On the other hand, when FALCK-HILLARP's fluorescent method was adopted, freshly resected human, rabbit, or guinea pig lung was used for investigation.

BIELSCHOWSKY's Staining Method (as modified by SUZUKI):

1) Fixation: The specimen is fixed in 20% neutral formalin for at least one week.
2) Preparation of section: 10–40 μ frozen sections are most suitable. When celloidin sections are to be made, BIELSCHOWSKY's method (modified by SUZUKI, and reformed by ODERA (1953)) is more suitable.
3) Preparatory treatment: a) Sections are kept in neutral formalin for one week or more. b) Sections will then be placed in a mixture of equal amounts of 5% sodium bicarbonate solution, neutral formalin, and 15% urotropin solution, for 30 min.
4) Washing: The material is washed in three 10-minute changes of distilled water.
5) Silver impregnation: After washing, the sections are placed in 20% silver nitrate solution for 1 hour at room temperature (20 minutes at 37°C, or 15 minutes at 50°C).
6) Washing: The sections are rinsed in distilled water for a few seconds.
7) Ammoniated silver nitrate bath: To 10 cc of 20% silver nitrate solution add a strong ammonia solution drop by drop until the sedimentation disappears. Then to 5 cc of this solution, again add 2 drops of strong ammonia. The sections are immersed in this final solution and left for 30 minutes in the dark.
8) Reduction: Put 10% tartaric acid-potassium bicarbonate solution in a small beaker or Petridish for ten sections are then picked up on a glass-rod at one time, put into the above solution and shaken gently for 30 seconds. The temperature of the reducing solution at this time should be 30°–40°C.
9) Washing: The sections are then washed in distilled water for 5 minutes.
10) Gold impregnation: The sections are then placed in a solution of 100 cc distilled water, 10 g ammonium rhodanilate, 10 g hydroquinone, to which 10 cc of 1% gold chloride is added. Gold impregnation and fixation occur simultaneously.
11) Mounting:

FALCK-HILLARP's Fluorescent Method (1962):

FALCK-HILLARP's fluorescent method uses sections fixed by formaldehyde gas after freeze drying under vacuum. By this method tissue catecholamine can be observed at the cellular level.

KAI and SAGAWA (1969) of the author's group used this fluorescent method in investigation of the sympathetic nerve supply of the lung. The postganglionic fibers of the sympathetic nerve are adrenergic fibers containing a large quantity of noradrenaline. For observation of these fibers in the lung the fluorescent microscope is used.

1) Preparation of specimen: Immediately after thoracotomy the lung is inflated to physiological size by increasing intrabronchial pressure. A portion of the lobe is resected. Using double forceps and cutting between them, a small wedge-shaped segment can be resected in the inflated condition.

The specimen thus prepared is immediately fixed in liquid nitrogen.

In the case of small animals (rabbit or guinea pig) these procedures are undertaken in vivo. For this purpose, KAI and SAGAWA adopted the rapid freezing method of STAUB, et al. (1962), as follows:

Under pentobarbital anesthesia, intratracheal intubation or tracheotomy is performed, and respiration is controlled.

Using an extensive and bilateral thoracotomy, the lung is exposed widely. When inflated to the physiological inspiratory phase, liquid nitrogen is poured into the thoracic cavity, freezing the lung instantaneously.

The lungs frozen as described are placed in a cryogenic chamber and cut in blocks (about 5 mm square) with a refrigerated razor blade. Several blocks are quickly wrapped with gauze and put into a vacuum container previously refrigerated by liquid nitrogen. The vacuum flask contains a drying agent (P_2O_5), and is connected to a vacuum lyophilizer.

2) Lyophilization: The vacuum lyophilizer developed by SHIMAMOTO and FUJIWARA (1965) is used. Pressure is reduced to 5×10^{-4} mm Hg. The container is placed in acetone which is refrigerated (dry ice) at minus 35–40°C. The temperature of the acetone should be maintained at minus 35–40°C.

It is necessary to perform all these procedures as quickly as possible.

Lyophilization is continued for 5 days; on the 6th day the acetone for refrigeration is removed. Room temperature is reached during the next 24 hours, and on the 7th day the pressure is returned to normal.

3) Treatment by paraformaldehyde-gas: After being returned to room temperature and normal pressure, the specimen is removed from the lyophilizer and moved as quickly as possible into a open glass container of paraformaldehyde. This tissue and container are then placed in a closed oven, and maintained at 80°C for 1 hour.

The paraformaldehyde vapor will permeate and fix the tissue, and at the same time cause oxidization of noradrenaline. The latter will form a fluorescent substance, as follows:

$$\text{noradrenaline} \xrightarrow{CH_2O} \text{6.7-dehydroxy-1.2.3.4-tetrahydroisoquinoline} \xrightarrow{CH_2O} \text{6.7-dihydroxy-3.4-dehydroisquinoline}$$

4) Embedding: The tissue is immediately placed in a container of paraffln-wax, at 60°C, connected to the lyophilizer and held for 30 minutes. The treatment in vacuo allows permeation of the paraffln into the tissue.

5) Preparation of section: The paraffin embedded block specimen, prepared as above, is cut into 6–15 μ sections. About 50 serial sections can be made from one block.

A section is flattened on a non-fluorescing glass slide; the glass is warmed until the paraffln melts and is then returned to room temperature. The section will adhere to the glass slide.

Several drops of a mixed solution of xylene and entellan (Merck) are placed on the section and a cover glass placed in position. Thus, deparaffining and mounting are carried out at the same time.

6) Observation and photographing: A fluorescent microscope (Nikon, Japan) and a 200W ultra electric pressure mercury lamp (Toshiba, Japan) as the source of the ultraviolet, are used to observe fluorescence.

In addition, it is necessary to use a BV excitationfilter (Nikon), a neutral filter, and Ratten 2B and Y-51 filters.

For ordinary observation it is desirable to use thicker sections, so that the course and distribution of the fibers can be seen clearly, but for simultaneously photographing it is necessary to make the section as thin as possible.

For color, ASA 100 Fuji-color film (Japan) or ASA 160 Ektachrome high speed film can be used. The exposure may require 3 or 4 minutes.

For black and white, Kodak Tri X is most suitable, using about 60 seconds exposure. When using these films it is recommended that findings be sketched when observed.

II. BRIEF HISTORY

A. Nineteenth Century

The nervous system of the lung has been studied, from both anatomical and histological standpoints, since the first half of the 19th century.

By the end of that century the following facts had been revealed.

1) On the anterior and posterior aspects of the hilum, anterior and posterior nerve plexuses are formed, mainly by the sympathetic and parasympathetic nerves. The nerve fiber bundles arising from these two plexuses run into the lung along the bronchi and blood vessels, and are distributed widely in the lung (BRAEUCKER, 1837).

2) In the submucous tissue of the bronchial wall a nerve plexus runs along the long axis of the respiratory tract (ISMEILOFF, 1873).

3) In the nerve fiber bundles distributing along the bronchi many small ganglion cells are observed (REMAK, 1844; VERSON, 1868; STIRLING, 1876).

4) In the membranous parts of the trachea and bronchi ganglion cells are observed, and nerve plexuses are observed between the bronchial mucus glands (FRANKENHÄUSER, 1879).

5) Of the nerve fibers in the lung, the myelinated nerves distribute to the bronchial mucous membrane and smooth muscle (STIRLING, 1876; KRAUSE, 1876); the non-myelinated nerve fibers are distributed to blood vessels and to bronchial mucous membrane (STIRLING, 1876; KRAUSE, 1876).

6) The nerve fibers accompanying the bronchial arteries give off branches to the smooth muscle or mucous membrane. Many nerve fibers and nerve endings are observed between the alveoli. The nerve plexuses surrounding the bronchial arteries are abundant as compared with those accompanying the pulmonary artery (BERKELEY, 1893).

7) The ganglia of the bronchial wall are composed of multipolar cells and belong to the sympathetic nervous system. The postganglionic fibers are extremely fine non-myelinated fibers and are distributed to bronchial muscles (ARNSTEIN and PLOSCHKO, 1897).

8) The nerve endings are bell-like or spiral (ARNOLD, 1863), glomerular (SMIRNOW, 1888), terminal lamina form (CUCCATI, 1888), or small and nodular in shape (RETZIUS, 1893).

B. Twentieth Century

Further detailed studies have continued, as noted in the following.

After REMAK (1844), BUDDE (1904) made a highly detailed study of the nerve ganglia of the lung. He stated as follows:

In the mammalian lung ganglion cells are observed on the bronchial walls, but not on the wall of the pulmonary arteries.

The number, shape and size of the sympathetic ganglia differ according to the animal form, and may be divided into the peribronchial and submucous ganglia according to location.

In mouse, guinea pig and dog, the ganglia are observed only in the region surrounding the bronchi, but in rabbit, hedgehog and human fetus they are observed in the region surrounding the bronchi, and in the submucous layer as well.

The peripheral distribution of the peribronchial ganglia differs from animal to animal, but the submucous ganglia are fewer in peripheral regions, and smaller in size.

The peribronchial ganglia are predominant in the region of the pulmonary vein and bronchi, as well as about the tracheal bifurcation and pulmonary artery and vein. The nerve bundles containing the ganglia belong to the bronchi, but not to the pulmonary artery or the vein.

PONZIO (1906): Later, PONZIO also performed the staining of the nervous systems of the lungs of the kitten, dog and human fetus. He used methylene blue and alum carmine staining methods, and issued the following report:

Numerous nerve fibers were observed around the bronchi and alveoli. Particularly in the region between the first and third order bronchi there were numerous nerve fibers, some of which reached the bronchial mucous membrane.

The bronchi of the fourth order were surrounded by nerve networks. From this region nerve fibers ran into the bronchial wall, and partly into the epithelium of the mucous membrane.

In the pulmonary parenchyma, many inter- and peri-alveolar plexuses were observed.

Parallel with the above histological investigations experiments on degeneration were performed as described in the following.

IKEGAMI and YAGITA (1907) investigated chromatolysis in nerve cells in the left nodose ganglion, after performing a left lower lobectomy in the dog. They stated that 12–13% of the nerve cells in this ganglion served as the origin of fibers which terminated in the lung.

MÖLLGAARD (1912) performed experiments on nerve degeneration using infant dogs and cats. He investigated chromatolysis in nerve cells after lung resection, classifying the nervous system of the lung as follows.

MOLHANT (1913) also investigated the chromatolysis which occurred after resection of a rabbit lung, and obtained results similar to those of IKEGAMI and YAGITA; he stated that bronchial muscles and pulmonary muscles (in the narrow sense) received innervation from the dorsal nucleus of the vagus nerve.

1. Sympathetic System

a. Nerve Fibers

These emerge from the lateral horn and reach the stellate ganglion via the white rami communicantes. The nerve fibers coming out from the above reach the lung of the same or the opposite side via the ansa subclavia and vagus nerves. His opinion was that these fibers were vasomotor nerves.

b. Afferent Nerve Fibers

These arise from the same or the opposite side of the lung and, via the ansa subclavia and the vagus nerve, reach the stellate ganglion. Further, via the rami communicantes, they reach Th_{II}–Th_{III} spinal ganglia. The nerve cell processes then enter the posterior roots of the spinal cord.

2. Parasympathetic System

a. Efferent Nerve Fibers

These nerve fibers leave the dorsal nucleus of the vagus nerve and, via the vagus nerve trunk, the nodose ganglion, and the pulmonary branch of the vagus nerve, reach the lung of the same side. There is a possibility that some nerve fibers may cross on the way and proceed to the opposite side.

These nerve fibers were classified into the bronchomotor and secretory nerves, and the former were further classified into bronchodilators or bronchoconstrictors.

b. Afferent Nerve Fibers

These nerve fibers leave the lung of the same or the opposite side and reach the nodose ganglion via the vague nerve, and then reach the sensory nucleus of the vague nerve or join the uppermost part of the tractus solitarius.

LARSELL and MASON (1921) performed the experiment of cutting one of the cervical vague nerves of the rabbit. Degeneration was evident in the pericellular neural networks of the lung of the operated side. The few normal nerve fibers that were observed in some regions they considered to have originated in the vagus nerve of the opposite side, and that the vagus nerve distributed not only in the lung of the same but also to the opposite side.

RASMUSSEN (1926) investigated the nerve pathways from pulmonary parenchyma to central nervous system, and devised a schema of nerve distribution. His results differed slightly from those of MÖLLGAARD.

Pathological changes in the nervous system in various chest diseases have been reported, *e.g.*, pulmonary tuberculosis (MILLER, 1918), FILATOWA and LAWRENTJEW (1932); and bronchiectasis (SUNDER-PLASSMANN, 1935).

A detailed study was made by LARSELL (1921) on peripheral nerve endings. The following is a summary of this study.

When using methylene blue staining, sensory nerve endings were observed in the epithelium of the intrapulmonary bronchi, particularly in the epithelium of the tracheal bifurcation, and in the outermost peripheral regions they were observed also on the alveolar walls. These endings were briefly classified according to position and function.

The stimulation of the nerve endings of the larger bronchi elicits the cough reflex. The endings of the peripheral small bronchi protect against intrusion of foreign bodies, causing reflectoric contraction of bronchial muscles. Nerve endings of the alveolar region are stimulated by expansion and contraction of this region and cause the Hering-Breuer reflex.

In the pulmonary artery and its branches an abundance of nerve fiber endings in the muscle cells of the tunica media is observed, whereas the distribution of nerve fibers in the pulmonary vein is sparse.

In the pulmonary artery and its branches an abundance of nerve fiber endings in the muscle cells of the tunica mammals, including studies of plexuses, ganglion cells, and nerve endings.

LARSELL and DOW (1935) investigated the innervation of lung and pleura. From these studies they concluded that the sensory nerve endings of the alveolar region of the human lung are chemoreceptors, which respond to changes in partial pressure of carbon dioxide.

The above investigations were on man or mammals. JONES (1926) performed detailed investigation on the distribution of the nerve endings and nerves of reptilian lungs, using methylene blue staining, with results as follows:

The sensory nerve endings observed in the epithelium of the bronchi and alveoli in snake and turtle can be classified as of two types.

One type is devoid of capsule, is composed of small nerve fibers and terminates in the epithelial cell layer; the other type is encapsuled and terminates in the subepithelial connective tissue. In the snake and the turtle specific intramuscular nerve endings are observed.

These nerve fibers are myelinated and originate in the peribronchial nerve plexus. In the muscles of the bronchial and atrial walls, motor nerve endings are observed.

On the bronchial wall around the hilum, ganglia of various sizes are observed. The ganglion cells are surrounded by pericellular networks; these are considered to represent the endings of myelinated nerves originating in the pulmonary plexus.

The postganglionic nerve fibers arising from the ganglion cells distribute to the bronchial walls and to intrapulmonary muscles.

In the vascular system of the lung, as with the bronchi, abundant nerve plexuses composed of fine nerve fibers are observed; the nerve fibers arising from these plexuses terminate in the smooth muscles of the tunica media. The capillaries of the lung are also innervated by nerve networks, which either run parallel with the capillaries or surround them.

Around the same time, GLASER (1927) carried out studies on the distribution of nerves and nerve endings to the bronchial walls and to the vascular walls in human and mammalian lungs. He used methylene blue, RONGALIT-WEISS', SCHULTZE-GROS' silver stainings etc.

Later OKAMURA (1937), investigated intrapulmonary nerve ganglia and nerve endings in human and animal lungs, using GOLGI's staining method. ARIMOTO and MIYAKEGAWA (1930) investigated, by CAJAL's method, the distribution of nerves in the lungs of turtle, pigeon and cat. They confirmed that nerve fibers are found on the alveolar wall and that ganglion cells occur in the pulmonary parenchyma.

Using CAJAL's method TAKINO (1932–1934) investigated the vasomotor nerves of various animals in detail.

TAKINO, together with EZAKI, carried out a comparative study of the innervation of the pulmonary blood vessels, and reported on the existence of blood pressure receptor areas.

TAKINO, in his research in relation to asthma, reported interesting findings on the pulmonary artery stem reflex and the pulmonary vein stem-left atrium reflex.

About the same time, SUNDER-PLASSMANN (1933) carried out his study on the sensory nerve endings of the bronchial wall, using BIELSCHOWSKY-GROS' method. His investigations concerned the clinical significance of the sensory nerve endings, especially in shock occurring during intrathoracic operations under local anesthesia. Several years after, he performed detailed histological studies on the innervation of the pulmonary parenchyma and capillaries.

The histological findings on the nervous system of the lung would seem to have been completed by the studies of SUNDER-PLASSMANN, but GAYLER (1934) performed similar researches with methylene blue staining. Adopting BIELSCHOWSKY's method as modified by SETO, HAYASHI (1937) also made systematic histological investigations on pulmonary innervation.

In the same year, NONIDEZ (1937) reported the observation of nerve endings at the openings of the pulmonary vein to the left atrium. Similar endings had been reported by Takino prior to this. TAKINO, et al. confirmed later (1950) by animal experiment that these endings participated directly in the Bainbridge's reflex.

In 1937, using CAJAL's method, MIYAKE studied pulmonary innervation as a part of histological researches on the blood vessels of the human fetus.

Following SUNDER-PLASSMANN, DIJKSTRA (1939) investigated the nervous system of the lung in detail, using BIELSCHOWSKY-GROS' method. Several years later, ELFTMAN (1943) using CAJAL-NONIDEZ' method, stained the nerve endings of the bronchi of the lungs of dogs; he found various types of endings, chiefly sensory in type. These investigators did not mention motor nerve endings.

Around the same time, SASAKI (1943) made observations on the innervation of the trachea of man, using BIELSCHOWSKY's method as modified by SETO.

As a result, it was disclosed that the centrifugal nerve endings were in the form of a terminal reticulum, and also that there were three types of centripetal sensory endings.

These were the specific nerve endings which are seen in the muscular or membranous parts of the trachea; simple glomerular type endings were found in the muscular tissues.

BRONKHORST and DIJKSTRA (1940) advanced a schema of innervation of the lung, based on DIJKSTRA's histological findings (1930).

Later their schema was helpful in the clinical researches of STURM (1948).

In his general remarks about the histology of the visceral sensory nervous system, SETO (1950) mentioned the sensory nerves of the lung; and UYEDA (1954), as a part of his study of innervation of the pulmonary circulation, performed histological studies on the sensory innervation of the pulmonary artery and vein.

In the next year, C. KIMURA (1954) using either BIELSCHOWSKY's method as modified by SETO, or EHRLICH's method for staining of medullary sheaths, investigated the sensory nerve innervation of the lung. They found afferent fibers in the vagus nerve from the lung to be more abundant than the afferent nerve fibers in spinal nerves. They stated that sensory nerve fibers were not observed to come from the opposite side.

MIZUKOSHI (1953) investigated histologically the innervation of human fetal lung, and SAITO (1955) made similar investigations on dog lung.

NAGAISHI and his associates carried out morphological and physiological studies of the lung, since 1948 as a part of their basic researches on chest surgery and chest diseases. Out of these researches, regarding the structure of the normal lung, they published a monograph (in Japanese) titled "The Structure of the Lung", describing the nervous system of the lung in Chapter IV of Vol. II, 1958.

Since then, KAI and SAGAWA of the present author's group (1969) have carried on studies of the sympathetic nerve supply of the lung, using FALCK-HILLARP's fluorescent method.

HIRSH and KAISER (1969) also published a book titled "The Innervation of the Lung".

The following is a summary of the contents of their text.

The vegetative nervous system, mainly composed of vagus nerves, goes into the lung from the tissue surrounding the bronchus at the hilum, and extends to the peripheral portions of the respiratory tract.

The vagus nerves are composed of many thick myelinated fibers, a few thin myelinated fibers, postganglionic non-myelinated fibers, and many ganglion cells.

Compared with the vagal fibers the sympathetic nerve fibers are finer and mostly non-myelinated, but they also contain many thin myelinated fibers.

Centrifugal and centripetal nerve fiber bundles are distributed in the lung, terminating in their respective nerve endings.

The centrifugal nerve fibers distribute mainly to the smooth muscle, and the centripetal fibers are widely distributed as sensory nerve endings.

The following types of sensory nerve endings are observed: 1) Fibers distributed in the bronchial epithelial layers, 2) Nerve endings (there are simple and complicated types) distributed in subepithelial tissues of the alveolar sacs, ducts, and bronchi, 3) Thick spinal nerve fibers distributed to the alveolar walls, and 4) Annular nerve fibers distributed in the smooth muscles of bronchi, parenchyma, and blood vessels.

In view of the structure and distribution of these centripetal nerve fibers, various sensory nerve reflexes (and other complicated functions) are considered to exist.

It is regrettable that only a few statements about the nervous system are found in the famous and widely appreciated books by MILLER (1947), and by HAYEK (1953 and 1970).

Embryological studies about the nervous system of the lung are rare; MÖLLGAARD'S (1912) is a singular exception.

He stated that the nervous system of the lung has two origins. In the same way as the lung is composed of two different systems, bronchial and vascular, the nervous system is also composed of two different systems.

From this point of view he considered that the bronchial system is innervated by the vagus nerve and the vascular system by the sympathetic nerves, the pulmonary parenchyma receiving joint innervation.

The most detailed and systematic investigation of nerve endings and nerve fibers of the lung is that of HAYASHI (1937), who used BILESCHOWSKY'S method (as modified by SETO).

Some researchers, such as DIJKSTRA (1939), are dubious about his work; however, according to investigations by the authors, the accomplishments of HAYASHI seem to be fairly credible.

As regards clinical researches on the nerve supply of the lung various reports have been made, *e.g.*, SAUERBRUCH (1932), OVERHOLT (1949), COURNAND (1950), and many others.

As previously mentioned, the clinico-pathological researches on the lung were made by STURM (1948) from the point of the vegetative nervous system.

As the result, many new interpretations were advanced regarding the role of the vegetative nervous system in atelectasis, pulmonary emphysema and bronchiectasis, etc.

However, most of these interpretations were made from clinical or physiological, and rarely from morphological viewpoints. The present author considers that further researches will be required, and on a proper histological basis.

III. DISTRIBUTION OF NERVOUS SYSTEM IN LUNG

Branches of the sympathetic, parasympathetic (vagus) and phrenic nerves are distributed in the lung.

The vagus nerve originates in the medulla oblongata, descends in the cervical tissues, and distributes in the thorax mainly to lung, heart and esophagus. The sympathetic nerves arise from the upper thoracic ganglia of the sympathetic chain and distribute similarly.

In the cervical and thoracic regions many anatomoses may occur in these nerve trunks.

On the anterior and posterior aspects of the hilum nerve plexuses are formed by mixed fibers.

Table 18 shows the relationship between these plexuses and the extra- and intrapulmonary nerves.

Peripherally, nerve fibers originating in the anterior and posterior pulmonary nerve plexuses are distributed in the lung, accompanying the bronchi and blood vessels.

The nerve bundles accompanying the bronchi contain many multipolar ganglia; each ganglion is made up of 2 to 10 ganglion cells.

In the regions surrounding the large bronchi ganglia are numerous, but they are less frequently found around the small peripheral bronchi. The large nerve bundles and ganglia are outside of rather than on the bronchial walls.

The existence of so many ganglion cells is one of the factors which make an understanding of the innervation of the lung rather difficult.

Whether the ganglion cells belong to the sympathetic or the parasympathetic system is still in question. A current interpretation is as follows:

The vagal efferent fibers are relayed by the ganglion cells in the lung; the afferent fibers do not show such relaying.

Most of the sympathetic nerves are efferent (motor), but the relay of nerve fibers by ganglion cells is not confirmed.

The above statements stem from the degeneration experiments of the nerves of LARSELL (1920), LARSELL and MASON (1921) and BRONKHORST and DIJKSRA, et al. (1940).

Table 18 Nervous system of the lung

Extrapulmonary portion	Hilar portion	Intrapulmonary portion
Sympthetic nerve	Anterior pulmonary nerve plexus	Peribronchial nerve plexus
Vagus nerve (para-sympathetic nerve)		Periarterial nerve plexus
Phrenic nerve	Posterior pulmonary nerve plexus	Perivenous nerve plexus

BRONKHORST and DIJKSTRA stated that the nervous system of the lung is classified into the centripetal (sensory) and centrifugal (motor, secretory, vasomotor) nerve fibers, innervating not only blood vessels but also bronchial muscle and bronchial mucous glands; the latter would better be called "Die allgemeine autonome Nervenbahnen". It was impossible specifically to classify these nerves by function, *e.g.*, secretory, motor, or vasomotor nerves. Both sympathetic and parasympathetic centrifugal nerve fibers are physiologically involved in regulating tissues and organs, and in this respect the lung is not an exception.

Figs. 244, 245, 246 and 247 show schemas of the nervous system of the lung. Among them Fig. 246 is adopted from that of STURM.

As will be seen from these figures, the lung receives innervation from the sympathetic, parasympathetic (vagus), and phrenic nerves; via these three nerve routes efferent nerve fibers (vegetative nervous system) and afferent nerve fibers (visceral sensory) can be considered to be distributed in the lung.

In relation to the above figures, NAGAISHI and INABA (1958) explained the distribution of nerves in the lung according to main functions, listing the following:

I. Afferent (Visceral Sensory).
  A) Distributed in the bronchial system:
    i) Intraepithelial nerves: Regulate cough reflex.
    ii) Sensory nerve endings distributed in the tunica propria of the mucous membrane and submucous tissue: Regulate the senses of touch and pain.
    iii) Sensory nerve endings distributed in bronchi and in intrapulmonary muscle: Relay the feeling of air hunger (*e.g.,* asthma).
    iv) Sensory nerve endings distributed in alveolar ducts and in alveolar interstices: Participate in the Hering-Breuer reflex.
    v) Specific sensory nerve endings distributed in the muco-muscular layer of the bronchi (Seto's type I which contributes to the baro-depressor reflex, Sunder-Plassmann's so-called "neuro-vegetative Rezeptorenfelder"): Decrease the blood pressure reflectively; may lead to cardiac arrest.
  B) Distributed in the vascular system:
    i) Sensory nerve endings distributed in the pulmonary artery: Participate in the pulmonary artery stem reflex (TAKINO), "Lungenentlastungs reflex" (SCHWIEGK).
    ii) Sensory nerve endings distributed in pulmonary veins: Induce reflex similar to the Bainbridge reflex (TAKINO, NONIDEZ).
    iii) Sensory nerve endings distributed in bronchial artery and vein: Regulate the sense of pain originating in blood vessels. However, there is a question about this point.
  C) Distributed in the pulmonary pleura: Sensory nerve endings which participate in the Hering-Breuer reflex.

II. Efferent (Vegetative, Autonomic).
  A) Distributed in the bronchial system:
    i) To bronchial mucus serous glands: Participate in mucus and fluid secretions.
    ii) To bronchial submucous tissue: Innervate the connective tissue cells of the submucosa and tunica propria.
    iii) To bronchial smooth muscle: Participate in the contraction and relaxation of bronchial and other muscles.
    iv) To pulmonary parenchyma: Participate in the contraction, dilation and permeability of alveolar epithelium, and possibly in innervation of the alveolar capillary.
  B) Distributed in the vascular system:
    i) Vasomotor nerves to the pulmonarry artery: Regulate the contraction and dilation of the pulmonary artery.
    ii) Vasomotor nerves to the pulmonary vein: Regulate the contraction and dilation of the pulmonary vein.
    iii) Vasomotor nerves to the bronchial artery and vein: Regulate the contraction and dilation of the bronchial vessels.
  C) To the pulmonary pleura: Distributed in the mesothelium of the pulmonary pleura, and to blood vessels: Participate in the permeability of the mesothelium, and regulate the contraction and dilation of capillaries. There is a question as to this point.

As a supplement to the above, it should be noted that the visceral sensory system of the lung is

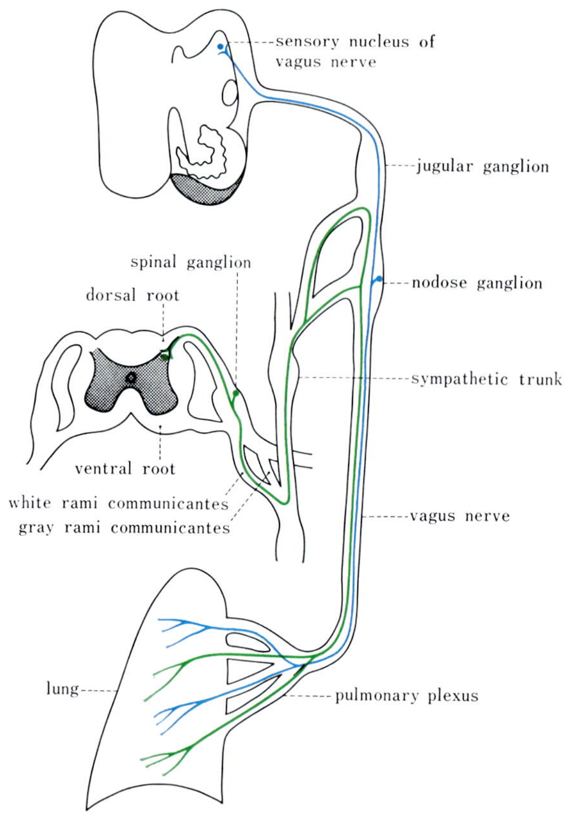

Fig. 244 Schema of the afferent innervation of the lung.
Blue: vagal nerve fibers, Green: sympathetic nerve fibers.

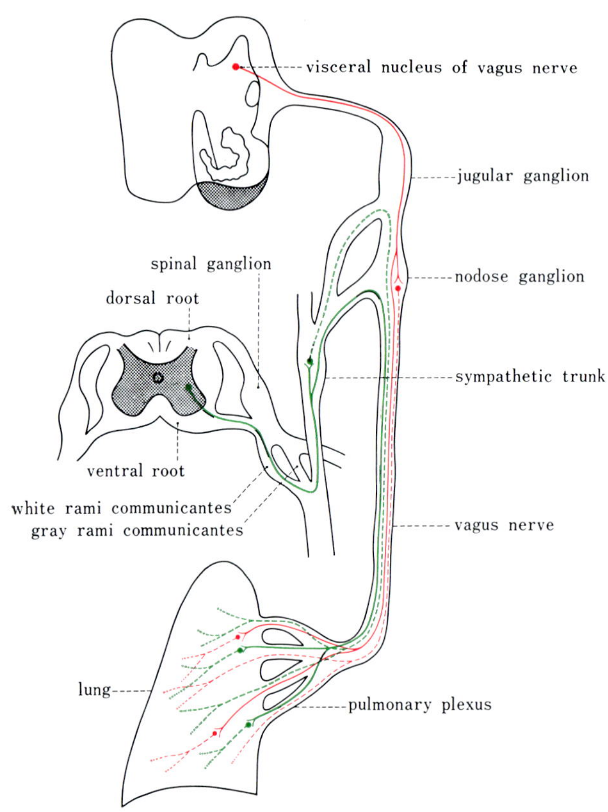

Fig. 245 Schema of the efferent innervation of the lung.
Red: parasympathetic preganlionic nerve fibers. Green: sympathetic preganglionic nerve fibers. Red (dotted): parasympathetic preganglionic nerve fibers. Green (dotted): sympathetic postganglionic fibers.

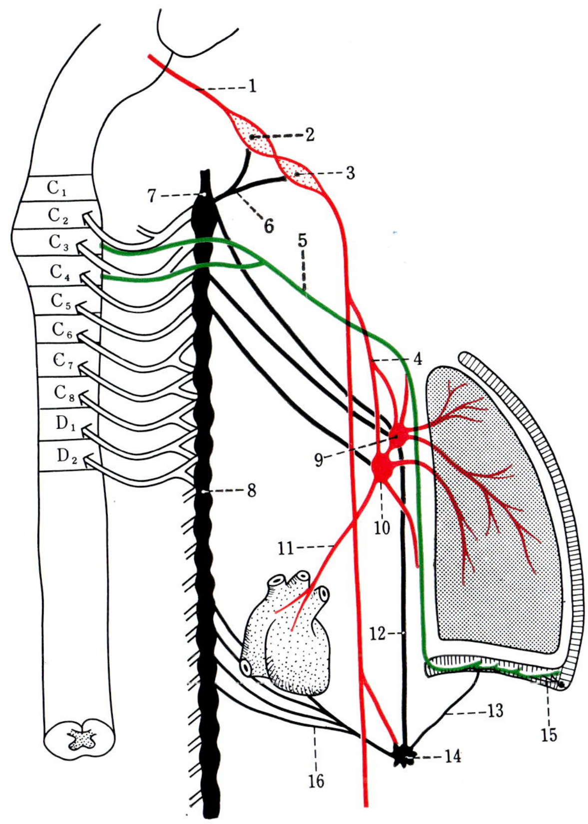

Fig. 246 Schema of the pulmonary innervation (STURM).

1. vagus nerve
2. jugular ganglion
3. nodose ganglion
4. rami pulmonales
5. phrenic nerve
6. rami communicantes
7. superior cervical ganglion
8. sympathetic trunk
9. anterior pulmonary plexus
10. posterior pulmonary plexus
11. pneumocardiac nerve
12. pneumogastric nerve
13. anastomosis of solar ganglion and phrenic nerve
14. caeliac plexus and solar ganglion
15. anastomosis of XII intercostal nerve and phrenic nerve
16. splanchnic nerve

composed of afferent nerve fibers distributed as mentioned above to bronchi, bood vessels, pulmonary parenchyma and pulmonary pleura, originating in specific sensory nerve endings.

These sensory nerve endings in addition to being far larger than the vegetative nerve fibers endings can also be definitely distinguished morphologically.

Most of these afferent nerve fibers run in the vagus nerve, reaching the sensory nucleus of the vagus in the medulla oblongata. Others enter posterior roots of spinal nerves. The latter run in the sympathetic nerves and reach the posterior roots of the spinal nerves via the rami communicantes.

In short, the visceral sensory nervous system of the lung is composed of the afferent nerve fibers, which relay intrinsic and extrinsic stimuli to the central nervous system. The vegetative nervous system is composed of efferent nerve fibers, which relay impulses from the central nervous system to the periphery.

As is well known, the vegetative nervous system is an efferent nervous system which regulates the secretion from glands, and the movements of organs and blood vessels, without regard to consciousness. The fibers of the sympathetic and parasympathetic nerves are histologically different from those of the sensory nerves; they terminate in a closed system which includes the terminal reticulum surrounding the tissue cells being innervated.

In the lung the efferent fibers distribute in the bronchi, pulmonary parenchyma and blood vessels, and provide vegetative innervation of the lung.

Supplement I: Distribution of Sympathetic Postganglionic Fibers

From the clinical standpoint it is extremely important to know the exact distribution of sympathetic and parasympathetic fibers in the lung. However, this has not yet exactly been demonstrated by any existing staining methods.

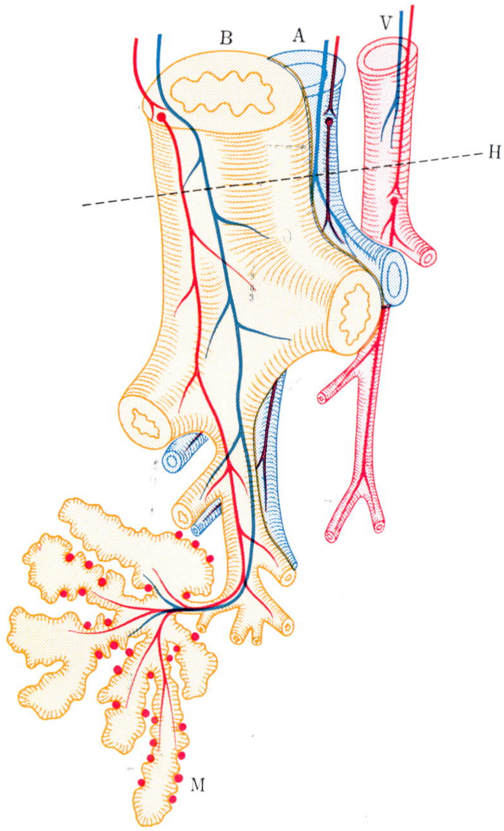

Fig. 247 Schema of the pulmonary innervation
V: pulmonary vein, A: pulmonary artery
B: bronchus, H: hilum, M: alveolar muscles
red: efferent nerve fibers
blue: afferent nerve fibers

Kai and Sagawa (1969) applied Falck-Hillarp's fluorescent method to the investigation of the post-ganglionic fibers of the sympathetic nerves, using guinea pig, rabbit and human lungs.

These are adrenergic fibers, containing large amounts of noradrenaline. When changed into a chemical substance on treatment with formaldehyde gas, and observed under the fluorescence microscope, yellow-green fluorescence can be seen. The location and distribution of the fibers can be determined by this method.

The following is a summary of the studies of Kai and Sagawa of the author's group.

As seen by previously used staining methods, innervation decreased in the following order: bronchi →pulmonary artery→pulmonary vein; however, the number of fluorescent fibers was in the order: pulmonary artery→bronchi→pulmonary vein. Particularly in the pulmonary vein, the number of fluorescent fibers is very few.

The differences disclosed will be, of course, a function of the specificity of the older and newer methods.

Postganglionic fibers of the parasympathetic nerve contain cholinesterase; its distribution can be observed in histochemical investigations.

The question as to whether the distribution of the vegetative nerve fibers is greater to bronchi or to pulmonary artery can be discussed upon detection of the postganglionic parasympathetic fibers, as stained selectively by such a method.

In the pulmonary artery, the postganglionic sympathetic fluorescent fibers run to peripheral regions, surrounding spirally the boundary surface between the adventitia and tunica media at intervals of 30–40 μ.

On the way the fibers anastomose with those of the bronchial wall by many rami communicates.

These fluorescent fibers are observed in some parts of the muscular artery in its entire length, but generally are not found in vessels of less than 100 μ internal diameter.

In the muscular arteries fluorescent fibers reach the tunica media, but this type of fiber is not observed in the inner coat.

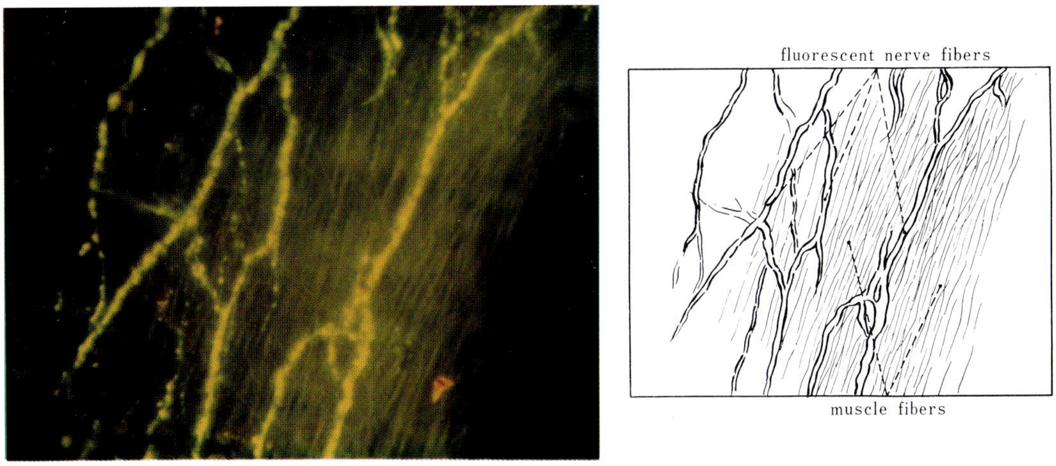

Fig. 248 Dot-like arrangement of the fluorescent nerve fibers in the longitudinal section of a pulmonary artery (1000 μ, inside diameter; rabbit)

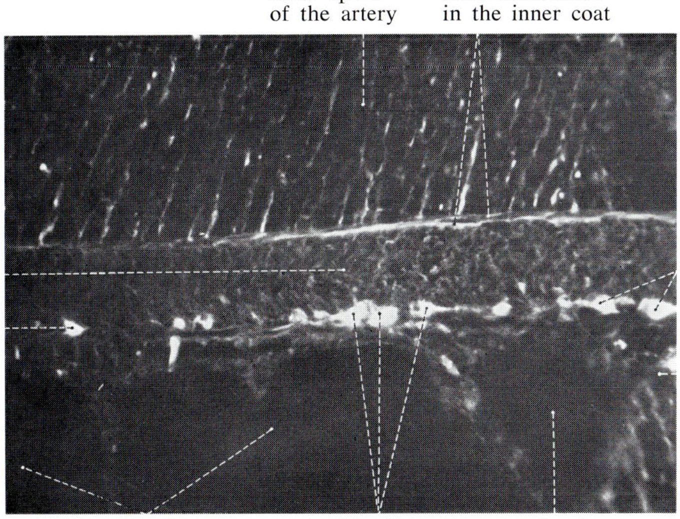

Fig. 249 Dot-like arrangement of the fluorescent fibers in the longitudinal section of a pulmonary artery (1000 μ, inside diameter; rabbit).

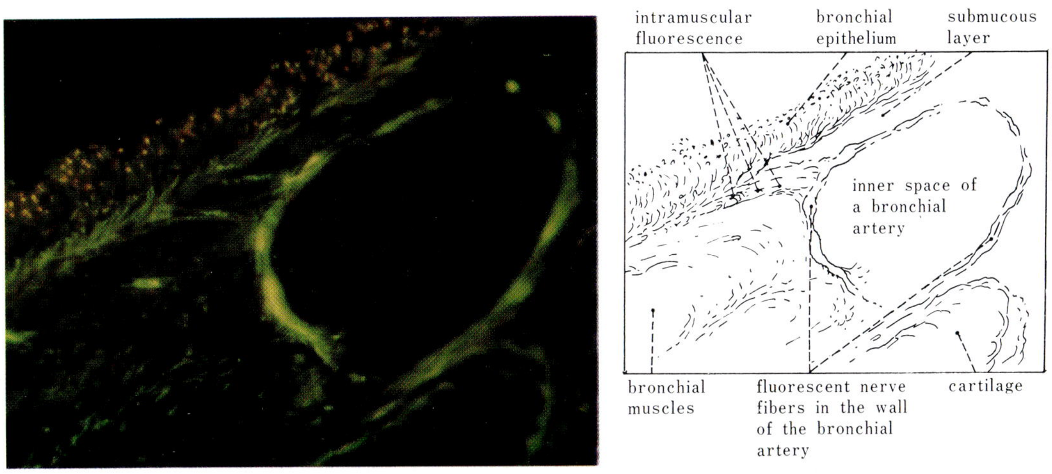

Fig. 250 Fluorescent nerve fibers in the bronchial wall (guinea pig).

Fig. 248 shows the wall of the pulmonary artery of a rabbit; the inside diameter is 1,000 μ. The fluorescent fibers form visible and numerous networks.

Fig. 249 shows a vertical section of a similar portion of the pulmonary artery of a rabbit. Between adventitia and tunica media a punctiform fluorescence is observed.

In the bronchi, fluorescent fibers are observed to be arranged as subchondral, extrachondral and subepithelial plexuses.

Contrary to findings using ordinary and customary staining methods, the distribution of fluorescent fibers is found to be far less extensive in the extrachondral as compared with the subchondral plexuses.

These plexuses are distributed mainly to smooth muscles.

Fluorescence is most distinguishable in the region surrounding the bronchial arteries running along the bronchial walls.

In the subepithelial layer of the bronchus, fluorescence is observed in the region corresponding to the portion where the subepithelial plexus exists.

Many anastomoses are observed between the fluorescent fibers of the plexus in the region surrounding the bronchial artery and the subchondral, extrachondral and subepithelial plexuses. The subepithelial plexuses appear to originate in the region surrounding the bronchial artery.

Fig. 250 shows the bronchial wall of a guinea pig. Fluorescence is observed in the bronchial muscles, but is more evident in the region surroundng the bronchial artery. In this figure, fluorescence is not found in the subepithelial tissues.

In the peripherial bronchi, where cartilage is lacking, there are peribronchial and subepithelial plexuses in which fluorescence can be observed. The intensity of fluorescence decreases as the bronchi become smaller.

When the walls of the bronchus and pulmonary artery are compared, it is generally considered that the bronchus shows a more plentiful innervation than does the pulmonary artery.

The bronchi appear to be more heavily innervated because the bronchi are accompanied by bronchial arteries which receive a more plentiful innervation by sympathetic nerves.

If the bronchial artery is removed from the bronchial wall there is found to be not much difference between the bronchus and the pulmonary artery.

Besides, in the peripheral bronchi which are devoid of cartilages fluorescent fibers seem to be fewer in number as compared with those in the accompanying pulmonary arteries.

Between the fluorescent fibers of the bronchial and pulmonary artery walls, evident anastomoses are observed.

The above findings are almost the same in guinea pig, rabbit, and man.

However in the pulmonary vein, depending on the kind of animals examined, evident differences are observed.

In rabbits, especially fluorescent fibers are observed in this view. In the pulmonary veins of guinea pig or man fluorescent fibers are also observed, but are less in quantity, than in the pulmonary artery.

A difference will also be seen according to the size of the veins. In the veins of 100–300 μ (internal dia.), fairly abundant fluorescent fibers are observed, but in veins larger than 500 μ, the fluorescent fibers are fewer, and in those smaller than 100 μ, no fluorescent fibers can be observed.

No anastomosing fibers exist between the fluorescent fibers of the pulmonary vein and those of the bronchus or the pulmonary artery.

Fig. 251 shows the fluorescent fibers of the pulmonary vein of 200 μ (internal dia.) of a guinea pig.

Fig. 252 shows the fluorescent fibers in the region surrounding a pulmonary vein of 150 μ (internal dia.) of a man.

Supplement II: Histological Studies of Nerve Endings

Histological studies of vegetative nerve endings are considered indispensable to an understanding of the innervation of the lung.

In addition to a consideration of past studies, the present author's opinion will be described.

The neuron theory of LANGLEY (1903, 1921) has been considered to be definitive; however, since the concept of "terminal reticulum" was reported for the first time by STÖHR (1928) and by REISER (1933), an epoch-making change was brought on our conception of the peripheral structure of the vegetative nervous system.

About the same time, BOEKE (1933–36) found similar fine reticular nerve endings and named these "sympathischer Grundplexus". BOEKE considered these nerve endings to be sympathetic in nature.

He also gave consideration to the relationship between the nerve endings and the tissue innervated, and stated

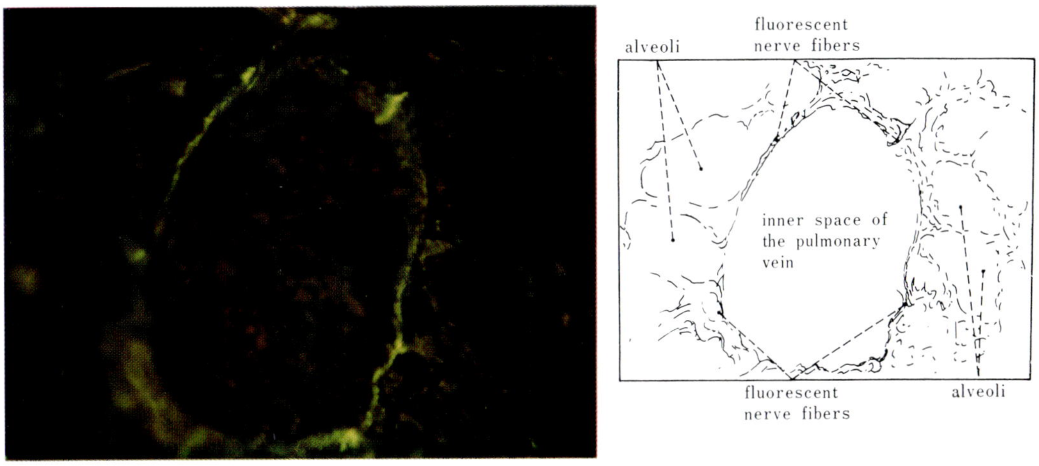

Fig. 251 Fluorescent nerve fibers in the wall of the pulmonary vein (guinea pig).

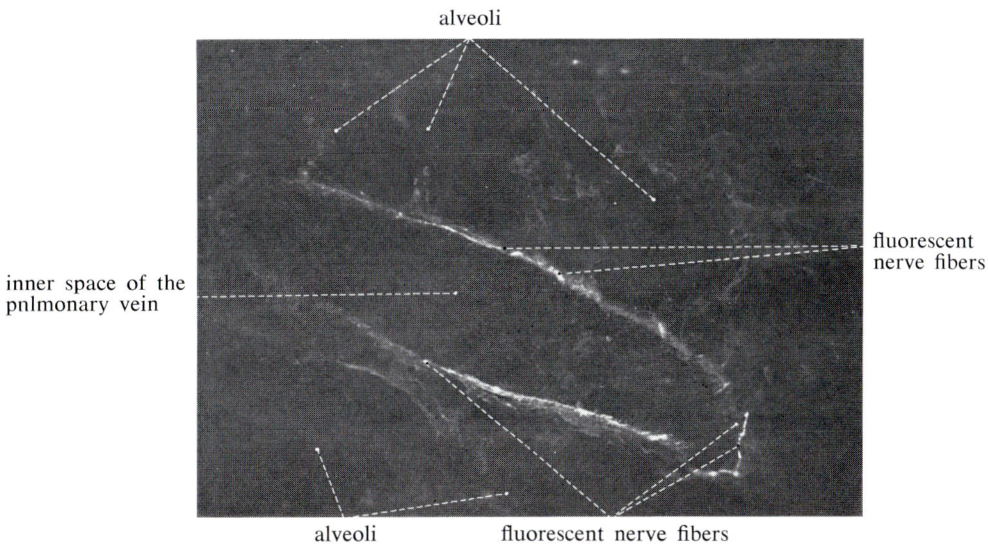

Fig. 252 Fluorescent nerve fibers in the wall of the pulmonary vein (man).

that the fine neurofibrils, *i.e.* "periterminal reticulum", originate in the "sympathischer Grundplexus", distribute to surrounding regions and supply the cells of the tissue innervated.

The "terminal reticulum" of SHÖHR is contrasted with the "sympathischer Grundplexus" of BOEKE as follows:

The endings of the vegetative nervous system are not free nerve endings but are composed of extremely fine neurofibril networks, spreading like cords wrapped by neuroplasm, and surrounding the cells of the tissue innervated.

This is called the "vegetatives Nervenendnetz", and corresponds to "sympathischer Grundplexus" (BOEKE), "Periterminales Netzwerk" (REISER), "kernhaltiges Terminalreticulum" (STÖHR), "Neuro-vegetativer Präterminalplexus" (SUNDER-PLASSMANN).

The "Neuroplasm Masse" which wraps this neurofibril network is also called "Leitplasmodium" and is observed to be nucleated. These are mainly SCHWANN's cell nuclei, but other easily stainable nuclei are also observed. The latter are called "interstitielle Zellen", "neurogene (nervöse) Nebenzellen", "Beizellen (Gleitzellen)". TTÖHR considered that these cells had some relation to the secretory capacity of the vegetative nervous system. Acetylcholine or epinephrine (fluid action substances) were considered to be secreted from these cells.

The neurofibrils, surrounded by neuroplasm, often appear cord-like in shape. In some instances fine neurofibrils, or veil-like or net-like networks, are observed.

STÖHR and REISER considered the former to be of a shape just prior to becoming nerve networks, and called this the "Präterminalreticulum".

They considered that the terminal reticulum anastomoses freely with other terminal reticula, and by such anastomoses the vegetative nervous system forms a huge closed nerve network.

The terminal reticulum is composed of sympathetic and parasympathetic fibers; in peripheral regions it is impossible to distinguish these by the usual histological methods.

The terminal reticula supply innervation to all fixed tissue cells, surrounding or penetrating the cell bodies.

The above is a summary of the theory of STÖHR and REISER.

BOEKE considered that these nerve networks consisted only of sympathetic fibers, and termed this the "sympathischer Grundplexus".

STÖHR, however, considered that the nerve network consist of both sympathetic and parasympathetic nerves. Since he could not prove the structure of the "Periterminalreticulum" of BOEKE, he adopted the name "nervöses Terminalreticulum".

In relation to STÖHR's theory, C. KIMURA (1954) claimed that if the vegetative nerve ending net belonged to both sympathetic and parasympathetic nerve systems, it would be impossible to show them as schematized by coloring distinctly in red (sympathetic) and blue (parasympathetic); rather these nerve ending networks must be shown in purple, the color of the mixture.

Regarding STÖHR's theory, many commentaries were made by investigators such as CAJAL (1906), MICHAILOW (1908), SUNDER-PLASSMANN (1933), BOEKE (1933–36), NONIDEZ (1936), FEYRTER (1950, 51), JABONERO (1953) and others.

MICHAILOW and NONIDEZ insisted that the terminal reticulum was not a nerve tissue but a substance similar to the lattice fibers of connective tissue.

FEYRTER agreed in general with the theory of STÖHR, but stated that besides the efferent nerve fibers, those of an afferent nature are also observed, and therefore, as a whole, the vegetative nervous system forms a closed circuit like the vascular system, and is similarly connected with cerebrospinal nerve endings.

As mentioned above, many researchers were in agreement with STÖHR's theory, SETO (1949, 51) and other colleagues advancing supportive results.

According to studies of the present authors, using BIELSCHOWSKY's staining method as modified by SUZUKI, the endings of the vegetative nervous system in the lung present a reticular appearance, and are obviously connected with nerve fibers originating in the hilum. Therefore, these terminal reticulums are not connective tissues, as mentioned by MICHAILOW and NONIDEZ, but are definitely to be regarded as nerve endings.

The authors' investigations, have not yet determined, however, that the entire vegetative nervous system forms a closed route similar to the vascular system. The author's opinion is rather negative about such a STÖHR's theory in the physiological point of view.

Regarding this and also the exact relationship of nerve endings to each cell, further detailed investigations are considered to be necessary.

For this purpose, application of the electron microscopy will also be in order.

IV. INNERVATION OF LUNG

A. Extrinsic Nerves

An outline of the extrinsic nerves of the lung is presented in Figs. 253 and 254.

1. Parasympathetic Nerve (Vagus)

As mentioned earlier, the vagus nerve originates in the dorsal nucleus of the vagus nerve of the medulla oblongata, and distributes in the periphery of the lung, forming anastomoses with sympathetic nerves in the cervical and thoracic regions.

a. Communications of Vagus and Sympathetic Nerves

Both sets of nerves are regularly connected by superior and inferior communicating branches, which connect the jugular and nodose ganglia with the superior cervical ganglia and sympathetic trunks.

Therefore, in the vagus nerve, afferent nerve fibers and efferent parasympathetic and sympathetic nerve fibers are found.

If the vagus nerve is severed peripherally both parasympathetic and sympathetic nerve fibers are divided simultaneously.

b. Trunk of Vagus to Hilum

The trunk of the vagus nerve, as shown is Fig. 255, descends in the posterior mediastinum and gives off the recurrent nerve. Via the inferior cardiac nerves it participates in the formation of the cardiac plexus.

Between the pulmonary plexuses, communication via the pneumocardiac nerves is observed.

Then, giving off tracheal and esophageal branches, the trunk of the vagus nerve gives rise to the anterior and posterior bronchial branches respectively.

The anterior, in two branches, formes the anterior pulmonary plexus.

The posterior, in four branches, formes the posterior pulmonary plexus.

The trunk of the vagus nerve expands in a ganglion-like shape in the region of the posterior bronchial branch.

c. Pulmonary Plexuses

On the anterior aspect of the hilum, as mentioned earlier, the anterior pulmonary nerve plexus is found. The posterior pulmonary nerve plexus is far larger than the anterior.

These plexuses communicate by means of fine nerve fibers.

The anterior pulmonary nerve plexus is connected on the anterior aspect of the tracheal bifurcation

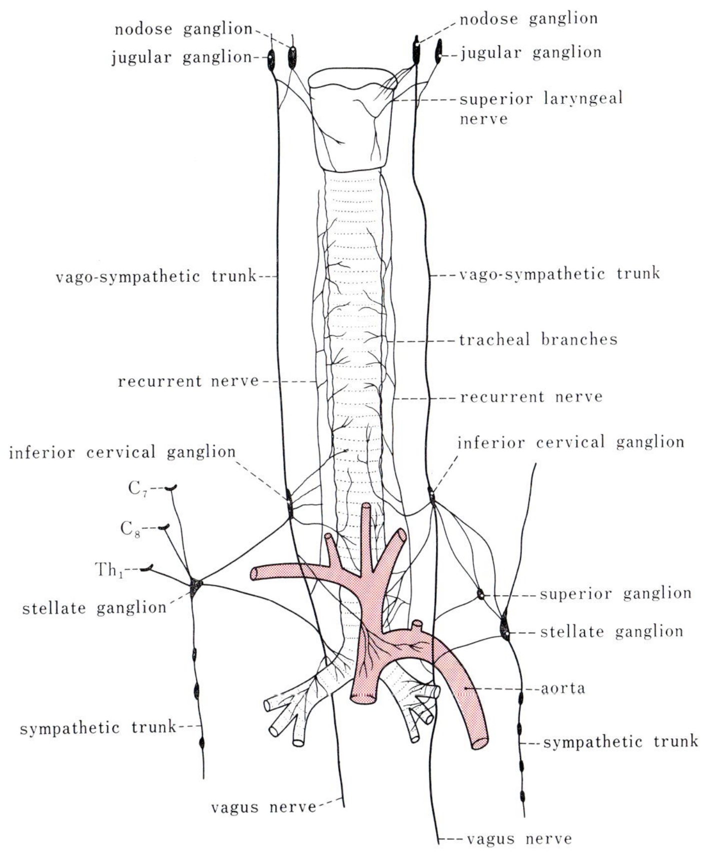

Fig. 253 Innervation of the trachea and the bronchi (frontal view).

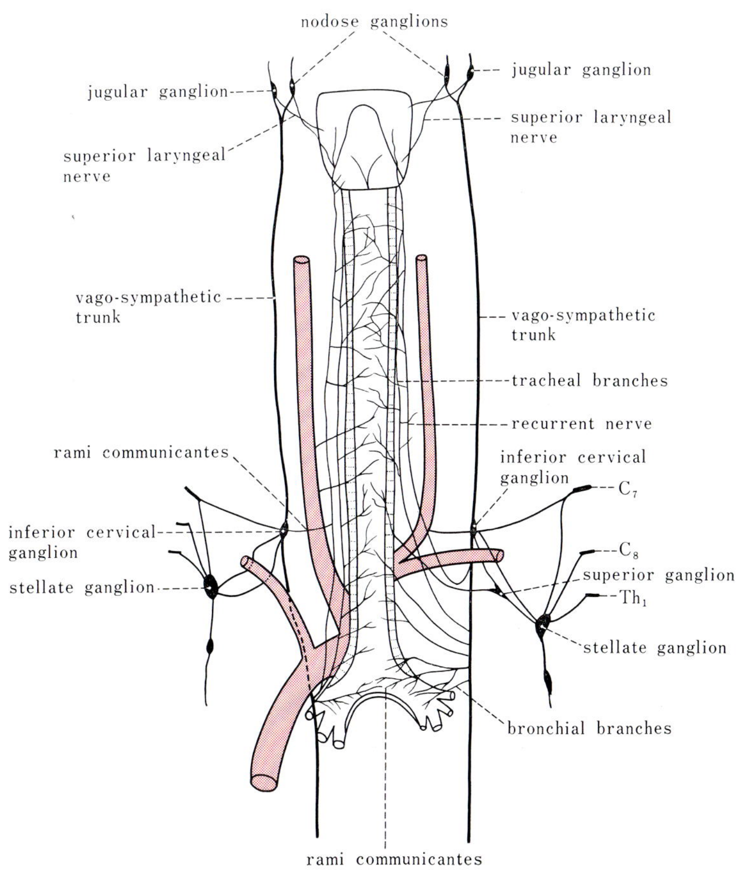

Fig. 254 Innervation of the trachea and bronchi (dog; dorsal view).

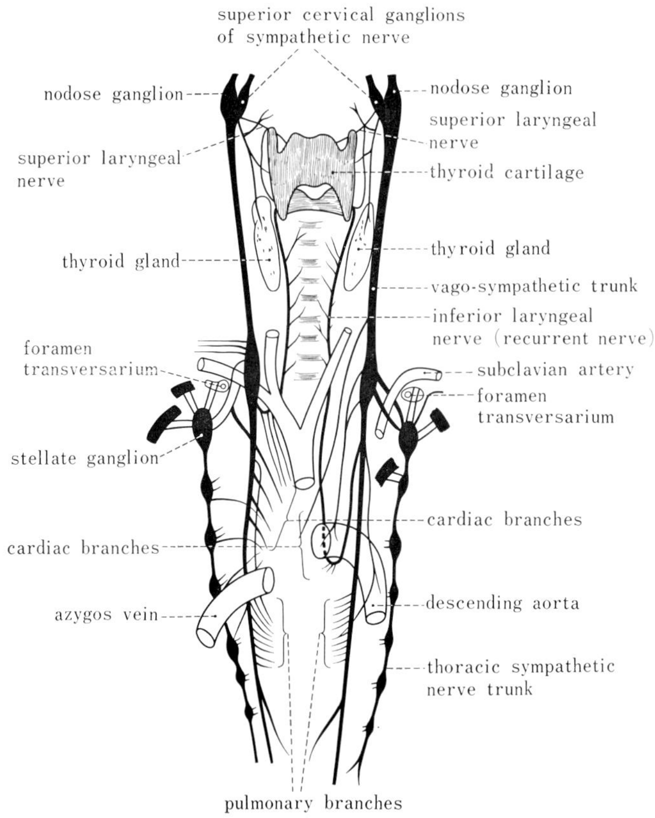

Fig. 255 Diagrammatic illustration of the sympathetic and vagal innervations (dog; SAMAAN).

with that of the opposite side, and the posterior pulmonary nerve plexuses are connected by the esophageal plexus and by nerve fibers on the posterior aspect of the tracheal bifurcation.

The pulmonary nerve plexuses receive many pulmonary nerve branches from the sympathetic nerve trunk of the same side.

The anterior pulmonary nerve plexus communicates with the cardiac plexus via the pneumocardiac nerves, and the posterior pulmonary nerve plexus communicates with the aortic plexus.

Thus the lung and the heart are in close relationship, from the standpoint of their innervation.

The nerve fibers emanating from the anterior and posterior pulmonary nerve plexuses are distributed to the lung along the bronchus, pulmonary artery aind vein. The posterior pulmonary nerve plexus is presumed to have a more important role in the innervation of the lung than has the anterior pulmonary nerve plexus.

d. Histological Findings

In the trunk of the vagus nerve peripheral to the nodose ganglion, myelinated and non-myelinated fibers are observed. The former are sensory, the latter vegetative.

KURE and OKINAKA (1950) investigated histologically the vagus nerve of the dog. The outline is as follows.

In trunk of the vagus, central to the nodose ganglion, large and small diameter myelinated nerve fibers are observed; the non-myelinated nerve fibers form discrete nerve bundles. Quantitywise, the small myelinated nerve fibers are the most numerous, followed by the large myelinated nerve fibers; the least numerous are the non-myelinated nerves.

In the trunk of the cervical sympathetic nerve, non-myelinated nerve fibers are increased in number; the small myelinated and non-myelinated nerve fibers are about the same in number, and the large myelinated nerve fibers are relatively few.

In the region of the thoracic trunk, *i.e.,* in the region of the stellate ganglion, similar observations have been made.

In branches to bronchi, to esophagus, and in the recurrent nerve the small myelinated and non-myelinated nerve fibers are found in almost equal ratio.

In pulmonary branches large and small myelinated nerve fibers are mingled. Non-myelinated nerve fibers are scattered as nerve fiber bundles, and are fewer in number.

The above results of KURE and OKINAKA (1950) are almost the same as those of MÜLLER (1910). Similar findings were reported by ASCHOFF and GOODHARDT (1909).

Sensory Nerve Fibers: The myelinated nerve fibers (sensory) arise from the nerve cells in the nodose ganglion. Most of these distribute to the lung of the same side, a small part to the opposite side.

Motor Nerve Fibers: The motor fibers arise from the dorsal nucleus of the vagus nerve, and in many instances are relayed at nodose ganglion.

2. Sympathetic Nerves

a. Routes to Hilum

As routes to the lung, three pathways are known: 1) Branches arising from the cardiac plexus communicate with the anterior pulmonary nerve plexus; 2) Branches from the inferior cervical ganglion or Th_I sympathetic ganglion run along the esophagus or the trachea and distribute to the anterior and posterior aspects of the bronchi; 3) Branches from Th_{I-V} sympathetic ganglia communicate directly with the pulmonary plexuses.

In common in the pathways is the contribution of the superior thoracic sympathetic ganglion to the innervation of the lung. The exact pathway differs in individual cases.

b. Communications of Sympathetic and Vagus Nerves

As noted previously, the sympathetic system anastomoses with all the plexuses in the thorax, with the pulmonary, aortic, and particularly with the cardiac plexuses.

c. Sympathetic Innervation

The sympathetic innervation of the lung is mainly efferent; however, according to MÖLLGAARD (1912), ROGER (1917), RASMUSSEN (1926) and FÖRSTER (1936) afferent pathways are also involved.

d. Segmental Innervation

The concept of segmental innervation of the lung was introduced by E. REINHARDT (1936).

He pointed out that the "peristatische Hyperämie" or pneumonia, which is apt to occur after cutting the anterior root of the spinal cord or the posterior roots of C_V–Th_{II} in the rabbit, appears in a horizontal dishape, and without regard to interlobar boundaries; he stated that this was a segmental reac tion caused by involvement of the sympathetic segmental innervation.

3. Phrenic Nerve

a. Origin

The phrenic nerve originates in C_{III}–C_{IV} or C_{II}–C_V spinal cord segments.

Other nerve fibers arising from C_{II}, C_{III} or C_V may form an accessory phrenic nerve.

The accessory phrenic nerve unites with the phrenic nerve within the thorax and extends to the diaphragm.

b. Communication between Phrenic and Sympathetic Nerves

Extensive communication occurs between the phrenic and sympathetic nerves. Regarding this there are many reports: the nerves are connected by the branches at the roots of the C_{III} and C_{IV} (MÜLLER, 1910): connections exist between the nerves in the inferior cervical region, the phrenic receives many nerve fine fibers from the inferior cervical and Th_1 sympathetic ganglions (LUSHUKA, 1853); the phrenic receives the sympathetic nerve fibers from the suprapleural plexus (FELIX, 1922).

In the thorax, the phrenic nerve connects with the pulmonary plexuses at the hilum and, after extending to the diaphragm, it receives additional sympathetic nerve fibers which distribute in the diaphragm.

In short, the phrenic nerve not only participates in innervation of the diaphragm, but also includes the nerve fibers belonging to the vegetative nervous system which distribute in that region.

c. Histological Findings

As mentioned previously, the phrenic nerve consists of myelinated and non-myelinated nerve fibers.

d. Branches to Lung

The phrenic nerve contribution to the innervation of the lung has frequently been discussed.

Some investigators denied such participation, but DONATI and VANUCCI (1930), UNGAR and GROSSIORD (1937), and FREERKSEN (1950) indicated the existence of such a role.

e. Segmental Innervation

The question of segmental innervation of the diaphragm has been also considered.

FUCHUS (1898) reported that the diaphragm of the rabbit receives its innervation from C_{IV}–C_{VII}, and that C_{IV} supplies the ventral, and C_{VI}–C_{VII} the dorsal, independently.

B. Intrinsic Nerves

1. Intrapulmonary Ganglia

a. Structure

The ganglia of the vegetative nervous system is classified into Types I, II and III by DOGIEL (1895). This classification is based on the shapes of processes of the ganglion cells making up the ganglion.

The Type I ganglion cell is called "Kronenzelle"(coronoid cell), the cell which has many short processes and a few long ones. With this type of cell, the short processes are ramified only in the "Amphycyter Mantel" (LENKOSSÈK) that surrounds the ganglion cell, whereas the longer ones perforate the mantel and communicate with other nerve fibers outside the ganglion.

On the other hand, in the Type II ganglion cells, both long and short processes penetrate the mantel and communicate with other nerve fibers.

Type III ganglion cell is called "Sternzelle".

Dogiel regarded it as a mixture of Types I and II, however, STÖHR (1928), REISER (1933) and SETO (1935) said that Type III need not be differentiated from Types I and II.

The above is a superficial classification of ganglia, but according to investigations by the present authors ganglion cells are not always so simply classified.

Most of the intrapulmonary ganglia consist of ganglion cells belonging to Dogiel's Type II. These are multipolar cells which have large type nuclei.

The long processes of these cells consist of large nerve fibers and are very few. The short processes consist of fine nerve fibers and are in large number.

The long processes communicate with other nerve fibers outside the ganglion, but the short process terminate in the region somewhat apart from the ganglion cells, and communicate with other nerve fibers only near the cell body.

There are the following two types in the endings of the processes of the ganglion cells. The most common ending forms terminal reticulum around the ganglion cell and communicates with many neighboring ganglion cells. The other, which is very rarely observed, cosists of nerve fibril nets in round or ovoid shapes. The so-called "Fortsatzlamellen" by SETO is an example of this type.

b. Functional Significance

It has been observed by REMAK (1844) and many other researchers, that the intrapulmonary ganglia is not of the spinal ganglion type of the cerebrospinal nervous system but is of the vegetative nervous system.

However, as to whether it belongs to the sympathetic nervous system or the parasympathetic nervous system has been discussed for a long time, and at the present stage there is no definite conclusion. Therefore it will be safer to take the standpoint that the sympathetic and parasympathetic systems are mixed.

c. Origin and Development

AREY (1942) stated that the initial evidence of development of the sympathetic nerves is observed in the 5 mm embryo; the nerve cells which will form sympathetic ganglia become isolated from the neural crest at about 7 weeks of embryonal life, and arrange in segmental form. The trunk of the sympathetic nerve is formed by ganglia arranged longitudinally in a chain-like manner. In addition to the chain of sympathetic ganglia, the pulmonary nerve plexuses form about one week later.

d. Distribution

Numerous various sized ganglia are observed on the tracheal wall.

The treachea receives nerve fibers from the recurrent nerve, a branch of the vagus nerve, and from sympathetic nerves. These nerve fibers form networks surrounding the trachea.

The nerve networks on the anterior aspect of the trachea are relatively coarse; in this region as shown in Fig. 256, a few ganglia are observed.

On the posterior aspect of the trachea, particularly on the membranous part, a plexus consisting of fine nerve networks is observed, accompanied by many ganglia. The ganglia in this region can be distinguished macroscopically.

Microscopically, many ganglion cells are observed among the nerve fibers, as shown in Fig. 257.

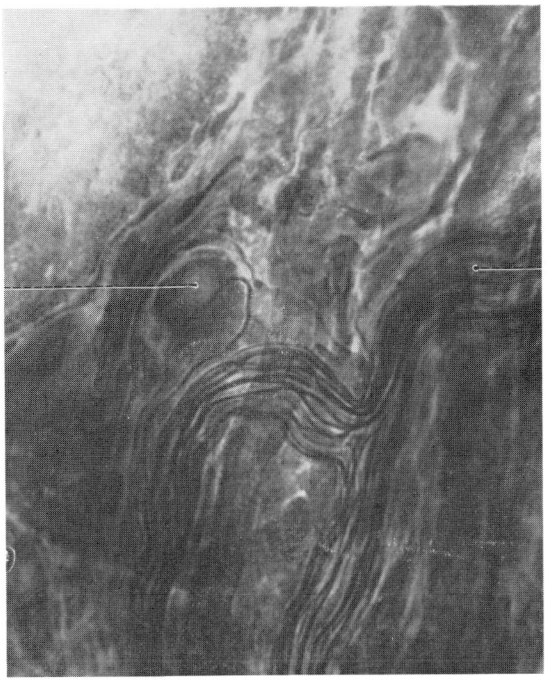

Fig. 256 Ganglion cell in the advantitia (man).

These ganglion cells are arranged like a chain, and are multipolar.

The nerve fibers originating in the ganglion cells of the tracheal wall can be classified into either of the following types:

1) Non-myelinated postganglionic fibers which are distributed to tracheal smooth muscle, and which regulate motor activity.

2) Small myelinated nerve fibers which terminate on the surface of ganglion cells as pericellular endings. The myelin sheath disappears before the endings are formed.

The ganglia distributed on the bronchi are located in the pulmonary nerve plexuses of the hilum and along the intrapulmonary bronchial walls.

As shown in Figs. 258 and 259, the ganglia of the bronchial walls are mainly observed in the extrachondral and subchondral nerve plexuses. Nerve networks connect the extrachondral and subchondral nerve plexuses, running along bronchial cartilaginous lamina.

The distribution of peribronchial ganglia differs in different animals, but in all cases the number and size of the ganglia decrease in the more peripheral regions.

The submucous ganglia are small in size as compared with the peribronchial, and their location is limited to the medium or large bronchi. The number of cells composing the ganglia is 3–10, as shown in Fig. 260.

The postganglionic processes arising from the ganglion cells of the subchondral nerve plexus are distributed, as are those of the extrachondral nerve plexus, to smooth muscles and bronchial glands.

No particular morphological difference is observed among the ganglion cells of these nerve plexuses.

The ganglia are covered with thick capsules of connective tissue, as shown in Fig. 261.

When the number of the ganglion cells is few (2–3), there is no specific capsule; these then are observed as isolated ganglion cells; these are few in number.

The ganglion cells of this type are, as shown in Fig. 262, Dogiel's Type I, in many instances.

In general, large ganglia are observed on the walls of large bronchi, and small ganglion on the walls of small bronchi; however, occasionally many small ganglia are observed on the walls of the large bronchi.

Whether or not ganglia occur on the walls of the pulmonary blood vessels is a question.

As to this point, various reports have been made. According to the authors' investigation, as shown in Figs. 263 and 264, ganglia are observed on the walls of pulmonary vein, and on the bronchial artery and vein, but not on the pulmonary artery, excepting the regions at its root.

The ganglia are not found on the blood vessels, but can be observed close to the walls, sending nerve fibers to the wall.

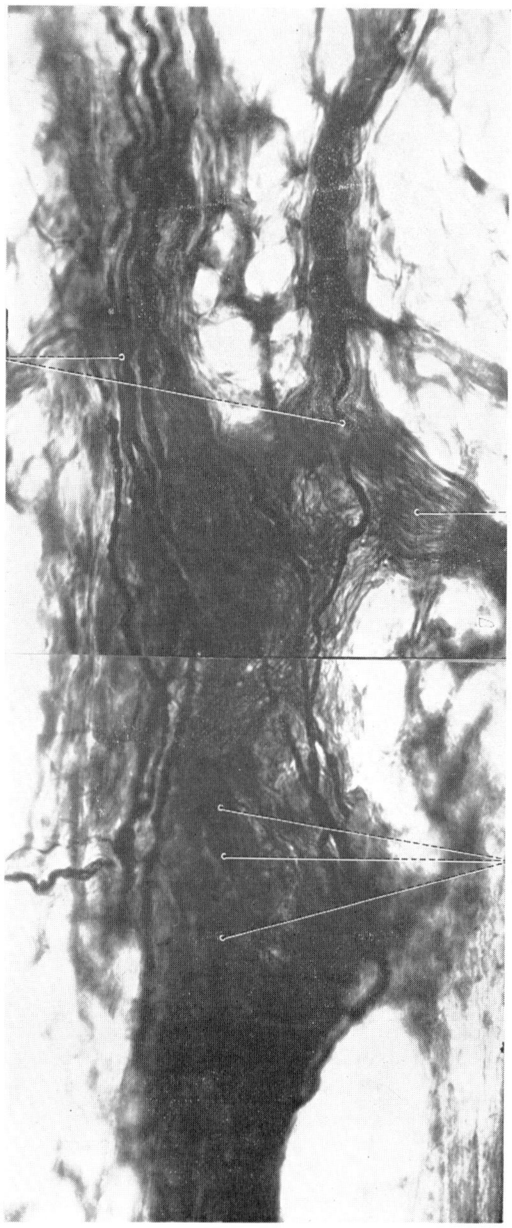

Fig. 257 Ganglion cell group and nerve plexus in the advantitia of the trachea (man).

ROMANOW (1904) reported on the observation of multipolar ganglion cells in the mediastinal pleura; KÖLLIKER (1902) and HAYASHI (1937) observed ganglion cells as occurring sporadically in the nerve networks of the pulmonary pleura. TAKINO (1933) also stated that ganglion cells occur in the connective tissue immediately under the pulmonary pleura, facing the mediastinum, in the bird. As for the authors, although detailed investigations have been carried out, ganglion cells were not found on either parietal or pulmonary pleura.

2. Intrapulmonary Nerve Plexuses

a. Bronchial

The nerve fiber bundles arising from the anterior and posterior pulmonary nerve plexuses run mainly along the bronchi, partly with the pulmonary blood vessels and particularly along the pulmonary arteries.

Each forms complicated plexuses and sends interconnected nerve fibers to the various tissues in the lung.

The plexuses of the bronchial walls are considered to be extensions of these on the tracheal wall, having divided at the bronchial cartilages.

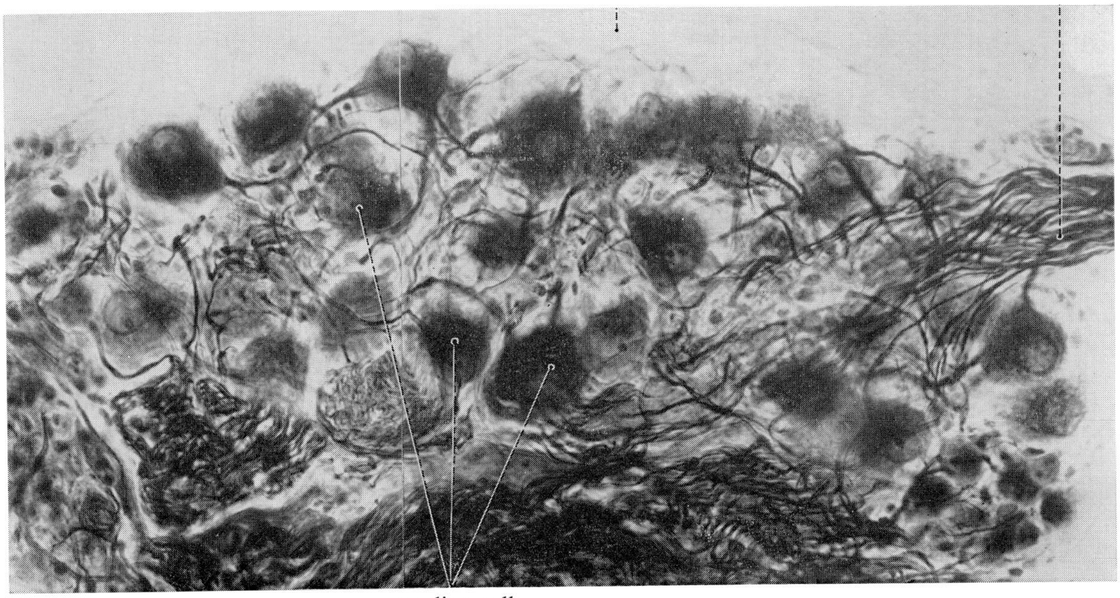

Fig. 258 Ganglia in the extrachondral plexus of the bronchial wall (man).

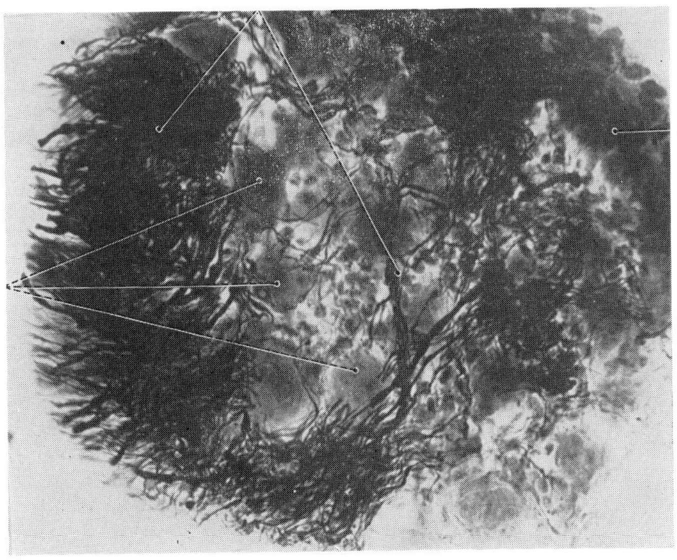

Fig. 259 Ganglia in the extrachondral plexus (man).

Extrachondral plexuses are observed in the connective tissue between bronchial cartilages and pulmonary parenchyma; these are composed of large nerve bundles of myelinated and non-myelinated nerve fibers, running along the longitudinal axis of the bronchus and interanastomosing. Fig. 265 shows an example.

Between these nerve fibers various sizes of ganglia and ganglion cells are observed, but the number decreases toward the periphery.

The extrachondral (peribronchial) nerve plexus serves as the origin of those intrapulmonary nerve bundles which innervate bronchi and pulmonary blood vessels.

As shown in Fig. 266, an extrachondral plexus is mainly composed of myelinated nerve fibers, but non-myelinated nerve fibers also contribute to its formation. Nerve fiber bundles consisting of non-myelinated fibers can also be observed.

The myelinated nerves to the bronchial walls can be classified as follows.

1) Large afferent fibers which run from bronchial epithelium and smooth muscles.

2) Small efferent fibers which form pericellular networks around ganglion cells. These can be considered to be preganglionic fibers of the vagus nerve.

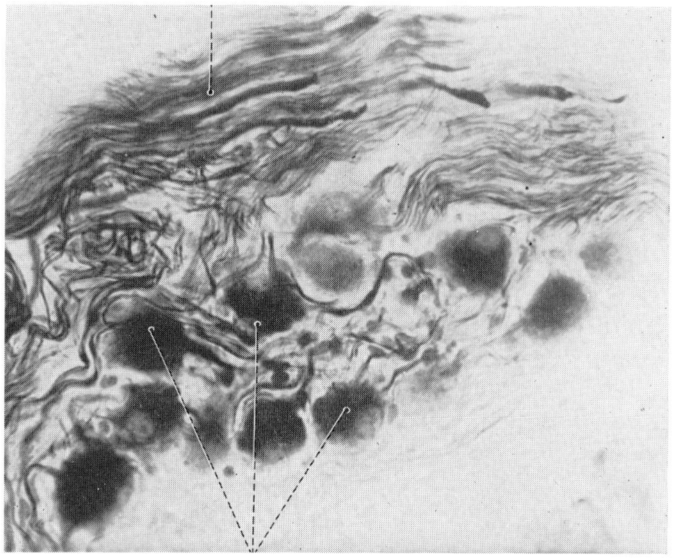

Fig. 260 Ganglia in the subchondral plexus of the bronchus (man).

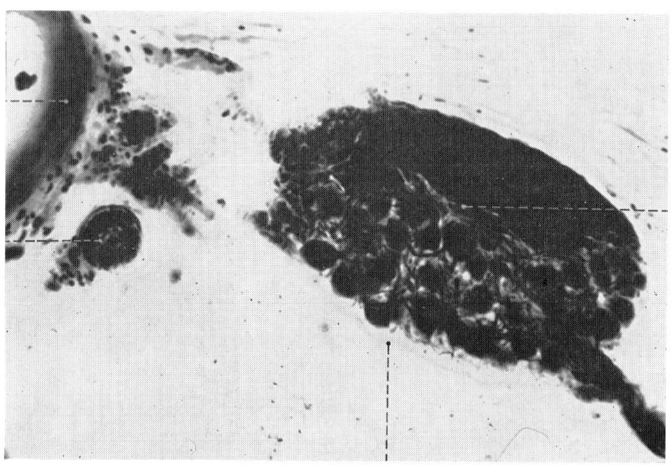

Fig. 261 Encapsulated giant ganglion in extrachondral plexus (man).

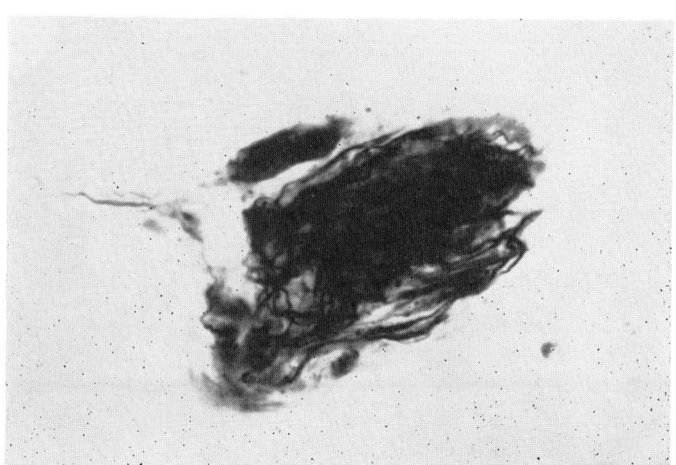

Fig. 262 Solitary ganglion cell in the bronchial wall (Dogiel's Type I, man).

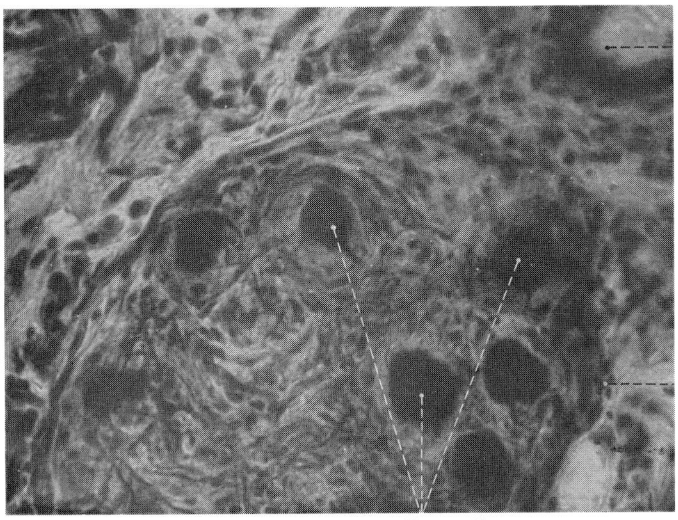

Fig. 263 Ganglion cells distributed near the pulmonary vein (man).

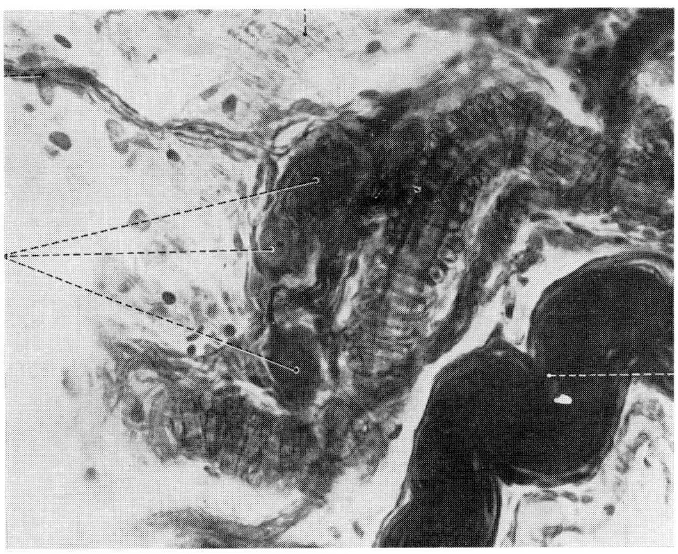

Fig. 264 Ganglion cells and nerve fibers distributed near the wall of the bronchial artery (man).

Numerous postganglionic non-myelinated nerve fibers arise from the ganglia of the extrachondral nerve plexus and form the motor or secretory nerve effectors to bronchial muscles and bronchial glands.

As shown in Fig. 267, the subchondral plexus, unlike the extrachondral, is observed to be deep in relation to the bronchial cartilages, *i.e.* in the connective tissue between cartilage and muscle.

The subchondral plexus is also called "subchondraler Plexus" (STÖHR), "sekundärer Plexus" (HAYASHI), or "submucosal plexus" (BUDDE).

The corresponding term, equivalent to "extrachondral", is "intrachondral"; however, the plexuses discussed here are beneath the cartilage, and therefore the term "intrachondral" or "enchondral" is not suitable, "subchondral" being more appropriate.

This subchondral plexus appears independent, but it is formed by nerve fibers arising from the extrachondral (peribronchial) plexus, which reached the subchondral layer via the intercartilaginous space. Compared with the extrachondral plexus the subchondral is on a smaller scale.

The ganglion cells in this region are sometimes isolated, but in many instances, 3–6 cells form a ganglion.

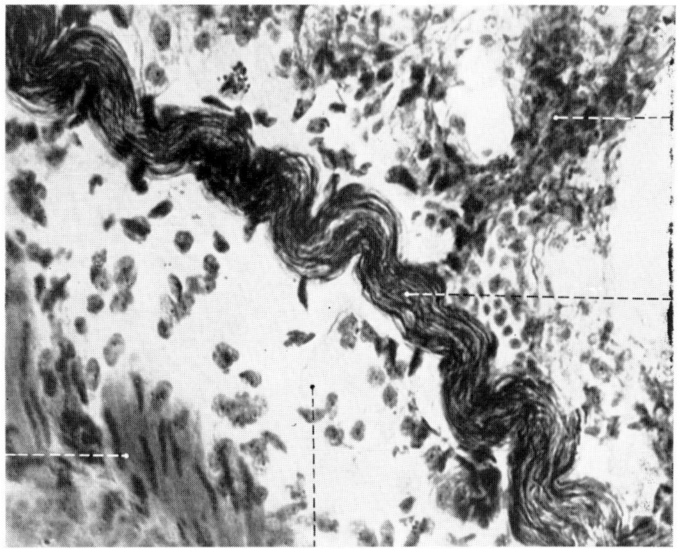

Fig. 265 Extrachondral plexus in the bronchus (man).

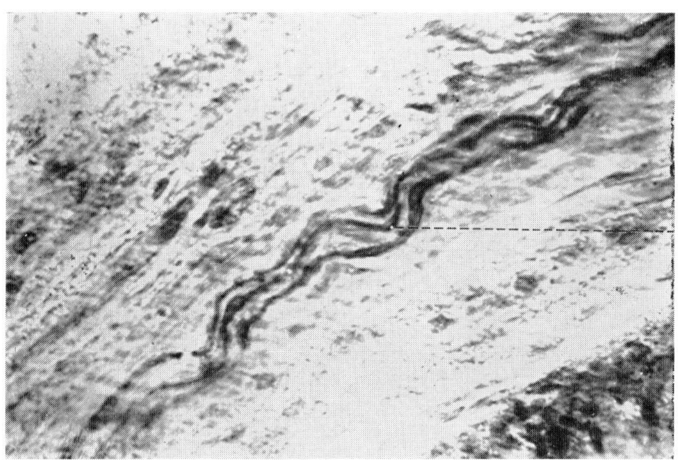

Fig. 266 Extrachondral plexus of the bronchial wall (man).

Besides the above-mentioned plexuses, other smaller ones are observed on the bronchial wall. These are the subepithelial nerve plexuses.

The subepithelial plexuses are found in the connective tissue between the mucous membrane and smooth muscles. The fine non-myelinated nerve fibers (and a few that are myelinated) which constitute these plexuses originate in the subchondral plexuses.

Fig. 268 serves as an example (stained by Bielschowsky's method as modified by Suzuki and so-called Sugamo myelin sheath method).

In the small bronchi, in which the walls are devoid of cartilages, the plexuses described merge into a single network, the components not being distinguishable.

b. Arterial

Differing from the peribronchial, the nerve plexuses are mainly composed of non-myelinated nerve fibers. Myelinated fibers can only be observed in small quantity on the wall of the large arteries, in the region of the hilum.

These nerve fibers form complicated plexuses, making anastomoses in the adventitia of the pulmonary artery.

On the walls of the pulmonary artery a few ganglion cells can be observed in the adventitia of the extrapulmonary vessel; in the intrapulmonary portions ganglia are observed in the region of the hilum.

The periarterial plexuses are remarkably developed in the region of the large pulmonary arteries near the hilum. The nerve fiber bundles which compose these plexuses decrease in size and in number peripherally; in the small peripheral arterials only a few nerve fibers are observed.

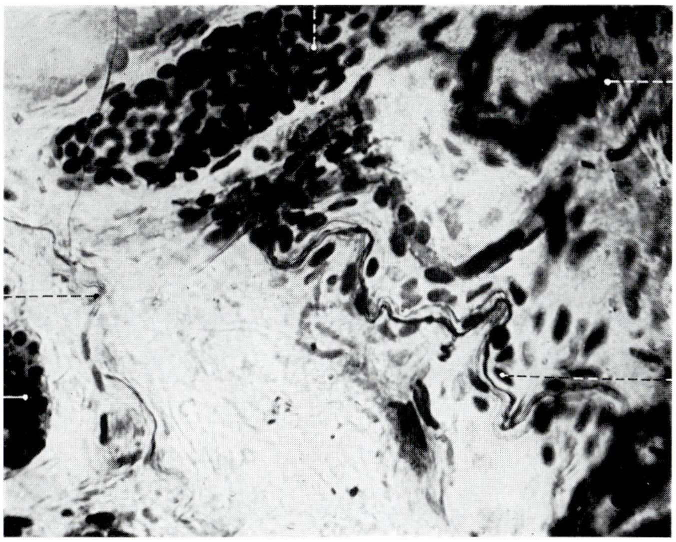

Fig. 267 Subchondral nerve plexus of the bronchus (man).

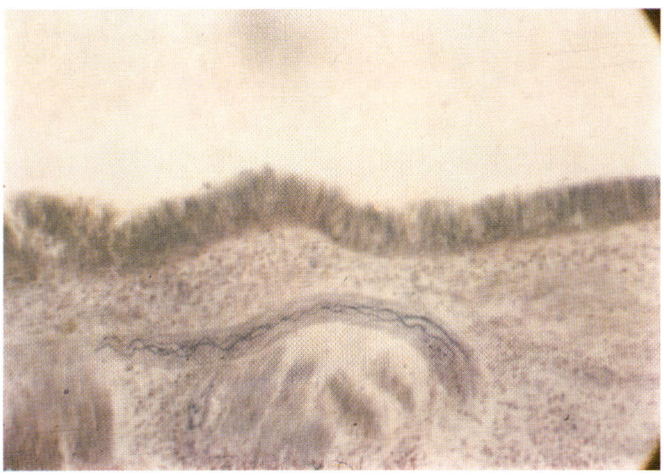

Fig. 268 Subepithelial plexus in the bronchus (man).

These nerve fibers are distributed to pulmonary arterial walls and to pulmonary parenchyma, meanwhile communicating with the peribronchial plexuses.

c. Venular

A few nerve fiber bundles are observed on the wall of the pulmonary vein, but existence of a perivenous plexus as mentioned by TAKINO (1932) or MIYAKE (1937) has not been corroborated.

3. Intrapulmonary Nerve Fibers

a. Afferent Nerve Fibers (Visceral Sensory Nervous System)

The sensibility of the lung is provided by fibers supplied by the vagus nerve or by posterior roots (Th_{I-V}) of the spinal cord. The latter are considered to represent a secondary pathway.

KIMURA and YAGITA (1954) severed these nerves in the dog and, as the result, reported that the innervation described was limited to the hilar region.

The nerve endings of afferent fibers are entirely different from those of the vegetative nervous system; the distinction can be made at a glance.

The sensory nerve fibers distributed in the lung, as shown above in Fig. 244, have their nerve cells in the spinal or in the nodose ganglion.

The afferent nerve fibers are large myelinated nerves which originate in variously shaped nerve endings. Occasionally, the nerve fibers are devoid of myelin sheath, in such cases the nerve fibers are larger than those of the vegetative nerve networks.

i) To Bronchial System: Intraepithelial nerve endings in the tracheal wall were first reported by ARNSTEIN and PLOSCHKO (1897), and were called "subepitheliales Endbäumchen".

These are afferent cerebrospinal nerves which pass along the vegetative nerve route. The nerve fibers bypass the ganglion cells in the tracheal wall.

These endings are seen primarily in the epithelium of the membranous part of the trachea, but frequently also in the epithelium of the cartilaginous part.

In dogs these nerve fibers take a simple course in most cases, very rarely showing complicated branchings.

A large myelinated nerve fiber is divided into several branches in the subepithelial layer, and distributes in the epithelium. Several terminal branches run parallel, expanding in the end in a nodular shape to form free endings; a single fiber, without forming branches, may distribute in the epithelium.

In man, unlike dog, the intraepithelial nerves are composed of relatively small nerve fibers and accompanying fibrillar networks.

The small nerve fibers which reach the subepithelial layer are divided into several branches; some show arborescent branchings as shown in Fig. 269, with endings of nodular or sharp shapes; some, as shown in Fig. 270, form nerve fibril networks of various shapes which terminate in free endings.

As shown in Fig. 271, relatively large fibers arise from the subepithelial nerve plexuses and extend to the submucous layer, then run between the epithelial cells and terminate in them. Some branch and some do not.

Whether or not the nerve endings actually terminate in the nuclei of epithelial cells is not yet evident.

The intraepithelial nerves are composed of myelinated nerve fibers. According to the authors' investigation (so-called Sugamo myelin sheath staining method) the myelinated nerve fibers emanate from the subepithelial plexus and run to the region immediately under the epithelium, lose their myelin sheaths, then ascend between the epithelial cells as the fine non-myelinated filaments to form free sensory nerve endings (Fig. 272).

As shown in Fig. 273, intraepithelial nerve endings are frequently observed in the mucous membrane of the lobar bronchi, but decrease in number toward the periphery. In the bronchi of less than medium size they are hardly observed.

When the intraepithelial nerves of the bronchial and tracheal walls are compared, the latter exceed the former in frequency. Peripheral to the lobar bronchi the frequency of intraepithelial nerves decreases rapidly.

The above findings coincide with the clinical observation that the cough reflex is strong in the trachea, tracheal bifurcation and extrapulmonary bronchus, and weaker in the intrapulmonary bronchus. It is almost certain that the tracheobronchial intraepithelial nerves participate in the afferent limb of the cough reflex.

FRÖHLICH (1949) remarked on "Helle Zellen" specific clear cells which could be considered as chemoreceptor (*e.g.*, ammonia, acetone, ether, etc.).

These cells are observed in the tracheobronchial mucous membrane of various animals. They can be distinctly distinguished from other columnar epithelium, by using specific morphological criteria.

A nerve fiber can be observed in the "Helle Zelle" cytoplasm. This nerve fiber terminates adjacent to the nucleus.

FRÖHLICH considered such nerve fibers to be afferent in character; stimulation of "Helle Zelle" would be relayed to the centrum.

ii) In Tunica Propria and in Submucosa: Although few in number, sensory nerve endings are observed in the tunica propria of the bronchi, in the submucosa and about the bronchial mucous glands. These endings are considered to participate in mediating the sense of touch and pain.

As regards this point, there is no detailed literature. However, the authors' investigations lead to some observations.

The sensory nerve endings which are seen in the tunica propria or submucosa are most often found in the membranous part of the trachea. They exist sparsely on the lateral or anterior wall.

As shown in Fig. 274, some of these terminate in simple free endings, large myelinated nerve fibers do not lose their myelin sheaths, and some, as shown in Fig. 275, entwine in glomerular shape.

These sensory nerve endings are observed in the regions from the trachea to the medium sized bronchi.

The authors also observed certain so-called "Schlingenterritorium" in the tracheal or bronchial submucosa.

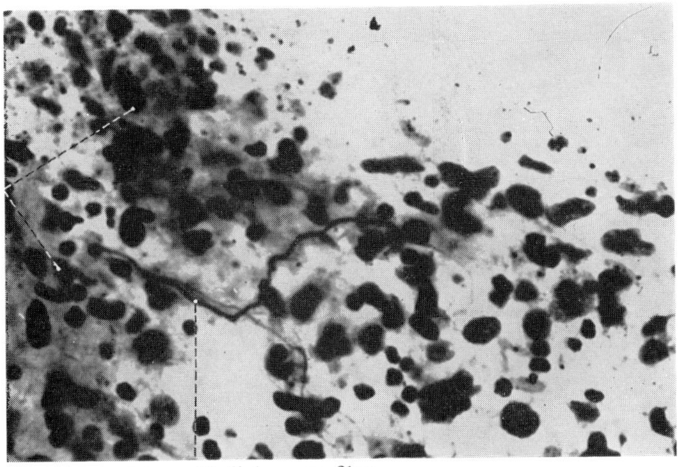

Fig. 269 Nerve ending in the epithelium of the membranous part of the trachea (man).

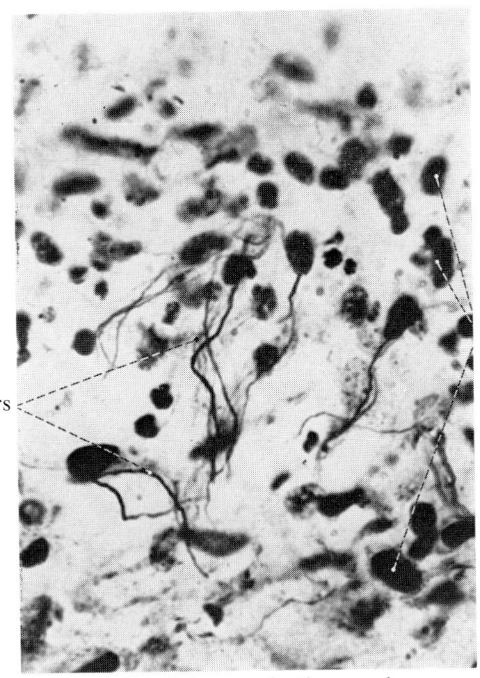

Fig. 270 Intraepithelial nerve in the membranous part of the trachea (man).

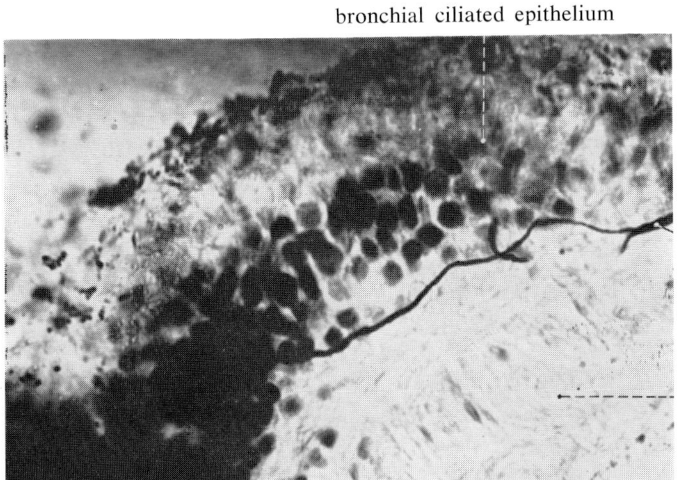

Fig. 271 Nerve ending in the epithelium of the intrapulmonary bronchus (man).

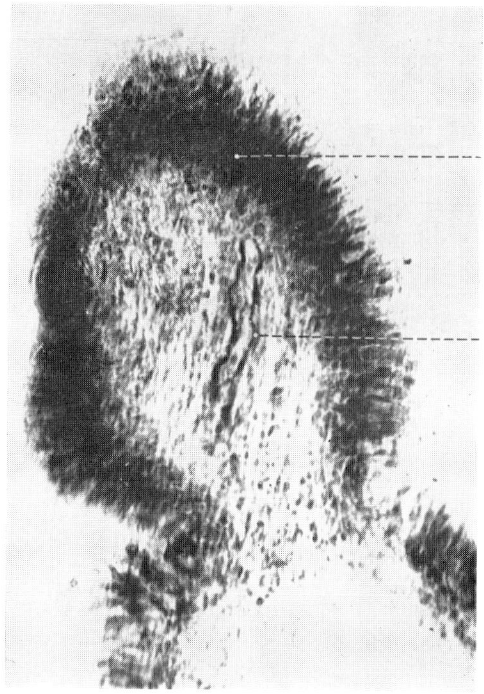

Fig. 272 Nerve ending in the epithelium of the bronchus (man).

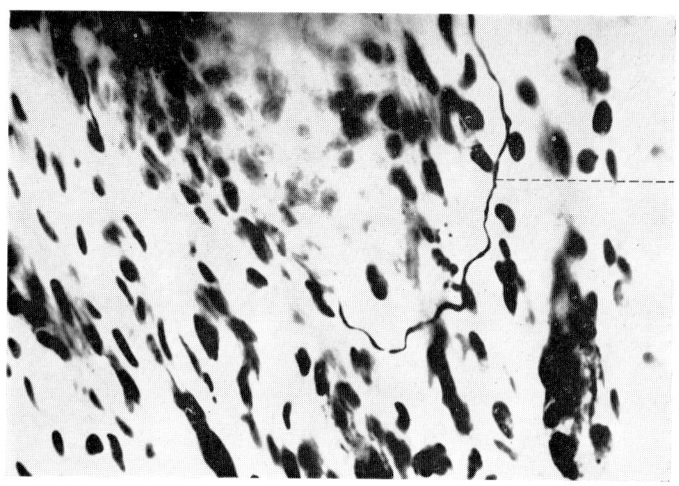

Fig. 273 Nerve ending in the epithelium of the intrapulmonary lobar bronchus (man).

These are generally considered to be parasympathetic receptors of spiral or glomerular shape, wrapped by so-called "Hüllplasmodium" which consists of neuroplasm. Up to the present, these have been observed in the esophagus, stomach, caudal end of the large intestine, and in the mucous membrane of the anus.

The nerve fibers comprising the "Schlingenterritorium" are, as shown in Fig. 276, composed of fine neuroplasm. Since the "interstitielle Zellen" of CAJAL (1906) and of SETO (1937, 51) and the "interkaläre Zellen" of FEYRTER (1950) are observed in their course, they are probably not afferent; rather they are probably of a vegetative character.

The sensory endings which are distributed in the mucosa or submucosa of the bronchi are observed to have a more complicated form, as compared with those of the trachea.

There are two types of nerve endings; one is of simple shape terminating in a pointed end (Fig. 277), the other exhibits relatively complicated arborescent branchings (Fig. 278). Neither type is too frequently observed, the distribution being limited to the walls of medium or large bronchi. From this fact, one can understand the absence of a sense of pain and sensibility in the lung.

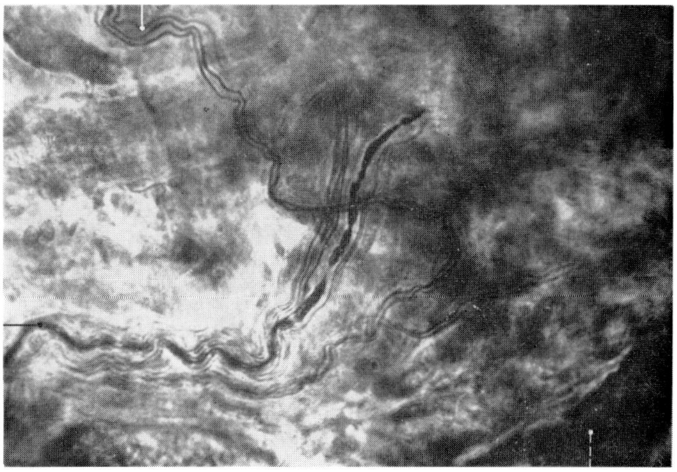

Fig. 274 Sensory nerve ending in the submucosa of the membranous part of the trachea (man).

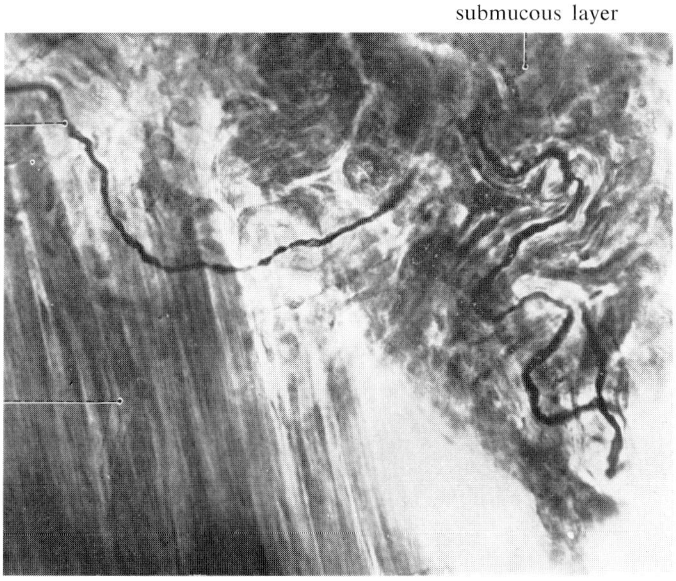

Fig. 275 Afferent nerve ending in the submucous layer of the trachea (man).

In general, the lung is considered to be insensitive to mechanical irritation.

Even if lung tissues are incised, or if the lung tissues are damaged by certain diseases, the pulmonary pleura or parenchyma is insensitive to pain. If inflammation or malignant tumors involve the lung, local pain will generally not be felt until involvement of parietal or mediastinal pleura occurs. However, in view of complaints at the time of bronchoscopy, or acknowledging the subjective symptoms of patients with lung cancer, it seems that the lungs are sensitive to certain kinds of abnormal stimulation. Some patients with tuberculosis who have cavities state that they actually feel the movement of sputa; some complain of unusual irritation in the lung at the time of hemoptysis. Or in severe bronchitis the patients may sometimes complain of slight pain in the lung. These symptoms are not the result of sensitiveness of the pulmonary parenchyma, however, but are rather the sensibility of the medium or large bronchi.

The above is evident from several clinical experiences, and from investigations made by the authors.

iii) In Smooth Muscle: The existence of sensory endings in tracheobronchial muscle was indicated by ARNSREIN and PLOSCHKO (1897).

They called these the "intramuskuläre Endbäumchen".

The extrachondral (peribronchial) or the subchondral nerve plexuses divide into large sensory nerve bundles; these nerve fibers perforate the intermuscular connective tissue and enter the bronchial muscles. Dividing into many branches, they run along the muscle fibers and terminate in free endings.

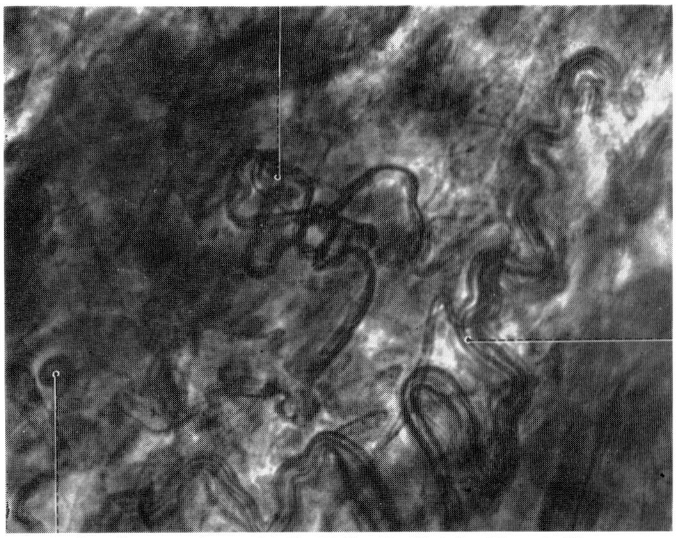

Fig. 276 "Schringenterritorium" in the submucous layer of the trachea (man).

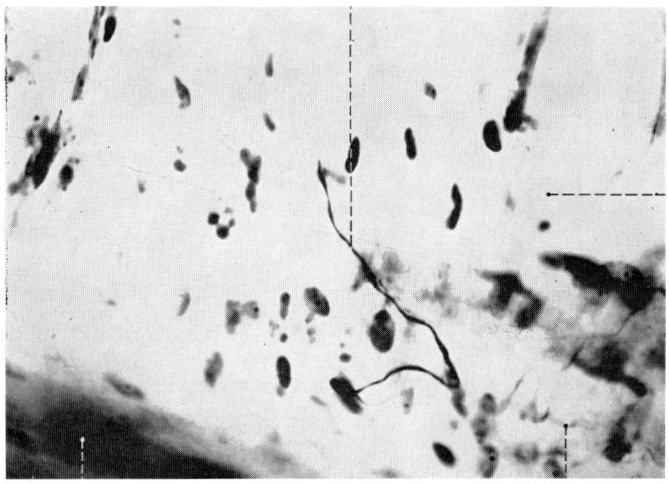

Fig. 277 Afferent nerve ending in the tunica propria of the bronchus (man).

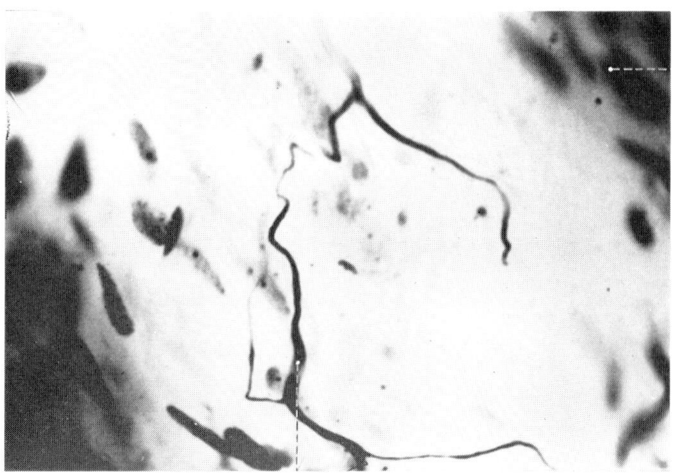

Fig. 278 Afferent nerve ending in the tunica propria of the bronchus (man).

These nerve endings are either extremely simple in shape, as shown in Fig. 279, or terminate in a fork-like shape, with several terminal branches, as shown in Fig. 280.

The authors' observations on sensory nerve endings in the tracheobronchial muscle are almost the same as these of DIJKSTRA (1939); however, we were unable to observe the smooth muscle nerve spindle ending described by LARSELL (1921, 23, 35). SUNDER-PLASSMANN (1938) assumed that the "smooth muscle nerve spindle" of LARSELL corresponded to his "neurovegetative Rezeptorenfelder".

The dyspnea during asthma has been ascribed to contraction of the bronchial muscle with resultant stenosis of the respiratory passages, and to insufficiency of the pulmonary circulation. TAKINO (1932–1949) denied the above mechanisms, stating that since oxygen inhalation at the time of an asthmatic attack did not relieve the feeling of air hunger, the dyspnea must involve irritation of the sensory nerve endings in the muscles, as the result of the contraction of the bronchial muscles.

The authors also consider that the sensory nerve ending in the bronchial muscle act to relay the feeling of air hunger, as stated by TAKINO.

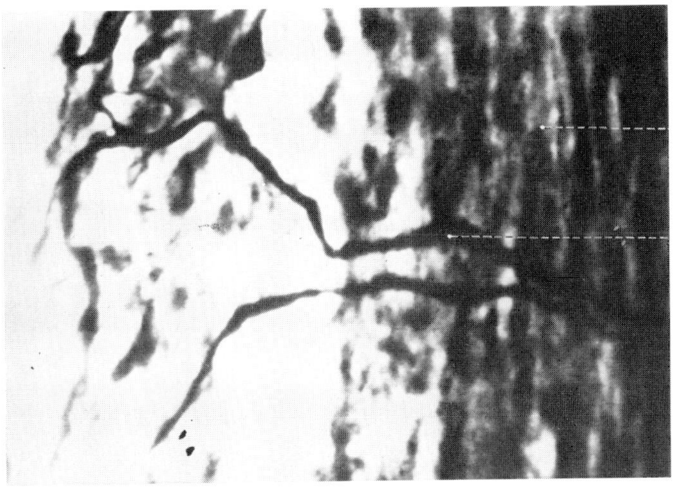

Fig. 279 Afferent nerve ending in the smooth muscle of the trachea (man).

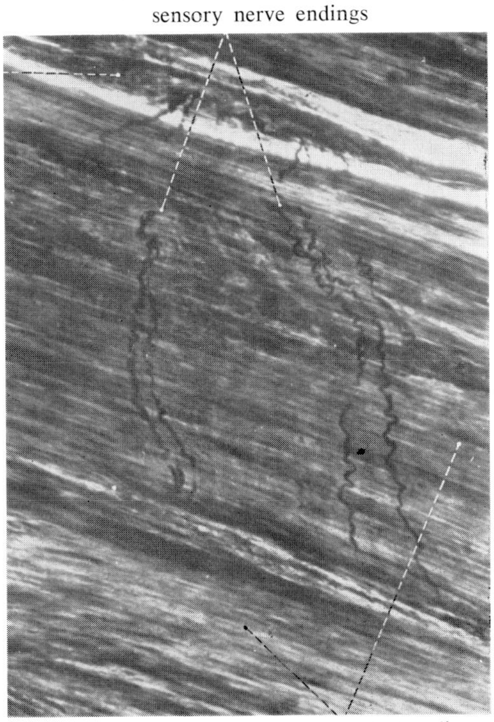

Fig. 280 Afferent nerve ending in the smooth muscle bundle of the trachea (man).

iv) In Pulmonary Parenchyma: As shown in Fig. 281, sensory nerve fibers run along the respiratory bronchioles; these nerve fibers form simple arborescent nerve endings in the alveolar interstices in dog and man.

Sensory nerve fibers in the pulmonary parenchyma run along the bronchial wall, sometimes extending from the alveolar duct to the alveolar wall, but as shown in Fig. 282, most frequently go directly into the peribronchial pulmonary parenchyma from the peribronchial plexus.

Our histological findings coincide with those on sensory nerve endings as mentioned by HAYASHI (1937), DIJKSTRA (1939) and YAGITA (1954). The complicated sensory nerve endings mentioned by LARSELL (1921, 35) or by ELFTMAN (1943) were not observed.

As to the sensory nerve endings in the pulmonary parenchyma, and particularly in the alveolar region, there remain some open question; electron microscopic investigations are considered to be necessary.

v) In Mucomuscular Layers of Trachea and Bronchi: SUNDER-PLASSMANN (1933) reported observations on the sensory nerve endings which participate in Hering's barodepressor reflex in the intrabronchial mucomuscular layer in man. He termed these the "neurovegetative Rezeptorenfelder".

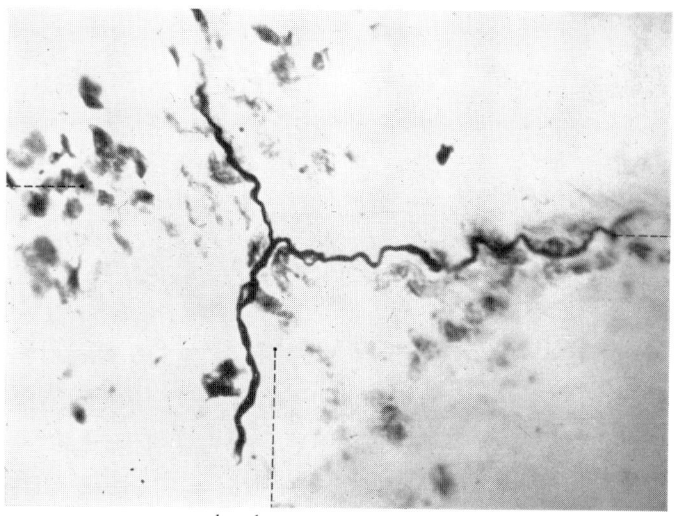

Fig. 281 Sensory nerve termination in the alveolar interstices (man).

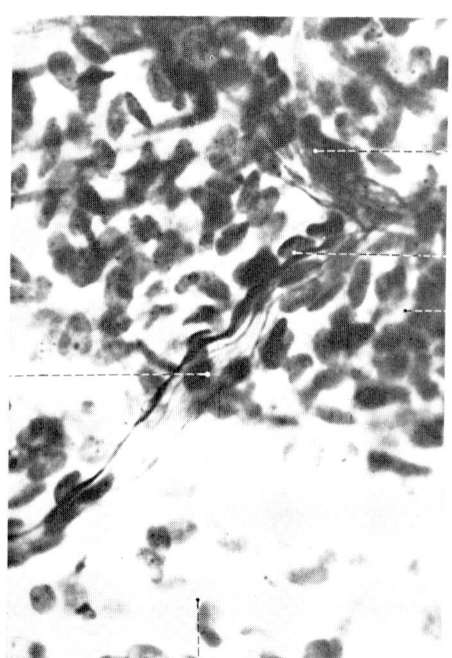

Fig. 282 Nerve fibers in the pulmonary parenchyma (man).

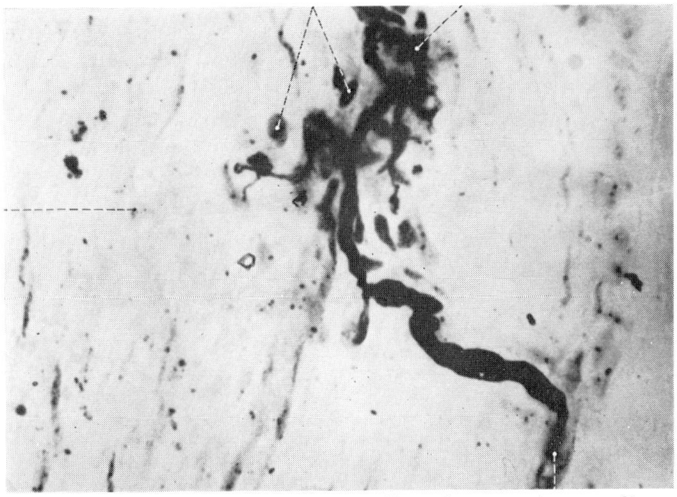

Fig. 283 Pressoreceptoric nerve ending (Type I) in the membranous part of the trachea (man).

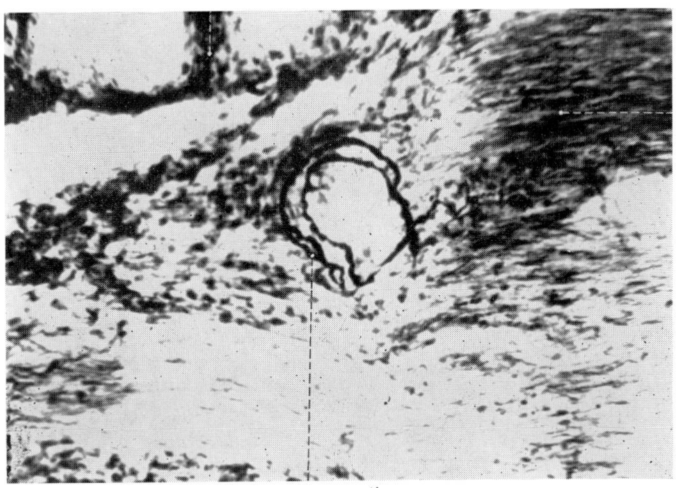

Fig. 284 Pressoreceptoric nerve ending (Type I) in the muscular layer of the trachea (man).

According to the authors' investigations, sensory nerve fibers are observed, as shown in Figs. 283 and 284, in the mucomuscular layers in man. These consist of one to three specific large myelinated nerve fibers, which spread in a palmate form, after dividing into numerous terminal branches. Each terminal branch expands to form small terminal networks consisting of fine fibrils. There findings are in accordance with those of SASAKI (1943) and ELFTMAN (1943).

These correspond to the sensory nerve endings (Type I) which participate in Hering's barodepressor reflex, as mentioned by SUNDER-PLASSMANN (1933) and SETO (1937).

In addition to the above, the authors observed nerve endings which belong to Type II.

As shown in Figs. 285 and 286, these nerve endings consist of several large myelinated nerve fibers, but are not always distributed in arborescent form. On not a few occasions they are arranged in an irregular shape.

The sensory nerve endings which regulate the barodepressor reflex are found in the mucomuscular layer of the membranous part of the trachea, but not on the lateral or ventral wall.

Their fine structure is the same as for the sensory nerves which regulate blood pressure (SUNDER-PLASSMANN, 1933, 38), and which are observed in the aortic arch or in the carotid sinus.

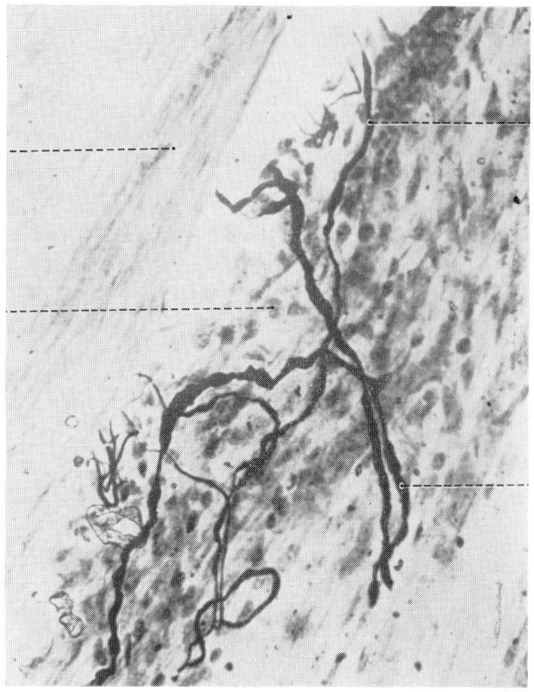

Fig. 285 Pressoreceptoric nerve ending (Type II) in the muscular layer of the trachea (man).

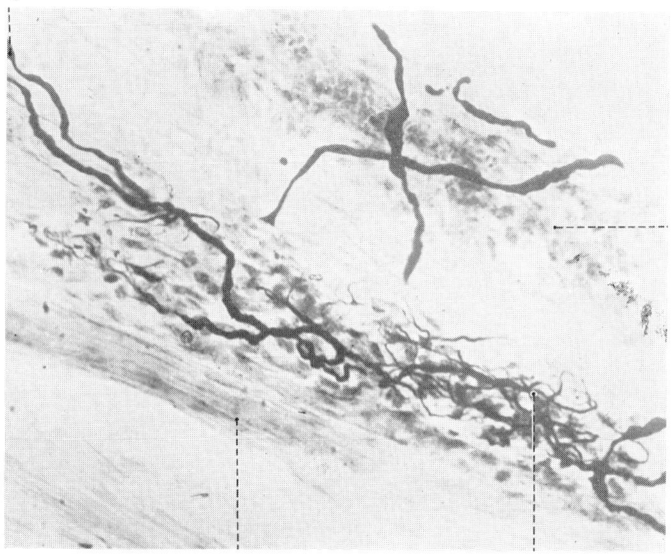

Fig. 286 Pressoreceptoric nerve ending (Type II) in the muscular layer of the trachea (man).

Figs. 287 and 288 show sensory nerve endings in the mucomuscular layer of an intrapulmonary bronchus of a dog. The myelinated nerve fibers arising from the extrachondral (peribronchial) nerve plexus are divided in the mucomuscular layer in arborescent form, and their terminal branches are as shown in Fig. 289. The networks consist of extremely fine nerve fibrils which terminate in free endings.

The histological findings are the same as for the sensory nerve endings which are seen in the aortic arch or carotid sinus (SUNDER-PLASSMANN, 1933), or for the sensory nerve endings which are found in the root of the superior vena cava, inferior vena cava and the pulmonary vein (NONIDEZ, 1937). According to SETO (1937), these nerve endings are said to correspond to the Type I sensory nerve endings which participate in the barodepressor reflex of HERING.

SUNDER-PLASSMANN considered that the neurovegetative receptors would be stimulated by dilation or contraction of the bronchi, and would influence the rhythm and depth of respiration in a manner similar to the func-

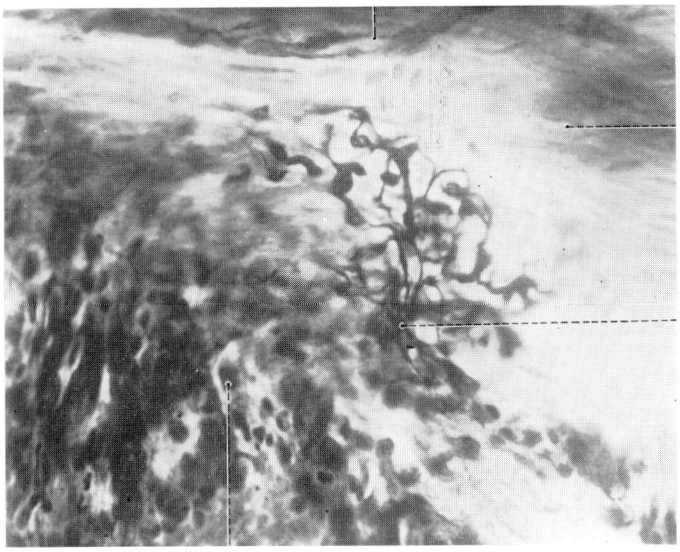

Fig. 287 Pressoreceptoric nerve ending in the muscular layer of the bronchus (man).

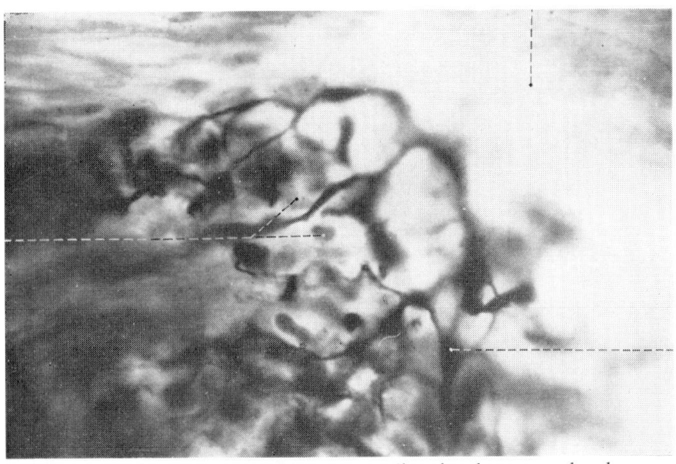

Fig. 288 Pressoreceptoric nerve ending in the muscular layer of the bronchus (man).

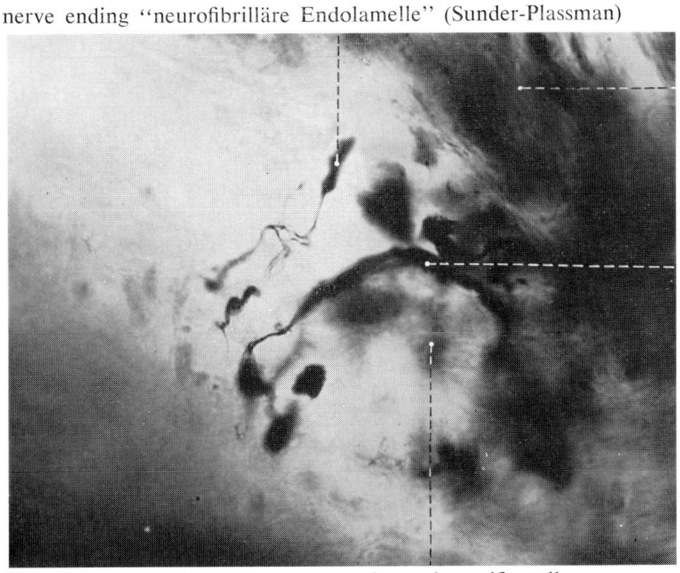

Fig. 289 Pressoreceptoric nerve ending in the muscular layer of the bronchus (man).

tion of the nerve endings which participate in and influence blood pressure, cardiopulmonary, and gastroenteric functions. He also noted that mechanical irritation in the intrapulmonary bronchus of dog in many instances caused cardiac arrest.

The authors have also noted that when a catheter is intubated into the intrapulmonary bronchus of a rabbit (without anesthesia), the pulse slows, and if the bronchial walls were pressed strongly by the catheter the heart beat and respiration would be markedly suppressed, occasionally resulting in cardiac arrest. These phenomena are considered to result from irritation of the neurovegetative receptors.

Similar experiences have been reported by NISSEN (1930) and by SAUERBRUCH (1932) in instances of bronchial ligature under local anesthesia.

vi) In Vascular System: The existence of the sensory nerve endings in the wall of the pulmonary artery was first reported by DOGIEL (1895).

Thirty-seven years later, SCHWIEGK (1935) reported that systemic blood pressure decreased upon ligation of the pulmonary vein at the hilum of a dog, or upon inserting a cannula into the pulmonary artery. SCHWIEGK termed this the "Lungenentlastungsreflex". However, his experiment was not one which gave direct stimulation to the baroreceptor area.

Prior to this, TAKINO (1933–1934) investigated serial sections by CAJAL's method, and reported existence of sensory nerve endings on the wall of the pulmonary artery.

Further, he showed that nerve endings of this type were similar to those of the carotid sinus or aortic arch. They were observed in the pulmonary artery of bat, rat, guinea pig, rabbit, dog, cat, cattle, pig, horse and man. TAKINO also defined the distribution of these baroreceptors.

Since considerable difference is seen in the frequency distribution of these sensory nerve endings on the wall of the pulmonary artery, according to the kind of animal, these nerve endings are considered to be functionally more significant in man, cattle and pig, as compared with other smaller animals that have fewer.

TAKINO and WATANABE (1937) observed that when electrical stimulus is applied to the wall of the pulmonary artery dropping of the blood pressure, or bradycardia occurred; these reflexes disappeared upon cutting the vagus and left depressor nerves.

TAKINO (1943) made further investigations on the nature of this reflex, using physiological methods; he termed this the "pulmonary artery (stem) reflex".

The existence of this reflex was confirmed later by PARIN (1947), UYEDA (1954), C. KIMURA (1954), COLERIDGE and KIDD (1960).

The routes of the reflex are as follows: sensory endings in the pulmonary artery stem → vagus nerve → medullary blood vessel and respiratory centers → vagus and sympathetic nerves → heart, and pulmonary and systemic blood vessels.

Besides the above, there are the following reports which deal with sensory endings in the wall of the pulmonary arteries.

MÜLLER (1910): In the pig, glomerular sensory endings are observed on the wall of the pulmonary artery.

LARSELL (1921): In the rabbit, sensory endings are found in the adventitia of the root of the pulmonary artery.

GLASER (1927): In the calf and man, ansa-like sensory endings are observed in the adventitia of the pulmonary artery.

LARSELL and DOW (1935): In the human infant, the sensory endings are found in the adventitia of the root of the pulmonary artery and also along arterial branches of the second order.

ELFTMAN (1943): Sensory endings were found predominantly in the adventitia of the larger branches of the pulmonary artery.

UYEDA (1954): Relatively large myelinated nerve fibers are observed on the wall of branches of the pulmonary arteries (up to 260 μ internal dia). These nerve fibers are variable in size, and bend and wind, terminating in the adventitia in ansa- or club-like endings.

NAGAISHI and INABA (1958) investigated the distribution of sensory endings in the pulmonary artery of man or dog using serial sections of extended or spread tissues, (stained by BIELSCHOWSKY's method, as modified by SUZUKI).

Fig. 290 shows the sensory endings which were observed in the adventitia.

The distribution of these nerve endings was limited to the region between the hilum and second order arterial branches of the pulmonary arteries.

The nerve endings in this region were, as shown in Fig. 291, morphologically similar to those observed by LARSELL, by GLASER, and by UYEDA. The free endings were nodular, glomerular, or ansaform in shape.

Morphologically the endings were somewhat different from those mentioned by TAKINO, but func-

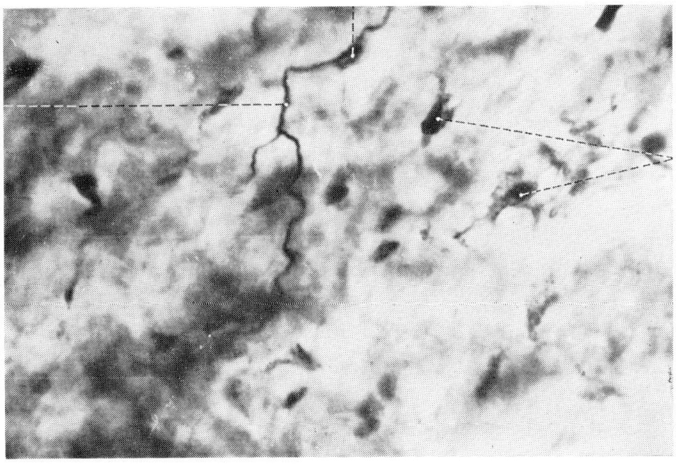

Fig. 290 Sensory nerve ending in the adventitia of the intrapulmonary portion of the pulmonary artery (man).

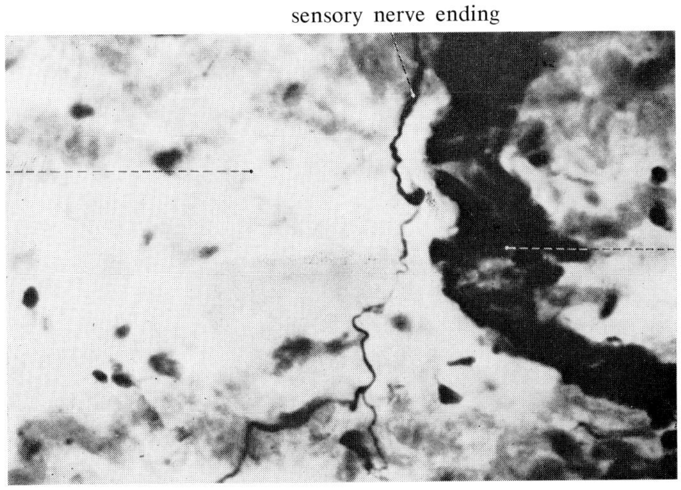

Fig. 291 Sensory nerve ending in the adventitia of the intrapulmonary portion of the pulmonary artery (man).

tionally they were considered to participate in the pulmonary artery (stem) reflex (Takino), that is "Lungenentlastungsreflex" (C. Schwiegk).

While investigating the nerve endings on the walls of the superior vena cava and inferior vena cava which participate in Bainbridge's reflex, Nonidez (1937) incidentally found similar nerve endings on the wall of the stem of the pulmonary vein.

According to Nonidez, the baroreceptor areas on the wall of the pulmonary vein stem, as shown in Fig. 292, are observed at the venous aperture of the left atrium, and on the posterior wall of the left atrium.

Nonidez classified these endings as of two types.

One type was represented by subendothelial nerve endings which were similar to the baroreceptors on the walls of the carotid sinus, aortic arch and subclavian arteries; the other type was the perimuscular nerve ending, which was found to be specific to the wall of the pulmonary vein.

The former endings were observed on both superior and inferior caval veins; they were found to be stimulated by an increase in the pulmonary venous pressure and were involved in the Bainbridge reflex, but the function of the latter was not known.

Nonidez did not mention sensory endings in the intrapulmonary pulmonary veins; however, Michelazzi (1937) stated distinctly that sensory endings did not occur in intrapulmonary pulmonary veins.

Takino (1933) investigated in detail the sensory nerve endings of the wall of the pulmonary veins, revealed their relationship to Bainbridge's reflex, and further found the existence of a pulmonary vein stem-left atrium reflex.

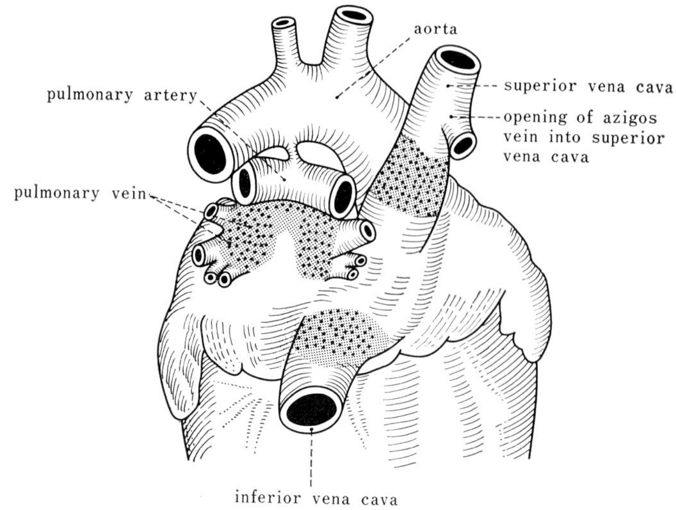

Fig. 292 Posterior view of the heart of a kitten showing location and approximate extent of the receptor areas (dotted) of the vein (NONIDEZ).

He proved the existence of baroreceptor nerve endings in the pulmonary vein of the pigeon and in various other animals (1933, 1934); then, together with WATANABE, he disclosed the existence of unipolar type sensory cells in the pulmonary vein stem of man (1937).

He conducted various other physiological experiments with WATANABE, from which they concluded that the afferent route for Bainbridge's reflex was mainly right vagus, whereas the afferent route for the pulmonary vein stem-left atrium reflex was mainly via left vagus.

ELFTMAN (1943) also observed baroreceptors in the pulmonary vein stem of the puppy, and UYEDA (1954) found baroreceptors in the adventitia of second order branches of the intrapulmonary pulmonary vein of the pig and guinea pig.

The authors (NAGAISHI and INABA, 1958) made detached extension and serial sections of the intrapulmonary pulmonary vein of man and dog. According to their investigation, sensory endings were not observed in the intrapulmonary pulmonary veins.

Although few in number, large myelinated nerve fibers are observed in the wall of the extrapulmonary pulmonary veins, as shown in Fig. 293.

As shown in Fig. 294, arborescent endings of these myetinated nerve fibers can be observed in the adventitia and also in the boundary regions between the tunica media and inner coats of the extrapulmonary pulmonary vein.

In short, by the authors' investigation baroreceptors can be observed in the extrapulmonary pulmonary veins, *i.e.* in the stem and hilar region, but not in the intrapulmonary tributaries.

Bainbridge's reflex is the response to stimulation of the sensory endings located in the walls of the pulmonary vein stem or atrium. Such stimulation results from expansion (stretching) of the venous wall due to increase in pressure in the pulmonary vein.

The pathway of Bainbridge's reflex is as follows:

Sensory endings in pulmonary vein stem→vagus nerve→medullary respiratory and vasomotor centers→vagus and sympathetic nerves→heart, and pulmonary and systemic peripheral blood vessels.

Myelinated nerve fibers are observed on the walls of bronchial arteries. These originate in the peribronchial nerve plexus or in the nerve fiber bundles which run along the bronchial arteries. In either case the nerves are distributed in the adventitia in nodular shaped endings. They have not been reported as occurring in the tunica media.

Similar sensory endings are observed on the wall of bronchial veins, but fewer than on bronchial arteries.

The sensory endings distributed to bronchial arteries and veins are considered to have the function of responding to various stimuli impinging on vascular walls.

b. Efferent Nerve Fibers (Vegetative Nervous System)

As mentioned earlier, the efferent innervation of the lung is provided by sympathetic and parasym-

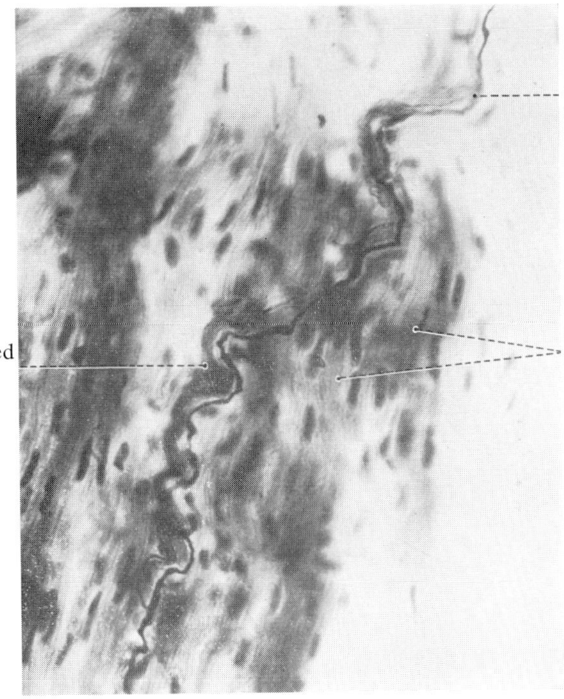

Fig. 293 Nerve fibers in the tunica media of the extrapulmonary portion of the pulmonary vein (man).

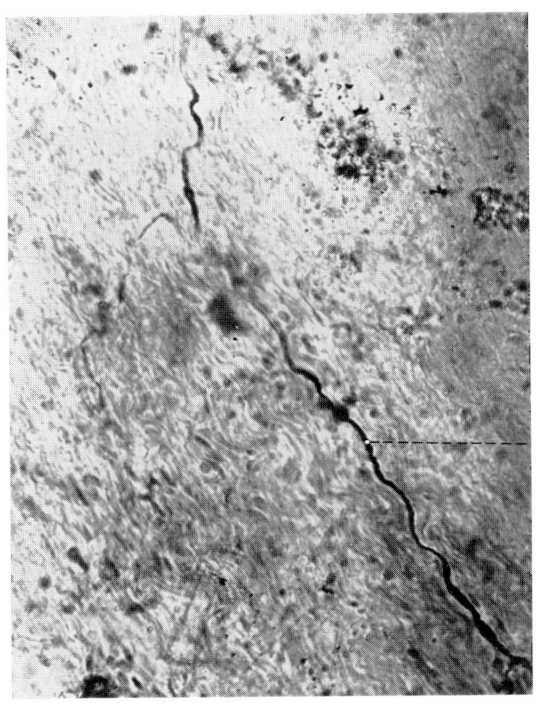

Fig. 294 Sensory nerve ending in the subendothelial layer in the extrapulmonary portion of the pulmonary vein (man).

pathetic nerves, which are mingled and distributed as a single system, and which terminate in recticular endings.

The vegetative nerves are not divisible or identifiable by their respective functions, *e.g.,* motor, vasomotor, or secretory, but rather the fibers have various functions according to distribution.

i) In Tracheobronchial System: After repeated branching and anastomosing the vegetative nerves of the tracheobronchial wall finally form preterminal nerves, extremely fine fibers, and, further peri-

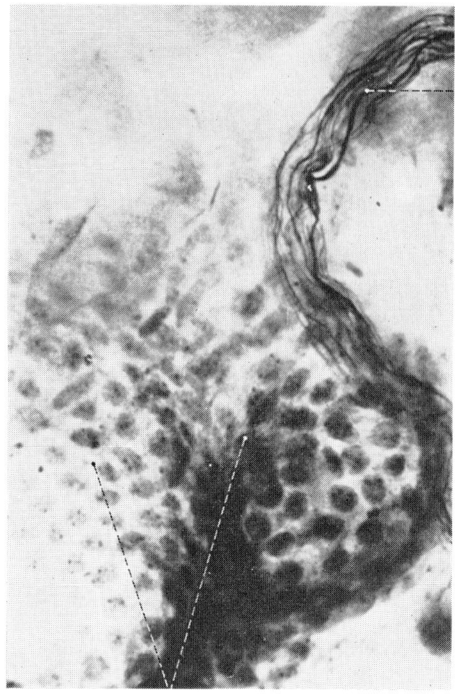

Fig. 295 Vegetative nerve fibers in the bronchial mucous gland (man).

pherally, a fine terminal reticulum. These terminal networks surround the perichondrium, smooth muscle, blood vessels, and tissue cells of the tunica propria.

Regarding the efferent nerves to bronchial mucous glands, there are reports by LARSELL (1921), LARSELL and DOW (1935), TAKINO and MIYANE (1936), HAYASHI (1937), DIJKSTRA (1938) and ELFTMAN (1943); however they are not all of the same opinion.

By the present author's investigations, it became clear that the nerve fibers which distribute to the bronchial mucous glands, as shown in Fig. 295, originate in the subchondral nerve plexus.

In other words, extremely fine non-myelinated nerve fibers extend from the subchondral plexus to the bronchial mucous gland, whence they enter the glandular cell group interstices.

Many of such nerve filaments are adjacent to the glandular cells and surround them, but in some instances, as shown in Fig. 296, fine nerve fibers are observed within the glandular cells. These are evidently the terminal reticulum of the vegetative nervous system.

Fig. 297 shows the terminal reticulum around the duct of a bronchial mucous gland.

Most of the nerve filaments observed in the bronchial mucous glands are considered to be postganglionic fibers of the vagus nerve.

MILLER (1918) pointed out the existence of ganglia in the bronchial mucous glands. His observation was made on a tuberculous lung in which a ganglion in the region studied showed specific changes and vacuolizations.

As already mentioned, besides the extrachondral and subchondral plexuses, there is a subepithelial plexus on the bronchial wall.

The subepithelial plexus is composed of many non-myelinated nerve fibers and a few that are myelinated. The nerve fiber bundles composing this plexus pass through the bronchial muscular layer from the subchondral plexus to reach the subepithelial tissues.

As shown in Fig. 298, this plexus forms preterminal networks in the region of the tunica propria and then forms an extremely fine terminal reticulum about connective tissue cells.

One must note, as shown in Fig. 299, that this terminal reticulum does not exclusively form the innervation of the tunica propria but, having close intercommunication with the nerve fibers to muscle and glandular cells, forms a closed reticular nervous system.

Between the terminal reticulum of the tunica propria and the connective tissue cells a close relationship is observed. Some fibers directly surround the connective tissue cells and some distribute in the cytoplasm.

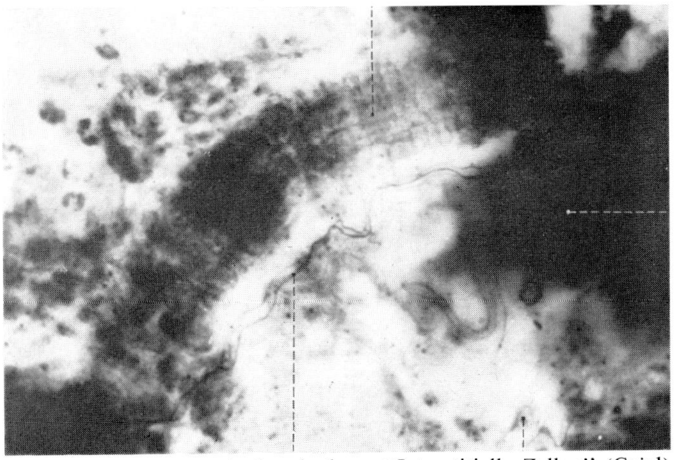

Fig. 296 Terminal reticulum in the bronchial mucous gland (man).

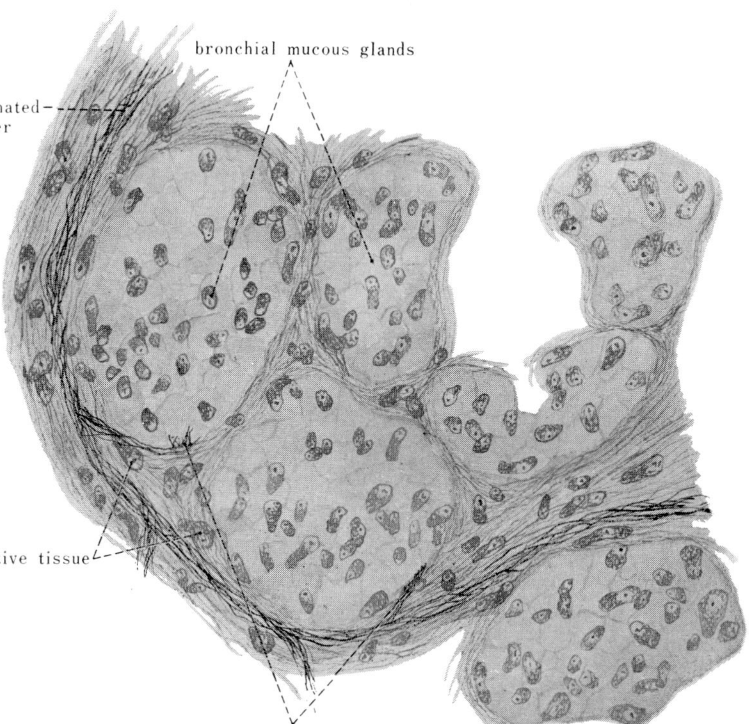

Fig. 297 Terminal reticulum of the bronchial mucous gland (man).

It provides an innervation not only to connective tissue cells of the tunica propria but also to perichondral and submucous connective tissue cells.

Regarding vegetative nerve endings in tracheobronchial muscles, PLOSCHKO (1897), LARSELL (1921), LARSELL and MASON (1921), GLASER (1927), LARSELL and DOW (1935), GAYLER (1934), HAYASHI (1937), DJIKSTRA (1939), ELFTMAN (1943), TAKINO (1950), and many other researchers have made reports.

According to the present author's investigations, as shown in Figs. 300 and 301, the nerve fibers originating in the subchondral and the extrachondral plexuses supply bronchial smooth muscles.

Most of these run parallel with the muscle fibers, as shown in Fig. 302, and divide into finer neurofibrils which have Schwann's nuclei, *i.e.,* they are preterminal fibers, as designated by REISER (1933).

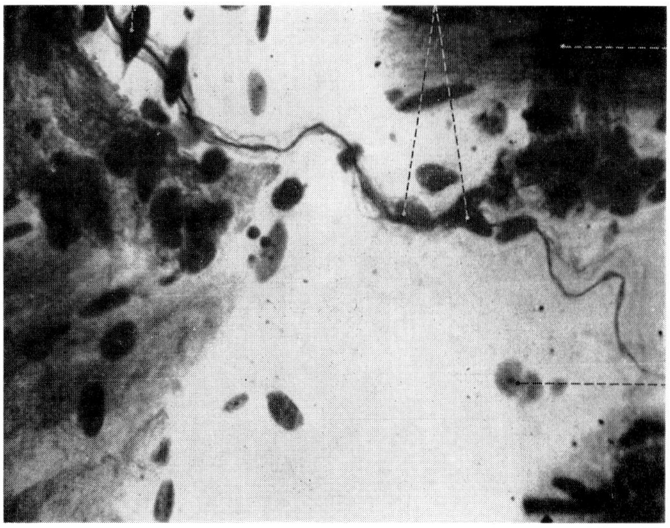

Fig. 298 Vegetative nerve fibers in the lamina propria mucosae of the bronchus (man).

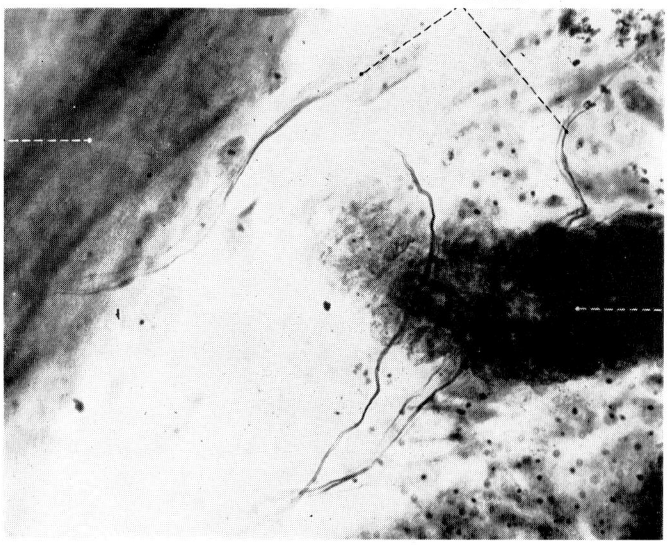

Fig. 299 Terminal reticulum in the propria mucosae and smooth muscle bundle of the bronchus (man).

Finally they give rise to very fine nerve endings which surround the muscle cells and function as the vegetative nerve supply.

The terminal reticulum which is found about the smooth muscle is generally ansaform, but sometimes, as shown in Fig. 303, it has a veil-like appearance.

The tracheobronchial muscles always maintain tonus, as do other organs such as the intestine.

This tension is regulated by the parasympathetic and sympathetic nerves. When the vagus nerve is cut the trachea and bronchi undergo dilation.

If the vagus is cut in the cervical region, and the peripheral end is electrically stimulated, the trachea and bronchi undergo contraction. Such contraction is most notable on the stimulated side, but slight contraction also occurs on the opposite; partial crossover of vagal fibers probably occurs in the pulmonary nerve plexuses. This was confirmed histologically by LARSELL and MASON (1921) in degeneration studies of the nerves in rabbits.

Also, according to DIXON and RANSON (1912), it is not an exceptional observation that a part of the vagus nerve crosses to the other side. In their experiments on the cat stimulation of the vagus nerve sometimes caused dilation of the bronchi, and sometimes strong stimulation of the cervical sympathetic nerves caused contraction of the bronchi.

By tests performed on guinea pigs by HEBB (1940), it was noted that stimulation of the sympathetic nerves frequently resulted in a remarkable contraction of bronchial smooth muscles.

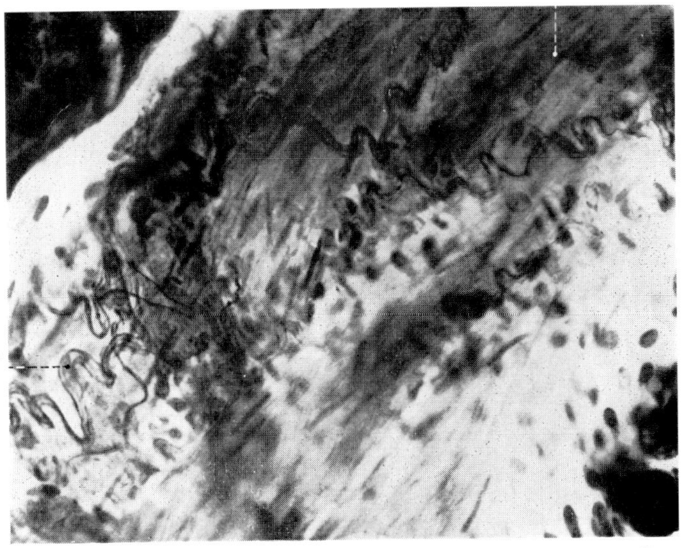

Fig. 300 Vegetative nerve fibers in the smooth muscle bundle of the bronchus (man).

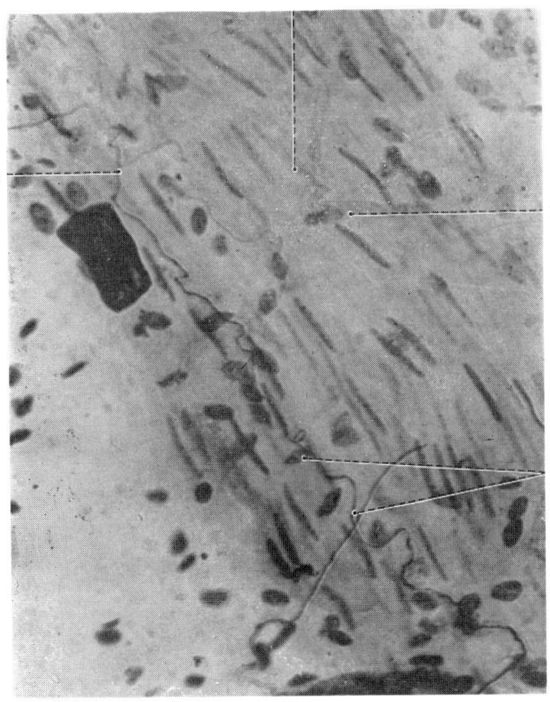

Fig. 301 Vegetative nerve fibers in the smooth muscle of the bronchus (man).

It is thus probable that, in some animals, some bronchial contracting nerves are contained in the sympathetic fibers distributed to bronchial smooth muscles.

With regard to the above, TAKINO (1950) suggested the possibility of a triple innervation of bronchial smooth muscle.

According to his theory, the sympathetic fibers (which participate in dilation of the bronchi) and vagal fibers are functioning antagonistically; however, other sympathetic contractile elements were believed to supply bronchial muscles.

By the authors' investigation, the bronchodilating fibers are sympathetic, originating mainly in inferior cervical ganglia or in superior thoracic sympathetic nerve trunks (Th_I-Th_{II}).

If, after cutting the cervical sympathetic nerve, electrical stimulation is given to the peripheral end, dilation of the bronchi on one or both sides may be observed. The dilation is most remarkable when the stimulation is given to the superior thoracic sympathetic nerve fibers.

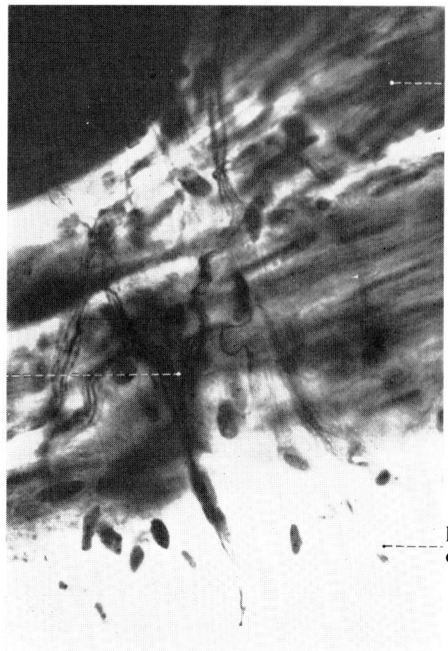

Fig. 302 Terminal reticulum in the bronchial smooth muscle bundles (man).

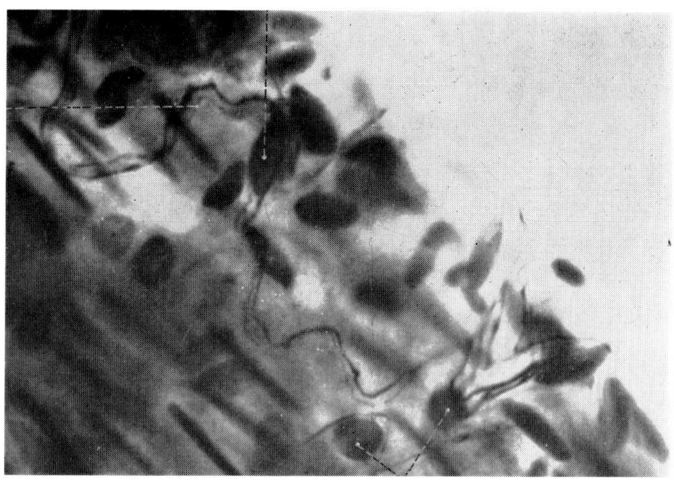

Fig. 303 Terminal reticulum in the bronchial smooth muscle bundles (man).

On the other hand, it is well known that drugs such as epinephrine, ephedrine, and atropine are effective in bronchial asthma, considered to be caused at least in part by spasm of bronchial smooth muscle.

Regarding this matter, DIXSON and RANSON (1912) carried out investigations on cats, and noted that when the bronchioles were more or less in the contracted condition, dilation would always be caused by epinephrine.

Acetylcholine is, in general, an agent which will cause contraction of bronchi, but according to the experiments of HEBB (1940), the contraction of the bronchus as the result either of direct stimulation of the vagus or by the use of acetylcholine, can be controlled by suitable doses of epinephrine, ergotamine, or atropine.

As will be seen from the above, bronchial smooth muscles are, in general, innervated antagonistically, by the dilating sympathetic and the contracting vagus nerves; however, some researchers consider that they are dually innervated by sympathetic nerves.

Regarding vegetative nerve endings in the pulmonary parenchyma, many reports have been made by investigators such as RETZIUS (1893), BERKELEY (1893), STÖHR (1928), ARIMOTO and MIYAKEGAWA (1930), LARSELL (1933), GAYLER (1934), LARSELL and DOW (1935), HAYASHI (1937), SUNDER-PLASSMANN (1938), and DIJKSTRA (1959), who agree that the non-myelinated nerves proceed from the peribronchial nerve plexus to the connective tissue of the interalveolar septa and thus reach the basal layers of the alveolar epithelium.

According to the present authors' investigations, nerve fibers go directly into the pulmonary parenchyma from the extrachondrial plexus of the bronchial walls.

As shown in Fig. 304, many of these extremely fine fibers run along the small blood vessels in the pulmonary parenchyma.

Some of the nerve fibers which run along the respiratory bronchiole or the alveolar duct pass directly to the alveolar walls.

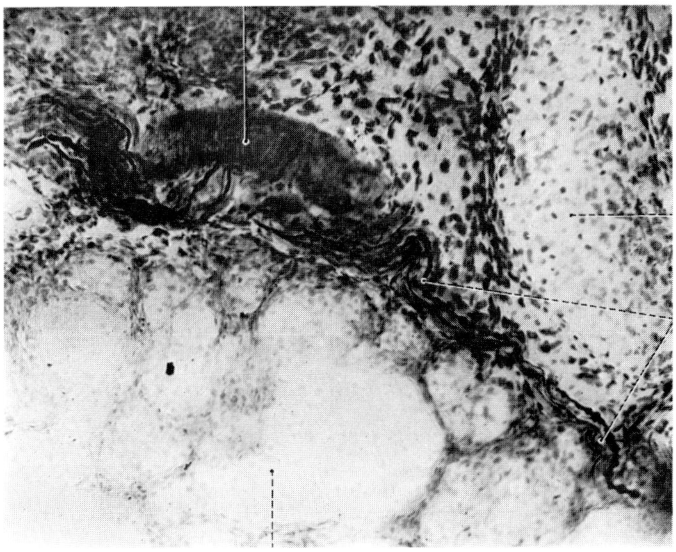

Fig. 304 Nerve fibers related to the arteriole (man).

According to previous reports, efferent nerve endings in the pulmonary parenchyma are in the form of nodose free endings; however, according to the author's investigations, all of these nerve endings are in the shape of a terminal reticulum.

The nerve fiber bundles in the pulmonary parenchyma, as reported by HAYASHI (1937), distribute in the connective tissue of the alveolar interstices, as shown in Fig. 305, and maintain a close relationship to nerve fibers of the vascular wall.

These nerve fibers are connected to each other in the form of a "Präterminalreticulum" (REISER), or "neurovegetative Präterminalplexus" (SUNDER-PLASSMANN); as the terminal reticulum consisting of fine neurofibrils they supply the vegetative innervation to the pulmonary parenchyma.

These terminal reticula in the pulmonary interstices distribute to the alveolar walls or to alveolar capillaries, as shown in Fig. 306.

HAYASHI (1937) stated that, although the terminal reticulum reached the portion immediately beneath the alveolar epithelium, endings were not observed in the cytoplasm of epithelial cells.

DIJKSTRA (1939) stated that, since Schwann's nuclei were missing in the schema of nerve fibers which was made by HAYASHI, he was dubious about HAYASHI's report. However, SUNDER-PLASSMANN (1938) had stated that the terminal reticulum which was distributed to the alveolar capillary also supplied alveolar epithelial cells. In investigating the relationship of the above, as shown in Fig. 307, he confirmed that extremely fine terminal reticulum distributed to each alveolar epithelial cells. SCHWANN's nucleus in this region is quite few and small.

From these findings SUNDER-PLASSMANN presumed that the permeability of the alveolar capillary of the human lung was regulated by the vegetative nervous system.

DIJKSTRA confirmed the existence of the centrifugal innervation which supplied the alveolar capillaries and interalveolar connective tissues; he did not mention the specific innervation of the alveolar epithelial cells.

As regards the author's investigation, the existence of a nerve supply to alveolar epithelial cells has not yet been confirmed.

ii) In Vascular System: As do the bronchi, the pulmonary arteries receive nerve fibers which originate in the nearby peribronchial nerve plexuses.

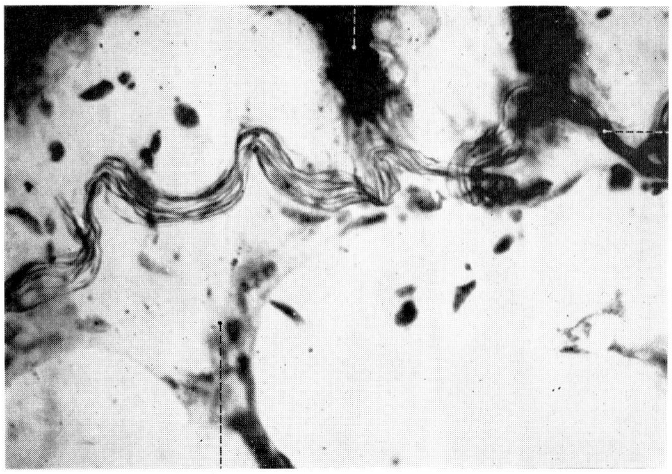

Fig. 305 Vegetative nerve fibers in the alveolar septum (man).

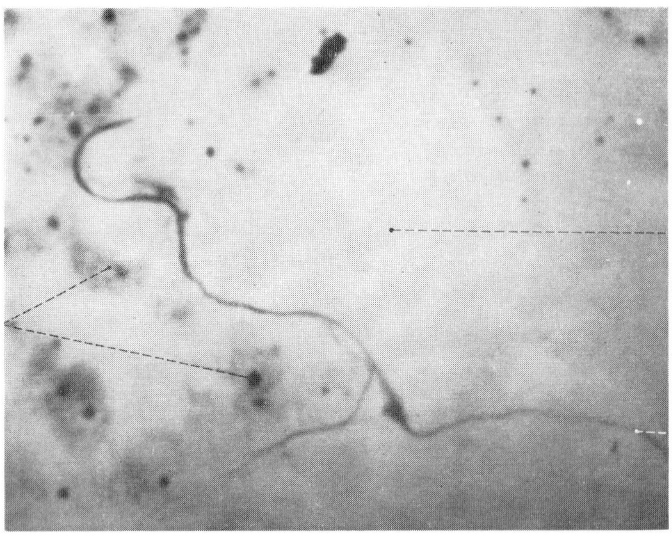

Fig. 306 Terminal reticulumin the alveolar septa (man).

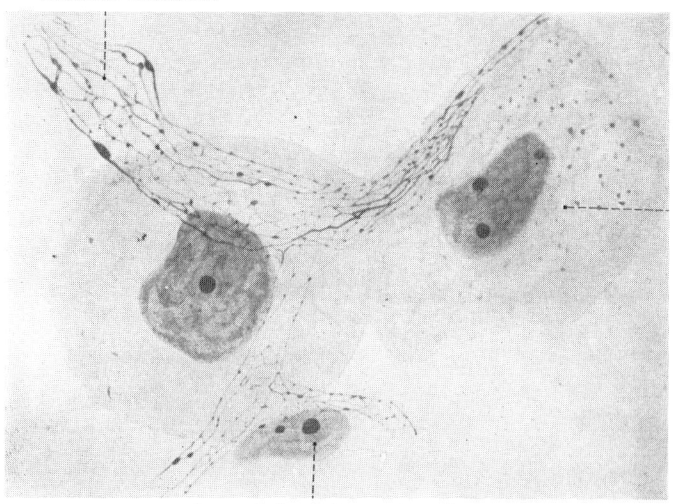

Fig. 307 Terminal reticulum in the alveolar cells (man) (SUNDER-PLASSMANN).

Regarding the motor innervation of the pulmonary artery, many researchers are carrying out studies of various kinds.

Particularly, Takino (1933) made investigations on various animals. He stated that in rabbit, dog, cat, guinea pig, mouse, and rat, the nerve fibers and nerve endings are observed to be most abundant on the extrapulmonary pulmonary artery. In the calf or horse the vasomotor innervation is said to be less rich.

Further, Takino performed comparative studies on the density of the vasomotor nerves in the pulmonary artery, as compared with other arteries in other regions. He stated that the innervation of the pulmonary artery was exceedingly poor as compared with systemic arteries, such as femoral, carotid or bronchial, etc.

Larsell (1923) and Larsell and Dow (1935) were of the same opinion.

Berkeley (1893), Kölliker (1896), Ponzio (1906), Larsell (1923), Jones (1926), Glaser (1927), Takino (1933), Larsell and Dow (1935), and Miyake (1937), stated that the nerve endings on the pulmonary arteries were of the simple nodular type; Boeke (1926), Stöhr (1928), Reiser (1933), Seto and Fukuyama (1936), Hayashi (1937), Sunder-Plassmann (1938), and Dijkstra (1939), stated that the vasomotor nerves ended in terminal reticula similar to those on the extrapulmonary vascular walls.

According to the authors' investigations (1958), nerve plexuses consisting of various sized fiber bundles were observed in the adventitia of the pulmonary arteries, and in relation to the peribronchial plexuses.

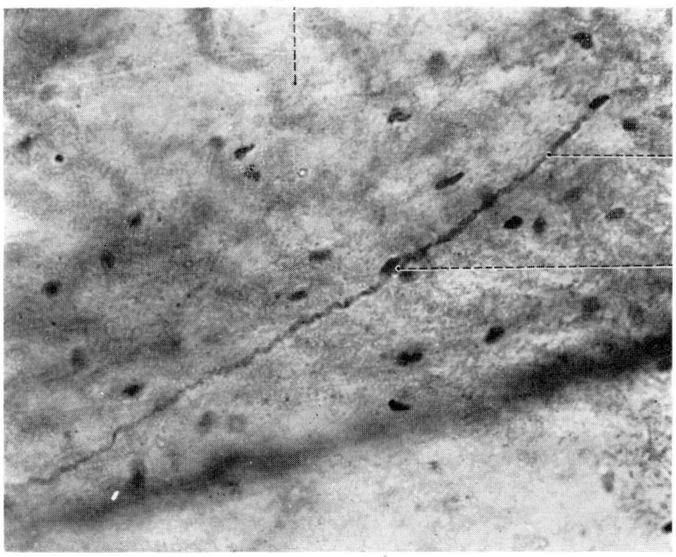

Fig. 308 Preterminal reticulum in the adventitia of the extrapulmonary part of the pulmonary artery (man).

The fine non-myelinated nerve fibers constituting the periarterial plexus divide in the adventitia, as shown in Fig. 308, into yet finer nerve fibers, which finally transit into the extremely fine preterminal reticulum.

As shown in Fig. 309, the preterminal reticulum in turn transits to the terminal reticulum (still finer neurofibrils), which distributes to the adventitia and also to the tunica media.

As shown in Fig. 310, this terminal reticulum originates in the non-myelinated nerve plexuses situated between the tunica media and the adventitia of the pulmonary artery.

As shown in Figs. 311 and 312, the terminal reticulums are the vegetative nerves to cells of the adventitia and of the tunica media.

In the pulmonary artery the terminal reticulum supplies the endothelial cells of the blood vessels, and has a close relationship to the perivascular cells of arterioles and capillaries, as shown in Fig. 313.

Sunder-Plassmann (1938) stated that the "neuro-vegetativer präterminaler Plexus" is connected in transit with the "nervöses Terminalreticulum", and between the terminal reticulum and each cell of the wall of the pulmonary artery a specific neural relationship is observed. This relationship is similar to that of the alveolar capillary of man, where the terminal reticulum surround each cell of the capillary and has close connections
capillary of man, where the terminal reticulum surround each cell of the capillary and has close connections
therewith.

Sunder-Plassmann stated also that the terminal reticulum provides innervation not only to alveolar capillaries but also to the alveolar epithelium; the present authors, however, were not able to adduce evidence of such findings.

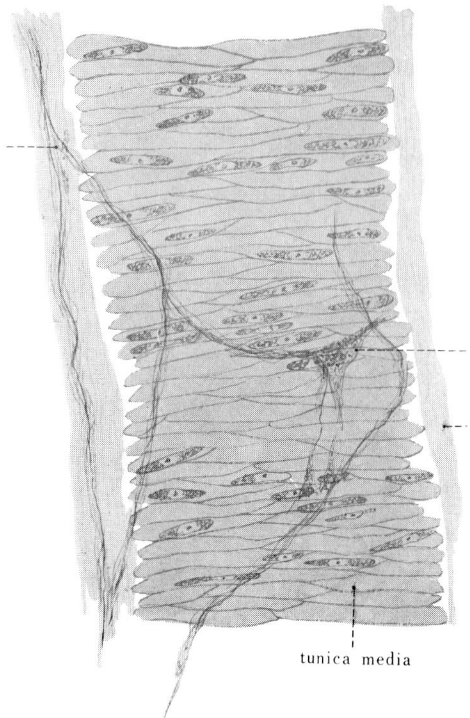

Fig. 309 Terminal reticulum in the adventitia and tunica media of the pulmonary artery (man).

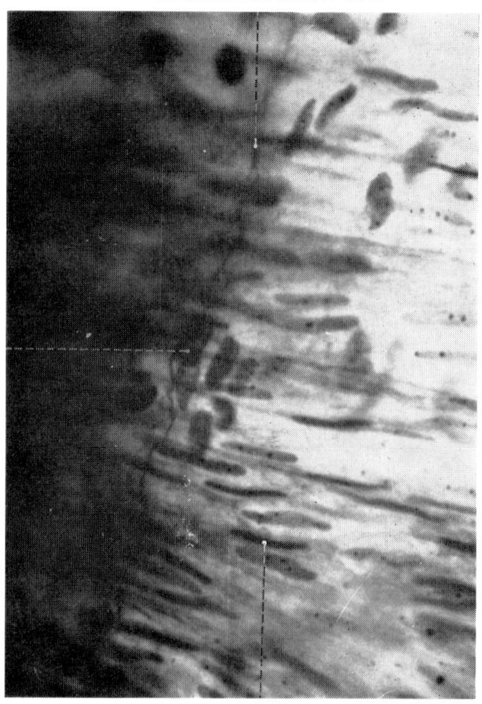

Fig. 310 Vasomotoric nerve fibers in the tunica media of the intrapulmonary portion of the pulmonary artery (man).

According to the author's investigation, the vasomotor nerves to the wall of the pulmonary artery are fewer than to the walls of systemic arteries, but the distribution of the terminal reticulum in each is similar.

Most of the terminal reticula distributing on the walls of the pulmonary artery run in the boundaries between adventitia and tunica media.

Efferent non-myelinated nerve fibers are observed also on the wall of the pulmonary vein; these originate in the perivenous nerve plexus of the hilum.

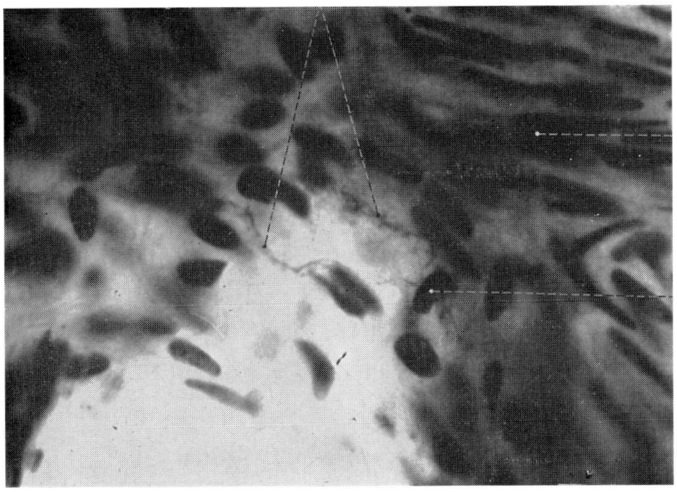

Fig. 311 Terminal reticulum in the tunica media of the intrapulmonary portion of the pulmonary artery (man).

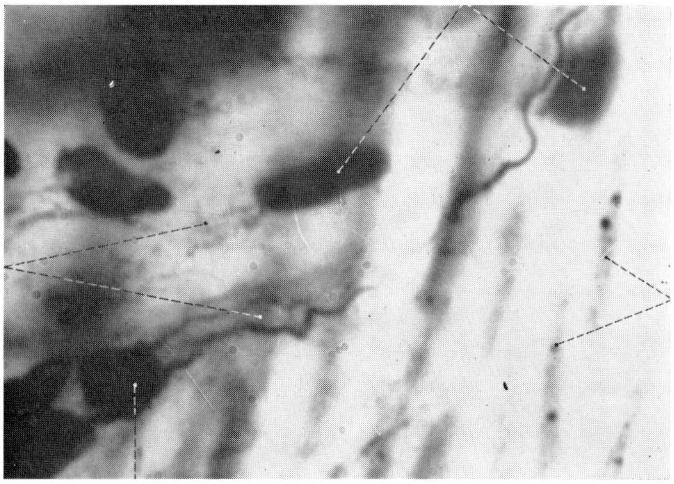

Fig. 312 Terminal reticulum in the tunica media of the pulmoary artery (man).

The vasomotor supply of the pulmonary vein is poorly developed as compared with that of the pulmonary artery.

The above was confirmed by Berkeley (1893), Larsell (1921), Glaser (1927), Takino (1933, 34) Larsell and Dow (1935), and Elftman (1943).

For example, Takino (1933) made detailed histological observation on the vasomotor innervation of the pulmonary artery and vein. The following is a summary of his study.

Vasomotor nerves to the pulmonary vein are abundantly observed on the tunica media of the large veins near the hilum; these nerve fibers and endings decrease in the periphery. Their development differs according to the kind of animals.

On the other hand, the vasomotor nerves to the intrapulmonary pulmonary arteries are observed to be fairly abundant in the periphery of the lung.

In small animals (rabbit, guinea pig, mouse, rat) the distribution of the vasomotor nerves to the pulmonary vein differs according to the extent of incorporation of heart muscle into the wall of the vessels. The wider the extension of the heart muscles, the wider the distribution of vasomotor nerves. However calves, pigs and birds are exceptions.

In man the vasomotor nerve fibers can be observed in the large intrapulmonary pulmonary veins, but compared with calves, colts, pigs and birds, the area of distribution in the tunica media is smaller. In dogs and cats the vasomotor nerve fibers can be observed only in the regions near the hilum, where the heart muscles are found to merge with the venous walls, and not in the more peripheral regions.

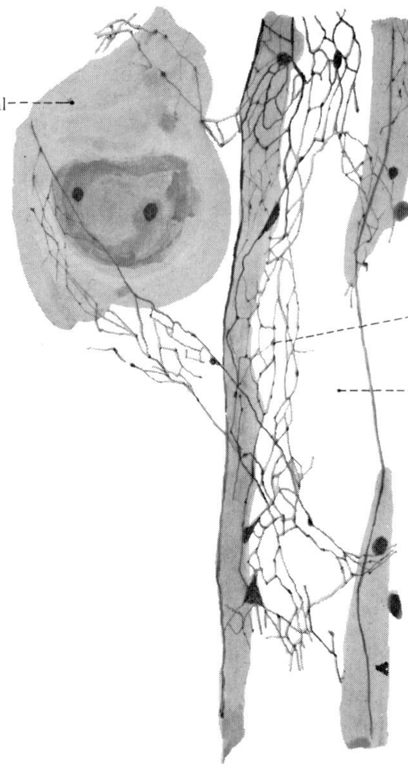

Fig. 313 Terminal reticulum of the alveolar capillary (man) (SUNDER-PLASSMANN).

Thus the pulmonary vein of man is more closely akin to that of the calf or pig, rather than to that of the dog or cat.

The authors' results (1958) on the dog and man differ slightly from those of TAKINO. Compared with the result of TAKINO, they observed a more abundant and widespread distribution of vasomotor nerves to peripheral regions. This difference may possibly be due to the adequacy of the staining method.

According to the study made by the authors, the vasomotor nerves and endings which distributed in the pulmonary vein were only a trace in the dog, but they were observed in adventitia and the media of veins of under medium size.

In man, the result was almost the same as for the dog. However, the authors found a far more abundant distribution of the nerves, especially in the region of the hilum. Indeed, the nerves were as abundant as for the pulmonary artery.

These vasomotor nerves originate in nerve fiber bundles, and include the postganglionic fibers of ganglion cells observed on the walls of pulmonary veins.

According to TAKINO (1933), the vasomotor nerves of the extrapulmonary pulmonary vein were said to arise from postganglionic fibers of ganglion cells on the left atrium.

Some differences are observed in the manner or style of distribution of nerve fibers and endings in the pulmonary vein and in the pulmonary artery.

For instance, large myelinated nerve fibers can be seen in the pulmonary artery at the hilar region; however in the pulmonary vein, as shown in Fig. 314, only the non-myelinated fibers are observed, and myelinated fibers are very scarce.

The quantity of the vasomotoric nerves distributing in the tunica media of the pulmonary vein corresponds to the quantity of the nerve fiber bundles which distribute in the adventitia.

As shown in Fig. 315 the nerve ending terminates in the smooth muscle cell of the tunica media. Like the pulmonary artery it is in the form of a terminal reticulum. Its innervation is similar to that of the pulmonary artery.

Fig. 316 shows the vasomotor nerve endings which are distributed in the pulmonary vein.

Compared with the pulmonary artery and vein, the bronchial artery and vein receive abundant innervation. This was pointed out by BERKELEY (1893), LARSELL (1921), TAKINO (1933), and LARSELL

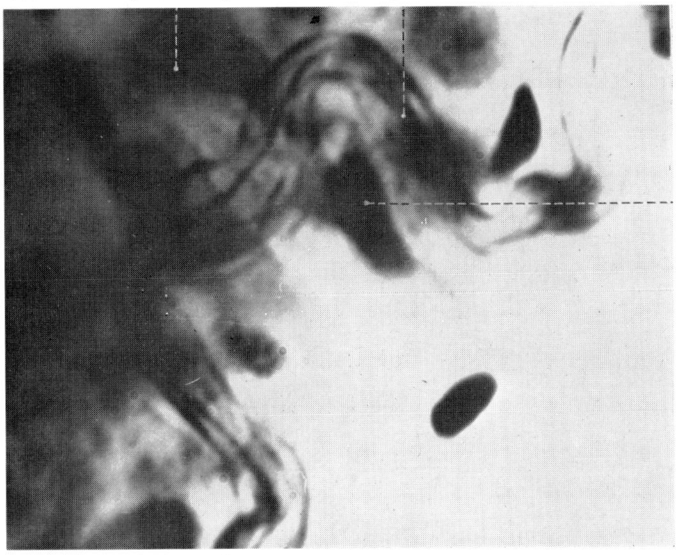

Fig. 314 Vegetative nerve fibers in the adventitia of the pulmonary vein (man).

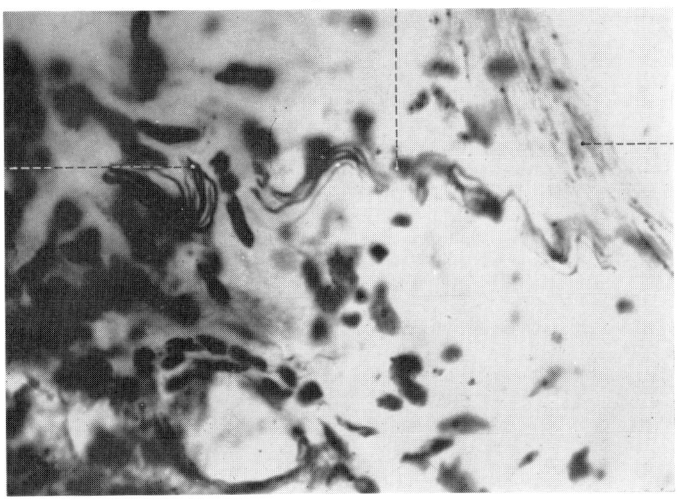

Fig. 315 Vegetative nerve fibers in the wall of the pulmonary vein originated in the peribronchial plexus (man).

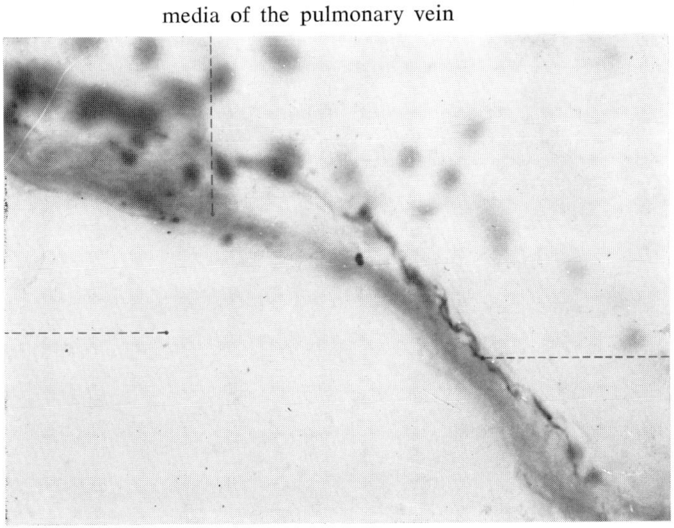

Fig. 316 Vegetative fibers in the tunica media of the intrapulmonary portion of the pulmonary vein (man).

and Dow (1935). Takino severally studied rats, rabbits, cats, dogs, birds, guinea pigs, calves, and pigs, and made histological studies on the innervation of the bronchial artery and vein.

Investigation by the authors (1958) also revealed an extremely abundant distribution of vasomotor nerves to the bronchial arteries, many nerve fibers forming plexuses surrounding the bronchial arteries and connecting closely with peribronchial plexuses.

As shown in Fig. 317, in the plexus surrounding the bronchial arteries a few ganglion cells are observed.

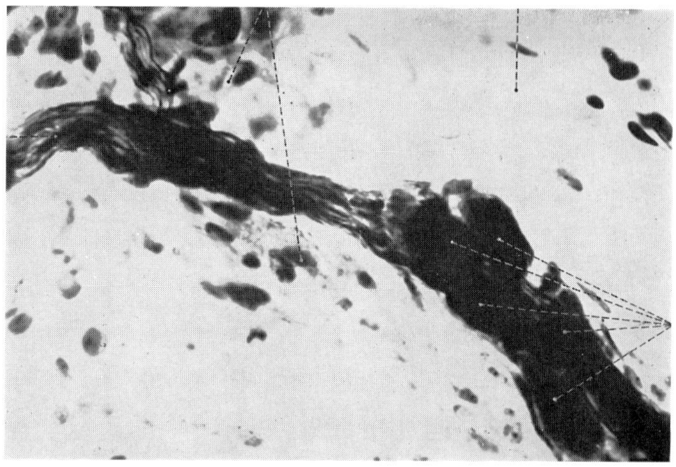

Fig. 317 Non-myelinated nerve fibers related to the bronchial artery (man).

The postganglionic fibers arising from these cells are distributed in the tunica media of the bronchial artery and terminate in and about the smooth muscle cells in the form of terminal reticulum.

Berkeley (1893) described free endings which terminate in nodose form either between smooth muscle cells or in nearby regions. Larsell (1921) was also of the same opinion, but according to the present authors' investigations, the nerve endings on the bronchial arteries are in the form of terminal reticulum. These differences in observations are perhaps dependent on adequacy of staining methods.

In short, the supply of vasomotor nerves to the bronchial arteries is relatively more plentiful than to the pulmonary arteries. As shown in Fig. 318, the vasomotor nerves can be observed equally abundantly, both centrally and peripherally. On this point the authors are entirely in agreement with Takino.

As shown above in Fig. 319, these vasomotor nerve fibers run along the bronchial arteries.

These vasomotor nerves originate in fiber bundles which compose the peribronchial plexus. As shown above in Fig. 263, the plexus includes scattered ganglion cells from which postganglionic fibers are given off for distribution to the bronchial arteries.

At the boundaries between adventitia and tunica media these nerve fibers form "präterminales Netzwerk" (Reiser) and transit to terminal reticulum, which surrounds the cells of the vascular wall.

The nerves which distribute in the bronchial artery mainly consist of non-myelinated nerve fibers but occasionally include myelinated (sensory) nerve fibers which distribute in the adventitia.

As mentioned earlier, the vasomotor and sensory nerves are observed as more abundant in the bronchial artery than in the pulmonary artery, particularly in the smooth muscle of the tunica media.

Incidentally, the distribution of vasomotor nerves to bronchial arteries resembles that to the extrapulmonary systemic arteries.

According to investigations by Takino (1933) and Miyake (1937) on the human fetus, the distribution of vasomotor nerves to the pulmonary artery is fairly abundant; when compared with that to the bronchial artery, however, it is actually far less. The difference in the density of distribution of the vasomotor nerves to these two arteries may also be observed for the respective capillaries.

As to the innervation of bronchial veins, histological investigations have not been carried out, other than that the authors' investigations have shown the situation to be the same as for the bronchial artery.

The nerve fibers arising from the peribronchial or perivenular plexuses distribute in the adventitia and the tunica media of the bronchial veins, and have terminals similar to those described for the bronchial arteries.

Fig. 320 is a schema showing an outline of the nervous system of the lung as described above.

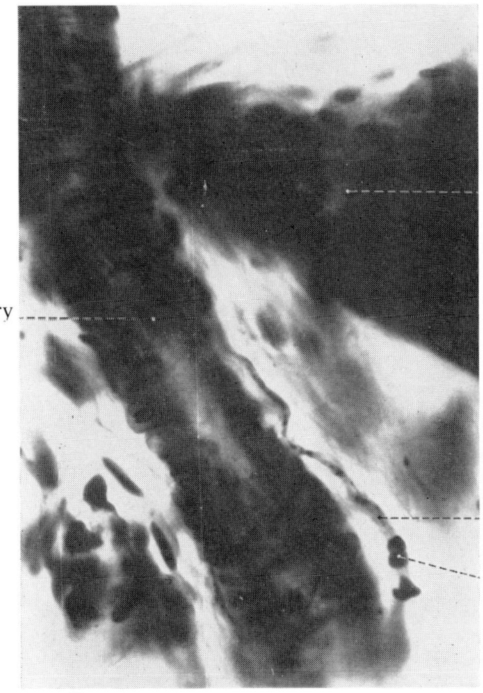

Fig. 318 Vasomotoric nerve fibers related to the bronchial artery (man).

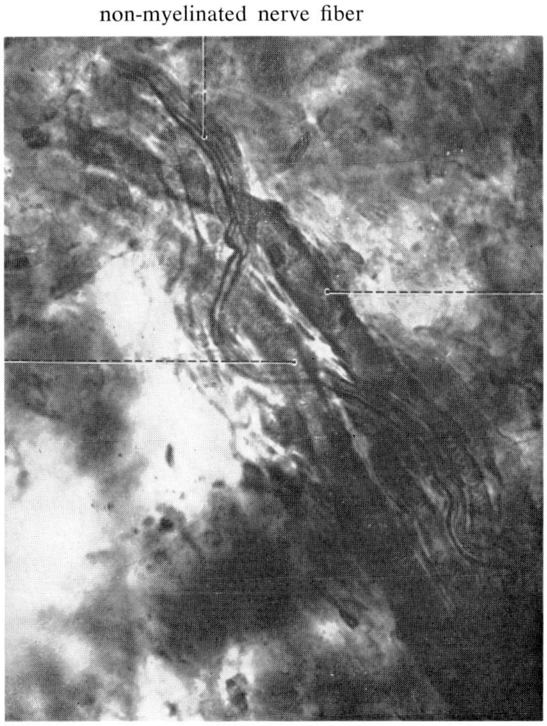

Fig. 319 Non-myelinated nerve fibers related to the bronchial artery and vein (man).

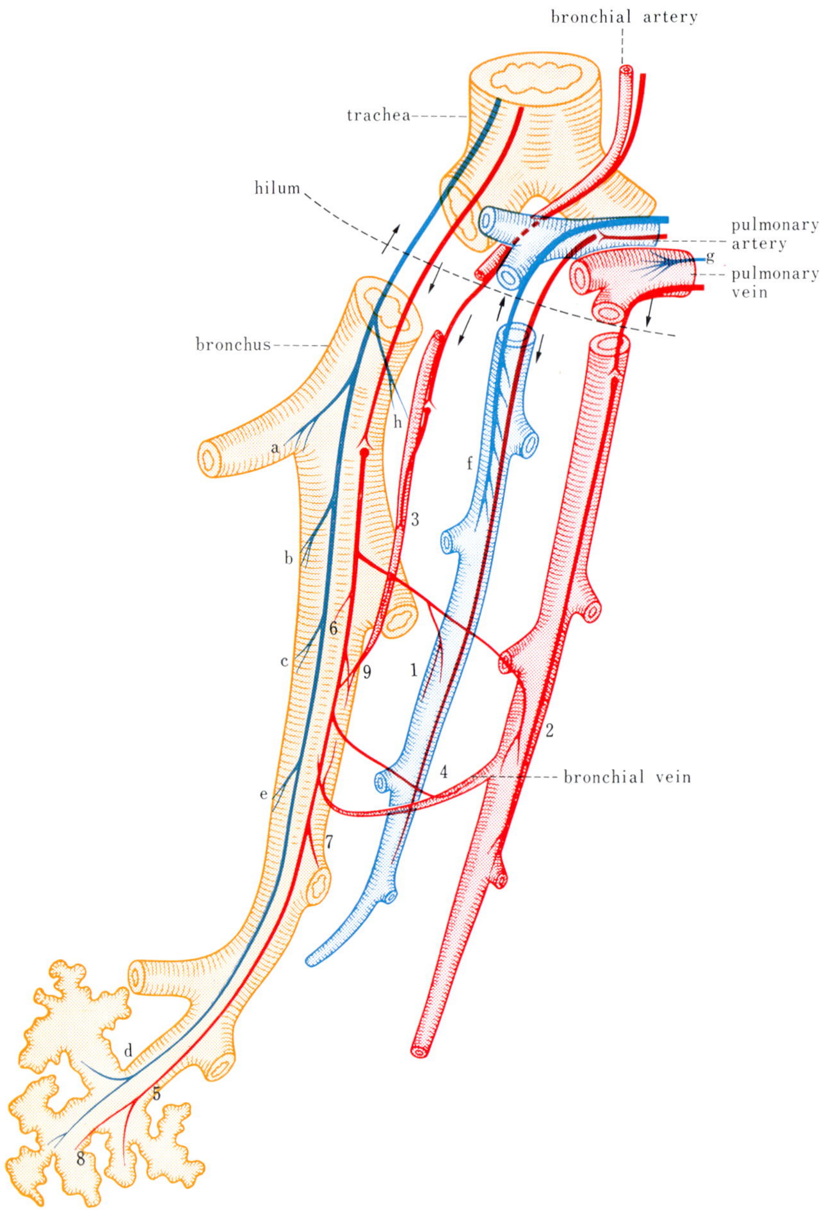

Fig. 320 Schema of the pulmonary innervation (man).

Red: efferent nerve fibers:

1. Vasomotoric nerve of pulmonary arteries
2. Vasomotoric nerves of pulmonary veins
3. Vasomotoric nerves of bronchial arteries
4. Vasomotoric nerves of bronchial veins
5. Motoric nerves of pulmonary blood capillaries
6. Motoric nerves of bronchial smooth muscles
7. Secretory nerves of bronchial mucous glands
8. Vegetative nerves of pulmonary alveoli
9. Vegetative nerves of submucous layer of the bronchus

Blue: afferent nerve fibers:

a. Intraepithelial nerves of bronchus
b. Sensory nerves of submucous layer of bronchi
c. Sensory nerves of bronchial smooth muscles
d. Sensory nerves of bronchial smooth muscles
e. Pressoreceptor nerves of bronchi
f. Pressoreceptor nerves of pulmonary arteries
g. Pressoreceptor nerves of pulmonary veins
h. Sensory nerves of bronchial arteries

V. INNERVATION OF PLEURA

A. Parietal Pleura

LUSCHKA (1863) was the first to report on the innervation of parietal pleura.

He stated that the nerve fibers which distribute in the parietal pleura originate in the intercostal, sympathetic, vagus and phrenic nerves.

BRAEUCKER (1920, 1926) investigated the parietal pleura of man. He stated that the parietal pleura was mainly innervated by the intercostal nerves, but in regions near the vertebra received branches of the sympathetic nerves, such branches being distributed in the mediastinal pleura. Further, the ventral part of the mediastinal pleura was innervated by the phrenic nerve or from nerve plexuses of nearby large blood vessels; the dorsal part was innervated by vagus nerves or by the nerve plexus surrounding the aorta.

The authors' investigations confirm the above findings.

1. Sensory Nerve Endings

DOGIEL (1903), ROMANOW (1904) and ROSSI (1931) reported on the histology of sensory endings in the parietal pleura.

According to their reports, some of the sensory endings are encapsulated, others are devoid of capsules. The nerve fibers which are regarded as vegetative form fine networks near the surface of the pleura.

The authors investigated the innervation of the parietal pleura in the dog.

After sacrifice by hemorrhage, segments of the thoracic wall or diaphragm are removed as quickly as possible, and fixed in 20% neutral formalin. After fixation for one week, the pleura is carefully separated from the thoracic wall and diaphragm with knife and forceps. Sections of the parietal pleura thus obtained are fixed in 20% neutral formalin for a further 2 or 3 months to insure adequate fixation. Sections are cut and stained using BIELSCHOWSKY's staining method as modified by SUZUKI or Sugamo myelin sheath staining method.

Myelinated and non-myelinated fibers are observed in the submesothelial layer of the parietal pleura, as shown in Fig. 321.

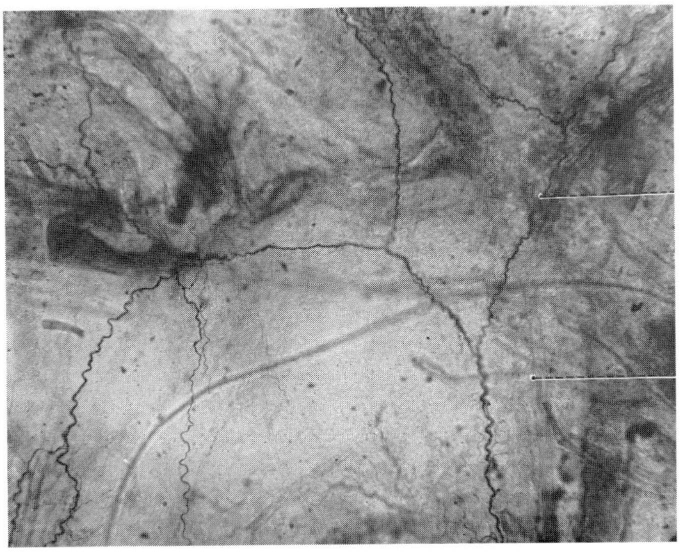

Fig. 321 Nerve plexus in the parietal pleura (man).

The myelinated fibers, considered to be afferent and sensory, form relatively large coarse networks, as shown in Fig. 322. These are accompanied by fine non-myelinated nerve fibers. After repeated bifurcations, these latter terminate in free endings, as mentioned by DOGIEL and ROMANOW.

As shown in Fig. 323, some of the nerve endings are composed of relatively simple shaped terminal branches with sharp or small nodular points. The others are, as shown in Fig. 324, of relatively complicated arborescent or glomerular shapes; in many cases, the myelin sheath is lost at the bifurcations of fibers.

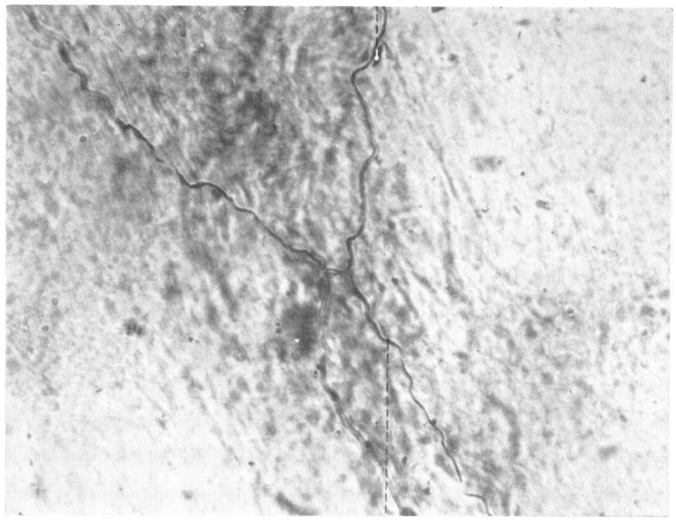

Fig. 322 Myelinated nerve fibers in the parietal pleura (man).

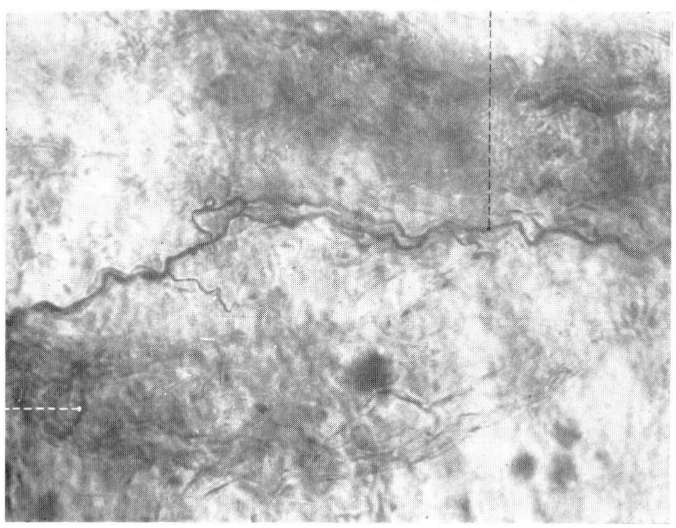

Fig. 323 Sensory nerve ending in the parietal pleura (man).

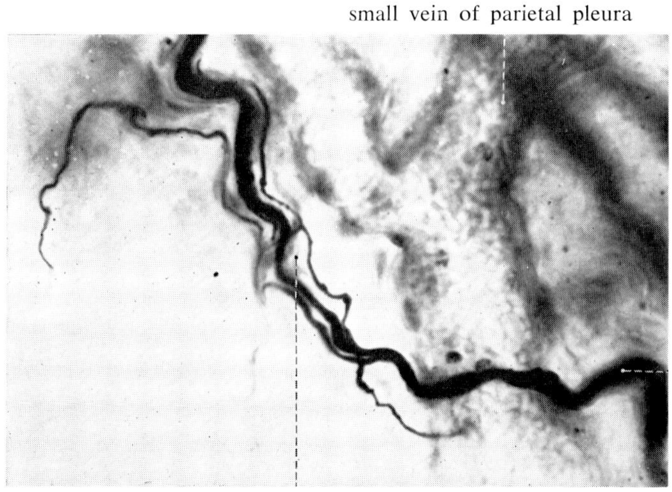

Fig. 324 Sensory nerve ending in the parietal pleura (man).

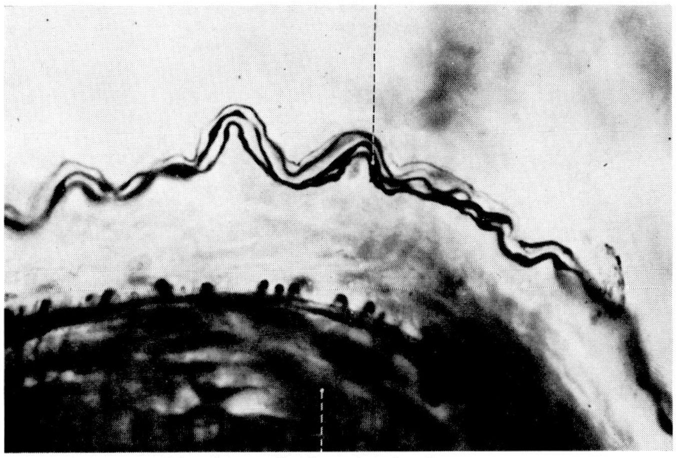

Fig. 326 Nerve fibers related to the blood vessel in the parietal pleura (man).

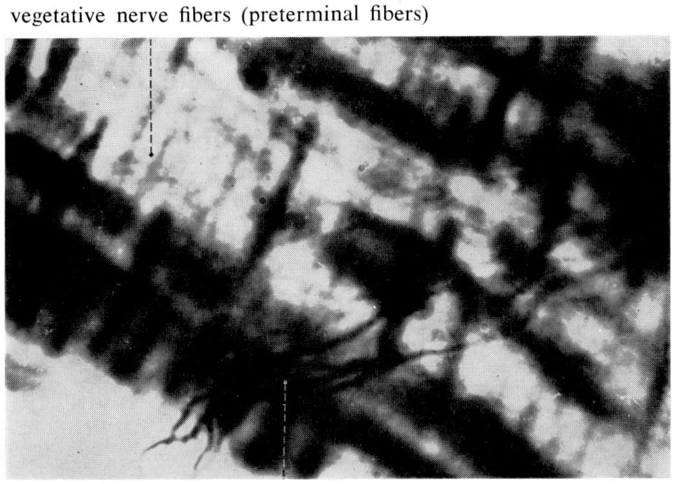

Fig. 327 Preterminal reticulum in the arterial wall of the parietal pleura (man).

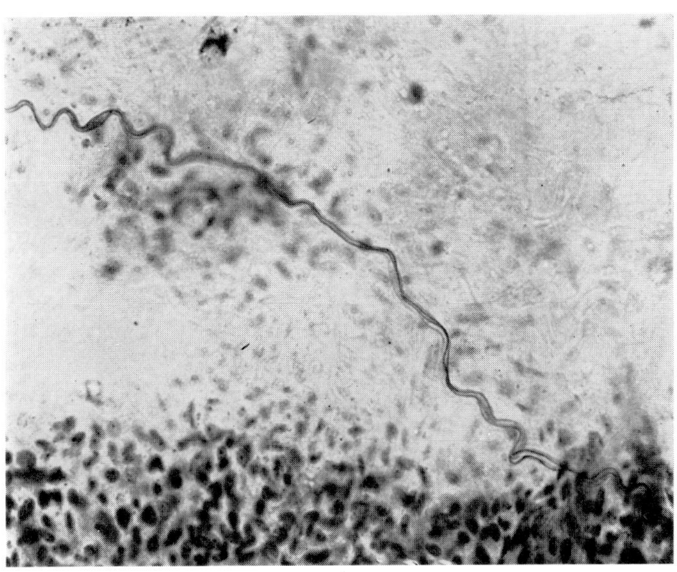

Fig. 328 Vegetative nerve fibers in the parietal pleura (man).

In summary, sensory endings are as follows:

1) Sensory endings which are devoid of capsules.
   i) relatively simple shaped free endings (above Fig. 323).
   ii) relatively complicated arborescent or glomerular shaped free ending (above Fig. 324).
2) Sensory endings, encapsulated, and small cone shaped sensory vesicles (Fig. 325 (a, b)).

These myelinated nerve fibers and nerve endings are most notably distributed to the costal pleura, followed by the diaphragmatic pleura and the mediastinal pleura, in terms of frequency of distribution.

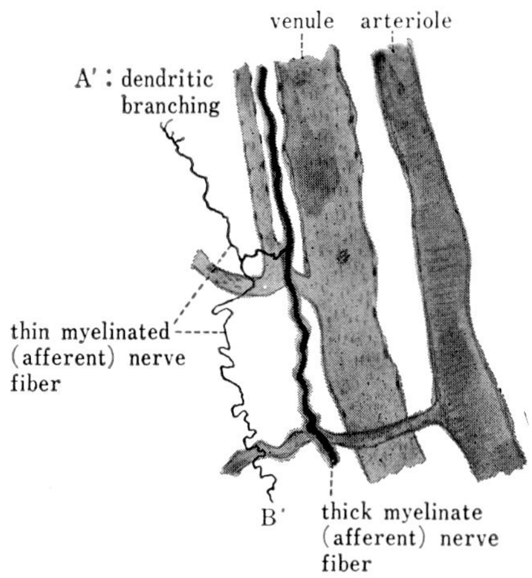

Fig. 325 a. Afferent myelinated nerve fibers related to the blood vessels in the paretal pleura.

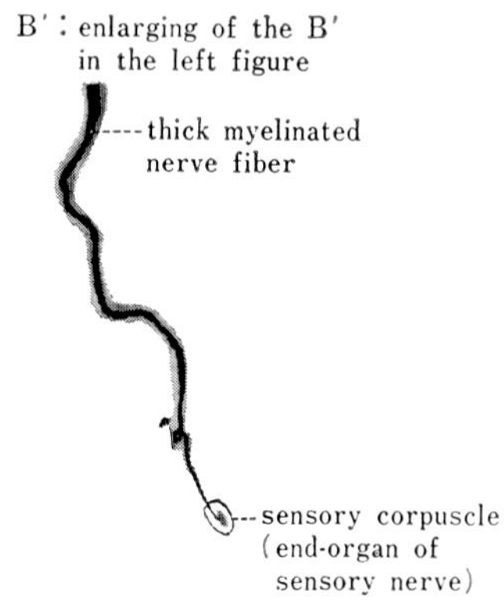

Fig. 325 b. Sensory nerve ending in the parietal pleura (man).

2. Vegetative Nerve Endings

The non-myelinated fibers of the parietal pleura can be distinguished as those that run along the blood vessels, and those that distribute to other parts.

The former, as shown in Fig. 326, ramify in so-called "Präterminales Netzwerk" (REISER), and distribute on the vascular walls in the form of the terminal reticulum, as shown in Fig. 327.

The latter, as shown in Fig. 328, do not take a typical terminal reticulum form, but in the form of preterminal reticulum spread on the pleural surface as loose networks.

3. Function

It was mentioned earlier that sensory fibers and endings are most abundant on the costal pleura, followed in frequency on the diaphragmatic pleura, and least on the mediastinal pleura.

This is quite understandable from clinical experience and physiological viewpoints.

In fact, the pulmonary and mediastinal pleuras are insensible or insensitive to stimulation, whereas the costal pleura is very sensitive.

After thoracoscopy under local anesthesia, UNVERRICHT (1934) stated that mechanical or electrical irritation of the costal pleura caused severe pain, but the costal pleura was insensitive to temperature changes, such as cold, etc. As for mechanical irritation, it was possible to distinguish the size and location of the stimulus, but a rubbing stimulus were not easily localized.

SIMENAUER (1927) also stated that the surface of the serous membrane of the costal pleura was relatively insensitive; on many occasions, rubbing was not an effective stimulus. Among the stimuli which caused a sense of pain he included electrical and mechanical irritations. As a response to these irritations, strong pain was perceived along the course of distribution of intercostal nerves.

As seen above, the parietal pleura is relatively sensitive to stimulation, and frequently responds to irritation. Cough (in pleurisy), syncope (in penumothorax), so-called pleural shock, respiratory insufficiency, tachycardia or syncope (on irrigation of the thoracic cavity against empyema), mydriasis, apnea and cardiac arrest, are all considered to result reflectively from pleural irritation.

TAKINO (1933) stated that some sensory endings of the arborescent type subserve the sense of pain, and others are involved in touch and cough reflexes.

As was seen in the experiment by UNVERRICHT (1934), the parietal pleura does not respond to temperature changes as such; temperature alteration may be perceived as pain.

When warmth is applied to the central region of the diaphragmatic pleura no special sensation results, but pressure or puncture applied to the region causes cervical or shoulder pain on the same side. When the central portion of the diaphragmatic pleura is stimulated, the pain may frequently be felt in the shoulder (scapular) region.

According to CAPPS (1911), when the central region of the diaphragmatic pleura is stimulated pain limited to the cutaneous distribution of C_{III}–C_{IV} will occur. When the periphery of the diaphragmatic pleura is stimulated uncomfortable sensations may be felt in the lower portion of the thorax, in the upper abdomen, or the upper part of the loins, which are supplied by the intercostal nerve.

In the case of pleurisy, pain may be felt in the region where the diaphragm joins the thoracic wall, or in the hypochondrium.

Inflammation of the diaphragmatic pleura will cause pain at the level of the lowest rib, and may spread to the epigastrium or to the nuchal or scapular regions. Pressure on the region where the diaphragm joins the thoracic wall may also elicit a cough reflex.

Since olden times, it has been stated that the mediastinal pleura is insensitive; however, although few in number, sensory nerve endings are observed on the mediastinal pleura.

Those who have inflammation affecting the mediastinal pleura sometimes complain of pain or pressure in the region of the sternum or related regions.

B. Pulmonary Pleura

The nerve fibers which distribute in the pulmonary pleura mostly arise from the pulmonary nerve plexus of the hilum.

Regarding this, BRAEUCKER (1927) stated that the pulmonary pleura is innervated not only by the pulmonary plexus but also by small nerve fibers from the bronchial branches which divided immediately before entering the lung.

1. Subpleural Plexus

The nerve fibers which distribute in the pulmonary pleura form a plexus of complicated shape, beneath the surface of the pleura. The distribution of these fibers shows evident differences according to the kind of animal.

The subpleural connective tissue extends into the pulmonary parenchyma, forms intrapulmonary septum, and divides the lung into many pulmonary lobules. These findings are observed in man, cattle and pig, but not in rabbit, cat or dog, in which the pulmonary pleura is particularly thin. The anatomical differences which are observed in various animals result in considerable variability in the distribution of the nerves in the interstitial layers of the pulmonary pleura.

For example, LARSELL and DOW (1935), HAYASHI (1937), and YAGITA (1954) stated that in man fiber bundles of various sizes, originating in the peribronchial plexus, reach and distribute on the pulmonary pleura along interlobular connective tissues. MILLER (1925) stated that in the dog or rabbit the plexus of the hilum, especially fibers originating in the periarterial plexus, distributed directly to the pulmonary pleura.

LARSELL (1935) stated that all the fibers distributing to the pulmonary pleura originated in the periarterial plexus, regardless of the kind of animal.

The nerve fibers originating in the plexus of the hilum and those originating in the intrapulmonary region, particularly in the peribronchial plexus to the pleura, running along the interlobular septum, form somewhat loose plexuses in the interstitial layer of the pulmonary pleura. HAYASHI (1937) designated this as the "subpleural plexus".

These plexuses are mainly composed of fine non-myelinated fibers, as shown in Fig. 329. They also sometimes contain myelinated fibers.

KÖLLIKER (1854) and HAYASHI (1937), observed ganglion cells in this nerve networks; however, the present authors, as well as others, could not coroborate their existence.

According to their investigations on the pulmonary pleura of man and dog, ganglion cells were not observed. The large myelinated nerve fibers composing the subpleural plexus distributed mainly along the surface of the interlobar pleura, however, they were not observed on the costal surface of the pulmonary lobes, as shown in Fig. 330.

2. Sensory Nerve Endings

Regarding the sensory endings of the pulmonary pleura, histological investigations were carried out by KÖLLIKER (1854), ROMANOW (1904), LARSELL (1923), HAYASHI (19931), MCLAUGHLIN (1933), LARSELL and DOW (1935) and YAGITA (1954). LARSELL in particular made systematic studies on pleural innervation in rabbit, dog and man.

According to LARSELL, myelinated and non-myelinated nerve fibers are observed in the pulmonary pleura of man, the former having free endings showing nodular expansions, as in the rabbit or dog. The latter have vasomotor nerves which run in the deep layers of the pleura, along the blood vessels.

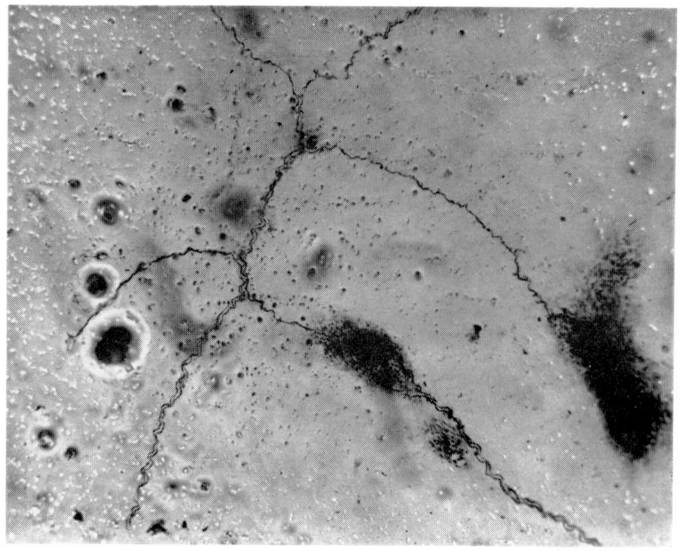

Fig. 329 Nerve plexus of the pleura near the hilum (man).

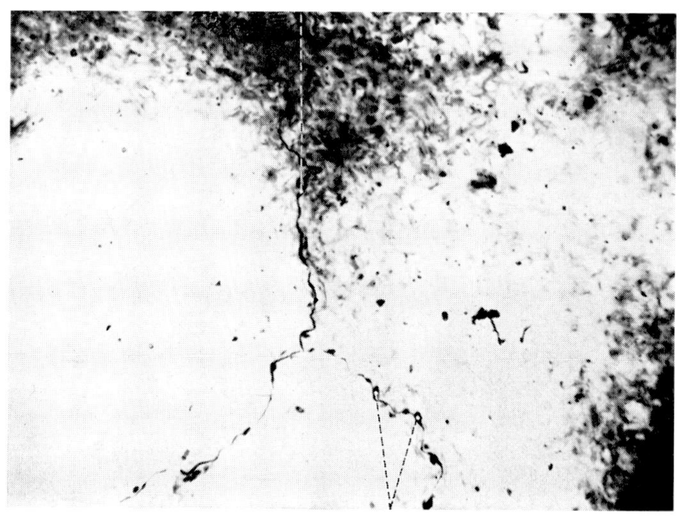

Fig. 330 Myelinated nerve fibers in the pulmonary pleura (man).

The sensory endings of man are quite similar to those of the dog, but those of the rabbit are somewhat larger. McLaughlin (1933) stated that small type sensory vesicles were observed in the pulmonary pleura of the cat; however, Larsell claimed that these could not be considered as sensory endings, in view of their shape.

In the author's investigations the sensory vesicles mentioned by McLaughlin were not observed in the pulmonary pleura.

Investigation by the present authors on the detached and stretched specimens of the pulmonary pleura of man and dog revealed that the myelinated nerve fiber of the pulmonary pleura run, as shown above in Fig. 329, from the hilum along the borders of the pulmonary lobes, particularly along their inner sides, and distribute in a coarse plexus in the submesothelial layer.

Large myelinated fibers, winding and bending irregularly, finally terminate in complicated arborescent shaped nerve endings, as shown in Fig. 331. Some show expansions resembling the leaves of a tree, and some end in simple sharp points.

Morphologically it is evident that these endings are those of sensory nerves; however, as to the origin of the nerve fibers, there are diversities of opinion.

Larsell (1923) presumed that many of the sensory nerves of the pulmonary pleura arise from the ganglia of the posterior roots of the spinal cord and, via the upper thoracic sympathetic nerve trunk the stellate ganglion and the inferior cervical ganglion, distribute in the pleura.

Möllgaard (1912) also presumed that they originated in the ganglia of the posterior roots of the spinal cord.

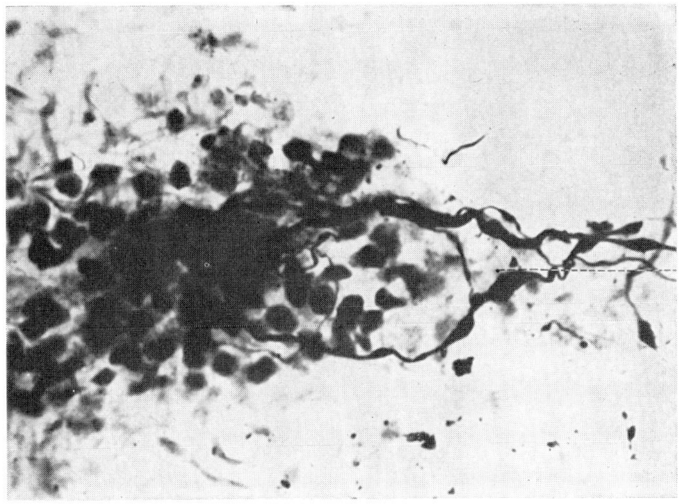

Fig. 331 Sensory nerve ending in the pulmonary pleura (man).

As explained above, almost all investigators considered that the sensory innervation of the pulmonary pleura originated in the ganglia of the posterior roots of the spinal cord; RASMUSSEN (1926) stated that the sensibility of the pulmonary pleura was supplied by the sympathetic nerves, the sensory fibers of the pulmonary pleura running to the posterior roots of the spinal cord of upper thoracic spinal nerves via the thoracic sympathetic nerve trunk.

Against this, YAGITA (1954) concluded that, since myelinated nerve fibers were observed to degenerate on the 5th day after cutting the vagus nerve, the sensibility of the pleura must be supplied by the vagus nerve.

3. Vegetative Nerve Endings

It was pointed out by ROMANOW (1904), LARSELL (1923), MCLAUGHLIN (1933), and LARSELL and DOW (1935), that the non-myelinated nerve fibers form networks on the pleural surface, particularly in the submesothelial layers.

According to the authors' investigations, the vegetative nerve fibers which distribute in the pulmonary pleura are observed on the mesothelial surface, as shown in Fig. 332. Some of these form relatively coarse networks, others run along the blood vessels, as shown in Fig. 333 and, giving off fine nerve fibers, distribute in the vessel walls.

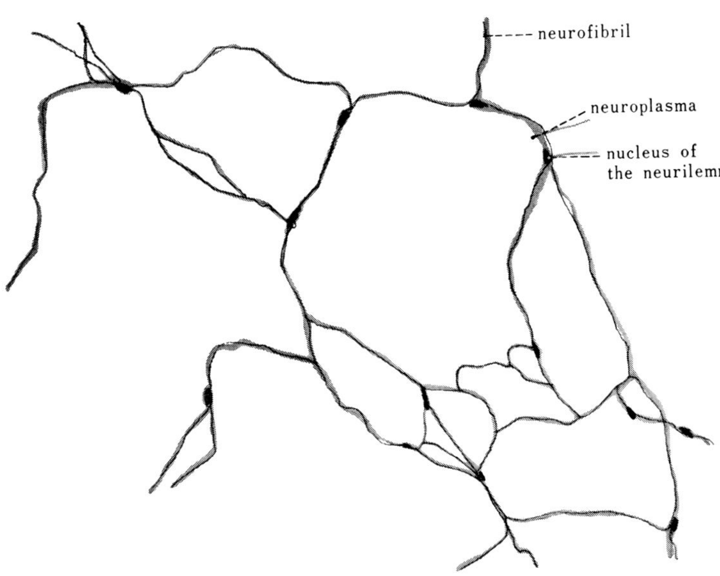

Fig. 332 Vegetative nerve network in the pulmonary pleura.

As shown in Fig. 334, these vegetative fibers surround the blood vessels of the pulmonary pleura and provide vasomotor regulation via the terminal reticulum; on the other hand, as shown in Fig. 335, some fibers spread and form networks on the surface. Such networks are composed of non-myeli-

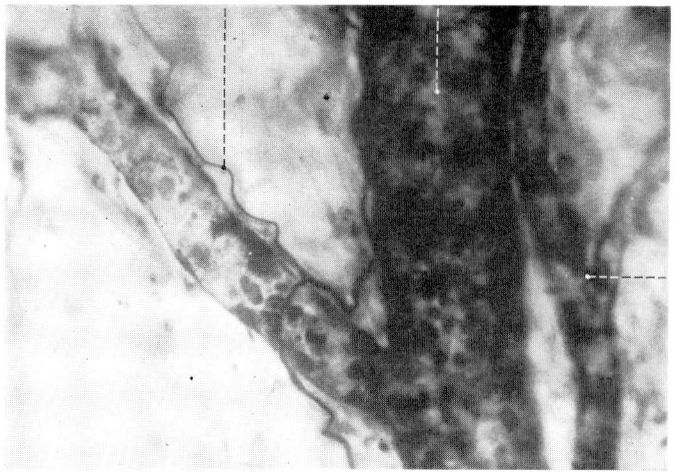

Fig. 333 Vasomotoric nerve fibers related to the blood vessel of the pulmonary pleura (man).

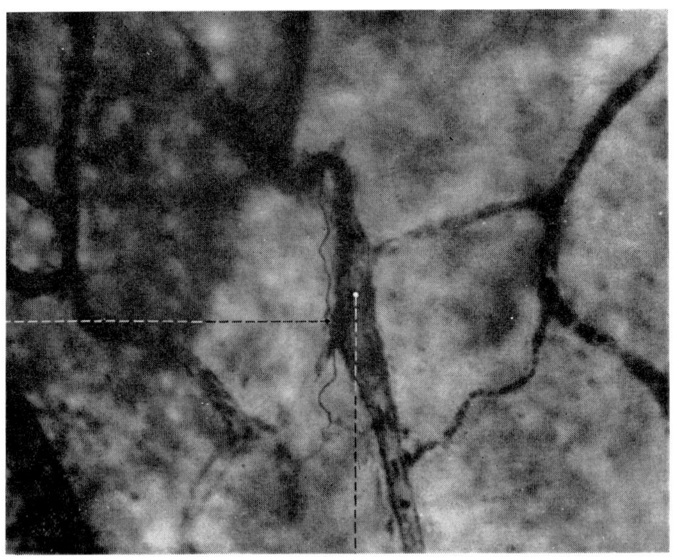

Fig. 334 Vasomotoric nerve fibers related to the blood capillaries of the pulmonary pleura (man).

nated fibers, which distribute widely on the pulmonary pleura immediately under the mesothelium in the form of "Plasmastrang" (STÖHR). In the networks, in addition to many Schwann's nuclei, interstitial nuclei of an oval shape are observed. In this case too, the nerve fibers distribute in net-like forms in the connective tissue of the blood vessels of the subpleural regions, terminating in closed forms.

4. Function

It is well known that the pulmonary pleura lacks sense of pain.

As mentioned earlier, UNVERRICHT (1934) investigated this with the thoracoscope and reported that, except for regions of the hilum, the pulmonary pleura hardly responds to mechanical or electrical irritations; cough reflex occurs only upon irritation of the hilum.

This is convincingly born out by our histological findings of the nerves of the pulmonary pleura.

However, in these investigations, a few sensory nerve endings were observed in the region of the hilum, on the border of the pulmonary lobe and the surface of the interlobar pleura.

How then will the function of such sensory endings be interpreted?

LARSELL (1923) succeeded in inducing a respiratory reflex by inflating a small rubber ball which had been inserted in the interlobar space, after interrupting bilaterally the vagus and the intercostal nerves of the dog. This reflex controls inspiration and also promotes expiration, but it does not occur when the rubber ball is put between either the diaphragm and lower lobe or the thoracic wall and the lobes.

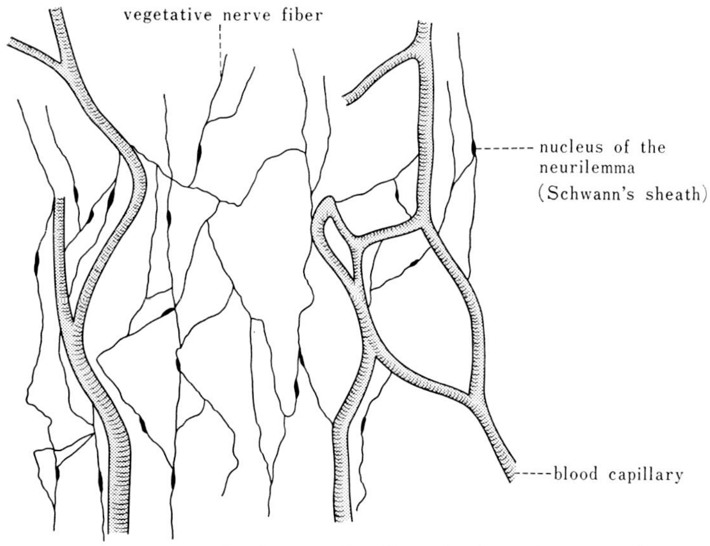

Fig. 335 Network of vegetative fibers in the pulmonary pleura.

From the above observations, LARSELL concluded that the sensory nerve endings in the margin of the lobe or the interlobar pleura responded to mechanical irritation.

Accordingly, the sensory endings which are distributed in the pulmonary pleura may respond to irritation involving the surfaces of the interlobar pleurae, upon extreme expansion of the lung.

However, since it was impossible to show these phenomena physiologically, LARSELL stated that in ordinary respiration the regulation of respiration occurs via the interpulmonary vagus nerves.

SAALFIELD (1933) presumed that an increasing irritation of the pulmonary pleura would reflexly influence the heart. SCHWIEGK (1935) denied the assumption that the sensory nerve endings in the pulmonary pleura contribute to the cardiac reflex. He proved that a cardiac reflex can be caused by increase of pulmonary artery pressures, not by inflation of the lung.

According to STURM (1948), many clinical observations are to be interpreted from the standpoint of the "pulmonary reflex". That is, many reactions which occur at the time of the pneumothorax are to be interpreted as pleuropulmonary reflexes caused by physical irritation of the pleura.

For example, atelectasis, such as may occur on occasion of an exudative pleurisy, is not caused by the pressure of the exudate alone, it cannot be understood without also considering the reflex factors. In such cases, even if bronchography is performed, obstruction in the bronchus will not be found.

ALEXANDER (1951) stated that when an inflammatory irritation takes place in the pleura the tonus of the lung will increase, resulting in contraction of the lung. It is said that, in patients who have already received an artificial pneumothorax, the intrathoracic pressure will decrease from 1/5 to 1/8 of normal at the time of an exudative pleurisy.

STURM (1948) reported that, if performing Jacobaeus' galvanocautery of pleural adhesions a mechanical irritation was delivered to the pulmonary pleura, a partial contractive depression could be observed by thoracoscope on the surface of the lung; however this reaction did not occur if the patient was pretreated by local anesthesia.

While resecting the lung under local anesthesia various pressure irritations were given to the surface of the lung; this caused localized and prolonged atelectasis in the affected region. These atelectases are hardly to be regarded as having been caused by stenosis of the bronchus, and cannot be explained without considering the existence of the pleuropulmonary reflex.

This phenomenon had not been observed in lung resections carried out under general anesthesia.

RASMUSSEN (1926), investigating the afferent route for the pleuropulmonary reflex, stated that the sensory fibers enter the thoracic sympathetic nerve trunk, reach the posterior roots of the upper thoracic nerves and, running into the spinal cord, join the motor reflex routes.

Chapter V. Muscular System

In this chapter the form and distribution of the muscular system of the lung will be described, in order to promote the understanding of physiological and clinical problems.

I. OUTLINE OF STRUCTURE

The muscular system of the lung is entirely composed of smooth muscle.

Morphologically, the muscle can be divided in three groups: bronchial, pulmonary (in a narrow sense), and interstitial.

The bronchial muscles are those which are distributed in the walls of the main bronchi to terminal bronchioles. These muscles surround the walls in an annular manner and, as the bronchi get smaller, run gradually into a spiral pattern.

The pulmonary muscle (in a narrow sense) indicates muscles which are distributed in the alveolar regions. In the respiratory bronchiole it surrounds spirally; in the alveolar duct it runs in a mere elongated spiral manner. In regions near the alveoli it occurs in net or bush-like forms, and surrounds the alveolar rings in sphincter-like formation uniting with the elastic fibers of the alveolar wall.

The interstitial muscle is distributed in the interstices of the lung. It differs here from that in the bronchial system and is divided into two groups; one distributes in the interstices proper, the other in the pulmonary pleura.

The muscular system of the lung receives its innervation from the nervous system, thus permitting a unified function.

Especially in the region of the respiratory bronchiole or the alveolar duct, it influences the inspiration and expiration of air to and from the alveoli by changing the caliber of respiratory passages.

Fig. 336 is a schema showing an outline of the muscular system of the lung.

Supplement: Materials and Methods

The authors (Nagaishi and Inaba, 1950) used fresh normal lungs of man, cattle, dog, rabbit and guinea pig, in their researches.

Especially in man, a portion of freshly resected lobe was used. The material was obtained from that (normal appearing) portion of a resected lobe which was farthest from the region of a pathological focus.

For the fixation of the specimen 10–20% neutral formalin was used.

For imbedding, paraffin or carbowax was used; in some cases celloidin or frozen section method was used. Sections were cut at 4–6 μ. Serial sections were obtained in an effort to reproduce the three-dimensional structure of muscle.

Baltisberger (1921) stated that the thickness of 10–15 μ was most suitable, but according to our experience it is better to make the section as thin as possible.

II. MUSCLES OF LUNG

As mentioned earlier, the muscles of the lung consist entirely of smooth muscles.

A. Tracheobronchial Muscle

Tracheal Muscle: The course and the location of tracheal muscles differ, according to the kind of animals and according to the region of the trachea under consideration.

In man strong muscle bundles connect the dorsal ends of the tracheal cartilages. The tracheal muscle in man is observed only in the membranous part. In the inferior portion of the trachea, near the bifurcation, annular muscles surround the entire circumference of the trachea.

In dog, the trachea is surrounded by strong annular muscles over its entire length.

The muscle of the membranous part of the trachea is composed of muscle bundles with many branchings and anastomoses.

The insertion of the muscle bundle varies in different animals, being sometimes on the internal aspect of the tracheal cartilages, sometimes on the external.

The insertion in man is internal; in dog or rabbit it is external.

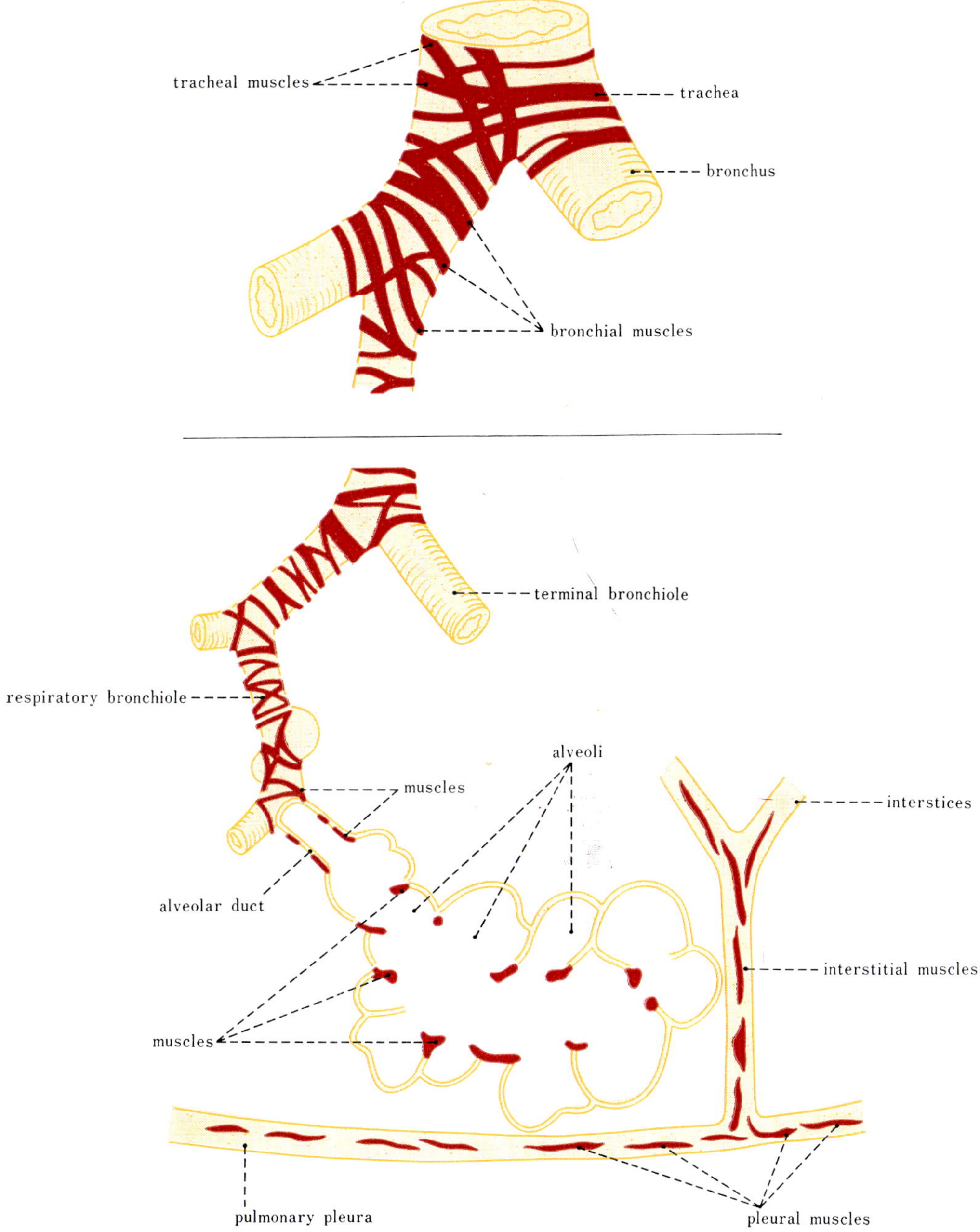

Fig. 336 Schema of the muscular system of the lung.

As mentioned earlier, the tracheal muscles are mainly those connecting the dorsal ends of the tracheal cartilages, and those running in an annular direction.

Willis (1676), Reisseisen (1822), Cramer (1947) and Luschka (1863), and v. Ebner (1899) reported observations of longitudinal muscles in the trachea; however, the authors consider that the longitudinal muscles referred to by them were not similar to those which are seen in the intestines, but were rather cross sections of annular muscles which, running obliquely, were interpreted as running longitudinally.

Bronchial Muscle: This term is used to designate muscles which are distributed on the bronchial wall, from the main bronchi to terminal bronchioles.

In man the muscles of the bronchi which have membranous parts are somewhat similar to those of the inferior portion of the trachea. In more peripheral regions annular or spiral muscles surround the circumference of the bronchi.

As shown in Fig. 337, these muscles are discontinuous; when compared with muscle of the intestine the continuity of the annular muscles is far from complete.

In dogs or rabbits, annular or spiral muscles are observed to surround the bronchi.

An abundant distribution of blood vessels is found in the bronchial muscles. As reported by Mischelazzi (1953) and Franzeschi (1953), the muscular cell is quite similar to that of the heart, to the extent that it contains an abundance of glycogen.

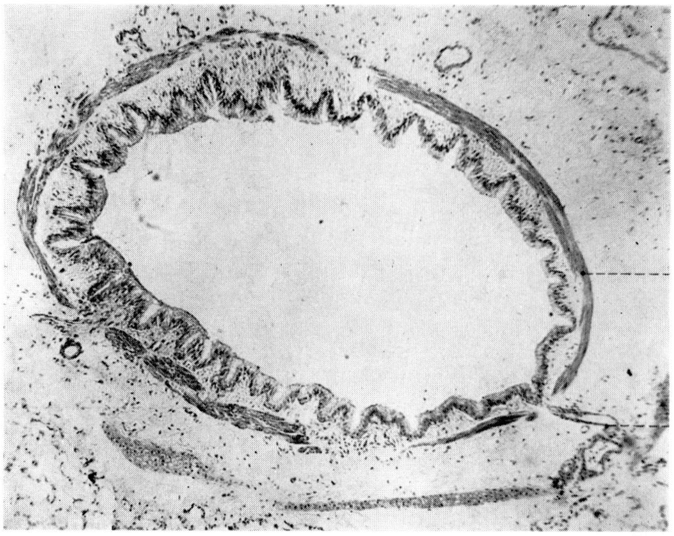

Fig. 337 Transverse section of the smooth muscle bundles of the bronchial wall (man).

Those muscles situated immediately beneath the tunica propria are perforated by many mucous gland ducts.

The bronchial muscles and cartilages are connected by the elastic fiber bundles. In the large bronchi the muscle insertion is at the dorsal extremity of the cartilages, but as the bronchi decrease in diameter it transits to the inner aspect of the cartilages, and in still further small bronchi the muscular layers become continuous.

As the bronchi get smaller, the muscle changes its course from annular to spiral. This tendency is increased in the more peripheral regions.

In the trachea, main bronchi, and lobar bronchi, mainly due to the contraction of the muscle of the membranous part, the lumen becomes smaller, but in the peripheral bronchus the lumen becomes smaller because of contraction of the annular muscles.

The bronchial lumen may be contracted, under various circumstances, into shelf-like folds in the mucous membrane. The arrangement of the ducts of the bronchial mucous glands in such cases will be radial to the bronchial lumen. When performing bronchography in the living body the bronchi in peripheral regions are sometimes observed to be as small as threads, by virtue of contraction of bronchial musculature.

When the contraction of the muscle becomes stronger, as stated by HAYEK (1953), the formation of the folds becomes even more evident, the surfaces of the mucus membrane folds touch each other and circulation of air may actually be suspended temporarily.

As regards the development of the bronchial muscles according to age, ENGEL and NEWS (1939) reported as follows:

The bronchial musculature is extremely thin in new-borns and infants; with the increase of age the muscles become thicker, but development ceases temporarily at 2 or 3 years of age. It resumes in the 4th year, and thereafter its development is completed in about the 5th year.

B. Pulmonary Muscle (in Narrow Sense)

The pulmonary muscles are those muscles which are distributed in the alveolar regions.

The course of muscle fibers gradually changes, in the respiratory bronchiole, from annular to spiral shapes; in the more peripheral regions it becomes bush- or net-like. The transition between the respiratory bronchioles and alveoli affects the course and shape of the muscles of the bronchial wall.

About the alveolar duct the course and distribution of muscle is similar to that for the respiratory bronchioles, but the quantity of muscle is far less.

Large muscle bundles are arranged in bush-like or net-like forms running spirally about the respiratory bronchioles. These muscle bundles are smaller at the level of the alveolar ducts, but at the alveolar ring, as shown in Fig. 338, the muscles become sphincter-like.

Thus, the structure and disposition of muscles in these regions is adapted to contraction and dilation of bronchial lumen.

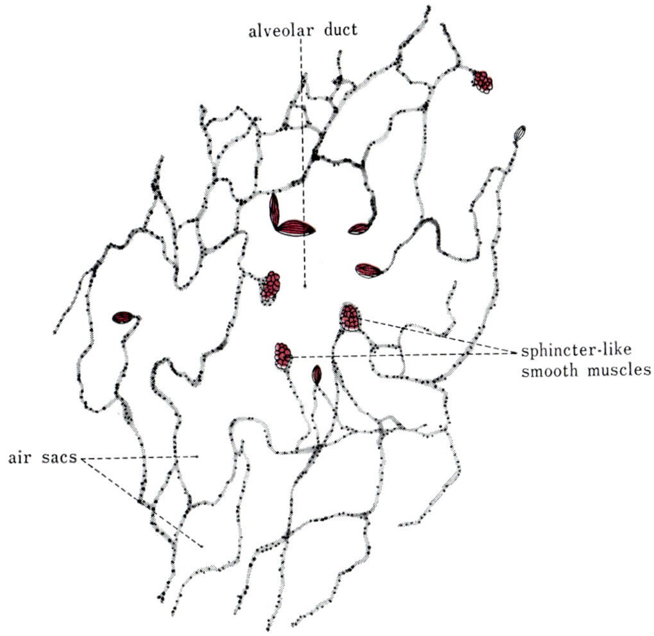

Fig. 338 Schema of the transverse section of the alveolar duct.

Such an arrangement of muscles, as described above, is not generally found in other organs. MASON (1933) and MILLER (1937), termed this arrangement the "geodesic network".

Regarding morbid changes in these muscles, there are reports by ORTH (1887), HARKAVAY (1924) and LUISADA (1934), etc.

For example, LUISADA reported on morbid changes in these muscles in pulmonary emphysema accompanied by bronchiectasis.

In our experience in cases of chronic pulmonary congestion or pulmonary emphysema, proliferation has been observed in these muscles.

Whether muscles exist in the regions peripheral to the alveolar ducts is still under discussion.

SCHULTZE (1871), KÖLLIKER (1881) and MILLER (1937) denied their existence, and BALTISBERGER (1921), LUISADA (1934), BRONKHORST and DIJKSTRA (1940) and HAYEK (1953) affirmed it. According to BALTISBERGER, the distribution of the muscles about the alveolar sacs was said to be correlated with the degree of development of the alveolar ducts.

The authors' investigations disclosed evidence sufficient to affirm the existence of muscles even in regions peripheral to the alveolar ducts.

The arrangement of muscles about the alveolar sacs, in general, is the same as for alveolar ducts, differing only in quality.

Ring-like sphincters are observed in each alveoli in the regions between respiratory bronchioles and alveolar sacs.

Fig. 339 shows such sphincter-like muscle bundles.

Fig. 340 shows the cross section of these muscle bundles and the alveolar interstices. The free edges of these look like club-form, as shown in Fig. 340.

The muscles in this region are a part of the muscles of the terminal bronchiole; they decrease in thickness along the transition from respiratory bronchioles to alveolar sacs. At the alveolar rings of small alveoli the muscles do not always surround the circumference, but are found to be partially lacking. The portion where the muscle is lacking is replaced by elastic fiber bundles.

ORSÓS (1936) termed this the "Musculo-desmoelastisches System".

In the central portion of this region, as shown in Fig. 341 (a,b), muscles and elastic fibers are observed, whereas in surrounding portions ordinary connective tissue fibers are found.

Whether or not muscular cells exist on the specific alveolar wall is under dispute:

RINDFLEISCH (1872), DUBREUIL and LAMARQUE (1919), BAUDRIMONT (1929), BRONKHORST and DIJKSTRA (1940) and HAYEK (1953) affirmed, but BALTISBERGER (1921), MÖLLENDORF (1941), MILLER (1947), and ENGEL (1948) denied the existence of muscle on alveolar sacs.

In general, the reports are considered to be negative; even the people who affirm the existence of alveolar muscles do not seem to consider the observation to be highly meaningful.

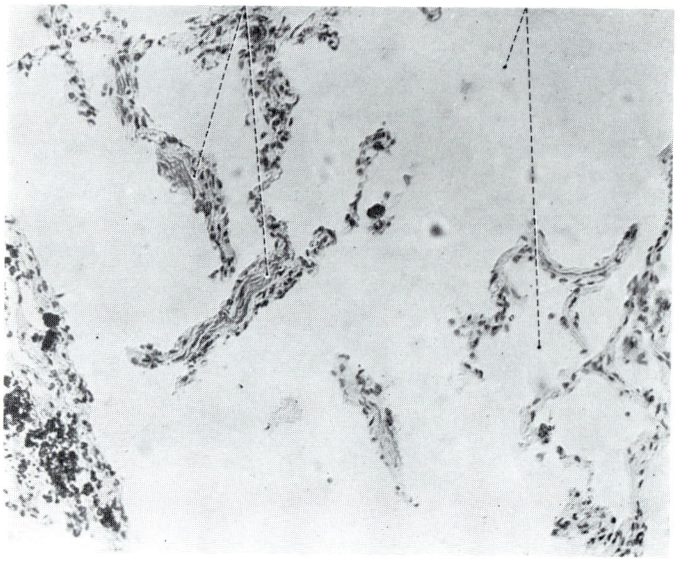

Fig. 339 Smooth muscles in the alveolar sacs (man).

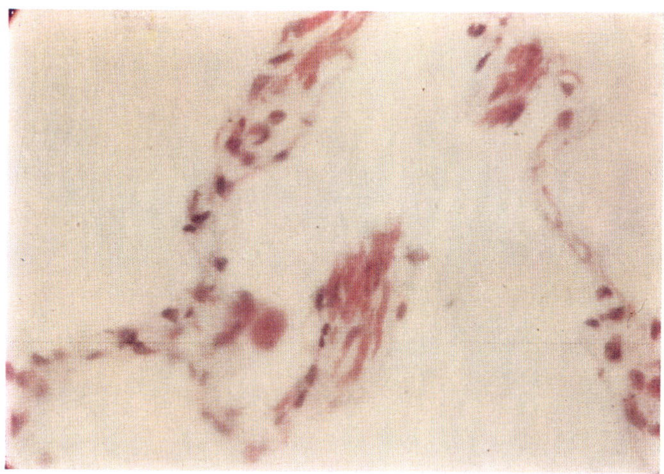

Fig. 340 Sphinctor-like smooth muscles of the alveolar ring (man).

According to the present authors' investigation on serial sections, as shown in Figs. 342 and 343, a few muscular cells were clearly observed on alveolar walls.

However such muscles were not observed in all samples of human lungs, but only in special cases in which the muscles were abnormally developed. Further, even in such cases, muscular cells did not exist about all the alveoli; the cells were few in number and, in some instances, single muscular cells were distributed on alveolar walls, not forming muscle bundles.

Fig. 344 shows the distribution of the muscles in the alveolar region.

A wide range of individual differences is observed in the muscles which distribute to the bronchi and the pulmonary parenchyma. Of all animals studied, the most abundant distribution of muscles was found in the guinea pig. Compared with other animals the lung of the guinea pig is difficult to inflate. The guinea pig is also particularly susceptible to anaphylaxis, which is considered to have some relation to the abundant distribution of muscles in the bronchi, pulmonary parenchyma and pleura.

C. Interstitial Muscle

This is a general term for muscles distributed in interstices of the lung.

These differ from muscles of the bronchial system. They can be divided into two groups, one distributed in the interstice, the other distributed in the pulmonary pleura.

The interstitial tissues of the lung mainly consist of connective tissues, forming septa between neighboring lobules or segments.

In a broad sense the pulmonary pleura also can be regarded as one of the interstitial tissues.

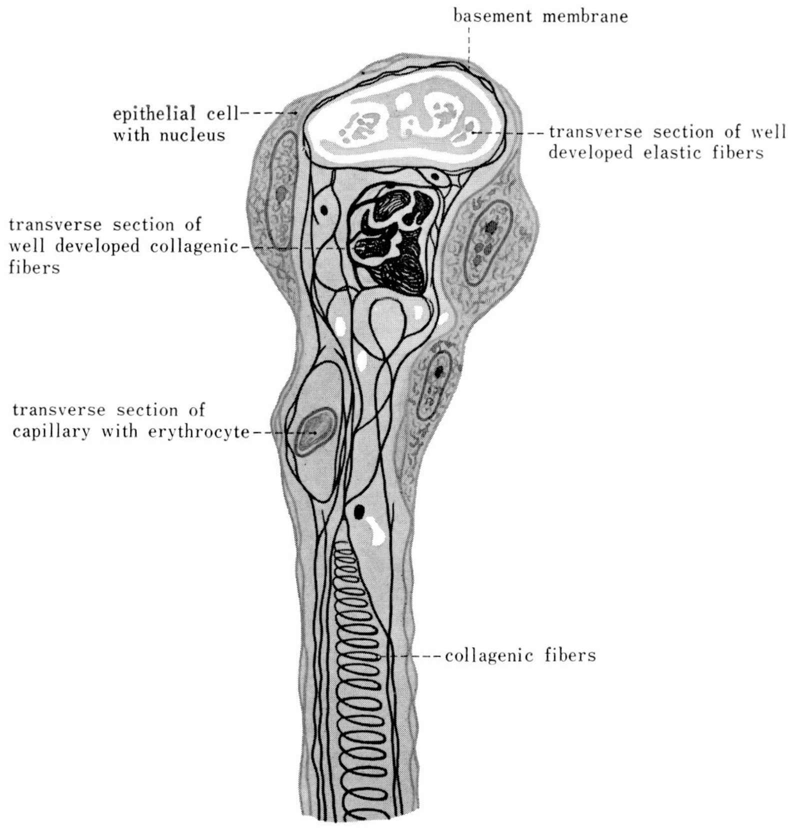

Fig. 341a Schema of the thin part of the alveolar ring (ORSÓS).

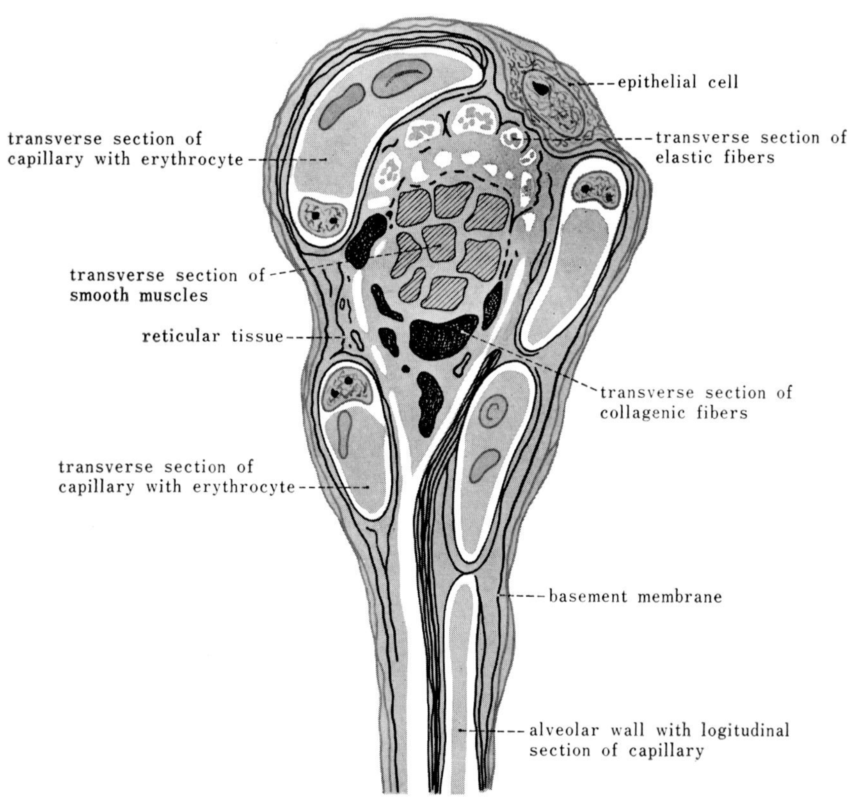

Fig. 341b Schema of the structure of the thick part of the alveolar ring (ORSÓS).

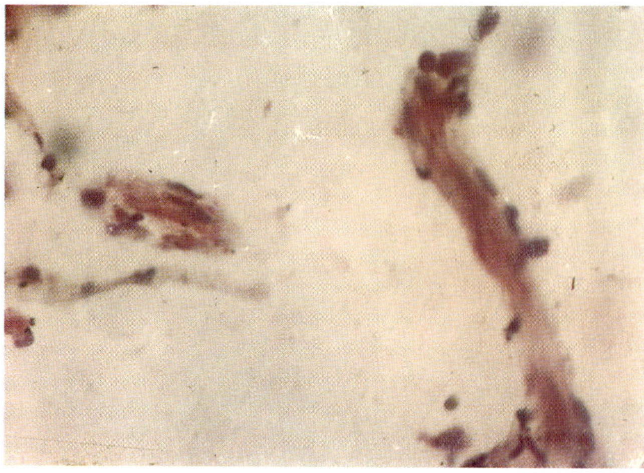

Fig. 342 Smooth muscles of the alveolar wall (man).

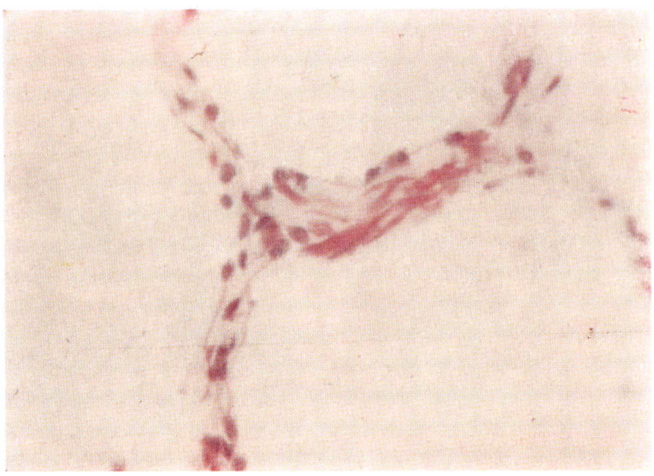

Fig. 343 Smooth muscles of the alveolar wall (man).

If the pulmonary pleura is considered in two components, the pleura and its subpleural tissues, the latter exactly corresponds to the interstitial tissues covering the lobule directly under the pleura.

The interstitial tissue of the lung consists chiefly of collagenic fibers, in which many elastic fibers and smooth muscles are distributed.

Muscle is distributed widely in the interstices of the lung. The arrangements are irregular, some crossing and some running parallel as large muscle bundles. Occasionally, as shown in Fig. 354, the muscles anastomose irregularly and form sheets.

BALTISBERGER (1921) termed these the "Muskelblätter" or "Gefensterte Membran".

These muscle bundles may be flat or may surround vessels.

Muscles surrounding lymph vessels run in the longitudinal direction, in single or multiple layers. These do not belong to the lymph vessel itself.

The course and distribution of interstitial muscle varies, depending on the region examined. For example, in a certain region the muscular sheet may run parallel in muscle bundles of two layers; in other regions, the muscular sheets may unite into a one-layer muscle bundle. Or again two muscular sheets may cross each other. When sectioned, this latter muscle will have a nodose or reticular appearance.

Muscle bundles in the interstices of the lung surround not only lymph vessels but also blood vessels and bronchi.

In the interlobular septum the direction of the muscle is irregular, neighboring muscle bundles running either parallel or anastomosing and crossing. The muscle bundles in these regions are observed in the connective tissue surrounding large blood vessels. Surrounding blood or lymph vessel bundles

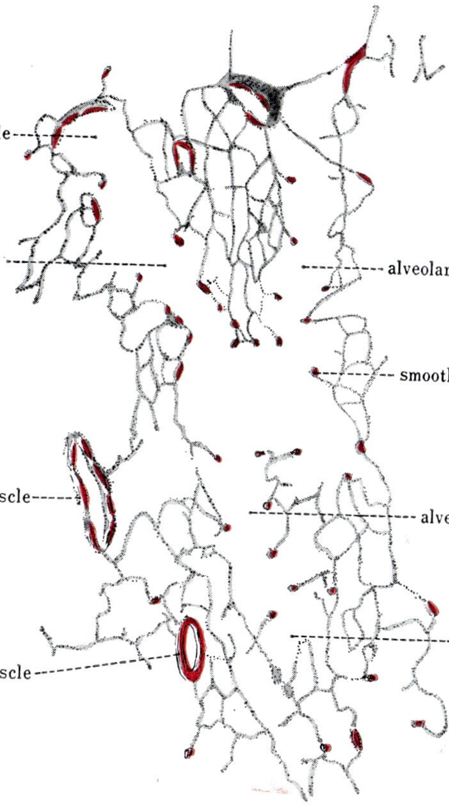

Fig. 344 Schema of the distribution of the smooth muscles in the alveolar region.

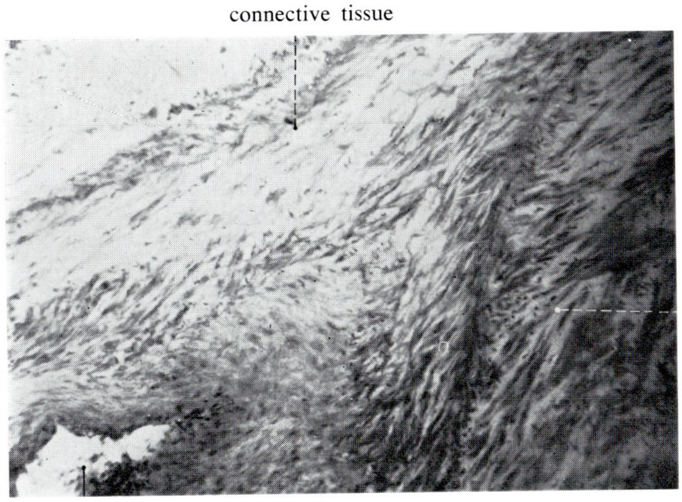

Fig. 345 Smooth muscles in the connective tissue of the lung (man).

run further peripherally, and transit into the muscular networks in the connective tissue of the alveolar septa.

Fig. 346 shows muscular cells in an alveolar septum.

Muscle in the pulmonary pleura is mainly observed in the interstitial layers.

The arrangement is not always regular, but in many instances, as shown in Fig. 347, is bush-like and extending along the pleura.

Some investigators are dubious about the conception that a specific muscle exists in the pleura; they believe that all muscles in pleura actually belong to the lymph or blood vessels. However, according to our investigation, specific muscle fibers are observed in subpleural connective tissues.

Individual differences are observed in man, and such muscle is not observed in all cases.

Remarkable differences also exist according to the kind of animal. Muscular fibers are found most

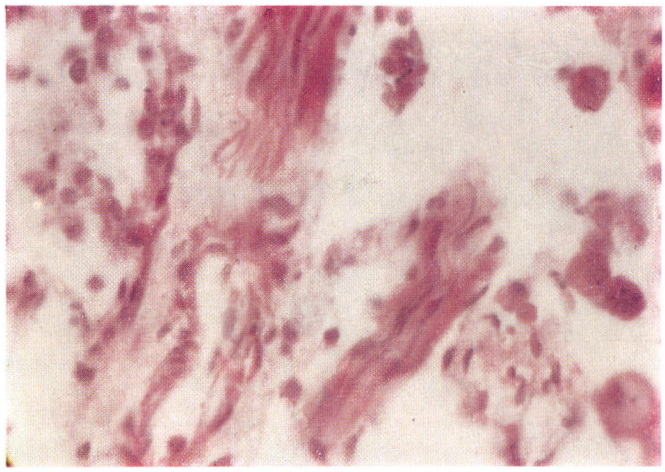

Fig. 346 Smooth muscles in the alveolar septum (man).

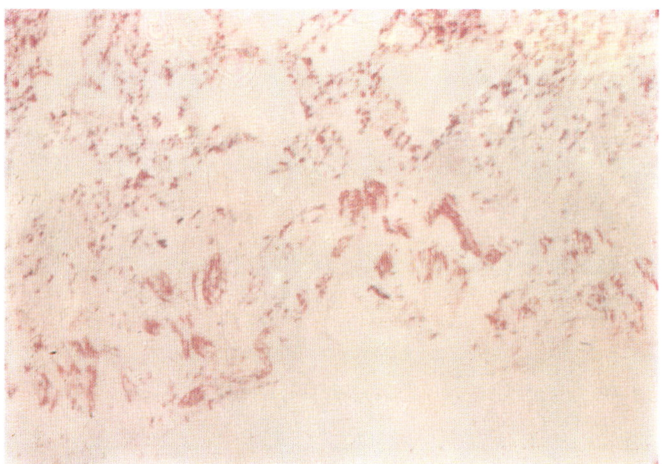

Fig. 347 Smooth muscles in pulmonary pleura (man).

abundantly in guinea pig pleura. The alveoli of guinea pigs are wrapped by muscle fibers which reach the pulmonary pleura, and which wrap about the pulmonary parenchyma like a sac.

III. FUNCTIONS OF PULMONARY MUSCLE

It was indicated by E. REINHARDT (1934), VERZAR and JEKER (1937), STURM (1943) and HAYEK (1953) that the pulmonary muscular system is under the control of the nervous system.

BRONKHORST and DIJKSTRA (1940) considered the role of the muscles in the alveolar region as important, and pointed out that the muscles in that region affect the tension of the pulmonary parenchyma, and particularly of the alveolar wall.

The muscles of the alveolar ring, in their sphincter-like arrangement, are considered to have an influence on the passage of air into the alveoli.

Muscle fibers, distributed along the alveolar ducts to alveoli, transit into the elastic fibers of the alveolar wall, as reported by v. EBNER (1899), GEHLEN (1940), STÖHR (1951) and HAYEK (1953). When the muscular fibers contract the alveolar wall becomes flattened, affecting its tension.

These alveolar muscles play a role as a part of the myoelastic "Spannmuskeln" or elastic tissue of the lung, as reported by MACKLIN (1922); according to NEERGAARD (1929) they are said to participate in altering the tension of the surface of alveoli.

BRONKHORST and DIJKSTRA (1940) included the interstitial muscles in the category of alveolar muscles, stating that the morphology and the surface tension of the alveolar wall change according to their state of contraction.

The muscular fibers which run spiral courses along the longitudinal axis of the respiratory bronchioles have functions in common with the alveolar muscles; by their contraction neighboring alveoli are approximated and compressed.

The above muscles, influenced by the nervous system, maintain the tension of the lung. Given extraordinary irritation, the tonus of the muscular system of the lung may increase extraordinarily, and an asthmatic condition may result.

Under what conditions does the tonus of the muscular system increase or decrease? Does the muscular system function only as a sustentacular form of elastic tissue, or does it entirely regulate the tension of the lung? These are interesting themes which are open for further studies.

Regarding this, ORSÓS (1936) stated that the effort to find a parallel between the elasticity of the lung and its elastic fibers is fundamentally wrong. He maintained that the elastic fibers play a role in preventing hyperextension of lung tissues. The muscles in the alveolar duct or the alveolar interstices were not considered to participate directly in the contraction of the lung.

It has been previously determined, both clinically and experimentally, that atelectasis may be caused by medication or by direct stimulation of nerves distributed in the lung by SEEMANN (1931), S. REINHARDT (1935), VERZAR (1937), STURM (1948) and ALEXANDER (1951). It is evident that in the occurrence of such "Kontraktionsatelectase" the muscles of the lung, under the innervation of the vegetative nervous system, play an important role. For example, VERZAR and JEKER (1937) pointed out that a physiological atelectasis may occur.

According to them, in normal animals which are put under absolute rest, at atmospheric pressure, many alveoli show atelectasis; this can be shown histologically.

It was further stated that if such animals were put under lowered pressure the collapsed alveoli would inflate immediately. Such a regulation of respiratory volume was considered to be under the control of the nervous system.

NIEDNER (1950) also observed that a localized spotty atelectasis was observed at the time of lung resection by thoracotomy. If the involved portion was fixed and studied histologically abundant muscular fibers were observed in the alveolar regions.

DIJKSTRA (1940) and DALY, et al. (1942) stated that histamine or acetylcholine induced contraction of the muscles of the lung, and decreased intrathoracic pressure.

Against the above, TROISIER, et al. (1940) made observations which showed that the muscular system of the lung was paralysed by large quantities of histamine, and that intrathoracic pressure was increased.

HAYEK (1953) investigated the role of the muscular system, and stated that when tonus was increased, the tension of the lung tissue was also increased, resulting in a decrease of lung volume.

For example, if a harmful irritative gas is inhaled the sensitive nerve endings of the mucous membrane of the respiratory system are irritated, and continuing contraction of the muscular system will occur.

As will be seen from the above, it is an unquestionable fact that the muscular system of the lung is an indivisible unit, exerting various influences on pulmonary function. However, the full range of such influences in health and disease is not yet known. Many interesting questions await future studies.

Chapter VI. Pulmonary Pleura

In this chapter the normal structure of the pulmonary pleura will be described, based on the result of studies performed by NAGAISHI and OKADA. Reference will also be made to certain pathological changes, and to permeability of the pleura to fluid, corpuscles or particles.

I. MACROSCOPIC STRUCTURE

The surface of the lung is covered continuously by a serous membrane called the pleura. The pleura is partly interlobar and extends into the fissures.

Normal pleura being extremely thin, lung tissue can be seen through the pleura, and the boundaries of neighboring lobules can be distinguished.

The pulmonary pleura has great elasticity and plays a certain role as a sustentacular tissue for the lung.

An extremely small quantity of serous fluid is present in the pleural cavity, making for smooth movement of the lung.

II. CLASSIFICATION OF LAYERS

The pulmonary pleura is classified into several layers as shown in Figs. 348 and 349.

Regarding the histology of the pleural layers there is not much difference of opinions among investigators; however, as to the classification, a divergence of opinions exists.

Table 19 presents a comparison of representative classifications of the pulmonary pleura.

As will be seen, the authors (1955) classified the pulmonary pleura into five layers, *i.e.,* mesothelial, submesothelial, external elastic, interstitial, and internal elastic.

Table 19 Classification of layers in the pulmonary pleura.

<table>
<tr><th>MILLER (1947)</th><th colspan="2">v. HAYEK (1953)</th><th colspan="2">NAGASAWA, YAMASHITA, OKADA, INABA, NAGAISHI (1955)</th></tr>
<tr><td>mesothelial layer</td><td rowspan="2">Endopleura</td><td>Deckschicht</td><td rowspan="2">pulmonary pleura</td><td>mesothelial layer</td></tr>
<tr><td>submesothelial layer</td><td>Bindgewebs-häutchen</td><td>submesothelial layer</td></tr>
<tr><td>elastic layer</td><td rowspan="2">Hauptschicht Gefässchicht</td><td rowspan="2"></td><td rowspan="2">subpleural tissues</td><td>external elastic layer</td></tr>
<tr><td>areolar layer</td><td>interstitial layer</td></tr>
<tr><td>basal membrane</td><td>Grenzmembran</td><td></td><td>alveolar wall</td><td>internal elastic layer</td></tr>
</table>

III. MICROSCOPIC STRUCTURE OF LAYERS OF PLEURA

Proceeding according to the above classification, the layers in the pulmonary pleura will be described in the order.

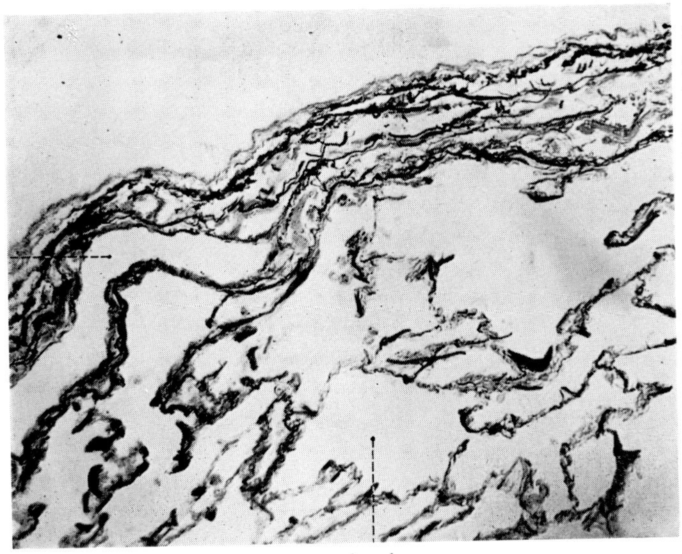

Fig. 348 Elastic fibers of the pulmonary pleura (human adult).

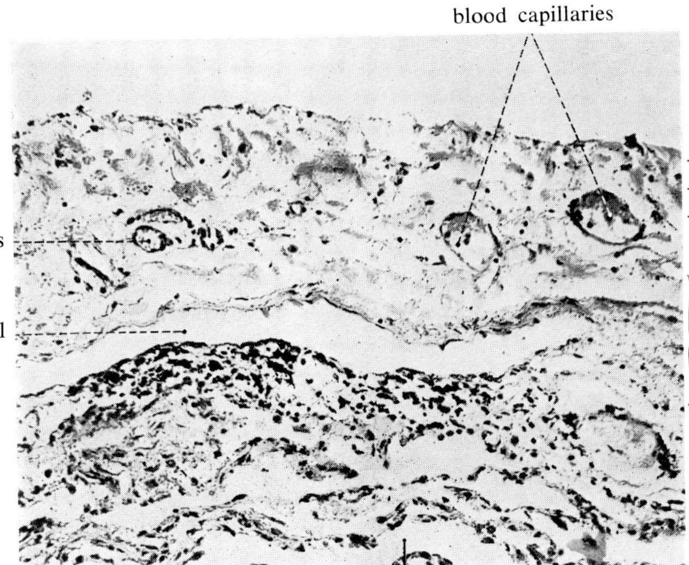

Fig. 349 Layers of the pulmonary pleura (human adult).

A. Mesothelial

As shown in Fig. 350 (a), (b) the mesothelial layer consists of single flat cells.

This layer was described as such by MILLER (1947) and was designated "Deckschicht" by HAYEK (1953).

The mesothelial cells are not notably varied in size, but the shape of each cell is not quite uniform. The nucleus is round or oval in shape and is situated in the center of the cell body.

According to SINAPIUS and VOLLHABER (1951), polymorphic nuclei are sometimes observed in normal lungs; the mesothelial cells are occasionally multinucleate.

HAYEK (1953) has stated that a small type of mesothelial cell can be observed in groups among numbers of larger mesothelial cells, and in that region infiltrations by lympocytes may be observed. The mesothelial cells could thus be classified roughly into two sizes of cells; however the authors' investigation did not corroborate such findings.

B. Submesothelial

The submesothelial layer is a thin layer consisting of connective tissues immediately under the mesothelial layer.

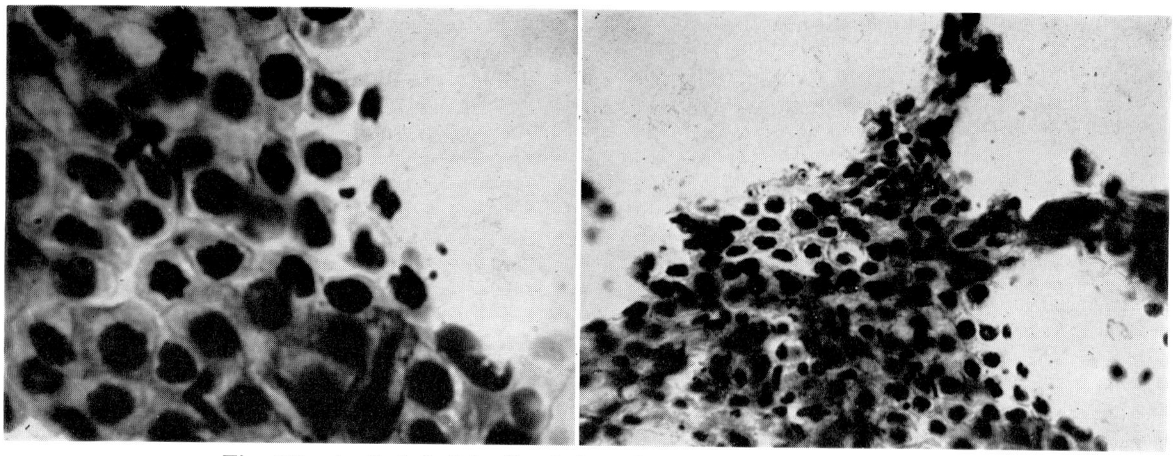

Fig. 350 a, b Endothelial cells of the pulmonary pleura (human adult).

This layer corresponds to the submesothelial layer as designated by MILLER (1947), or "Das Bindegewebshäutchen" (HAYEK, 1953) or "Das intrapleurale Bindegewebe" (TAKEDA 1955).

Anthracosis is not observed in this layer.

C. External Elastic Layer

This is the layer situated immediately under the submesothelial layer; it is formed of an abundance of elastic fibers.

It variously corresponds to "limitante elastique superficielle" (LETULLE, 1924); "elastic layer" (MILLER, 1947); "internal lamina elastica" (CROXATTO and SAMPIETRO, 1951); "internal elastic layer" (SEKIGUCHI, 1955), or "lamina fibroelastica externa" (TAKEDA, 1955).

In the deepest layer of the pulmonary pleura another layer consisting of elastic fiber is observed. LETULLE (1924) termed this the "limitante elastique profonde".

The authors distinguish between these two layers by terming that closer to the pleural cavity as the external elastic layer, and that closer to the lung tissue as the internal elastic layer.

Incidentally, CROXATTO and SAMPIETRO (1951) and SEKIGUCHI (1955) have used these same terms in the opposite sense.

YANAGIHARA (1959), studying in human, stated that the external elastic layer of the pulmonary pleura develops in the 4th month of fetal age as a layer consisting of extremely small elastic fibers; development thereafter is slow; after birth it can be observed for the first time as large bundles of elastic fibers.

In man and other mammals the elastic layers, as shown in Figs. 351–355, consist of several elastic fibers which run parallel with the pleural surface; the extent of development varies somewhat depending on the kind of animals.

When elastic fiber staining is performed on the detached and stretched specimen of pulmonary pleura, it is seen that the elastic fibers which in normal section appear to be running parallel with the pleura run, in fact, in many directions.

The elastic fibers make anastomoses and form complicated networks.

D. Interstitial Layer

This is the layer situated between the external and the internal elastic layers.

This layer corresponds to the "areolar layer" (MILLER, 1947); "subpleural tissue" (CROXATTO and SAMPIETRO, 1951); or "subpleural connective tissue" (TAKEDA, 1955).

The authors have termed this the interstitial layer because the tissue in this region closely resembles the interlobular connective tissue; the collagenic fibers of the former are continuous with the latter.

The authors generally regard those layers situated closer to the surface than the external elastic layer as the pulmonary pleura proper, and have considered the external elastic layer and interstitial layers to form the subpleural connective tissues.

The interstitial layer can roughly be divided into a portion closer to the pleural surface, which is riched in lymph vessels. The former is a more vascular layer; the latter is more fibrous.

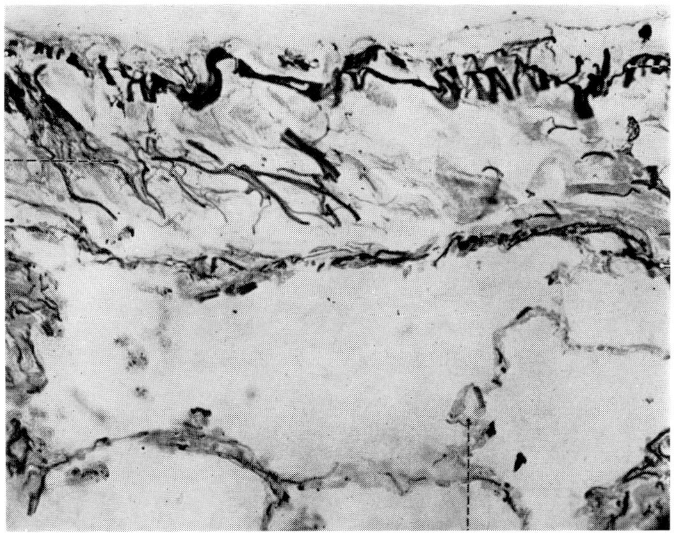

Fig. 351 Elastic fibers of the pulmonary pleura (man).

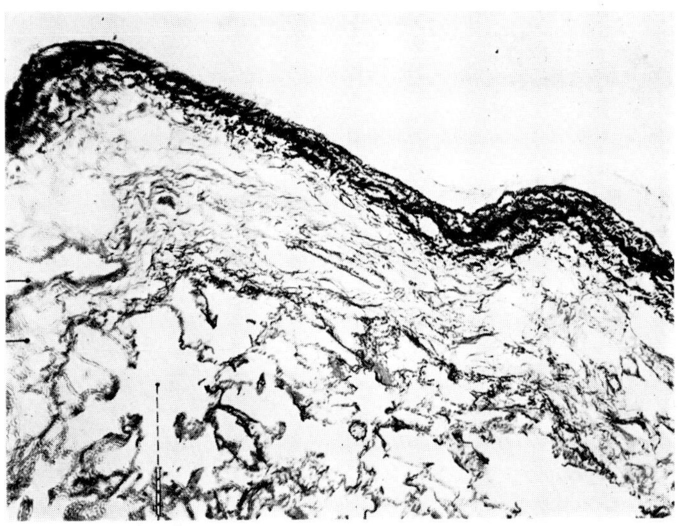

Fig. 352 Elastic fibers of the pulmonary pleura (cattle lung).

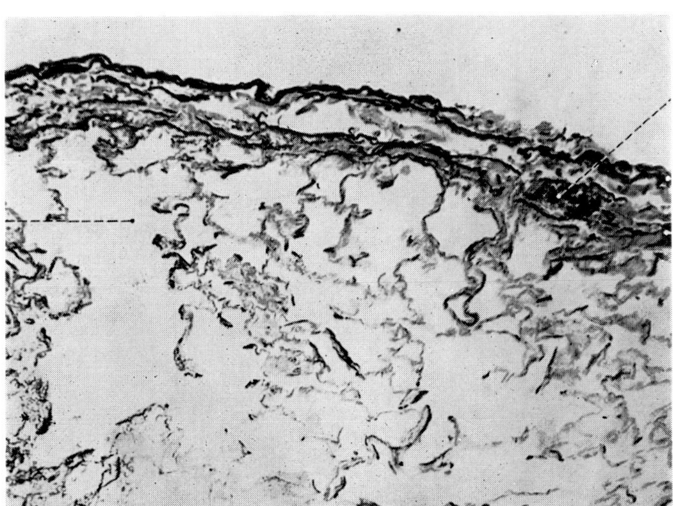

Fig. 353 Elastic fibers of the pulmonary pleura (dog lung).

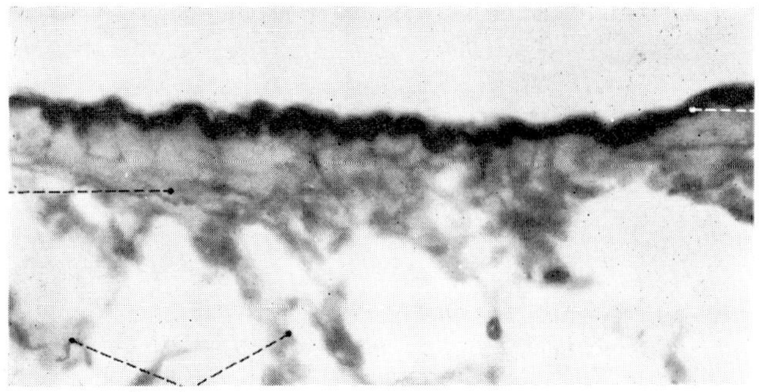

Fig. 354 Elastic fibers of the pulmonary pleura (guinea pig).

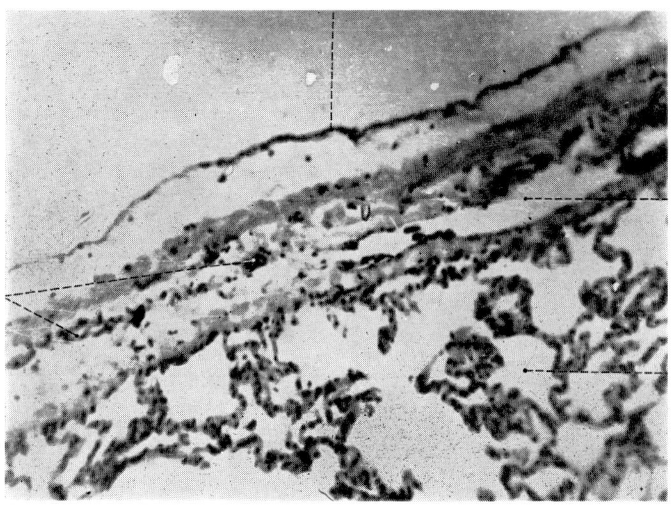

Fig. 355 Blood and lymph vessels in the interstitial layer (cattle lung).

Fig. 358, as will be shown later, illustrates the relationship between these layers.

When ablating the pleura from the lung, separation frequently occurs between the vascular and the fibrous layers, where the connective tissue is relatively loose.

Abundant collagenic fibers are observed in the fibrous layer.

These fibers run mostly parallel with the pleural surface; some elastic fibers from the external and internal elastic layers are observed to interweave with the collagenic fibers.

As shown by Miller (1947), in the guinea pig smooth muscle fibers are observed in the interstitial layers. Fig. 356 shows these muscle fibers.

In the pulmonary pleura of man, abundant smooth muscles are sometimes observed. As to whether these are normal components of the pleura, or whether they belong to the vascular system, a diversity of opinions exists.

E. Internal Elastic Layer

This is the layer which is closest to the pulmonary parenchyma.

This layer corresponds to "limitante elastique profonde" (Letulle, 1924), "deep layer" (Croxatto and Sampietro, 1951), "Grenzmembran" (Hayek, 1953).

The internal elastic layer consists of relatively few elastic fibers. As shown in Fig. 357, these fibers are related to the alveolar walls.

Takeda (1955) considered that most of the fibers belong to the subpleural tissues, but that some also belong to the alveolar wall. Many other researchers consider that this layer belongs entirely to the alveolar wall.

While both perforating the interstitial layer and connecting with the external elastic layer, part of the elastic fibers of the internal elastic layer transit into the elastic fibers of the alveolar wall. Therefore the elastic fibers in this region contain these belonging to the subpleural connective tissue and those belonging to the alveolar wall; the authors consider that most of the internal elastic layer should be regarded as belonging to the alveolar wall.

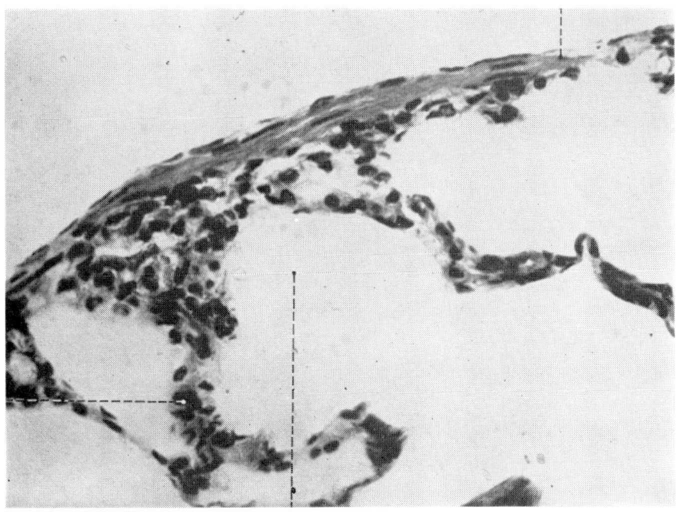

Fig. 356 Smooth muscles of the pulmonary pleura (guinea pig).

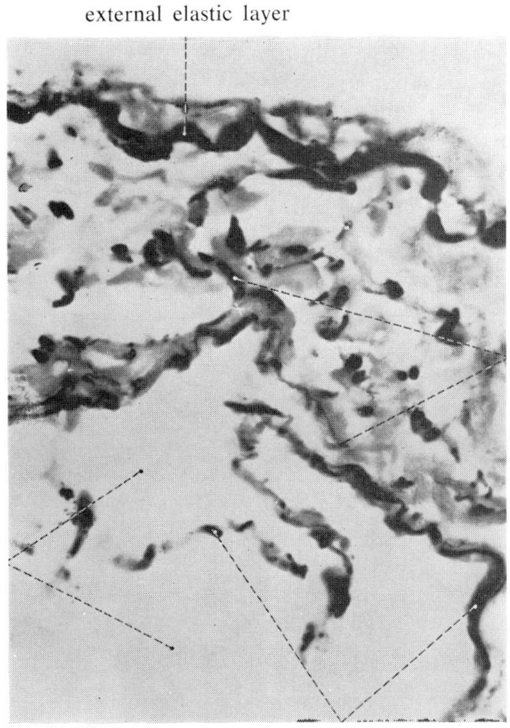

Fig. 357 Elastic fibers of the pulmonary pleura and the alveolar septa (human adult).

According to YANAGIHARA (1959), in the fetus the sequence of development of the internal elastic layer corresponds to that of the elastic fibers of the alveolar wall. From this point of view, the above interpretation can be considered as correct.

Figs. 358 and 359 show the schematized structure of the pulmonary pleura.

IV. PASSAGE OF FLUIDS AND PARTICLES THROUGH PLEURA

Whether the extremely small amount of serous fluid found in the normal pleural cavity arises from the pleura is still without definite answer.

Under normal conditions it is certain that the pleura does not permit passage of fluid, corpuscles or gases from surrounding tissues.

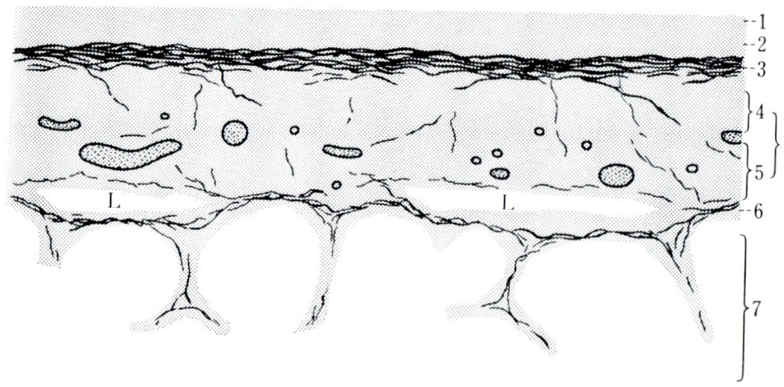

Fig. 358 Schema of the pulmonary pleura.
dotted: blood vessels, L: lymph vessels
1. mesothelial layer, 2. submesothelial layer
3. external elastic layer, 4. fibrous layer
5. vascular layer, 6. internal elastic layer
7. alveoli, I: interstitial layer

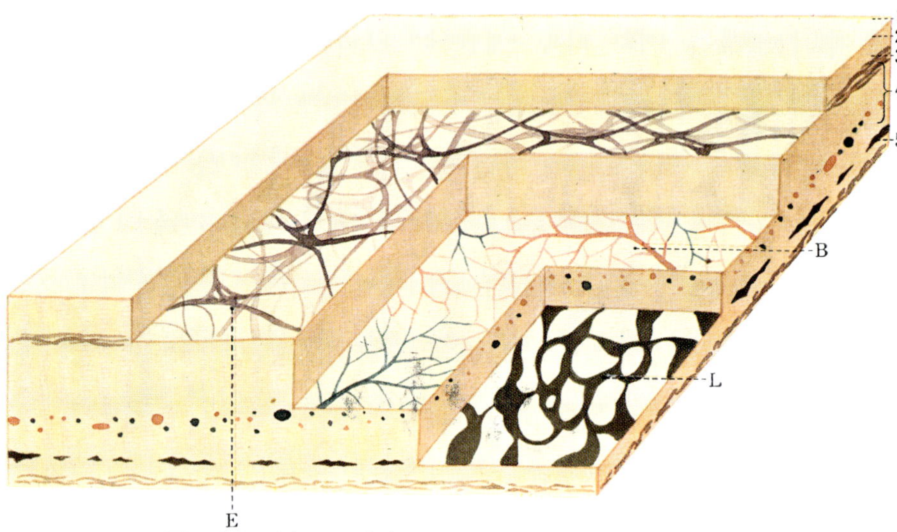

Fig. 359 Schema of the structure of the pulmonary pleura.

1. mesothelial layer
2. submesothelial layer
3. external elastic layer
4. interstitial layer
5. internal elastic layer

B: blood capillary net
E: elastic fiber net
L: lymph vessel net

However, in abnormal conditions the pleura will be unduly permeable. The accumulation of fluids (pleural effusion) is a case in point.

Even under otherwise normal conditions if fluids, corpuscles, or gases are insufflated into the pleural cavity, these substances will pass the pleura.

Regarding the permeability of the pulmonary pleura to body fluids or to corpuscles, various experimental investigations have been carried out.

It has been reported by BRATIANO and BRATIANU (1928) and by FUJIMORI (1950), that the various substances which enter the pleural cavity are absorbed into the blood or lymph vessels via the pleura.

KARSNER and SWANBECK (1920, 21) in particular have investigated the sites of absorption. They stated that the removal of corpuscles from the pleural cavity is accomplished by phagocytosis; the absorptive function was most evident in the mediastinal and pulmonary pleura, and was least evident in the parietal pleura. On the contrary, WADSWORTH (1922) stated that the parietal pleura, in its capacity for absorption, was more effective than the pulmonary pleura.

From the result of investigations carried out by OGO (1934), who insufflated India ink into the pleural cavity, the parietal and the mediastinal pleura were found to be permeated by particles of India ink; the pulmonary pleura was not thusly permeated.

TSUBOUCHI (1950) stated that beneath the mediastinal or parietal pleura there are regions where the fibers show a morphologically specific arrangement, inferring that corpuscles are absorbed into the pleural cavity from said sites. However, according to the authors' investigations, such a finding was not observed for the pulmonary pleura.

The specific region showing such a structure was observed in the parietal pleura, and constitutes a part of the "extravascular fluid pathway system" or "Extravaskuläre Saftbahnensystem" (KIHARA, 1950). KIHARA termed this morphological specialization the "Membrana cribriformis" or "Macula cribriformis".

Judging from the above it is conceivable that the pulmonary pleura lacks the ability to act as a pathway for the absorption of particulate materials.

Regarding the permeability of the pulmonary pleura, GROVER (1901) showed that transbronchially insufflated India ink appeared in the pleura cavity. HAYEK (1953) also presumed that the body fluid can transit into the pleural cavity from the pulmonary parenchyma, via the pulmonary pleura.

In normal lung, subpleural anthracosis does not extend to the submesothelial layer of the pleura; the authors are of the opinion that the excretion of certain particulate materials from the pulmonary parenchyma into the pleural cavity is doubtful.

HIRAKAWA (1925) also was unable to obtain experimental evidence to show that a dye insufflated into the lung would enter the pleural cavity via pleural transit.

In short, regarding the absorption of substances in the pleural cavity by the parietal pleura, there still remain a few unanswered questions.

When pleurisy occurs exudation may begin in the pulmonary pleura and collect in the pleural cavity; when the pleurisy resolves the exudate may be absorbed through the parietal pleura.

When the progress of pleurisy or empyema is unduly prolonged, the lining layers bounding the pleural cavity may become thickened, and absorption of fluid or exudate may be prevented.

When an exudate is absorbed an adhesion may form, depending on the conditions extant.

According to MOCKEBERG (1903), and CROXATTO and SAMPIETRO (1951), the mesothelial cells of the pulmonary pleura will be replaced by interstitial cells at the time of inflammation, thus contributing to the formation of pleural adhesions.

If pleural adhesions develop new lymph pathway will be formed between the thoracic wall and the lung; inflammatory changes or malignant cells of the lung and pleura may be transmitted through this pathway.

The route of development of the pericostal tuberculosis named by INOKO and TORIKATA is an example of this pathway.

KAUFMANN (1931), S. TAKECHI and Y. AOYAGI (1943) investigated separately about the mechanism of lymphatogenous development of the pericostal tuberculosis, and pathogenesis and surgical treatment of this disease were clarified by AOYAGI and TAKEUCHI (1943). About the details of this research was described by AOYAGI on the Japanese compendium of Surgery (1956).

According to NAGAISHI and N. MAEKAWA (1947) when performing thoracoplasty for pulmonary tuberculosis, lymph nodes showing anthracotic or tuberculous changes are sometimes observed in the intercostal spaces.

The mechanism of their development is also considered to be similar to that of the pericostal tuberculosis.

When pleural adhesions are widespread, movements of the thorax or diaphragm may be impeded and restrictive ventilatory insufficiency may develop to a greater or lesser degree.

In cases exhibiting pleural callosity the impedance will be especially marked, and thoracic and abdominal respirations will be severely disturbed.

Regarding the influence of pleural callosity and the effect of decortication of the lung on pulmonary functions, detailed investigations have been carried out.

Table 20 shows certain influences of pleural callosity on pulmonary function (SAGAWA and NAGAISHI, 1955).

When the lung is put in an extended position for a long time due to pleural callosity, the function of the pleura as a sustentacular tissue will act inversely, and become a cause of abnormal pneumatic changes in the bronchoalveolar system.

Table 20 Influences of pleural scars on the pulmonary function (SAGAWA and NAGAISHI, 1955).

indexes	normal values	values in case of pleural scars
air velocity index	1.0	1.10
dead space	<25	28
venous admixture	< 8	19
diffusion coefficient	10–12	9
% vital capacity	94	50
max. breath. capacity	90	54
O_2-removal	>30.0	27.1
arterial O_2-saturation	>96.0	93.3
ratio of residual volume	<30	54
N_2-clearance	< 2.5	2.9
pulmon. art. pressure	<15.0	18.4
total pulm. vascul. resistance	<200	266

REFERENCES

GENERAL

BERTALANFFY, F. D.: Respiratory Tissue (Structure, Histophysiology, Cytodynamics). International Review of Cytology. Vol. 16, Academic Press, Inc., New York, 1964.

BRAUS, H.: Anatomie des Menschen. 2, Berlin, 1924.

COMROE, J. H., Jr.: Physiology of Respiration. Year Book Medical Publishers, Chicago, 1965.

EBNER, V. v.: Köllikers Handbuch der Gewebslehre des Menschen. 6 Aufl., Bd. iii, Leipzig, 1899.

ENGEL, S.: The Child's Lung. E. Arnold and Co., London, 1947.

——: Die Lunge des Kindes. Stuttgart, 1950.

——: Lung Structure. C. C. Thomas, Springfield, 1962.

FELIX, W.: Topographische Anatomie des Brustkorbes, der Lunge und der Pleura. In: Sauerbruchs Chirurgie der Brustorgane. Bd. 1, Berlin, 1928.

GERLACH, J.: Handbuch der Gewebslehre. 9 Aufl., Wien, 1860.

HAYEK, H. v.: Die menschliche Lunge. Springer-Verlag, 1 Aufl., Berlin·Göttingen·Heidelberg, 1953, und 2 Aufl., Berlin·Heidelberg·New York, 1970.

HENLE, J.: Handbuch der systematischen Anatomie des Menschen. Bd. 2, Braunschweig, 1871.

KIYONO, K.: Die vitale Karminspeicherung. Gustav Fischer, Jena, 1914.

KÖLLIKER, A.: Mikroskopishce Anatomie oder Gewebslehre des Menshen, Leipzig, 1854.

MERKEL, F.: Atmungsorgane. In: Bardelebens Handbuch der Anatomie des Menschen. Bd. 6, Jena, 1902.

MILLER, W. S.: The Lung. Second Edition, First Printing, C. C. Thomas, Springfield, 1947.

NAGAISHI, C., NAGASAWA, N., YAMASHITA, M., OKADA, Y. and INABA, N.: The Structure of the Lung (in Japanese). Igaku Shoin Ltd., Tokyo, Vol. 1, 1957; Vol. 2, 1958.

NAGAISHI, C.: Histology of the Lung. In: "New Histology" edited by NISHIMURA and SHIMIZU (in Japanese). Igaku Shoin Ltd., Tokyo, First Ed., 1962; Second Ed., 1970.

——: Anatomy of the Respiratory Tract (in Japanese). In: Tracheoesophagology ed. by Japan Society of Bronchoesophagology, Igaku Shoin Ltd., Tokyo, 1968.

——: Die Struktur der Lunge. In: "Klinik der Lungenkrankheiten" herausgegeben von KNIPPING und RINK. F. K. Schattauer-Verlag, Stuttgart, 1964.

——: The Structure of the Lung (in Japanese). In: "Thoracic Surgery" edited by Kimoto and Shinoi, Vol. 1, Igaku Shoin, Tokyo, 1966.

——: Anatomy and Histology of the Lung (in Japanese). In: Current Encyclopedia of Surgery, Vol. 30 A, edited by KIMOTO, et al., Nakayama Shoten, Tokyo, 1968.

OKAJIMA, K.: Anatomy. Vol. 1 (in Japanese). Tohodo, Tokyo, 1942.

OPPEL, A.: Lehrbuch der vergleichenden Mikroskopischen Anatomie. 7 Aufl., Jena, 1905.

PERNKOPF, E.: Topographische Anatomie des Menschen. Urban and Schwarzenberg, Wien, 1943.

POLICARD, A.: Le Poumon. Masson, Paris, 1938.

SCHLUZE, F. E.: Die Lungen. In: Strickers Lehre von d. Geweben. Leipzig, 1871.

SCHULZ, H.: Die submikroskopische Anatomie und Pathologie der Lunge. Springer-Verlag, Berlin· Heidelberg · New York, 1959.

STÖHR, Ph., Jr.: Lehrbuch der Histologie und der Mikroskopischen Anatomie. Springer-Verlag, Berlin · Göttingen · Heidelberg, 1951.

SUGAYAMA, S.: Studies on Blood and Tissues (in Japanese). Vol. 3, Nankodo, Tokyo, 1952.

TOLDT, C.: Lehrbuch der Gewebslehre. 3 Aufl., Stuttgart, 1881.

WATERS, A. T. H.: The Anatomy of the Human Lung. London, 1860.

WEIBEL, E. R.: Morphometry of the Human Lung. Springer-Verlag, Berlin · Heidelberg · New York, 1963.

BRONCHOALVEOLAR SYSTEM

ADDISON, T.: Observation on pneumonia and its consequences. Guy's Hosp. Res., S. 2, *1*: 365, 1843.

ADDISON, W.: Observations on the anatomy of the lungs. Medicochir. Trans., 1841.

——: On the ultimate distribution of the air passages and the formation of the air cells of the lung. Phil., Trans., 1842.

ADRIANI, A.: 1847. cit. from W. S. MILLER.

AEBY, C.: Der Bronchialbaum der Säugetiere und des Menschen. Leipzig, 1880.

AKAZAKI, K.: Epithelial covering of the alveolar wall (in Japanese). Nisshin Igaku, *32*: 930, 1943.

——: Reticuloendothelial system and its related tumors (in Japanese). Saishin Igaku, *7*: 5, 1952.

ALLEN, v.: Kollaterale Respiration zwischen Lungen Läppchen. Zschr. Anat., *98*: 453, 1932.

AMANO, S.: Hematology (in Japanese). Maruzen, Tokyo, 1948.

APPLETON, A. B.: The arteries and veins of the lung. J. Anat., *79*: 97, 1945.

ASCHOFF, L.: Die elastischen Systeme des Tracheobronchialbaum. Atti Congr. internat, Patologi. Turin, 1912.

——: Das retikulo-endotheliale System. Erg. inn. Med. Kinderheilk., *26*: 1, 1925.

——: Bemerkungen zur Physiologie des Lungengewebes. Zschr. ges. exp. Med., *50*: 52, 1926.

——: Über den Lungenacinus. Frankf. Zschr. Path., *48*: 499, 1935.

ATWELL, S. W.: Major anomalies of the tracheobronchial tree, with a list of the minor anomalies. Dis. Chest, *52*: 611, 1967.

AZZOPARDI, A. and THULBECK, W. M.: The histochemistry of the non-ciliated bronchiolar epithelial cell. Amer. Rev. Resp. Dis., *99*: 516, 1969.

BARBER, V. C. and BOYDE, A.: Scanning electron microscopic studies of cilia, Zschr. Zellforsch., *84*: 269, 1968.

BARGMANN, W. and KNOOP, P. A.: Vergleichende elektronenmikroskopische Untersuchungen der Lungenkapillaren. Zschr. Zellforsch., *44*: 263, 1956.

——: Elektronenmikroskopische Untersuchungen an der Reptilien und Vögellungen. Zschr. Zellforsch., *54*: 541, 1961.

BAZIN, P. A. E.: Sur la structure intime du poumon. Compt. rend. Acad. Roy. Sc., Paris, 1832.

BENNETT, H. S. and LUFT, J. H.: s-Collidine as a basis for buffering fixatives. J. biophys. biochem. Cytol., *6*: 113, 1959.

BENSCH, K., SCHAEFER, K. E. and VVERY, M. E.: Granular Pneumocytes. Electron microscopic evidence of their exocrinic function. Science, *145*: 1318, 1964.

BENSLEY, R. D. and BENSLEY, S. H.: Studies on the lining of the alveolus of normal lungs of adult animals. Anat. Rec., *64*: 41, 1935.

BERDEL, H.: Nouveaux élements. De histologie hormale. 6 ed., Paris, 1903.

BERTALANFFY, F. D. and LEBLOND, C. P.: The continuous renewal of the two types of alveolar cells in the lung of the rat. Anat. Rec., *115*: 515, 1953.

BERTALANFFY, F. D.: The modern concept of respiratory tissue structure. Acta cytol., *5*: 385, 1961.

BLÜMCKE, S. and MORGENROTH, K., Jr.: The stereo ultrastructures of the external and internal surfaces of the cornea. J. Ultrastr. Res., *18*: 502, 1967.

BOATMAN, E. S. and MARTIN, H. B.: Electron microscopy of the alveolar pores of Kohn. Amer. Rev. Resp. Dis., *88*: 799, 1963.

BOCKENDAHL, A.: Über die Regeneration des Trachealepithels. Arch. mikros. Anat., 24, 1885.

BOLANDE, R. P. and KLAUS, M. H.: The morphologic demonstration of an alveolar lining layer and its relationship to pulmonary surfactant. Amer. J. Path., *45*: 449, 1964.

BOREN, H. G.: Alveolar fenestra. Amer. Rev. Resp. Dis., *85*: 328, 1962.

BOYDE, A. and STEWART, A. D. G.: Scanning electron microscopy of the surface of developing mammalian dental enamel. Nature, *198*: 1102, 1963.

BOYDE, A. and LESTER, K. S.: Electron microscopy of resorbing surface of dental hard tissues. Zschr. Zellforsch., *83*: 538, 1967.

BOYDEN, E. A.: The intrahilar and related segmental anatomy of the lung. Surg., *18*: 706, 1045.

——: Segmental Anatomy of the Lungs. The Blackiston Division, McGraw-Hill Book Co., New York·Toronto·London, 1955.

——: Notes on the development of the lung in infancy and early childhood. Amer. J. Anat., *121*: 749, 1967.

——: The pattern of the terminal air spaces in a premature infant of 30–32 weeks that lived nineteen and a quarter hours. Amer. J. Anat., *126*: 31, 1969.

BREMER, J. L.: The lung of the oppossum. Amer. Journ. Anat., *3*: 67, 1904.

BROCK, R. C.: Anatomy of the bronchial tree. Oxford University Press, New York, 1946.

——: Nomenclature of broncho-pulmonary anatomy. Internat. nomenclature accept. by the Thorax Society. Thorax, *5*: 5, 1950.

BROOKS, R. E.: Concerning the nomenclature of the cellular elements in respiratory tissue. Amer. Rev. Resp. Dis., *94*: 112, 1966.

BUCKINGHAM, S., MCNARY, W. F., Jr. and SOMMERS, S. C.: Pulmonary alveolar cell inclusions. Their development in the rat. Science, *145*: 1192, 1964.

BUCKINGHAM, S., HEINEMANN, H. O., SOMMERS, S. C. and MCNARY, W. F.: Phospholipid synthesis in the large pulmonary alveolar cell. Amer. J. Path., *48*: 1027, 1966.

BUSINCO, A.: Struttura del polmone. Monit zool. ital., Suppl. 44, 1933.

CAMPICHE, M. A.: Les inclusions lamellaires des cellules alvéolaires dans le poumon du raton. J. Ultrastr. Res., *3*: 302, 1960.

CAMPICHE, M. A., GAUTÉER, A., HERNANDES, E. I. and REYMOND, A.: An electron microscopic study of the fetal development of human lung. Pediatrics, *32*: 976, 1963.

CARLETON, H. M.: Studies on epithelial phagocytosis. Proc. Roy. Soc., London, ser. B *114*: 513, 1934.

CARSON, S., GOLDHAMER, R. and CARPENTER, R.: Mucus transport in the respiratory tract. Amer. Rev. Resp. Dis., *93* (Pt. 2 of No. 3): 86, 1966.

CHAMBERS, R. and RÉNYI, G. S.: The structure of the cells in tissues as revealed by microdissection. I. The physical relationship of the cells in epithelia. Amer. J. Anat., *35*: 1925.

CHARCOT, J. M.: Maladies des Poumon, 1887.

CHRZONSZCZEWSKY, N.: Über das Epithel der Lungenbläschen der Säugetiere. Würzburger med. Zschr., *4*: 1863.

——: Zur Lehre von den Lungenepithel. Arch. pathol. Anat. u. Physiol. *35*: 165, 1866.

CHURCHILL, E. D. and BELSEY, R.: Segmental pneumonectomy in Bronchiectasis. The lingula segment of the upper lobe. Ann. Surg., *109*: 481, 1939.

CLARA, M.: Vergleichende Histologie des Nierenglomerulus und der Lungenalveole nach Untersuchungen beim Menschen und beim Kaninchen. Zsch. mikrosk. anat. Forsch., *40*: 147, 1936.

——: Zur Histobiologie des Bronchialepithels. Zschr. mikr.-anat. Forsch., *41*: 321, 1937.

CLARKE, J. A. and SALSBURY, A. J.: Surface ultramicroscopy of human blood cells. Nature, *215*: 402, 1967.

CLEMENTS, J. A., BROWN, E. S. and JOHNSON, R. P.: Pulmonary surface tension and the mucus lining of the lung. J. Appl. Physiol., *12*: 262, 1958.

CLEMENTS, J. A.: Surface phenomena in relation to pulmonary function. Physiologist, *5*: 11, 1962.

CLEMENTS, J. A., NELLENBOGEN, J. and TRAHAN, H. J.: Pulmonary surfactant and evolution of the lungs. Science, *169*: 603, 1970.

COLBERG, A.: Beiträge zur normalen und pathologischen Anatomie der Lungen. Dtsch. Arch. klin. Med., *2*: 1866.

COSSLETT, V. E.: Scanning microscopy with electrons and X-rays. J. Electr. Microsc., *16*: 51, 1967.

DAIDO, S.: Electron microscopic studies of the pulmonary adenoma (in Japanese). Kyodai Kekken Kiyo, *9*: 164, 1961; and *12*: 65, 1966.

DALHAM, T.: Effect of cigarett smoke on ciliary activity. Amer. Rev. Resp. Dis., *93* (Pt. 2 of No. 3): 108, 1966.

DIVERTIE, M. B. and BROWN, A. L.: The pulmonary alveolar macrophage. Medical Clinics of North America, *48*: 1049, 1964.

——: The fine structure of the normal human alveolocapillary membrane, J. Amer. Med. Assoc., *187*: 938, 1964.

DIVERTIE, M. B., BROWN, A. L. and HARRISON, E. G.: Pulmonary alveolar proteinosis. Two cases studied by electron microscopy. Amer. J. Med., *40*: 351, 1966.

DOGLIOTTI, G. and AMPRINO, R.: Action de Chimiques sur la cellule epithelial pulmonaire. Comp. rend. Soc. Biol., *170*: 1344, 1920.

——: Ricerche sulla struttura dell'alveolo. Arch. ital. Anat., *30*: 1, 1932.

DRASCH, O.: 1880. cit. from W. S. MILLER.

——: 1881. cit. from W. S. MILLER.

EBE, T.: Light and electron microscopic studies on experimental pneumonitis induced by Blasticidin-S, with special reference to the regeneration of alveoli. Arch. Histol. Jap., *30*: 149 ,1969.

EBERTH, C. J.: Der Streif über das Epithel der Lungenbläschen. Arch. Pathol. Anat. u. Physiol., *24*: 503, 1862.

EBNER, V. v.: In Kölliker-v. Ebners Handbuch der Histologie. 1902.

ECHLIN, P.: Pollen. Scientific American, *218*: 80, 1968.

ECHLIN, P., CHAPMAN, B., GODWIN, H. and ANGOLD, R.: The fine structure and development of the pollen of Helleborus foetidus L. 6th Internat. Congr. Electr. Microsc., Kyoto, 1966.

ELENZ, E.: Über das Lungenepithel. Würzburger nat.-wissensch. Zschr., *5*: 1863.

EWART, W.: The Bronchi and Pulmonary Blood Vessels. London, 1889.

FAUCETT, D. W.: Membranes of cytoplasm. Lab. Invest., *10*: 1162, 1961.

FLINT, J. M.: The development of the lung. Amer. J. Anat., *6*: 1, 1907.

FOOT, N. C.: The macrophages of the loose connective tissue. J. Med. Res., *40*: 353, 1919.

——: The endothelial cell in experimental tuberculosis. J. Exp. Med., *32*: 513, 1920

——: Studies on endothelial reactions: Origin of pulmonary "dust cell". Amer. J. Path., *3*: 413, 1927.

——: In: Pathology in Surgery. J. B. Lippincott Co., Philadelphia, 1945.

FRANKENHÄUSER, K.: Untersuchungen über den Bau der Tracheobronchialschleimhaut. St. Petersburg, 1879.

FUJITA, T.: Observation of living body sample (rabbit tongue and appendix) through scanning electron microscope. JEOL News Japan Electron Optics Co., Ltd. 7B: 4, 1969.

GALEN, C.: De usu partium corporis humani. Omnia quae extant, in latinum sermonem conversa. Frobenianae Editione, bib. VI., cap. III, Basil, 1562.

GERLACH, J.: Handbuch der Gewebslehre. 9 Aufl., Wien, 1860.

GIRALDES, J. A.: Note sur la termination des bronches. Bull. de la Soc. Anatom., 1839.

GMELICH, J. T., BENSCH, K. and LIEBOW, A. A.: Cells of Kultshitzky type in bronchioles and their relations to the origin of peripheral carcinoid tumor. Lab. Invest., *17*: 88, 1967.

GOCO, R. V., KRESS, M. B. and BRANTIGAN, O. C.: Comparison of mucus glands in the tracheobronchial tree of man and animals. Ann. N.Y. Acad. Sci., *106*: 555, 1963.

GOUGH, J. and WENTWORTH, J. E.: Sections of entire organs mounted on paper. J. Roy. Microsc., *69*: 231, 1949.

GOUGH, J. and LEOPOLD, J. G.: Techniques used in the study of lung pathology. The anatomy of emphysema, Ciba Foundation Symposium on Pulmonary Structure and Function. ed. by Reuck, A. V. S., and O'Conner, M., Little, Brown and Co., Boston, 1962.

GREEN, J. G., BROWN, A. L. and DIVERTIE, M. B.: Fine structure of suamous cell carcinoma of the lung. Mayo Clin. Proc., *44*: 85, 1969.

GRONIOWSKI, J. and DJACZENKO, W.: Die Feinstruktur des Lungengewebes nach dem Beginn der Atmung. Zschr. Zellforsch., *53*: 639, 1961.

GRONIOWSKI, J. and BICZYSKOWA, W.: Structure of the alveolar lining film of the lungs. Nature, *204*: 745, 1964.

——: Electron microscopic studies on alveolar lining film of the lungs. 6th Internat. Congr. Electr. Microsc., Kyoto, 1966.

GROSS, J. and SCHMITT, F. O.: Structure of human skin collagen as studied with electron microscope. J. Exp. Med., *88*: 555, 1947.

GROSS, J.: Structure of elastic tissue as studied with electron microscope. J. Exp. Med., *89*: 699, 1949.

GROSS, P., PFITZER, E. A. and HATCH, T. F.: Alveolar clearance. Its relation to lesion of the respiratory bronchiole. Amer. Rev. Resp. Dis., *94*: 10, 1966.

GUIEYSSE-PELLISSIER, M. A.: Modification et lésions des céllules épithéliales pulmonaires. Acad. Soc., Paris, *170*: 1411, 1920.

HAGIHARA, T., UCHIYAMA, T. and ARIYAMA, Y.: So-called non-respiratory lung function (in Japanese). Nihon Kyobu Rinsho, *30*: 225, 1971.

HANSEMANN, D.: Über die Poren der normalen Lungenalveolen. Arch. mikroskop. Anat. Entwickl.-gesch., *55*: 337, 1900.

HATASA, K. and NAKAMURA, T.: Electron microscopic observations of lung alveolar epithelial cells of normal young mice, with special reference to formation and secretion of osmiophilic lamellar bodies. Zschr. Zellforsch., *68*: 266, 1965.

HATTORI, S., MATSUDA, M. and WADA, A.: An electron microscopic study of pulmonary adenomas in mice (in Japanese). Gann, *56*: 275, 1965.

HATTORI, S. and TAKENAGA, A.: Ultrafine structure of the bronchoalveolar system with reference to aging phenomenon (in Japanese). Nihon Kyobu Rinsho, *28*: 874, 1969.

HAUSER, G.: Über die Entstehung des fibrösen Infiltrates bei der croupösen Pneumonie. Beitr. path. Anat. u. allg. Path., *15*: 1894.

HAYAKAWA, M.: Über die epitheloiden Histiozyten nach Hamazaki. Nihon Byorigakkaishi, *19*: 202, 1929.

HAYEK, H. v.: Über flimmertragendes und sezernierendes Bronchial-Epithel. Arch. exp. Path., 1952.

——: Cellular structure and mucus activity in the bronchial tree and alveoli. Ciba Foundation Symposium on Pulmonary Structure and Function. ed. by REUCK, A. V. S., and O'CONNER, M., Little, Brown and Co., Boston, 1962.

HELLER, A. und SCHRÖTTER, v.: Die Carina tracheae. Denkschr. Akad. Wien., math.-nat. Kl. 1897.

HERRENHEISER, G. und KUBAT, A.: Systematische Anatomie der Lungengefässe. Ztsch. Anat. u. Entwickl.-gesch., *105*: 570, 1936.

HOLMA, B.: Scanning electron microscopic observation of particles deposited in the lung. Arch. Environ. Health (Chicago), *18*: 330, 1969.

HUSTEN, K.: Über den Lungenacinus und den Sitz der acinösen phthisischen Prozesse. Beitr. z. Path. Anat. u. z. allg. Path., *68*: 1921.

IKEDA, SI.: Bronchofiberscopy. In: Broncho-esophagology. ed. by Japan Broncho-Esophagological Society, Igaku Shoin Ltd., Tokyo, 145, 1968.

IKEDA, SI and YANAUCHI, N.: Flexible fiberscope. (in Japanese), Nihon Kikan-Shokudoka Gakkai Kaiho, *19*: 54, 1968.

IRAVANI, J.: Physiologie und Pathophysiologie der Cilientätigkeit und Schleimtransportes im Tracheobronchialbaum, Pneumonologie, *144*: 93, 1971.

ISHIKO, S.: Electron microscopic studies on the lining tissue of pulmonary alveoli and so-called dust cells (in Japanese). Kyodai Kekken Kiyo, 7, Suppl. III: 191, 1959.

ITAGI, K.: Electron microscopic observation of pulmonary alveolar structure. Acta. Tub. Jap., *5*: 1, 1956.

——: Electron microscopy of the alveoli (in Japanese). Kokyu to Junkan, *4*: 400, 1956.

——: Electron microscopic observation of pulmonary alveolar structure of laboratory mammals. Acta Tuberc. Jap., *6*: 75 and 91, 1957.

JACKSON, C. L. and HUBER, J. F.: Correlated applied anatomy of the bronchial tree with a system of nomenclature. Dis. Chest., *9*: 319, 1943.

KARRER, H. E.: The ultrastructure of mouse lung. General architecture of capillary and alveolar walls. J. biophys. biochem. Cytol., *2*: 241, 1956 and Exp. Cell. Res., *10*: 237, 1956.

——: Electron microscopic study of bronchiolar epithelium of normal mouse lung. Exp. Cell Res., *10*: 238, 1958.

——: The ultrastructure of mouse lung. The alveolar macrophage. J. Biophys. Cytol., *4*: 693, 1958.

——: Vierte Int. Konf. Elektronenmikroskopie, 1958 verhandl. Berlin, 1960.

KIKKAWA, Y., MOTOYAMA, E. K. and COOK, C. D.: The ultrastructure of the lungs of lambs. The relation of osmiophilic inclusions and alveolar lining layer to fetal maturation and experimentally produced respiratory distress. Amer. J. Path., *47*: 877, 1965.

KIKKAWA, Y., MOTOYAMA, E. K. and GLUCK, L.: Study of the lungs of fetal and newborn rabbits. Amer. J. Path., *52*: 177, 1968.

KINOSHITA, Y., OGIMA, I., et al.: Agricultural drug pneumonitis (in Japanese). Nihon Naikagaku Zasshi, *57*: 1219, 1968.

KIYONO, K. and MAJIMA, U.: Pathologic-histological studies on pneumonia (in Japanese). Kyoto Igaku Zasshi, *17*: 1920.

KIYONO, K., SUGIYAMA, S., et al.: The Vital Staining (in Japanese). Tokyo, 1933.

KISCH, B.: Electron microscopic investigation of the lungs (Capillaries and specific cells). Exp. Med. Surg., *13*: 101, 1955.

——: Specific cells and other cells of osmiophilic enclosure. Exp. Med. Surg., *15*: 101, 1957.

——: Electron microscopy of the lungs in acute pulmonary edema. Exp. Med. Surg., *16*: 17, 1958.

——: The so-called basement membrane of the capillaries of the lung. Exp. Med. Surg., *23*: 133, 1965.

KLAUS, M., REISS, O. K., TOOLEY, W. H., PIEL, C. and CLEMENTS, J. A.: Alveolar epithelial cell mitochondria as source of the surfaceactive lung lining. Science, *137*: 750, 1962.

KLÄRNER, P. and GIESEKING, R.: Zur Ultrastruktur des Lungentumors der Maus, Zschr. Krebsforsch., *64*: 7, 1960.

KLEINERMAN, J.: Reparative processes of the lung in 10th Hahnemann Sympos. New York, Grune and Stratton, 77, 1964.

KOHN, H. N.: Zur Histologie des indurierenden Pneunonie, Münch. me. Wschr., *40*: 42, 1893.

KÖLLIKER, A.: Zur Kenntnis des Baues der Lunge des Menschen. Verhandl. physik. -med. Ges., Würzburg, n. F., *16*: 1, 1881.

KOZU, K., et al.: Branching of the main bronchi (in Japanese). Nihon Kikan-Shokudoka Gakkai Kaiho, *2*: 2, 1951.

KRAMER, R. and GLASS, A.: Bronchoscopic localisation of lung abscess. Amer. Otorhinolaryng., *41*: 1212, 1932.

KUNO, K. and STAUB, N.: Acute mechanical effects of lung volume changes on artificial microholes in alveolar walls. J. Appl. Physiol., *24*: 83, 1968.

LAGUESSE, E., et D'HARDEVILLER, A.: Sur la topographie du lobule pulmonaire. Bibliog. Anatomique, 1898.

LANG, F. T.: The relation of lung tissue to tuberculous infection in vitro. J. Infec. Dis., *37*: 1925.

——: Gewebskulturen der Lunge. Arch. exp. Zellforsch., *2*: 1926.

——: Alveolarphagocyten. Virchows Arch. path. Anat., *275*: 1929.

LEREBOULLET, A.: 1838. cit. from MILLER.

LIEBOW, A. A.: Recent advances in pulmonary anatomy. Ciba Foundation Symposium on Pulmonary Structure and Function. ed. Reuck, A. V. S., and O'Conner, M., Little, Brown and Co., Boston, 1962.

LIN, G.: Selective Bronchography of the Segmental Bronchi (in Japanese). revised by C. NAGAISHI, Igaku Shoin Ltd., Tokyo, 1958.

LINSER, P.: Über den Bau und die Entwicklung des elastischen Gewebes in der Lunge. Anat. Hefte, *13*: 1900.

LOESCHKE, H.: Die Morphologie des normalen und emphysematösen Acinus der Lunge. Beitr. path. Anat. u. allg. Path., *68*: 213, 1921.

LOOSLI, C. G.: Interalveolar communications in

normal and in pathological mammalian lungs. Arch. Path., *24*: 743, 1937.

——: The structure of the respiratory portion of the mammalian lung with notes on the lining of the frog lung. Amer. J. Anat., *62*: 375, 1938.

LOOSLI, C. G. and POTTER, E. L.: The prenatal development of the human lung. Anat. Rec., *109*: 320, 1951.

LOOSLI, C. G. and BAKER, R. F.: The human lung: Microscopic structure and diffusion. In: Ciba Foundation Symposium on Pulmonary Structure and Function. ed. REUCK, A. V. S. and O'CONNER, M., Little, Brown and Co., Boston, 1962.

LOW, F. N.: Electron microscopy of the rat lung. Anat. Rec., *113*: 437, 1952.

——: The pulmonary alveolar epithelium of laboratory mammals. Anat. Rec., *117*: 241, 1953.

——: The extracellular portion of the human blood air barrier and its relation to tissue space. Anat. Rec., *139*: 105, 1961.

LUFT, J. H.: Improvements in epoxy resin embedding methods. J. biophy. biochem. Cytol., *9*: 409, 1961.

MACKLIN, C. C.: Pulmonary alveolar epithelium. J. Thorac. Surg. 6, 1936.

——: Alveolar pores and their significance in the human lung. Arch. Path., *21*: 202, 1936.

——: The pulmonary alveolar mucoid film and the pneumocytes. Lancet, *266*: 1099, 1954.

MAJIMA, U.: Pathohistological study on pneumonia (in Japanese). Kyoto Igaku Zasshi, *17*: 974, 1920.

MALPIGHI, M.: 1679. cit. from MILLER.

MANDL, L.: Anatomie microscopique. Paris, 1857.

MARTIN, H. B.: The effect of aging on the alveolar pores of Kohn in the dog. Amer. Rev. Resp. Dis., *88*: 773, 1963.

MAXIMOW, A. A.: Über undifferenzierte Blutzellen und mesenchymale Keimlayer im Erwachsenen Organismus. Klin. Wschr., *5*: 2139, 1926.

McDONALD, L. W., PEASE, R. F. W. and HAYES, T. L.: Scanning electron microscopy of sectioned tissue. Lab. Invest., *16*: 532, 1967.

MÉTRAS, H.: L'arbre bronchique. Vigot, Paris, 1948.

MEYRICK, B. and REID, L.: The alveolar wall. Brit. J. Dis. Chest., *64*: 121, 1970.

MILLER, W. S.: The arrangement of the elastic fibers in the bronchi and lung. J. Anat. Physiol. *40*: 162, 1906.

——: The epithelium of the lower respiratory tract. In: Special Cytology., New York, 1932.

MIZUTANI, A.: Scanning electron microscopy of the bronchus and adnexes of rats. Kyodai Kyobuken Kiyo, *2*: 163, 1969.

MOLESCHOTT, J.: De Malpighianis pulnonum vesicula. Heidelberg, 1845.

MÖLLENDORF, F. v.: Handbuch der mikroskopischen Anatomie des Menschen, 1928.

——: Lehrbuch der Histologie. 23 Aufl., Jena, 1933.

——: Über die Lungenkonstruktion. Zsch. Anat. III: 224, 1941.

MONTGOMERY, G. L.: Healing of experimental wounds of lung. Brit. J. Surg., *31*: 292, 1944.

MÜLLER, A.: Zur vergleichenden Histologie der Lungen der Haussäugetiere. Arch. mik. Anat., *69*: 1907.

NAGAISHI, C. and NAGASAWA, N.: Bronchoalveolar system. In: Nagaishi's monograph "The Structure of the Lung", Vol. I (in Japanese). Igaku Shoin Ltd., Tokyo, 1957.

NAGAISHI, C. and OKADA, Y.: The structure of the bronchoalveolar system with special reference to its fine structure. Acta Tuberc. Jap., *10*: 20, 1960.

NAGAISHI, C. OKADA, Y., ISHIKO, S. and DAIDO, S.: Electron microscopic observation of the pulmonary alveoli. Exp. Med. and Surg., *22*: 81, 1964.

——: Electron microscopic observations of the human lung cancer. Exp. Med. and Surg., *23*: 177, 1965.

NAGAISHI, C.: Relationship between alveolar pores and pulmonary emphysema (in Japanese). Kokyu to Junkan, *18*: 593, 1970.

NAGASAWA, N., YAMASHITA, M. and NAGAISHI, C.: Three-dimensional and microscopic studies of the normal and tuberculous Lungs using resin casts (in Japanese). Kekkaku Kenkyu, *2*: 1, 1952.

NAGASAWA, N., YAMASHITA, M., OKAMOTO, H. and NAGAISHI, C.: Indication for pneumothorax in the light of construction of bronchial system, esp. of pulmonary lobules (in Japanese). Nihon Geka Hokan, *2*: 1, 1953.

NAKAMURA, T., TAKIZAWA, T. and MORONE, T.: Anatomic changes in lung parenchyma due to aging process. Dis. Chest, *52*: 518, 1967.

NAKANOIN, T.: Experimental cholesterinsteatosis and vital staining. Hokuetsu Igakukai Zasshi, *32*: 100, 1917.

NARATH, A.: Die Bronchialbaum der Säugetiere und des Menschen. Stuttgart, 1901.

NEIL, J. H.: Anatomy of bronchial tree. Brit. Med. J., *1*: 495, 1939.

NELSON, H. P.: Postural drainage of lungs. Brit. Med. J., *2*: 251, 1934.

NICOLAS, A.: Organes de la respiration in traité d'anatomie humaine. t. 4, Paul Poirier, Editor, Paris, 1898.

NIDEN, A. H. and YAMADA, E.: The fine structure of Clara cell in the mouse lung. J. Electron Microscopy, *14*: 139, 1962.

——: The fine structure of Clara cell in the mouse lung. J. Electr. Microsc., *14*: 139, 1965.

——: Some observation on the fine structure and function of the nonciliated bronchiolar cells. 6th Internat. Congr. Electr. Microsc., Kyoto, 1966.

NIDEN, A. H.: Bronchiolar and large alveolar cell in pulmonary phospholipid metabolism. Science, *158*: 1323, 1967.

NISHIMARU, K.: Studies on Body Fluid Circulation (in Japanese). Igaku Shoin Ltd., Tokyo, 1952.

NISHIUCHI, I.: Morphological studies on the acinus and the acinous caseous foci (in Japanese). Kyodai Kekken Kiyo, *7*: 60, 1959.

NOWELL, J. A. and TYLER, W. S.: Scanning electron microscopy of the surface morphology of mammalian lungs. Amer. Rev. Res. Dis., *103*: 313, 1971.

OGAWA, C.: Contributions to the histology of the respiratory spaces of the vertebrate lungs. Amer. J. Anat., *27*: 333, 1920.

——: The finer ramifications of the human lung. Amer. J. Anat., *27*: 315, 1920.

——: Histological studies on respiratory spaces of the vertebrate lungs. Kyoto Igaku Zasshi, *14*: 6, 1917.

OKA, H.: Primary complex. Tokyo Igakukai Zasshi, *43*: 208, 1929.

OKADA, Y., DAIDO, S. and ISHIKO, S.: Morphological studies of induced pulmonary tumors in mice with special reference to their cytogenesis. Acta Tuberc. Jap., *11*: 73, 1962.

OKADA, Y., ISHIKO, S., DAIDO, S., et al.: Comparative morphology of the lung with special reference to alveolar epithelial cells: I. Lung of the amphibia. Acta Tuberc. Jap., *11*: 63, 1962.

——: Comparative morphology of the lung with special reference to the alveolar lining cells. II. Lung of the reptilia. Acta Tuberc. Jap., *12*: 1, 1962.

——: Comparative morphology of the lung with special reference to alveolar epithelial cells. III. Lung of the bird. Acta Tuberc. Jap., *14*: 89, 1965.

OKADA, Y. and GENKA, K.: Histological and electron microscopic observation on the adenomatous hyperplasia of the alveolar epithelial cell in the human lung. Acta Tuberc. Jap., *16*: 48, 1966.

OKADA, Y., IKEDA, SA., KITANO, M., GENKA, K. and YAMAMOTO, H.: Scar cancer of the lung (in Japanese). Nihon Kyobu Rinsho, *26*: 39, 1967.

OKADA, Y. and NAGAISHI, C.: Transmission and scanning electron microscopies of normal lung (in Japanese). Nihon Kyobu Rinsho, *28*: 861, 1969.

OKADA, Y.: The ultrastructure of the Clara cell in the bronchiolar epithelium. Kyodai Kyobuken Kiyo, *3*: 1, 1969.

OKADA, Y., AKAMINE, Y., IKEDA, SA., IZUMI, T. and KAI, T.: Electron microscopy of pulmonary alveolar proteinosis. Nihon Denshikenbikyo Gakkaishi, *3*: 699, 1971.

OPPEL, A.: Atmungsapparat. In: Lehrbuch der vergleichenden mikroskopischen Anatomie. 6 Teil, Jena, 1905.

ORSÓS, F.: Über das elastische Gerüst der normalen und emphysematösen Lunge. Beitr. path. Anat., Allg. Path., *41*: 95, 1907.

OTSUKA, K.: Morphological studies on the obstructive atelectasis (in Japanese). Kyodai Kekken Kiyo, *8*: 374, 1959.

OVERHOLT, R. H., WOOD, F. M. and RAMSAY, B. H.: Segmental pulmonary resection. J. Thor. Surg., *19*: 207, 1950.

OYAMADA, A., GASUL, B. M. and HOLINGER, P. H.: Agenesis of the lung. Amer. J. Dis. Child., *85*: 182, 1953.

PATTLE, R. E.: The lining layer of the lung alveoli. Brit. Med. Bull., *19*: 41, 1963.

PEARSE, R. F. W. and HAYES, T. L.: Scanning electron microscopy of biological material. Nature, *210*: 1049, 1966.

PEIRCE, C. B. and STOCKING, B. W.: The roentgenological anatomy of the chest. II. Amer. Rev. Tuberc., *39*: 516, 1939.

PISO-BORME: 1869. cit. from A. OPPEL.

POLICARD, A., et GALY, P.: Le vacuome de la cellule du poumen. C. R. Soc. Biol., *103*: Paris, 1930.

——: Les bronches., Paris, 1945.

POLICARD, A.: Reactions pulmonaires aux poussieres. Bull. Histol. appl., *25*: 71, 1948.

POLICARD, A., COLLET, A. and PREGERMAIN, S.: Electron microscopic studies on alveolar cells from mammals. Electron Microscopy. Almqvist and Wiksell, Stockholm, 244, 1957, and Acta Anat., *30*: 624, 1957.

POLICARD, A., COLLET, A. and MORTIN, J. C.: La surface d'echange air-sang dans le poumon des oiseaux, Zsch. Zellforsch., *57*: 37, 1962.

PUMP, K. K., DUNN, H. G. and MEUWISSEN, H.: A study of the bronchial and vascular structures of the lung. From a case of ataxia-telangiectasia. Dis. Chest, *47*: 473, 1965.

PUMP, K. K.: Morphology of the acinus of the human lung. Dis. Chest, *56*: 126, 1969.

RAMSEY, B. H.: The anatomic guide to the intersegmental plane. Surg., *25*: 533, 1949.

REISSEISEN, F. D.: Über die Struktur, die Verrichtung, und den Gebrauch der Lungen., Berlin, 1808.

RHODIN, J. A. G.: Ultrastructure and function of the human tracheal mucosa. Amer. Rev. Resp. Dis., *93* (pt. 2 of no. 3): 1, 1966.

RIBBERT, H.: Zur Anatomie der Lungenentzündungen. Forschr. d. Med. *12*: 1894.

RINDFLEISCH, E.: Die Muskulatur der kleinen Bronchien und des Lungenparenchyms. Zbl. med. Wissenschaften, *5*: 65, 1872.

ROMANOVA, L. K.: Regenerative hypertrophy of the lungs in rats after simultaneous removal of the entire left lung and of the diaphragmatic lobe of the right lung. Bull. exp. biol. Med., *50*: 100, 1960.

ROSSIGNOL, H.: 1846. cit. from MILLER.

RUSAKOFF, A.: Die Gitterfasern der Lunge. Beitr. pathol. Anat. allg. Patho., *45*: 476, 1909.

SAKAMOTO, S.: Study on caseous pneumonia by vital staining. Osaka Igaku Zasshi, *16*: 201, 1917.

SASAKAWA, K., et al.: Electron Microscopy. Honda Shoten, Kyoto, 1951.

SAUERBRUCH, F.: Chirurgie der Brustorgane. Bd. I, 1930.

SAWADA, H.: Pulmonary surfactant (in Japanese). Kokyu to Jyunkan, *17*: 264, 1969.

SCANNEL, J. G.: An anatomic approach to segmental resection. J. Thorac. Surg., *18*: 64, 1949.

SCHLIPKÖTER, H. W.: Elektronenoptische Untersuchungen ultradünner Lungenschnitte. Dtsch. Med. Wschr., *79*: 1858, 1954.

SCHULTZ, E.: 1850. cit. from W. S. MILLER.

SCHULZ, H.: Über den Gestaltwandel der Mitochondrien in Alveolarepithel unter CO_2- und O_2-Atmung. Naturwissenschaften, *43*: 205, 1956.

——: Die Pathologie der Mitochondrien im Alveolarepithel der Lunge. Beitr. pathol. Anat., *119*: 45, 1958.

——: Die submikroskopische Anatomie und Pathologie der Lunge. Springer Verlag, Berlin. Heidelberg, 1959.

——: Some remarks on the sub-microscopic anatomy and pathology of the blood-air pathway in the lung. Ciba Foundation Symposium on Pulmonary Structure and Function. ed. by REUCK, A. V. S., and O'CONNER, M., Little, Brown and Co., Boston, 1962.

SCHULZE, F. E.: Die Lungen. In: Strickers Lehre von den Geweben. Leipzig, 1871.

SCHULZE, W.: Untersuchungen über das Ligamentum pulmonale. Dtsch. Zschr. Chir., *239*: 34, 1933.

SEEMANN, G.: Histobiologie der Lungenalveole. Jena, 1931.

SENDA, N. and TOYOTA, M.: Alveolar lining layer (in Japanese) Igaku no Ayumi, *63*: 808, 1967.

SHIMADA, H.: Structure and pathology of the alveolus (in Japanese). Nihon Byori Gakkai Zasshi, *52*: 1, 1963.

——: Light and electron microscopic studies on the structure of the pulmonary alveolus and its pathology (in Japanese). Trans. Soc. Path. Jap., *52*: 1, 1963.

SHIOZAWA, M.: Segmental Resection of the Lung (in Japanese). Vol. I and II, Bunkodo, Tokyo, 1954 and 1955.

SMITH, F. and BOYDEN, E. A.: Segmental bronchi of right lower lobe. J. Thorac. Surg., *18*: 195, 1949.

STÖHR, PH.: Lehrbuch der Histologie und der mikroskopischen Anatomie. Springer Verlag, Berlin·Göttingen·Heidelberg, 1915.

STURM, A.: Zur klinischen Pathologie der Lunge. Stuttgart, 1948.

SUTNICK, A. I., SOLOFF, L. A. and SETH, R. S.: Influence of alveolar collapse upon surface activity of lung extracts. Dis. Chest, *53*: 257, 1968.

SVOBODA, D. J.: Ultrastructure of pulmonary adenomas in mice. Cancer Res., *22*: 1197, 1962.

SWIGART, R. H. and KANE, D. J.: Electron microscopic observations of pulmonary alveoli. Anat. Rec., *118*: 57, 1954.

TAKAGI, B. and YASUDA, H.: Ultrastructure of the normal lungs of the rats (in Japanese). Nihon Byorigakkaishi, *45*: 443, 1956.

TAKAHASHI, T.: Bronchial branching and pulmonary segment (in Japanese). Kyobu Geka, *4*: 6, 1952.

TAMARU, K.: A few problems of the alveolar structure of rabbit (in Japanese). Kaibogaku Zasshi, *28*: 1, 1953.

TIERNEY, D. F.: Pulmonary surfactant in health and disease. Dis. Chest, *47*: 247, 1965.

TODD, R. B. and BOWMAN, W.: The Physiological Anatomy and Physiology of Man. Vol. II Respiration. 1859.

TOKUNAGA, J., FUJITA, T. and INOUE, H.: Application of the scanning electron microscopy to medicine (in Japanese). Igaku no Ayumi, *68*: 485, 1969.

TOMITA, A.: Epitheloid cell in alveolus. Osaka Igakukai Zasshi, *17*: 747, 1918.

TURNER, W.: An introduction to Human Anatomy. Part ii, Edinburgh, 1877.

TYLER, W. S. and PANGBORN, J.: Laminated membrane surface and osmiophilic inclusions in avian lung epithelium. J. Cell Biol., *20*: 157, 1964.

UJI-IYE, T.: Fundamental studies on segmental resection (in Japanese). Kyobu Geka, *5*: 6, 1952.

VERSON, E.: Kehlkopf und Trachea. In: Strickers Handbuch der Lehre von den Geweben des Menschen und der Tiere. Leipzig, 1871.

WALLER, C. and BJÖRKMAN, G.: 1882, cit. from W. S. MILLER.

WATSON, J. H. L. and BRINKMAN, G. L.: Electron microscopy of the epithelial cells of normal and bronchitic human bronchus. Amer. Rev. Resp. Dis., *90*: 851, 1964.

WEIBEL, E. R., KISTLER, G. S. and TONDURY, G.: A stereologic electron microscopic study of "tubular myelin figures" in alveolar fluids of rat lungs. Zschr. Zellforsch., *69*: 418, 1966.

WEIBEL, E. R. and GIL, J.: Electron microscopic demonstration of an extracellular duplex lining layer of alveoli. Resp. Physiol., *4*: 42, 1968.

WILLIS, T.: 1676. cit. from W. S. MILLER.

WOODSIDE, G. L. and DALTON, A. J.: The ultrastructure of lung tissue from new-born and embryo mice. J. ultrastr. Res., *2*: 28, 1959.

YAMADA, Y.: Comparative histological studies on the alveolar epithelium of vertebrates (in Japanese). Kaibogaku Zasshi, *28*: 1, 1953.

YAMASHITA, H.: Studies on pulmonary segments (in Japanese). Kyobu Geka, *4*: 6, 1951.

——: Atlas of X-ray Finding of the Lung (in Japanese). Igaku Shoin Ltd., Tokyo, 1956.

YAMASHITA, H. and ISHIKAWA, E.: Pulmonary segment (in Japanese). Kekkaku Kenkyunoshimpo 5 and 6, 1954.

YAMORI, T. and SASAKI, M.: Electron Microscopic cytopathology of the Respiratory System (in Japanese). Iwanami, Tokyo, 1967.

YAMORI, T.: Ultrastructure of bronchoalveolar system (in Japanese). Symposium, 9 Nihon Kyobu Shikkan Gakkai, 1969.

YASUDA, H.: Electron microscopic cyto-histopathology. IV. A study of normal adult and fetus lung in mammals as revealed by electronmicroscopy. Acta Path. Jap., *8*: 189, 1958.

YOSHIDA, S. and ARAI, T.: Metabolism of fatty substances with reference to the surfactant (in Japanese). Kokyu to Jyunkan, *17*: 379, 1969.

ZIMMERMAN, K. W.: 1900. cit. from W. S. MILLER.

ZENKER, R., HEBERER, G. and LÖHR, H. H.: Die Lungenresektion. Anatomie. Indikationen. Technik. Springer, Heidelberg, 1954.

VASCULAR SYSTEM

ADACHI, B.: Das Arterien System der Japaner. Kyoto, 1931.

——: Das Venen System der Japaner. Kyoto, 1933.

ALLEN, D. M. v.: Collaterale Respiration. Zschr. Anat. Entwickl.-Gesch., *98*: 453, 1932.

AOKI, S.: Bronchial artery (in Japanese). Kokyu to Junkan, *2*: 259, 1954.

——: Pathological studies on the healing mechanism of the pulmonary tuberculosis (in Japanese). Kekkaku Shinryo, *6*: 319, 1954.

AOKI, S., YOSHIMURA, M. and HISADA, T.: Studies on the bronchus, bronchial artery and pulmonary artery using resin casts. Nihon Ishikai Zasshi, *32*: 695, 1954.

APPLETON, A.: Segments and blood vessels of the lung. Lancet, *2*: 592, 1944.

ARMSTRONG, J. B. und CUDKOWITZ, L.: Die pathologische Anatomie der Bronchialarterien. Erg. ges. Tuberk.- u. Lungen-Forsch., *14*: 191, 1958.

BERRY, J. L. and DALY, I. de B.: The relation between the pulmonary and bronchial vascular systems. Proc. Roy. Soc., S. B. London, *109*: 319, 1931.

BERRY, J. L., BRAILSFORD, J. F. and DALY I. de B.: The bronchial vascular system in the dog. Proc. Roy. Soc., *109* (B): 214, 1932.

BERRY, J. L.: The relation between bronchial and pulmonary circulations in human lung, investigated by radioopaque injections. J. Exp. Physiol., *24*: 305, 1935.

BJÖRK, V. O.: Circulation through an atelectatic lung in man. J. Thorac. Surg., *26*: 533, 1953.

BLOOMER, W. E., HARRISON, W., LINDSKOG, G. E. and LIEBOW, A. A.: Respiratory function and blood flow in the bronchial artery after ligation of pulmonary artery. Amer. J. Physiol., *157*: 317, 1949.

BOLT, W. und RINK, H.: Selektive Angiographie der Lungengefässe bei Lungentuberkulose. Schweiz. Zschr. Tuberk., *8*: 380, 1951.; *10*: 8, 1953.

BOLT, W. FORSSMANN, W. und RINK, H.: Selektive Lungenangiographie, Georg Thieme, Stuttgart, 1957.

BOLT, W.: Lungenangiographie. In: Handbuch der Tuberkulose, herausgegeben v. Hein, Kleinschmidt, u. Ühlinger, Georg Thieme, Stuttgart, 1957.

——: Lungenangiographie. Forschungsberichte des Landes Nordrhein-Westfalen, Nr. 1032, Köln, Opladen, 1961.

——: Lungenangiographie. Klinik der Lungenkrankheiten, herausgegeben v. Knipping u. Rink, Schattauer, Stuttgart, 1964.

BÜCHERL, E.: Über die Bronchialgefässe. Klin. Wschr. *30*: 961, 1952.

CALMETTE, A.: Tubercle Bacillus Infection and Tuberculosis in Man and in Animals. trans. by W. Soper, and G. Smith, 191, Baltimore, 1923.

CAMARRI, E. and MARINI, G.: La circulation bronchique. J. Fr. Méd. Chir. Thor. *20*: 191, 1966.

CAULDWELL, E. W., SICKERT, R. G., LININGER, R. S. and ANSON, B. J.: The bronchial arteries. An anatomic study of 150 human cadavers. Surg. Gynec. and Obst., *86*: 395, 1948.

CHRISTELLER, E.: Functionelles and anatomisches bei der angeborenen Verengerung und dem angeborenen Verschluss der Lungenarterie, insbesondere über die arteriellen Kollateralbahnen bei diesen Zuständen. Virchows Arch. *223*: 40, 1917.

CLARA, M.: Die arterio-venösen Anastomosen der Vögel und Säugetiere. Ergeb. Anat. u. Entw. Gesch., *27*: 249, 1927.

——: Die arterio-venösen Anastomosen. Springer, Wien, 1956.

CLARKE, J. A.: An X-ray microscopic study of the vasa vasorum of normal human pulmonary arteries. Thorax, *19*: 561, 1964.

——: An X-ray microscopic study of the postnatal development of the vasa vasorum in the pulmonary trunks and arteries. Thorax, *20*: 348, 1965.

COCKETT, F. B. and VASS, C. C. N.: A comparison of the role of the bronchial arteries in bronchiectasis and in experimental ligation of the pulmonary artery. Thorax, *6*: 268, 1951.

COHNHEIM, J. und LITTEN, M.: Über die Folgen der Embolie der Lungenarterien. Arch. Anat. Physiol., *65*: 99, 1875.

COLBERG, A.: 1863 and 1866, cit. from MILLER.

COLOMBUS, R.: 1559, cit. from MILLER.

CUDKOWICZ, L. and ARMSTRONG, J. B.: Observations on the normal anatomy of the bronchial arteries. Thorax, *6*: 343, 1951.

CUDKOWICZ, L.: Human Bronchial Circulation in Health and Disease. Williams and Wilkins, 1968.

DAS, M. M. and CHATTERJEE, B. P.: Bronchial arteries, pulmonary arteries and bronchopulmonary anastomoses. J. Indian Med. Ass., *53*: 325, 1969.

DELARUE, J.: Les dispositifs de la circulation artérielle bronchique et leur adaptations aux états pathologiques. J. Fr. Méd. Chir. Thor., *23*: 221, 1969.

EDWARDS, J. E.: Classification of pulmonary hypertension and anatomy of the postnatal and fetal pulmonary vascular bed. Pulmonary Circulation ed. by W. Adams and I. Veith, Grune and Stratton, New York·London, 1959.

ELLIS, F. E., GRINDLAY, J. H. and EDWARDS, J. E.: The bronchial arteries. Surg., *30*: 810, 1951.

FARRAR, J. F., BLOMFIELD, J. and REYE, R. D. K.: The structure and composition of the maturing pulmonary circulation. J. Path. Bact., *90*: 83, 1965.

FERENCZ, C. and GRECO, J.: A method for the three-dimensional study of pulmonary arteries. Dis. Chest, *57*: 428, 1970.

FEYRTER, F.: Über die pathologische Anatomie, der Lungenveränderungen beim Keuchhusten. Frankf. Zschr. Path., *35*: 213, 1927.

FLORANGE, W.: Anatomie und Pathologie der A. bronchialis. Ergebn. allg. Path. path. Anat., *39*: 151, 1960.

GALEN, C.: 1562, cit. from MILLER.

GHOREYEB, A. A. and KARSNER, H. T.: A study of the relation of pulmonary and bronchial circulations. J. Exp. Med., *18*: 500, 1913.

——: Veins of the Lungs. Medicina, Tomo IV, núm. 3, Salamanca, 1959.

HALES, S.: Statistical Essays. London, *2*: 66, 1733.

HALES, M. R. and LIEBOW, A. A.: Collateral circulation to the lungs in congenital pulmonic stenosis, Bull. Internat. A.M. Museums, *28*: 1, 1948.

HALL, H. L.: A study of the pulmonary circulation by the transillumination method. Amer. J. Physiol., *72*: 446, 1925.

HAYEK, H. v.: Über verschlussfähige Arterien in der menschliche Lunge. Anat. Anz., *89*: 216, 1939.

——: Über die Kurzschlusskreislauf. Zschr. Anat., *110*: 412, 1940.

——: Über die funktionelle Anatomie der Lungengefässe. Verh. dtsch. Ges. Kreisl. Forsch., *17*: 17, 1951.

HLASZ, N. A., HALLORAN, K. H. and LIEBOW, A. A.: Bronchial and arterial anomalies with drainage of the right lung into the inferior vena cava. Circulation, *14*: 826, 1956.

HURWITZ, A., CALABRESI, M., COOK, R. W. and LIEBOW, A. A.: An experimental study of the venous collateral circulation of the lung. Amer. J. Path., *30*: 1085, 1954.

INOUE, S.: Comparative anatomical studies on the bronchial vascular systems of the dog, goat and rabbit (in Japanese). Kyodai Kekken Kiyo, *7*: 263, 1959.

ISHIBASHI, Y.: Vascular system of the lungs (in Japanese). Saishin Igaku, *8*: 30, 1953.

——: Distribution of Pulmonary Blood Vessels. Kekkaku Shinsho XI, 1954.

JACKSON, C. L. and HUBER, J. F.: Correlated applied anatomy of the bronchial tree and lungs with a system of nomenclature. Dis. Chest, *9*: 319, 1943.

JOANNIDES, M.: The structure of the normal lung. A. M. A. Arch. Int. Med., *47*: 19, 1931.

JONES, E. L.: Quantitative histological study of the medical thickness of the pulmonary trunk and muscular pulmonary arteries in the velvet monkey. J. Path., *99*: 181, 1969.

KLINE, J. L., STERN, H., BLOOMER, W. E. and LIEBOW, A. A.: Application of induced bronchial collateral circulation to coronary arteries by cardiopneumonoplexy. I. Anatomical Observations. Amer. J. Path. *32*: 663, 1956.

KOBAYASHI, K., TONOMURA, S. and YAZAKI, J.: Cardiopulmonary angiography (in Japanese). Kekkaku Kenkyu no Shimpo, *27*: 329, 1959.

KONASCHKO, P. J.: Über Anastomosen zwischen der A. pulmonalis und der Aa. bronchiales. Zschr. Anat. Gesch., *78*: 136, 1926.

KOVÁTS, F. und ZSEBÖK, Z.: Röntgenanatomische Grundlagen der Lungenuntersuchung. Verlag der Ungarischen Akademie der Wissenschaften, Budapest, 1959.

KUBAT, H.: Systematische Anatomie der Lungengefässe. Fortschr. Röntgenstr., *53*: 178, 1936.

LAPP, H.: Beziehungen der Arteria bronchialis und pulmonalis. Verh. path. Ges., 1950; Verh. Ges. Kreisl. Forsch. 1951.

——: Über die Sperrarterien der Lunge und die Anatomosen Zwischen A. bronchialis und A. pulmonalis. Über ihre Bedeutung, insbesondere für die Entstehung des hämorrhagischen Infarktes. Frankf. Zschr. Path., *26*: 537, 1951.

LEE, G. de J. and DUBOIS, A. B.: Pulmonary capillary blood flow in man. J. Clin. Invest., *34*: 1380, 1955.

LEIBOW, A. A., HALES, M. R. and LINDSKOG, G. E.: Enlargement of the bronchial arteries, and their anastomoses with the pulmonary arteries in bronchiectasis. Amer. J. Path., *25*: 211, 1949.

LIEBOW, A. A., HALES, M. R., BLOOMER, W. E., HARRISON, W. and LINDSKOG, G. E.: Studies on the lung after ligation of the pulmonary artery. Amer. J. Path., *26*: 177, 1950.

LIEBOW, A. A., HALES, M. R., BLOOMER, W. E. and LINDSKOG, G. E.: The genesis of collateral circulation of the lung. Yale Journ. of Biol., *22*: 6, 1950.

LIEBOW, A. A., HALES, M. R. and BLOOMER, W. E.: Relation of bronchial to pulmonary vascular tree. In: "Pulmonary Circulation" ed. by W. ADAMS and I. Veith, Grune and Stratton, New York • London, 79, 1959.

MACGREGOR, R. G.: Examination of the pulmonary circulation with the microscope. J. Physiol., *80*: 65, 1934.

MANABE, S.: Distribution of the vascular system of the lung (in Japanese). Nihon Gekagakkai Zasshi, *51*: 6, 71, 1950–1951.

MARCHAND, P., GILGOY, J. C. and WILSON, V. H.: An anatomical study of the bronchial vascular system and its variation in disease. Thorax, *5*: 207, 1950.

MARCHETTIS, D. de: 1656, cit. from MILLER.

MATSUO, K.: Blood supply for the encapsulated caseous foci in the collapsed lung (in Japanese). Hai, *1*: 451, 1954.

MEESEN, H.: Zur pathologischen Anatomie des Lungenkreislaufs. Verh. dtsch. ges. Kreislauf., *17*: 25, 1951.

MERKEL, H.: Zur Histologie der Lungengefässe. Beitr. Path. Anat., *105*: 176, 1940–1941.

——: Zur Struktur und Funktion des Lungenkreislaufes. Zschr. Kreisl.-Forsch., *38*: 705, 1949.

MILLER, W. S.: The arrangement of the bronchial blood vessels. Anat. Anz., *28*: 432, 1906.

MILLOY, F. J., WRAGG, L. E. and ANSON, B. J.: The pulmonary arterial supply to the upper lobe of the left lung. Surg. Gynec. and Obst., *126*: 811, 1968.

MIYAKE, S.: Histological study of the pulmonary vascular system of the human fetus (in Japanese). Nihon Naibunpitsu Zasshi, *11*: 1381, 1937.

MIZUGUCHI, M.: Histological studies on the pulmonary blood vessels (in Japanese). Igaku Kenkyu, *22*: 60, 1952.

NAGAISHI, C.: Pulmonary circulation with reference to venous admixture. Jap. Circul. J., *20*: 1, 1956.

NAGAISHI, C. and YAMASHITA, M.: Vascular system of the lung. In: Nagaishi's monograph "The Structure of the Lung" Vol. I (in Japanese). Igaku Shoin Ltd., Tokyo, 1957.

NAGAISHI, C.: The structure of the vascular system of the lung. Relationship between pulmonary and bronchial vascular systems (in Japanese). Naika, *2*: 4, 1958.

NAKAMURA, T.: Pulmonary circulation in silicosis (in Japanese). Sogo Igaku, *12*: 469, 1955.

——: Bronchial blood vascular system (in Japanese). Kokyu to Junkan, *3*: 1, 1955.

——: Pulmonary circulation in silicosis. Jap. Circul. J., *19*: 513, 1956.

NAKAMURA, T. and TAKIZAWA, T.: Bronchial vascular system and pulmonary circulation (in Japanese). Saishin Igaku, *9*: 757, 1954.

NAKAMURA, T., TAKIZAWA, T. and KATORI, A.: Studies on Bronchial Vascular System (in Japanese). Igaku Shoin Ltd., Tokyo, 1958.

NAKATA, K., NAGAI, S., HARA, K. and SAKAEDA, T.: Microscopic observation on living mice organs by means of our unique transillumination. Nihon Byorigakkaishi, *43*: 615, 1954.

NAKAYAMA, Y.: Studies on the peripheral parts of the pulmonary blood vessels. Yokohama Shidai Kiyo, *22*: 1954.

NEWTON, T. H. and PREGER, L.: Selective bronchial angiography. Radiology, *84*: 1043, 1965.

OLIVEROS, G. L.: Arterias y venas pulmonares. Su relación con la anatomia bronquial segmentaria III. Supplemento Archivo Espanol de Morfologia, Valencia, 1951.

OMOCHI, SA. and JINNO, M.: Relation of the bronchial artery to the pulmonary artery (in Japanese). Osaka Igakukkai Zasshi, *36*: 661, 1937.

OUDET, P., REY, PH., MORAND, G., et al.: Les deux types dánastomoses artérielles bronchopulmonaires dans le poumon pathologique. J. Fr. Méd. Chir. Thor., *23*: 289, 1969.

PRUNE, D. M.: Lower accessory pulmonary artery with intralobar sequestration of lung. J. Path. Bact., *58*: 457, 1946.

PUMP, K. K.: The circulation in the peripheral parts of the human lung. Dis. Chest., *49*: 119, 1966.

RAMOS, J. G.: On the dynamics of the lung capillary circulation. Amer. Rev. Tbc., *71*: 822, 1955.

REISSEISEN, F. D.: 1808 and 1822, cit. from MILLER.

RÉMY, J., WALLAERT, C., et VOISIN, C.: Lártériographie bronchique sélective. Technique nouvelle d'investigation physiopathologique et diagnostic en pneumologie. Journ. Fr. Méd. Chir. Thor., *23*: 269, 1969.

REUCK, A. V. S. and O'CONNOR, M. (eds.): Ciba Foundation Symposium on Pulmonary Structure and Function. Little, Brown and Co., Boston, 1962.

RINK, H.: Lungenkreislauf und Lungenkollaps. Beitr. Klin. Tuberk., *110*: 79, 1953.

——: Arteriovenöse Anastomosen. In: "Lungenzirkulation" herausgegeben von H. Rink, Schattauer Verlag, Stuttgart·New York, 1970.

——: Lungenzirkulation: Ergebnisse angiographischer und szintigraphischer Untersuchungen. Schattauer, Stuttgart·New York, 1970.

ROBERTSON, B.: The normal intrapulmonary arterial pattern of the human late fetal and neonatal lung. A microangiographic and histologic study. Acta Paediat. Scand., *56*: 249, 1967.

——: The intrapulmonary arterial pattern in normal infancy and in transposition of the great arteries. Acta Paediat. Scand. Suppl., *184*: 1, 1, 1968.

ROEDER, T. and ROEDER, F.: Beobachtungen an Lungencapillaren. Zschr. ges. exp. Med., *80*: 540, 1932.

RUYSCH, F.: 1732. cit. from W. S. MILLER.

——: F.: 1721. cit. from ZUCKERKANDL.

SCHMIDT, M. B.: 1898. cit. from H. v. HAYEK.

SCHOBER, R.: Selektive Bronchialisangiographie. Fortschr. Röntgenstr., *101*: 337, 1964.

SHIOZAWA, M.: Segmental Resection. Vol. I and II, Bunkodo, Tokyo, 1954 and 1955.

SÖMMERING, S.: 1808. cit. from W. S. MILLER.

SPAIN, D. M.: Structural Effect on the Pulmonary Vascular Tree. In: "Pulmonary Circulation" ed. by W. Adams and I. Veith, Grune and Stratton, New York·London, 1959.

STAUB, N. C.: Microcirculation of the lung utilizing very rapid freezing. Angiology, *12*: 469, 1961.

TAKAHASHI, U.: Pathohistological studies on the pulmonary and bronchial vascular systems in pulmonary tuberculous lung (in Japanese). Kyodai Kekken Kiyo, *7*: 189, 1959.

TAKIZAWA, T.: Sperrartery and bronchial artery (in Japanese). Saishin Igaku, *10*: 2665, 1955.

——: Fundamental studies on collateral circulation of the lung (in Japanese). Nihon Jyunkanki Zasshi, *20*: 215, 1956.

TANAKA, M.: On the bronchial artery (in Japanese). HAI, *1*: 504, 1954.

——: Studies on bronchial artery (in Japanese). Hiroshima Igaku *7*: 77, 1954.

TOBIN, C. E.: The bronchial arteries and their connections with other vessels in the human lung. Surg. Gynec. Obst., *95*: 741, 1952.

——: Arteriovenous shunts in the peripheral pulmonary circulation in the human lung. Thorax, *21*: 197, 1966.

TÖNDURY, G. und WEIBEL, E. R.: Anatomie der Lungengefässe. Ergeb. ges. Tuberk.- Lung. Forsch., *14*: 60, 1958.

UCHINO, F.: Morphological studies on pulmonary vascular system (in Japanese). Nihon Byori Gakkai Zasshi, *44*: 229, 1955.

VÁZQUEZ V., E.: Circulation bronchial. Modifications consecutivas a la ligadura unilateral de la arteria y venas pulmonares. Neumol. Cir. Tórax, *25*: 321, 1964.

VERLOOP, M. C.: The arteria bronchiales and their anastomoses with the arteria pulmonalis in the human lung. Acta Anat., *5*: 171, 1948.

——: Arteriae bronchiales and their anastomosis with the arteria pulmonalis in the human lung. A microanatomical study. Acta Anat., *5*: 171, 1958.

VIDONE, R. A. and LIEBOW, A. A.: Anatomical and functional studies of the lung deprived of pulmonary arteries and veins, with an application in the therapy of transposition of the great vessels. Amer. J. Path., *3*: 539, 1957.

WAGENVOORT, C. A. and WAGENVOORT, N.: Age changes in muscular pulmonary arteries. Arch. path., *79*: 524, 1965.

WATANABE, K.: Microscopic observation of the peripheral portion of the pulmonary vascular system in living animals (in Japanese). Kyodai Kekken Kiyo, *7*: 243, 1959.

WATZKA, M.: Über Gefässsperren und arteriovenöse Anastomosen. Zschr. mikr.- anat. Forsch., *39*: 521, 1936.

WEIBEL, E. R.: Morphometry of the Human Lung. Springer, Berlin·Göttingen·Heidelberg, 1963.

WOOD, D. A. and MILLER, M.: The role of the dual pulmonary circulation in various pathologic conditions of the lung. J. Thorac. Surg., *7*: 49, 1938.

WRIGHT, R. D.: The blood supply of abnormal tissues in the lungs. J. Path. Bact., *47*: 489, 1938.

WYATT, J. P., BURKE, D. R. and HANLON, C. R.: Morphologic study of canine lungs after ligation of the pulmonary veins. Amer. J. Path., *29*: 291, 1953.

YAMASHITA, H.: Studies on pulmonary segments (in Japanese). Kyobu Geka, *8*: 6, 1951.

YAMASHITA, H. and ISHIKAWA, E.: Pulmonary segments. Kekkaku Kenkyu no Shimpo, *5*: 3, 1954; *6*: 10, 1954.

YAMASHITA, M. and NAGAISHI, C.: Studies on bronchial vascular system. Its relation to pulmonary vascular system (in Japanese). Hai, *1*: 458, 1954; *1*: 476, 1954.

YAMASHITA, M. and NAGASAWA, N.: Studies on the genesis of bronchiectasis, with reference to the ligation of pulmonary and bronchial arteries (in Japanese). Nihon Kyobugeka Gakkai Zasshi, *2*:

YAZAKI, J.: Selective angiography of the segmental arteries (in Japanese). Kyodai Kekken Kiyo, *7*: 160, 1959.

ZIMMERMAN, K.: Der feinere Bau der Blutkapillaren. Zsch. Anat. Entwickl.-Gesch., *68*: 29, 1923.

ZUCKERKANDL, E.: 1881. cit. from W. S. MILLER.

——: 1883. cit. from W. S. MILLER.

LYMPHATIC SYSTEM

AKIYAMA, T.: Histo-embryological study of the lung of a human fetus (in Japanese). Handai Igakkai Zasshi, *4*: 309, and *4*: 315, 1952.

ALBERTS-SCHÖNBERG: Die Röntgendiagnostik. Hamburg, 1919.

ALTSCHULE, M.: Acute Pulmonary Edema. Grune and Stratton, New York, 1954.

AMANO, S.: Tuberculosis, its Phases and Structure. Nagai Publisher, Osaka, 1947.

ANEZYRIS, N., SAWAS-DIMOPOULOU, C., DONTAS, N. and SAMARAS, V.: Thoracic lymph node scintiscan as a diagnostic test in mediastinal malignant enlargement. Dis. Chest., *59*: 372, 1971.

ARCHBALD, E. and BROWN, A. L.: Dangers of introducing iodized oil into the tracheobronchial system. J.A.M.A., *88*: 1310, 1927.

ARNOLD, E. and BROWN, A. L.: Dangers of introducing iodized oil into the tracheobronchial system. J.A.M.A., *88*: 1310, 1927.

ARNOLD, J.: Über das Vorkommen lymphatisches Gewebes in der Lungen. Virchows Arch. Anat. path. Anat., *80*: 315 and 326, 1880.

——: Untersuchung über Staubinhalation und Staubmetastase. Leipzig, 1888.

ASCHOFF, L.: Die lymphatischen Organe. Med. klin. Beih. *1*: 1926.

——: Über die lymphatischen Organe. Verh. anat. Ges., *46*: 152, 1938.

BALTISBERGER, W.: Glatte Muskulatur der menschlichen Lunge. Zschr. Anat., *61*: 249, 1921.

BARTELS, P.: Das Lymphgefässsystem. In: Bardelebens Handbuch d. Anatomie, Bd. 3, Fischer, Jena, 1909.

BAUM, H.: Das Lymphgefässsystem. In: Bardelebens Handbuch d. Anatomie. Bd. 3, G. Fischer, Jena, 1909.

——: Das Lymphgefässsystem des Rindes. Berlin, 1912.

——: Das Lymphgefässsystem des Hundes. A. Hirschwald, Berlin, 1918.

——: Die Lymphgefässe des Pferdes, Rindes, Hundes und Schweins. Zschr. Anat. u. Entwickl. *78*: 714, 1926.

BEITZKE, H.: Über lymphogene Staubverschleppung. Virchows Arch., *254*: 625, 1925.

BERG, H. F., CHRISTOPHEREN, W. M., ISAACS, A. M. and BRYANT, J. R.: Localization of radioactivity in regional lymph nodes. Arch. Surg., *67*: 228, 1953.

BERNARD, C.: Leçons sur le effets des substances toxiques et medicamenteuses., Paris, 1857.

BESREDKA, A.: Infection et vaccination par voie tracheale. Ann. de l'Inst. Pasteur, *34*: 361, 1920.

——: Láction des sérums par la voie respiratoire, Ann. de l'Inst., Pasteur, *34*: 51, 1920.

BOKU, S.: Genesis of lymphaticus in rabbits (in Japanese). cit. from Kihara's Genesis and development of lymphoid tissues. Ketsuekigaku Togikai Hokoku, *6*: 1, 1954.

BORCHARDT, H.: Über die Einatmung verschiedener Kohlenstaubarten. Virchows Arch., *271*: 366, 1929.

BRYANT, J. R., BERG, H. F. and CHRISTOPHERSEN, W. M.: Localization of radioactivity in lung and lymph nodes. J. Thorac. Surg., *26*: 221, 1953.

BURDON-SANDERSON, J.: Recent researches in tuberculosis. Edinburgh Med. J., *15*: 1, 1870.

CHARLETON, H.: Pulmonary lesions produced by the inhalation of dust. J. Hygiene, *22*: 1924.

COLIN, G.: Traité de physiologie comparée des animaux. 2 ed. Vol. 2, J-B. Bailliére et Fils, Paris, 1873.

CORNET, G.: Die Tuberkulose. Wien, 1907.

COURTICE, F. C. and SIMMONDS, W. J.: Absorption from the lungs. J. Physiol., *109*: 103, 1949.

COURTICE, F. C. and PHIPPS, P. J.: The absorption of fluid from the lungs. J. Physiol., *105*: 186, 1946.

CRUIKSHANK, W.: The Anatomy of the Absorbing Vessels of the Human Body., London, 1970.

CUNNINGHAM, R. S.: On the development of the lymphatics in the lungs of the pig. Contrib. to Embryol., *4*: 45, 1916.

D'AUNOY, R.: Antibody production after intratracheal injection of antigen. J. Inf. Dis., *30*: 347, 1922.

DRINKER, C. K. and FIELD, M. E.: Lymphaticus, Lymph and Tissue Fluid. Williams and Wilkins Co., Baltimore, 1933.

DRINKER, C. K., WARREN, M. F. and MACHANAHAN, M.: The absorption of protein solution from the pulmonary alveoli. J. Exp. Med., *66*: 449, 1937.

DRINKER, C. B. and YOFFY, J. M.: Lymphatics, Lymph and Lymphoid Tissue. Harvard Univ. Press, Cambridge, 1941.

DRINKER, C. K.: Pulmonary Edema and Inflammation. Harvard Univ. Press, Cambridge, 1945.

DRINKER, C. K. and HARDENBERG, E.: Absorption from the pulmonary alveoli. J. Exp. Med., *86*: 7, 1947.

DRINKER, C. K. and FIELD, M. E.: Pulmonary Edema. Harvard Univ. Press, Cambridge, 1950.

EBNER, V. v.: In: Köllikers Handbuch der Gewebslehre des Menschen. 6 ed. *3*: 304, 1899.

——: Von der Respirationsorgane. In: Köllikers Handbuch der Gewebslehre des Menschen, 7 Aufl., W. Engelmann, Leipzig, 1902.

ENGEL, J.: 1859. cit. from W. S. MILLER.

ENGEL, S.: Die Topographie der bronchialen Lymphknoten und ihre präparatorische Darstellung. Beitr. Klin. Tbk., *64*: 468, 1926.

——: The origin of the pulmonary lymph system. Acta anat. (Basel) *29*: 229, 1957.

FLEINER, W.: Resorption d. corpusculäre Elemente durch Lunge und Pleura. Virchows Arch., *112*: 97, 1888.

FLINT, G. J.: The development of the lungs. Amer. J. Anat., *6*: 1, 1906.

FOX, J. P.: The permeability of the lungs to antibiotics. J. Immnol., *31*: 7, 1936.

FRANKE, F.: Über die Lymphgefässe der Lunge, zugleich ein Beitrag zur Erklärung der Baucherscheinung bei Pneumonie. Dtsch. Zschr., *119*: 107, 1912.

FRANKENHÄUSER, K.: Tracheobronchialschleimhaut. Diss. Dorpat, 1879.

FUJIMOTO, B.: Zur Behandlung der Lungentuberkulose durch Kalkinhalation. Dtsch. med. Wschr. 51 Jahng., *50*: 2072, 1925.

GEROTA, D.: Zur Technik der Lymphgefässinjection. Eine neue Injectionsmasse der Lymphgefässe. Polychrome Injection. Anat. Anz., *12*: 216, 1896.

GHON, A.: Der primäre Lungenherd bei Tuberkulose der Kinder. Berlin u. Wien, 1912.

GHON, A. and POTOTSCHNIG, G.: Über den Unterschied im pathologisch-anatomischen primär Lungen und primär Darminfektion bei der Tuberkulose der Kinder. Beitr. kl. Tbk., *40*: 87, 1919.

GILLIAN, L. A. and COCKLIN, R. E.: Removal of foreign substances by the lymphaticus of the snake lung. Amer. J. Physiol., *123*: 598, 1938.

GRAY, H.: Anatomy of the human body. 25th ed., C. Mayo Goss, Philadelphia, 1948.

GROSS, F.: Über die alveoläre Reaktion der Lunge gegenüber Russ, Quarzstaub und Tuberkelbazillen und die hier herrschenden Lokalisationsgesetze. Ztschr. path. Anat. u. allg. Path., *76*: 374, 1927.

GUIEYSSE-PELLISSIER, A.: Modification et lesions de céllules epithéliales pulmonaires dues aux gaz suffocants. Compt. rend. Acad. Soc., Paris, *170*: 1411, 1920.

HAGIHARA, H.: Genesis of lymph in the lung, and distribution and structure of the pulmonary lymphaticus (in Japanese). Hiroshima Igaku, *4*: 110, 1951.

HAGIHARA, T.: Absorption of the substances through the wall of respiratory system. Igaku no Ayumi, *68*: 498, 1969.

HARVEY, D. F. and ZIMMERMAN, H. M.: Studies on the development of human lung. I. The pulmonary lymphatics. Anat. Rec., *61*: 203, 1935.

HASE, H.: Lymphapparatus in human lungs (in Japanese). Osaka Jyoshiidai Zasshi, *2*: 11, 1948.

HAYEK, H. v.: Periarterielle Lymphräume. Anat. Anz., *89*: 209, 1940.

——: The human lung (Übersetzung und Erweiterung des Buches), New York, Hafner Publ. Co., 1960.

HELLER, A. und SCHRÖTTER, v.: Die Carina Tracheae. Denkschr. d. math.-naturus. Kl. d. Kais. Akad. d. Wissensch., *64*: 1897.

HELLMANN, T.: Das Lymphgefässe, Lymphknötchen und Lymphknoten. In: Möllendorfs Handbuch d. mikrosk. Anat. d. Menschen, VI/I, Springer, Berlin, 1930.

——: Lymphknoten. In: Möllendorfs Handbuch d. mikrosk. Anat., Bd. II, Teil 1, 1936.

HEUBNER, W.: Über Inhalation zerstäubter Flüssigkeiten. Zschr. ges. exp. Med., *10*: 267, 1920.

HEUER, G.: The development of lymphatics in the small intestine of the pig. Amer. J. Anat., *9*: 93, 1909.

HIRAKAWA, K.: Experimental studies on resorption, secretion and excretion. On the permeability of the alveoli of the lung (I–II). Acta schol. Med. Univ. Kioto, *8*: 197, 1925 and *8*: 279, 1925.

HORII, I.: The structure of the lymph node (in Japanese). Ketsuekitogikai Hokoku, *6*: 45, 1954.

HORII, I. and TAMAKI, Y.: Studies on the Lymphocytes. Rinshoigaku Bunko 125, Nihonigaku Shuppan Ltd., Tokyo·Kyoto, 1951.

HUNTINGTON, G. S. and MACCLURE, C.: The anatomy and development of the jugular lymph sac in the domestic cat. Amer. J. Anat., *10*: 177, 1910.

INS, A. v.: Einige Bemerkungen über das Verhalten des inhalierten Staubes in den Lungen. Virchows Arch., *73*: 151, 1878.

ITO, H.: Zur operativen Behandlung der Perikostaltuberkulose. Dtsch. Zschr. Chir., *185*: 124, 1924.

ITO, W., SEKI, I. und NAKAZAWA, F.: Studien über den kolloidosmotischen Druck des Blutes bei normalen und pathologischen Zuständen. Tohoku J. Exp. Med., *14*: 254, 1929.

IWASE, K.: Experimental and clinical studies of the intrabronchial insufflation of chemotherapeutic agents using P^{32} and C^{14} labelled IHMS as tracers (in Japanese). Kyodai Kekken Kiyo, *7*: 146, 1959.

JONES, F. E.: The permeability of the lining of lower respiratory tract for antibodies. J. Exp. Med., *40*: 73, 1924.

——: The effects of the intrabronchial administration of foreign serum. J. Exp. Med., *40*: 63, 1924.

JOSSIFOW, G. W.: Das Lymphgefässsystem des Menschen. G. Fischer, Jena, 1930.

KAMPMEIER, O. F.: The distribution of valves and the first appearance of definite direction in the drainage of lymph in the human lung. Amer. Rev. Tbc., *81*: 360, 1928.

KAWAHARA, M.: Über die Durchlässigkeit der Wirbeltierlunge für corpusculäre Elemente. Pflügers Arch. ges. Physiol., *206*: 352, 1924.

KIHARA, T.: Lymphatics of the lung and the pleura (in Japanese). Kyoto Igakkai Zasshi, *26* (6): 18, 1924.

KIHARA, T. and TESHIMA, G.: Das Lymphgefässsystem des Shimpansen. Folia Anat. Japonica., *13*: 33, 1935.

KIHARA, T.: Das extravaskuläre Saftbahnensystem (in Japanese). Ketsueki Togikai Hokoku, *3*: 118, 1950.

——: Distribution and development of lymphoid tissues (in Japanese). Ketsuekigaku Togikai Hokoku, *6*: 1, 1954.

——: Das Extravaskuläre Saftbahnensystem. Okajimas Folia Anat. Japonica, *28*: 601, 1956.

——: Das tiefe Lymphgefässsystem der Japaner. Zschr. Dtsch.-Japanisches Kulturinstitute Kyoto, 1963.

KIHARA, T., Jr.: Study on reticulum fibers. Kyodai Kaibogaku II Ronbunchu, 1953.

KITA, R.: Clinical Pathology of Pulmonary Tuberculosis (in Japanese). Bunkodo, Tokyo, 1953.

KLEIN, E.: The Anatomy of the Lymphatic System. Vol. II, London, 1875.

KNAUFF, H.: Das Pigment der Respirationsorgane, Virchows Arch., *39*: 442, 1867.

KÖLLIKER, A.: Mikroskopische Anatomie od. Gewebslehre d. Menschen., Leipzig, 1854.

KRAUSE, A. K.: The localization of tuberculous infection in the rabbit, with particular reference to that in the lungs. Amer. Rev. Tbc., *14*: 243, 1926.

KUTSUNA, M.: Die Lymphgefässe in der Lunge. Folia Anat. Japonica, *13*: 385, 1935.

KÜTTNER, C.: Die Abscheidung des indigo-schwefelsäuren Natrons in die Gewebe der Lunge. Zbl. med. Wissensch., *42*: 816, 1875.

KYLIN, E.: Studien über den kolloidosmotischen Druck. Arch. exp. Path. Pharmakol., *161*: 91, 1931.

LAQUEUR, E.: Über künstlich erzeugtes (osmotisches) Lungenödem und über Resorption in der Lunge. Münch. Med. Wschr. Jahrg., *43*: 1221, 1919.

LAQUEUR, E. and MAGNUS, R.: Über Kampfgasvergiftungen. V. Experimentalle und theoretische Grundlagen zur Therapie der Phosgenerkrankung. Zschr. ges. exp. Med., *13*: 200, 1921.

LEEDS, S. E., UHLEY, H. N., SAMPSON, J. J., et al: A new method for measurement of lymph flow from the right duct in the dog. Amer. J. Surg., *98*: 211, 1959.

LEEDS, S. E., REICH, S., UHLEY, H. N., SAMPSON, J. J. and FRIEDMAN, M.: The pulmonary lymph flow after irradiation of the lungs of dogs. Dis. Chest, *59*: 203, 1971.

LEVADITI, C.: Ectodermoses neurotropes., Paris, 1922.

LEWIS, F. T.: The development of the lymphatic system in rabbits. Amer. J. Anat., *5*: 95, 1905.

LUBENEAU, C.: Experimentelle Staubinhalationskrankheit der Lungen. Arch. Hygiene, *63*: 391, 1907.

LÜDERS, C.: Über das Vorkommen von subpleuralen Lymphdrüse. Dissert., Kiel, 1892.

MAGNUS, G.: Die Darstellung der Lymphwurzeln in menschlichen und tierischen Geweben, ihr Verhalten im serösen Häuten und ihre Bedeutung für deren Pathologie. Dtsch. Zschr. Chir., *175*: 138, 1922.

MARASCHIO, P.: Lymphgefässe der Lunge. Anat. Anz., *90*, 1940.

MASCAGNI, P.: 1787, cit. from W. S. MILLER.

MATHIS, M. E., HOLMAN, E. and REICHERT, F. L.: A study of the bronchial, pulmonary and lymphatic circulations in the lungs under various pathologic conditions experimentally produced. J. Thorac. Surg., *1*: 339, 1932.

MAXIMOW, A. A. and BLOOM, W.: A Textbook of Histology. 6th ed. W. B. Sanders Co., Philadelphia and Boston, 1952.

MENEELY, G. R.: Transbronchial inhalation of radioactive gold colloid in lung of dog, distribution studies, servival and pathology. Amer. J. Med. Sc., *225*: 172, 1953.

MENKES, B.: Röntgendarstellung der Blut-und Lymphgefässe an der Leiche und an Lebenden Mittels Umbrather und Throtrast. Fortschr. a. d. G. d. Röntgenstr., *46*: 571, 1932.

MERKEL, F.: Atmungsorgane. In: Bardelebens Handbuch der Anatomie des Menschen. Bd. 6, Jena, 1902.

MILLER, W. S.: The distribution of lymphoid tissue in the lung. Anat. Rec., *5*: 99, 1911.

MORI, K.: Running direction and valve of pulmonary lymphatics originated in bronchial wall, and their relation with subpleural lymphatics (in Japanese). Kyoto Igakkai Zasshi, *37*: 1851, 1940.

MORIWAKI, H.: Histological study of lymphatic system in man. IV. (in Japanese). Kyoto Igakkai Zasshi, *40*: 1510, 1943.

MOST, A.: Die Topographie des Lymphgefässapparates d. menschlich. Körpers. Biblioth. med. Abt. C., 1908.

MUNKA, V.: Das Lymphgefässsystem der Lungen vom Standpunkt ihrer Segmentstruktur. Biologické Práce. Biol. Arbeiten des wiss. Kollegium f. Biologie d. Slow. Akad. d. Wiss. IX/4, 1963.

NAGAISHI, C. and OKADA, Y.: Topographic-anatomy and nomenclature of the hilar lymph nodes (in Japanese). Nihon Rinsho Kekkaku, *16*: 723, 1957.

——: Lymphatic system of the lung. In: Nagaishi's monograph "The Structure of the Lung" Vol. II (in Japanese). Igaku Shoin Ltd., Tokyo, 1958.

——: Relations between the structure of the lymph vessels of the lung and the genesis and development of some pulmonary diseases. Transactions of the Vth Inte. Congr. Dis. Chest, Tokyo, 430, 1958.

NAGAISHI, C.: Some problems on fine structure of the lung, Saishin Igaku, *14*: 12, 1959.

NAGAISHI, C. and OKADA, Y.: Some problems on lymphatogenous metastasis of lung cancer (in Japanese). Nihon Kyoburinsho, *24*: 397, 1965.

NAGASAWA, N., YAMASHITA, M., OKADA, Y. and INABA, N.: Some problems on the structure of the pleura. (in Japanese), Hai, *2*: 111, 1955.

NISHIKAWA, T.: Fate of the inhaled charcoal powder (in Japanese). Kyoto Igakkai Zasshi, *37*: 1779, 1940.

——: Structure, distribution and significance of the pulmonary lymphoid tissues (in Japanese). Kyoto Igakkai Zasshi, *37*: 1497, 1940.

——: Absorption of coaldust from the respiratory tract in rabbits suffering from pneumonia (in Japanese). Kyoto Igakkai Zasshi, *38*: 194, 1941.

NOTHNAGEL, H.: Zur Resorption des Blutes aus dem Bronchialbaum. Virchows Arch., *71*: 414, 1877.

OGO, M.: Characteristics of the subpleural lymphatics (in Japanese). Nihon Gekahokan, *11*: 1091, 1934.

——: Über das Vorkommens von lymphatischen Gewebe unter der Lungenpleura des Menschen. Folia Anat. Japonica, *8*: 325, 1935.

OKA, H.: Supplementary reports on primary complex in pulmonary tuberculosis (in Japanese). Tokyo Igakkai Zasshi, *43*: 208, 1929.

OKADA, Y., SAGAWA, Y., NAKA, T., WATANABE, K., et al.: Microscopic and electron microscopic observation of experimentally produced pulmonary edema. Kokyu to Jyunkan, *6*: 201, 1958.

OKADA, Y. and NAGAISHI, C.: Studies on the structure of the pulmonary lymphatics (in Japanese). Kekkaku Kenkyu no Shimpo, *24*: 365, 1959.

OPPEL, A.: Atmungsapparat. In: Lehrbuch d. vergl. mikr. Anatomie, 6 T., Jena, 1905.

OTANI, T. and TAKAWA, O.: The demeanour of intrapulmonary lymphaticus to the infection of whooping cough bacilli. Kyoto Igakkai Zasshi, *40*: 794, 1943.

OTANI, T. and ARISHIGE, Y.: Study of age difference of lymphatics (in Japanese). Nisshin Igaku, *39*: 233, 1952.

OTTAVIANI, G.: Ricerche anatomiche sui vasi linfatici el polmone umano. Morph. Jahrb., *82*: 453, 1938.

PARFENOVA, J. P.: The lymphatic network within the limits of the pulmonary lobules. Doklad An (USSR), *72*: 613, 1590.

PEIPER, E.: Über die Resorption durch die Lungen. Zsch. klin. Med., *8*: 293, 1884.

PERL, L. and LIPMAN, H.: Experimenteller Beitrag zur Lehre von der Lungenblutung. Virchows Arch. Path. Anat., Physiol. u. kl. Med., *51*: 552, 1870.

PERNKOPF. E.: Topographische Anatomie., Wien, 1937.

POLICARD, A.: Sur quelques caractéres histophysiologiques des formation lymphoides bronchiques. Bull. Histol. Appl., *27*: 118, 1950.

——: Le poumen. 2 éd., Massen and Cie, Paris, 1955.

PUMP, K. K.: The circulation in the peripheral

parts of the human lung. Dis. Chest, *49*: 119, 1966.

——: Lymphatics of the human pulmonary alveoli. Preliminary report. Dis. Chest, *58*: 140, 1970.

QUALLS, G., CURTIS, H. J. and MENEELY, G. R.: Rate of uptake of fluid from lung measured with radioisotopes. Comparison of rapid rate for water with slower rate for saline. Amer. J. Physiol., *172*: 22, 1953.

RANKE, K. E.: Primäraffekt, sekundäre u. tertiäre Stadien der Lungentuberkulose, auf Grund von histologischen Untersuchung der Lymphdrüsen der Lungenpforte. Dtsch. Arch. kl. Med., *119*: 201, 297 u. *129*: 224, 1916.

RANVIER, L.: Morphologie et dévelopment des vaisseau lymphatique chez les mammiféres. Arch. d'Anat. Microsc., *1*: 69, 1897.

RICH, A. R.: The Pathogenesis of Tuberculosis., C. C. Thomas, Springfield, 1951.

ROSENTHAL, D. S. and WEG, J. G.: Intrapulmonary lymph node presenting as a solitary pulmonary nodule. Dis. Chest, *51*: 336, 1967.

ROUVIÉRE, H.: Anatomie der lymphatiques de l'homme., Masson et Cie, Paris, 1932.

——: Anatomy of the Human Lymphatic System., Edwards Brothers Inc., Michigan, 1938.

RUDBECK, O.: 1653. cit. from W. S. MILLER.

RUPPER, H.: Experimentelle Untersuchung über Kohlenstaubinhalation. Virchows Arch., *72*: 14, 1878.

SABIN, F. R.: The lymphatic system in human embryos, with a consideration of the morphology of the system as a whole. Amer. J. Anat., *9*: 43, 1909.

——: Der Ursprung und die Entwicklung des Lymphgefässsystems. Erg. Anat. Entwickl., *21*: 1, 1913.

SAGAWA, Y., YOKOYAMA, T. and IWATA, A.: Pulmonary circulation in pulmonary tuberculosis (in Japanese). Kekkaku Kenkyu no Shimpo, *9*: 81, 1955.

SAGAWA, Y.: Pathogenesis of acute pulmonary edema in pulmonary surgery (in Japanese). Nihon Kyobugekagakkai Zasshi, *6*: 569, 1958.

——: Studies on pulmonary edema using rapid freezing method (in Japanese). Kyobu Shikkan, *8*: 1186, 1964.

SAGE, H. H. and GOZUN, B. V.: Lymphatic scintigrams. Cancer, *11*: 200, 1958.

SAGE, H. H., KIZILAY, D. and MIYAZAKI, M.: Lymph node scintigrams. Amer. J. Roentgenol., *84*: 666, 1960.

SAKAMOTO, S.: Studies of the caseous pneumonia by means of vital staining (in Japanese). Osaka Igakkai Zasshi, *16*: 201, 1916.

SAPPEY, P. C.: Anatomie, physiologie, pathologie des vaisseaux lymphatiques concidérés chez l'homme et les vertébrés. Adrien Delahaye, Paris, 1874.

——: Traité d'anatomie des criptive., Paris, 1888.

SASAMOTO, H.: Pulmonary circulation. Sogo Igaku, *9*: 524, 1952.

SCHAFFER, J.: Lehrbuch der Histologie., Leipzig, 1933.

SCHOTTELIUS, M.: Experimentelle Untersuchungen über die Wirkung inhalierter Substanzen. Virchows Arch., *73*: 524, 1878.

SCHULZ, R. Z., WARREN, M. F. and DRINKER, C. K.: The passage of rabbit virulent type III pneumococci from the respiratory tract of rabbits into the lymphatics and blood. J. Exp. Med., *68*: 251, 1938.

SCHWARZ, P.: Einbrüche tuberkulösen Lymphknoten in das Bronchialsystem und ihre pathologische Bedeutung. Beitr. kl. Tbk., *103*: 182, 1950.

——: The role of the lymphatics, in the development of bronchogenic tuberculosis. Amer. Rev. Tbc., *67*: 440, 1953.

SEHRWALD, E.: Über die percutane Injection von Flüssigkeiten in die Trachea, deren Verbreitung in der Lunge und Wirkung auf Lunge und Gesammtorganismus. Dtsch. Arch. kl. Med., *39*: 162, 1886.

SENDA, Y.: Electron microscopic studies on the structure of the bronchoalveolar system and the absorption of solid particles or tubercle bacilli via respiratory tract (in Japanese). Nihon Geka Hokan, *6*: 1433, 1958.

SEWELL, W. T.: The phagocytotic properties of the alveolar cells of the lung. J. Path. and Bact., *22*: 40, 1918.

SHDANOW, D. A.: Röntgenologische Untersuchungen des Lymphgfässsystem des Menschen und der Tiere. Fortschr. a. d. G. d. Röntgenstr., *46*: 680, 1932.

——: Die Kollaterallymphwege der Brusthöhle des Menschen. Anat. Anz. *82*: 417, 1936.

SHESTOPAL, A.: Über die Durchlössigkeit der Froschlunge für gelöste und körnige Farbstoffe. Virchows Arch., *75*: 199, 1879.

SHIDA, T.: Distribution of lymph nodes in chest (in Japanese). Nagasaki Igakkai Zasshi, *10*: 317, 1932.

SHIMAZAKI, H.: Anatomical study of the lymphatic system in chest (in Japanese). Kaibogaku Zasshi, *4*: 786, 1931.

SICARD, J. A. et FORESTIER, J.: Methods générale d'exploration radiologique par l'huile iodée (Lipiodol), Bull. et. Mée. Soc. méd. hôp. Paris, *46*: 463, 1922.

SIKORSKY, J.: Über die Lymphgefässe der Lungen. Zbl. med. Wissensch., *8*: 817, 1870.

SIMER, P. H.: Drainage of pleural lymphatics. Anat. Rec., *113*: 269, 1952.

SLAVJANSKY, K.: Experimentelle Beiträge zur Pneumokoniosis-Lehre. Virchows Arch. path. Anat. Physiol. and kl. Med., *48*: 326, 1869.

SOMMERBRODT, J.: Hat das in die Luftwege ergossene Blut ätiologische Bedeutung für die Lungenschwindsucht? Virchows Arch. path. Anat. Physiol. and kl. Med., *55*: 165, 1872.

SOYKA, J.: Über die Wanderung corpusculärer Elemente im Organism. 3 Jahrg., 25: 247, 1878.

STAUB, N. C. and STOREY, W. F.: Relation between morphological and physiological events in the lung studied by rapid freezing. J. Appl. Physiol., *17*: 381, 1962.

STEELE, J. D.: The Solitary Pulmonary Nodule. C. C. Thomas, Springfield, 1964.

STEINERT, R.: Untersuchungen über das Lymphsystem der Lunge, zugleich ein Beitrag zur Frage der Topographie der bronchialen Lymphknoten. Beitr. kl. Tbk., *68*: 497, 1928.

Sternberg, C.: Lymphknoten. In: Handbuch der pathologischen Anatomie, Bd. I Abt. 1, 13,1926.

Stöhr, Ph. and Kölliker, A.: Zur Kenntnis des Baues der Lunge des Menschen. Verhandl. d phys. med. Gesell. zu Würzburg, 1881.

Stöhr, Ph. Jr.: Lehrbuch der Histologie und der mikroskopische Anatomie des Menschen. Gustav Fischer, Jena, 1951.

Sukiennikow, W.: Topographische Anatomie der bronchialen und trachealen Lymphdrüsen. Berl. klin. Wschr., *40*: 316, 347, 369, 1903.

Suzuki, T.: Intratracheal insufflation of antigen (in Japanese). Eiseigaku-Densenbyogaku Zasshi, *18*: 62, 1932.

Taplin, G. V., et al.: Pulmonary distribution of radioactive particles in rabbits after inhalation and intravenous injection. Ann. Allergy, *9*: 703 and 726, 1951.

Tasaka, S.: Problems on intravenous catheterisation and pulmonary circulation. Kokyu to Junkan, *1*: 3, 1953.

Tei, J. (Chung, Ch.-M.): Absorption of corpuscular elements through the peritoneum (in Japanese). Kyoto Igaku Zasshi, *34*: 541, 636, 697, 1937.

——: Die Stomata auf der peritonealen Fläche des Zwerchfells und ihre Beziehung zu den Lymphgefässen. Nihon Geka Hokan, *14*: 876, 1937.

Teshima, G.: Das Lymphgefässsystem des Macacus. Folia Anat. Japonica, *13*: 251, 1935.

——: Phenomena in lymphatics caused by the absorption of foreign bodies into the peritoneum (in Japanese). Nihon Geka Hokan, *9*: 585,, 1932.

——: Das Lymphgefässsystem des Lemurs. Folia Anat. Japonica, *13*: 289, 1935.

Tobin, C. E.: Lymphatics of the pulmonary alveoli. Anat. Rec., *120*: 625, 1954.

——: Human pulmonic lymphatics. An anatomic study. Anat. Rec., *127*: 611, 1957.

——: Pulmonary lymphatics with reference to emphysema. Amer. Rev. Res. Dis., *80*: 50, 1959.

Toldt, C.: Atmungsapparat, In: Lehrbuch der Gewebslehre, 3 Aufl., Stuttgart, 1888.

Tomita, T.: Epitheloid cells in the alveolar space (in Japanese). Osaka Igakkai Zasshi, *17*: 747, 1918.

Torii, T.: Anatomical studies of the pulmonary and bronchial lymphatic systems (in Japanese). Jyuzenkai Zasshi, *36*: 381, 1931.

Trivelim, A. and Rossi, R.: Scintigraphic technique to evaluate the lymphatic drainage of normal and neoplastic breast. Int. Contra Cancrum, *20*: 1834, 1969.

Turner, W.: An Introduction to Human Anatomy. Part 2, Edinburgh, 1877.

Umeda, S.: Anatomical studies on the lymphatic system of the lung (in Japanese). Kekkaku, *7*: 705, 1929.

Walske, B. R.: The solitary pulmonary nodule. Dis. Chest, *49*: 302, 1966.

Wassermann, F.: Fettorgan und lymphatisches System. Zschr. Zellforsch., *3*: 235, 1926.

——: Fettorgan und lymphatisches System. Sitzgsber. Ges. Morph. u. Physiol. Münch., 42, 1933.

Watanabe, S.: Pulmonary edema and pulmonary congestion. Kokyu to Junkan, *3*: 205, 1955.

Weg, J. G. and Harkleroad, L. E.: Aberrations in pulmonary function due to lymphangiography. Dis. Chest, *53*: 534, 1968.

Willis, T.: 1673. cit. from W. S. Miller.

Winternitz, M. C. and Smith, G. H.: Preliminary studies on intratracheal therapy. Collected studies on the pathology of war gas poisoning. Yale Univ. Press, New Haven, 1920.

Wywodzoff, D. W.: Die Lymphwege der Lunge. Wiener Med. Jahrg., *11*: 3, 1866.

Yamagata, T.: X-ray Schema of Infant Tuberculosis, I. Shindan to Chiryosha, Tokyo, 1954.

Yoffey, J. M. and Courtice, F. C.: Lymphatics, Lymph and Lymphoid Tissue. Cambridge, Harvard Univ. Press, 1956.

Yoshida, F.: Experimental study on the excretion of the inhaled staubs (in Japanese). Kokumin Eisei, *4*: 743, 1926.

Zimmerman, K. W.: Der feinere Bau der Blutcapillaren. Zschr. Anat. Entwickl., *68*: 29, 1923.

NERVOUS SYSTEM

Adams, W. E.: The Comparative Morphology of the Carotid Body and Carotid Sinus. C. C. Thomas, Springfield, 1958.

Alexander, H.: Übergang zur Frage der Lungenatelektase, unter besonderer Berücksichtung der Tuberkulose. Beitr. kl. Tbk., *104*: 422, 1951.

Altenähr, E.: Untersuchungen über die Feinstruktur der vegetativen Innervation der Rattenlunge. Zschr. mikros.-anat. Forsch., *72*: 439, 1965.

Araki, J.: Patho-morphological studies of the peripheral nervous system (in Japanese). Nihon Byorigakkai Zasshi, *44*: 35, 1955.

Arey: Developmental Anatomy: A Textbook and Manual of Embryology. Philadelphia and London, 1942.

Arimoto, R. and Miyakegawa, R.: Histological studies on the nerve distribution of the lung (in Japanese). Kyoto Furitsu Idai Zasshi, *4*: 737, 1930.

Arnold, J.: Zur Histologie der Lunge. Virchows Arch. Path. Anat. Physiol. u. kl. Med., *28*: 433, 1863.

Arnstein, C.: Zur Morphologie der sekretorischen Nervenendapparatate. Anat. Anz., *10*: 410, 1895.

Arnstein, C. and Ploschko, A.: Die Nervenendigungen und Ganglion der Respirationsorgane. Anat. Anz., *13*: 258, 1897.

Asai, N., et al.: Effect of unilateral hypoxia on the distribution of pulmonary blood flow in man. Acta Tuberculosea Japonica, *16*: 1, 1966.

Aschoff, L. and Goodhardt, G.: Vorkommen von Paraganglion in peripherischen Stamm des N. vagus. Dtsch. med. Wschr., *35*: 1461, 1909.

Berkeley, H.: The intrinsic pulmonary nerves in mammals. J. comp. Neur., *3*: 107, 1893.

——: The intrinsic pulmonary nerves in mammals. Johns Hopkins Hosp. Reports, *4*: 72, 1893.

Blessing, M. H. and Hora, B. J.: Glomera in der Lunge des Menschen. Zschr. Zellforsch., *87*: 562, 1968.

BLÜMCKE, S.: Experimentell-morphologische Untersuchungen über die efferente bronchiale Innervation. I. Der Plexus peribronchialis. Beit. Path. Anat., *137*: 239, 1968.

——: Lunge und vegetatives Nervensystem. Beit. klin. Tuberk., *138*: 229, 1968.

BOEKE, J.: Noch einmal das periterminale Netzwerk, die Struktur der motorischen Endplatte und die Bedeutung der Neurofibrilla. Zschr. mikr.-anat. Forsch., *7*: 95, 1926.

——: De-und Regeneration des peripheren Nerven systems. Dtsch. Zschr. Nervenhk., *115*: 1930.

——: Some observation on the structure and innervation of smooth-muscle fibers. Journ. comp. Neur., *56*: 1933.

——: Innervationsstudien. I–IV. Zschr. mikr.-anat. Forsch., *33*: 23, 47, 233, 276, 1933.

——: V. Zschr. mikr.-anat. Forsch., *34*: 330, 1933.

——: VI. Zschr. mikr.-anat. Forsch., *35*: 551, 1934.

——: VII–VIII. Zschr. mikr.-anat. Forsch., *38*: 554, 594, 1935.

——: IX. Zschr. mikr.-anat. Forsch., *39*: 477, 1936.

BRÄUCKER, W.: Der Brustteil des vegetativen Nervensystems und seine klinisch-chirurgischen Bedeutung. Beitr. klin. Tbk., *66*: 1, 1926.

BRONKHORST, W. and DIJKSTRA, C.: Das neuromuskuläre System der Lunge. Anatomische und physiologische Untersuchungen über die Lungenmuskulatur und ihre Bedeutung für die Klinik der Tuberkulose. Beitr. Klin. Tbk., *94*: 445, 1940.

BROWNLEE, R. T., FISK, R. L. and COUVES, C. M.: Function and morphology of the canine lung. Two years following immediate or delayed reimplantation. Dis. Chest, *55*: 310, 1969.

BUDDE, M.: Untersuchungen über die sympathischen Ganglien in der Lunge bei Säugetieren und beim menschlichen Fetus. Anat. Hefte, *23*: 211, 1904.

CAJAL, R. S.: Die Struktur der sensiblen Ganglien des Menschen und der Tiere. Erg. Anat. u. Entwickl., *16*: 177, 1906.

CAPPS, T. A.: An experimental study of the pain sense in the pleural membrane. Arch. Int. Med., *8*: 717, 1911.

——: 1932. cit. from KUNTZ.

COLERIDGE, J. C. and KIDD, C.: Electrophysiological evidence of baroreceptors in the pulmonary artery of the dog. J. Physiol., *150*: 319, 1960.

COMROE, J. H., Jr.: The location and function of the chemoreceptors of the aorta. Amer. J. Physiol., *127*: 176, 1939.

——: The functions of the lung. Harvey Lect., *48*: 110, 1952; 144, 1953.

——: The peripheral chemoreceptors. In: W. O. Fenn and H. Rahn's Handbook of Physiology. Sec. 3, Respiration, Vol. 1 (Wash. D. C.: Amer. Physiol. Soc.): 557, 1964.

——: Physiology of Respiration. Year Book Medical Publ., Inc., Chicago, 1965.

——: The main functions of the pulmonary circulation, *33*: 146, 1966.

CORRODI, H. and JONSON, G.: Fluorescence method for the histochemical demonstration of monoamines. 4. Histochemical differentiation between dopamine and noradrenaline in models. J. Histochem. Cytochem., *13*: 484, 1965.

COURNAND, A.: Some aspect of the pulmonary circulation in normal man and in chronic cardiopulmonary diseases. Circulation, *2*: 641, 1950.

CUCCATI, G.: 1888. cit. from P. STÖHR.

DALY, I. D. B. and HEBB, C.: Pulmonary and Bronchial Vascular Systems. E. Arnold Ltd., London, 1966.

DAWES, G. S. and COMROE, J. H.: Chemoreflexes from the Heart and lungs. Physiol. Rev., *34*: 167, 1954.

DAWES, G. S.: Reflexes originating in the pulmonary circulation. In: "Pulmonary Circulation". edited by Adams, W. and Veith, I., Grune and Stratton, New York·London, 1959.

DEJOURS, P.: Chemoreflexes in breathing. Physiol. Rev., *42*: 335, 1962.

DIJKSTRA, C.: Über die Innervation der Lunge. Beitr. klin. Tbk., *92*: 445, 1939.

DIXON, W. E. and RANSON, F.: Bronchodilator nerves. J. Physiol., *45*: 415, 1912.

DOGIEL, A. S.: Zur Frage über die Ganglien der Darmgeflechte bei den Säugetieren. Anat. Anz., *10*: 517, 1895.

——: Nervenendigungen in der Pleura des Menschen und der Säugetiere. Arch. mikr. Anat. u. Entwickl., *62*: 244, 1903.

DONATI, V.: 1930. cit. from H. v. Hayek.

ELFTMAN, A. G.: The afferent and parasympathetic innervation of the lungs and trachea of the dog. Amer. J. Anat., *72*: 1, 1943.

FALCK, B. and HILLARP, N-A., THIEME, G. and TORP, A.: Fluorescence of catecholamines and related compounds condensed with formaldehyde. J. Histochem. Cytochem., *10*: 348, 1962.

FALCK, B.: Observations on the possibilities of the cellular localization of monoamines by a fluorescence method. Acta Physiol. Scand., *56* (Suppl.): 197, 1962.

FARBER, S.: Neuropathic pulmonary edema. Arch. Path., *30*: 180, 1940.

FELIX, W.: Anatomische experimentelle und klinische Untersuchungen über den Phrenicus und über die Zwelchfellinnervation. Dtsch. Zschr. Chir., *171*: 283, 1922.

——: Lebensnerven und Lebenstrieb., Springer, Berlin, 1931.

FEYRTER, F.: Über der Bauplan der nervösen Peripherie. Virchows Arch., *318*: 1, 1950.

——: Über die Pathologie der vegetativen nervösen Peripherie und ihren ganglionären Regulationsstätten. W. Haudrich, Wien, 1951.

FILATOWA, A. G. and LAWRENTJEW, B. I.: Über die pathologische Histologie der Nerven und Ganglien bei Kehlkopf- und Lungentuberkulose. Virchows Arch., *286*: 1, 1932.

FISHER, A. W. F.: The intrinsic innervation of the pulmonary vessels. Acta anat., *60*: 481, 1965.

FÖRSTER, O.: 1936. cit. from A. STURM.

FRANKENHÄUSER, K.: Untersuchungen über den Bau der tracheobronchial Schleimhaut, Med. Diss. Dorpat., St. Petersburg, 1879.

FREERKSEN, E.: Vegetative Nervensystem und Lunge. I. Beitr. klin. Tbk., *103*: 384, 1950.

FRÖHLICH, F.: Die "Helle Zelle" der Bronchialschleimhaut und ihre Beziehungen zum Problem der Chemorezeptoren. Frankfurter Zschr. Path., *60*: 517, 1949.

FUCHS, R. F.: 1898. cit. from H. v. HAYEK.

GAYLOR, J. B.: Intrinsic nerve mechanism of the human lung. Brain, *57*: 143, 1934.

GESELL, R.: The chemical regulation of respiration. Physiol. Rev., *5*: 551, 1925.

GLASER, F.: Die intraneurale Nerven der Blutgefässe in der Lunge. Zschr. Anat. Entwickl.-gesch., *83*: 327, 1927.

——: Die Nerven der Bronchialwand. Zschr. Anat. Entwickl.-gesch., *83*: 332, 1927.

HAYASHI, S.: Mikroskopische Studien zur Innervation der Lunge. Manshu Igaku Zasshi, *27*: 37, 1937.

HEBB, C. O.: Bronchomotor responses to stimulation of the stellate ganglion and to injection of acetylcholin in isolated perfused guinea pig lungs. J. Physiol., *99*: 57, 1940.

HERING, E. and BREUER, J.: Die Selbststeurerung der Atmung durch den Nervus Vagus. Sitzber. Akad. Wis. Wien Math.-naturw. Kl. (abt. II), *57*: 672 and *58*: 909, 1868.

HEYERS, W.: Beitrag zur Morphologie des Glomus pulmonale. Frankfur. Zschr. Path., *72*: 616, 1963.

HIRSCH, E. F., et al.: The innervation of the mammalian lung. III. Regression of the intrinsic nerves and of their afferent receptors following thoracic sympathectomy, cervical vagotomy or thoracic stripping of vagus. Arch. Surg., *96*: 149, 1968.

——: Innervation of the mammalian lung. Arch. Path., *85*: 51, 1968.

HIRSCH, E. F. and KAISER, C. G.: The Innervation of the Lung. C. C. Thomas, Springfield, 1969.

HIRT, A.: Die anatomischen Grundlagen des symp. und parasymp. Nervensystems. Schweiz. Med. Jb. 1931.

HONJIN, R.: On the nerve supply of the lung of the mouse with special reference to the structure of the peripheral vegetative nervous system. J. Comp. Neurol., *105*: 587, 1943.

INABA, N.: Studies on nervous and muscular system of lung. Some problems of pulmonary circulation in reference to its histologic findings (in Japanese). Kyodai Kekken Kiyo, *5*: 237, 1957.

ISMAILOFF: 1873. cit. from P. STÖHR.

IWAMA, Y.: Untersuchungen über den peripheren Bau des Nervus Vagus. Folia anat. jap., *3*: 215, 281, 1925, and *6*: 129, 1928.

JABONERO, V.: Der anatomische Aufbau des peripheren Neurovegetativensystems. Acta Neuroveg. Suppl., *4*: 1, 1953.

JONES, A. C.: Innervation and nerve terminations of the reptilian lung. J. Comp. Neur., *40*: 371, 1926.

KAI, T. and SAGAWA, Y.: Distribution of adrenergic nerve fibers in the lungs of the rabbit, guinea pig and man, as demonstrated by Falck-Hillarp's fluorescence method (in Japanese). Kyodai Kyobuken Kiyo, *2*: 225, 1969.

KATO, M. and STAUB, N. C.: Response of small pulmonary arteries to unilateral hypoxia and hypercapnia. Circulation Res., *19*: 426, 1966.

KIMURA, C.: Double innervation theory of the visceral sensible nervous system (in Japanese). Nihon Rinsho, *11*: 85, 1953.

——: The problems of adbominal pain. Nihon Geka Hokan, *22*: 59, 1953.

——: Visceral sensible nervous system and vegetative nervous system (in Japanese). Saishin Igaku, *9*: 604, 1954.

KNOCHE, H. und BLÜMCKE, S.: Neurorezeptorareale der Arteria pulmonalis. Zschr. Zellforsch., *62*: 514, 1964.

KNOCHE, H.: Beitrag zur Gefässversorgung der aorticopulmonalen Glomera. Zschr. mikr.-anat. Forsch., *74*: 283, 1966.

KODANOFF, D. und GÜROWSKI, A.: Morphologie der Rezeptoren des Atmungs- und Verdauungssystem beim Menschen. Gustav Fisher, Jena, 1963.

KOELLE, G. B.: The elimination of enzymatic diffusion artifacts in the histochemical localization of cholinesterases and a survey of their cellular distributions. J. Pharmacol., *103*: 153, 1951.

KÖLLIKER, A.: Handbuch der Gewebslehre des Menschen. Leipzig, 1902.

KRAHL, V. E.: The glomus pulmonale. Its location and microscopic anatomy. In: Ciba Foundation Symposium on Pulmonary Structure and Function, ed. A. V. S. de Reuck, and M. O'Conner, Little, Brown Co., Boston, 1962.

KRAUSE, C. FR. TH.: Handbuch der menschlichen Anatomie, Hannover, 1876.

KURE, K.: Vegetative Nervous System (in Japanese). 2 ed., Kokuseido, Tokyo, 1935.

KURE, K. and OKINAKA, S.: The autonomic Nervous System (in Japanese). Isho Shuppan, Tokyo, 1950.

KURUCZ, J.: A contribution to the innervation of the pulmonary artery. Acta anat., *34*: 305, 1958.

LANGLEY, J. N.: Das sympathische und verwandte nervöse Systeme der Wirbeltiere (autonomes nervöses System). Erg. Physiol., *2* II Abt.: 818, 1903.

——: The Autonomic Nervous System, Part I, W. Heffer and Sons Ltd., Cambridge, 1921.

——: Das autonome Nervensystem. I Teil, 1922.

LARSELL, O. and MASON, M. L.: Experimental degeneration of the vagus nerve and its relation to the nerve termination in the lung of the rabbit. J. Comp. Neur., *33*: 509, 1921.

LARSELL, O.: Nerve terminations in the lung of rabbit. J. Comp. Neur., *33*: 105, 1921.

——: The ganglia, plexuses, and nerve terminations of the mammalian lung and pleura pulmonalis. J. Comp. Neur., *35*: 97, 1923.

——: Nerve ending in the human pleura pulmonalis. J. Comp. Neur. *61*: 407, 1935.

LARSELL, O. and DOW, R. S.: The innervation of the human lung. Amer. J. Anat., *52*: 135, 1935.

LIEBOW, A. A.: Recent advances in pulmonary anatomy. Ciba Foundation Symposium on Pulmonary Structure and Function, eds. A. V. S. de Reuck, and M. O'Conner, Little, Brown and Co., Boston, 1962.

LILJESTRAND, A.: Neural control of respiration. Physiol. Rev., *38*: 691, 1958.

LUSCHKA, H.: 1853. cit. from H. v. HAYEK.

——: 1863. cit. from W. BRÄUCKER.

MCLAUGHLIN, A. I. G.: Nerve and nerve endings in the visceral pleura of the cat. J. Physiol., *80*: 101, 1933.

MICHELAZZI: Sur l'innervation des veins. Arch. Ital. Biol., *91*: 101, 1937.

MICHAILOW, S.: Die feinere Struktur der sympathetischer Ganglion der Harnblase bei den Säugetieren. Arch. mikr. Anat., *72*: 554, 1908.

MILLER, W. S.: A study of the nerves and ganglia of the lungs in a case of pulmonary tuberculosis. Amer. Rev. Tbc., *2*: 123, 1918.

MIYAKE, S.: Histological studies of the vegetative nervous system in patient of bronchial asthma (in Japanese). Nihon Naibunpitsugakkai Zasshi, *13*: 802, 1937.

——: Histological studies of the human pulmonary vasomotor Nerves in human fetus (in Japanese). Nihon Naibunpitsugakkai Zasshi, *13*: 4, 1937.

MIZUKOSHI, T.: Histological studies on the innervation of the lung of human embryo. Tohoku J. Exp. Med., *58*: 223, 1953.

MOLHANT: 1910. cit. from H. v. HAYEK, and 1913. cit. from P. STÖHR.

MÖLLGAARD, H.: Studien über das respiratorische Nervensystem bei den Wirbeltiere. Acta Physiol. Scand., *26*: 315, 1912.

MÜLLER, L. R.: Beiträge zur Anatomie, Histologie und Pathologie des Nervus vagus, zugleich des Herzens, der Bronchen, des Magens. Dtsch. Arch. klin. Med., *101*: 421, 1910.

MURAO, H.: Nervous regulation of the bronchial vascular system. Jap. Circulation J., *22*: 855, 1965.

NAGAISHI, C. and INABA, N.: Nervous system of the lung. In: Nagaishi's "The Structure of the Lung", Vol. II (in Japanese). Igaku Shoin Ltd., Tokyo, 1958.

NAGASAWA, N., YAMASHITA, M., OKADA, Y., INABA, N. and NAGAISHI, C.: Some problems related to the structure of the pleura (in Japanese). Hai, *2*: 111, 1955.

NIEDNER, F. F.: Beiträge zur Kenntnis von neurovegetativen Lungenreaktionen; Beobachtungen andere Lunge bei intrathorakalen Operationen. Acta Neuroveg., *1*: 353, 1950.

NIGRO, S. L., et al.: The innervation of the mammalian lung. Regression of the intrinsic nerves and other sequelae in the reimplanted lung. Arch. Surg., *96*: 138, 1968.

NISSEN, R.: 1930. cit. from SUNDER-PLASSMANN.

NONIDEZ, J. F.: The nervous "terminalreticulum". Anat. Anz., *82*: 348, 1936.

——: Identification of the receptor areas in the venae cavae and pulmonary vein which initate reflex cardiac acceleration (Bainbridge's reflex). Amer. J. Anat., *61*: 203, 1937.

OBERHOLZER, R. J. H. and TOFANI, W. O.: The neural control of respiration. In: H. W. Magoun's Handbook of Physiology. Sec. 1 Neurophysiology, Vol. II (Wash. D.C.: Amer. Physiol. Soc.), 1960.

OKAMURA, C.: Die Ganglien der Wand der Bronchien und Alveolen. Zschr. mikr.-anat. Forsch., *41*: 267, 1930.

OLSEN, C. R., et al.: Motor control of pulmonary airways studied by nerve stimulation. J. Appl. Physiol., *20*: 202, 1965.

OVERHOLT, R. H.: The Technique of Pulmonary Resection. C. C. Thomas, Springfield, 1949.

PAINTAL, A. S.: Vagal afferent fibers. Ergebn. Physiol., *52*: 74, 1963.

PLOSCHKO, A.: Die Nervenendigungen und Ganglien der Respirationsorgane. Anat. Anz., *13*: 12, 1897.

PONZIO, F.: Le termination nervore nel pulmone. Anat. Anz., *28*: 74, 1906.

RASMUSSEN, A. T.: The pathways for nervous reflexes from the parenchyma of the lung. Amer. Rev. Tbc., *13*: 545, 1926.

REINHARDT, E.: Beiträge zur Kenntnis der Lunge als neurovasculäres und neuromusculäres Organ nach Beobachtungen an der Lunge des lebenden Kaninchens. Virchows Arch. path. Anat. Physiol. und kl. Med., *292*: 322, 1934.

——: Die Topik der lobären Pneumonie als Beweis ihrer Entstehung im Zentralnervensystem. Verh. dtsch. path. Ges. *66*: 222, 1936.

REISER, K. A.: Über die Endausbreitung des vegetativen Nervensystems. Zschr. Zellforsch., *17*: 610, 1933.

——: Über die Nerven der Darmmuskulatur. Zschr. Zellforsch., *22*: 675, 1934.

——: Der Nervenapparat im Processus vermiformis nebst einigen Bemerkungen über seine Veränderungen bei chronischer Appendicitis. Zschr. Zellforsch., *15*: 761, 1932.

REMAK, R.: 1844. cit. from W. S. MILLER.

RETZIUS, G.: Zur Kenntnis der Nervenendigungen in der Lungen. Biol. Untersuch. N.F., *5*: 41, 1893.

RODBARD, S. and HARASAWA, M.: A pulmonary-bronchomotor reflex. Fed. Proc., *19*: 96, 1960.

ROGER: 1917. cit. from W. BRÄUCKER.

ROMANOW, A.: 1904. cit. from H. v. HAYEK.

ROSSI, F.: L'innervazione della pleura. Arch. Zool. Ital., *16*: 701, 1931.

SAALFIEDL, E. V.: Herzreflex pulmonalen Ursprungs. Pflügers Arch., *231*: 33, 1933.

SAGAWA, Y.: Study of the vagal pulmonary edema using rapid freezing (in Japanese). Kyobu Shikkan, *8*: 1186, 1964.

SAITO, M.: Supplement to the observations on the innervation of the lung in dog. Arch. Hist. Jap., *9*: 41, 1955.

SASAKI, Y.: Microscopic observations of the nervous distribution in human larynx (in Japanese). Tohoku Igakkai Zasshi, *32*: 569, 1943.

——: Nervous distribution in human trachea (in Japanese). Tohoku Igakkai Zasshi, *32*: 595, 1943.

SAUERBRUCH, F.: 1932. cit. from P. SUNDER-PLASSMANN.

SCHWIEGK, H.: Lungenentlastungsreflex. Pflügers Arch., *236*: 206, 1935.

SETO, H.: Über zwischen Aorta und Arteria pulmonalis gelegene Herzparaganglien. Zschr. Zellforsch., *22*: 213, 1935.

——: Mikroskopische Studien zur Innervation des menschlichen Herzens. Arb. Anat. Inst. Tohoku Univ., *19*: 1, 1936.

SETO, H. and FUKUYAMA, U.: Zur Innervation der Speicheldrüsen des Igels. Manshu Igaku Zasshi, *25*: 177, 1936.

SETO, H.: Über die afferenten Nerven im Aortenbogen und in Herzen beim Menschen im Hinblick auf den Aorten-und Herzreflex. Arb. Anat. Inst. Tohoku Univ., *20*: 1, 1937.

——: Silver impregnation for the nervous system being used in our laboratory. Tohoku J. Exp. Med., *54*: 1, 1951.

——: Human Sensibility (in Japanese). Igaku Shoin Ltd., Tokyo, 1957.

SHIMAMOTO, K. and FUJIWARA, M.: Fluorescence histochemical demonstration of cathecholamine and serotonin. Saishin Igaku, *22*: 100, 1967.

SIMENAUER, E.: Die Sensibilität von Pleuren, Perikard und Peritoneal Überzug des Diaphragma mit der besonderen Berücksichtung des Nervus phrenicus. Zschr. Tbk., *48*: 273, 1927.

SMIRNOW, A.: Über Nervenendknäuel in der Froschlunge. Anat. Anz., *3*: 258, 1888.

SPENCE, H. and LEOF, D.: The innervation of the human lung. J. Anat. Lond., *98*: 599, 1964.

STANULA, H.: Zur Kenntnis der Lungendetektomie. Thorax-u. vaskuläre Chir., *16*: 204, 1968.

STAUB, N. C. and STOREY, W. F.: Relation between morphological and physiological events in lung studied by rapid freezing. J. Appl. Physiol., *17*: 381, 1962.

STAUB, N. C. and KATO, M.: Effect of alveolar hypoxia on pulmonary vascular resistance. J. Appl. Physiol., *19*: 1084, 1964.

STERNSCHEIN, E.: Anastomosen zwischen Vagus und Sympathicus bei der Katze. Zschr. Anat. Entwickl.-gesch., *64*: 441, 1922.

STIRLING, WM.: Nervous apparatus of the lung. Brit. Med. J., *2*: 401, 1876.

——: On the nerves of the lung. J. Anat., *16*: 96, 1882.

STOECKENIUS, W.: An electron microscopic study of myelin figures. J. Biophys. and Biochem. Cytol., *5*: 491, 1959.

STÖHR, P. Jr.: Lehrbuch der Histologie. Gustav Fischer, Jena, 1928.

——: Mikroskopische Anatomie des vegetativen Nervensystems. Springer, Berlin, 1928.

——: Mikroskopische Studien zur Innervation des Magen-Darmkanals (II). Zschr. Zellforsch., *16*: 123, 1932.

——: (III). Zschr. Zellforsch., *21*: 243, 1934.

——: Beobachtungen und Bemerkungen über die Endausbreitung des vegetativen Nervensystems. Zschr. Anat., *104*: 133, 1935.

——: Lehrbuch der Histologie und der mikroskopischen Anatomie des Menschen. Springer, Berlin, 1951.

STURM, A.: Die klinische Pathologie der Lunge in Beziehung zum vegetativen Nervensystem. Stuttgart, 1948.

SUNDER-PLASSMANN, P.: Untersuchungen über den Bulbus carotides bei Mensch und Tier im Hinblick auf die Sinusreflex nach H. E. Hering. Zschr. Anat., *93*: 567, 1930.

——: Über nervöse Rezeptorenfelder in der Wand der intrapulmonalen Bronchien des Menschen. Dtsch. Zschr. Chir., *240*: 249, 1933.

——: Neurovegetative Rezeptorenfelder. Zschr. ges. Neurol. Psychiat., *147*: 414, 1933.

——: Über pathologische Veränderungen des intramuralen Ganglienapparates bei Bronchiektasie. Arch. Klin. Chir., *183*: 166, 1935.

——: Der Nervenapparat der menschlichen Lunge. Dtsch. Zschr. Chir., *250*: 705, 1938.

——: Die nervöse Abhängigkeit von Schilddrüse und Nebenniere. Dtsch. Zschr. Chir., *245*: 756, 1935.

——: Zur Basedowproblem. Dtsch. Zschr. Chir., *250*: 543, 1938.

SUZUKI, K.: Technical notes on making microscopic sections. IV. Cerebral nerves (in Japanese). *5*: 184, 1952.

——: V. Cerebral nerves (in Japanese). *6*: 58, 1953.

TAKINO, M.: Über die Innervation der Lungengefässwand, besonders über das Vorkommen der Ganglienzellen an der Gefässwand der Venae pulmonales und über die Verbreitungszustände der Lungenblutgefässnerven bei der Fledermaus. Acta Schol. Med. Univ. Kioto, *15*: 303, 1932.

——: Über die Innervation der Blutgefässe der Lunge beim Vögel (Taube und Haushuhn), besonders über das Vorkommen der Ganglienzellen in order an der Wand der Venae und Arteriae pulmonales und über die Verbreitung der Blutgefässnerven daselbst. Acta Schol. Med. Univ. Kioto, *15*: 308, 1933.

——: Vergleichende Studien über die histologische Struktur der Arteriae und Venae pulmonales, die Blutgefässnerven der Lunge und die Nerven der Bronchien bei verschiedenen Tierarten, besonders über die Beziehung der Blutgefässnerven zu den glatten Muskeln der Blutgefässe. Acta Schol. Med. Univ. Koto, *15*: 321, 1933.

TAKINO, M. und EZAKI, S.: Über die Besonderheiten der Arteriae und Venae pulmonales bei verschiedenen Tieren, besonders beim Menschen. Acta Schol. Med. Univ. Kioto, *17*: 1, 1934.

TAKINO, M. und MIYAKE, S.: Über die Besonderheiten der Arteriae und Venae pulmonales bei verschiedenen Tieren, besonders beim Menschen. Die funktionelle Bedeutung des Muskelwülste (sog. Sperrvorrichtung der Venae pulmonales). Acta Schol. Med. Univ. Kioto, *18*: 226, 1936.

TAKINO, M. und WATANABE, S.: Über das Vorkommen der Ganglienzellen von unipolaren Typus in der Lunge des Menschen und Schweines. Acta Schol. Med. Univ. Kioto, *19*: 317, 1937.

——: Über die Bedeutung des Ligamentum arteriosum bzw. des Ductus Botalli und der Ansatzstelle desselben an der Pulmonalwand (A. pulm.) als Blutdruckzügler bei verschiedenen Tierarten. Archiv für Kreislaufforsch, *11*: 18, 1937.

——: Über das Vorkommen von Astklappen in die Lungenvenen des Schweines. Morpholog. Jb., *18*: 479, 1937.

TAKINO, M., et al.: Über die Astklappen in die Lungenvenen. 1. Mitteilung. Kalb. Acta Schol. Med. Univ. Kioto, *22*: 321, 1939.

——: Über die Astklappen in die Lungenvenen. 2. Mitteilung. Mensch. Acta Schol. Med. Univ. Kioto, *22*: 330, 1939.

TAKINO, M.: Pathology of pulmonary circulation (in Japanese). Nihon Rinsho Jyunkanki Zasshi, *6–8*: 1, 1940.

TAKINO, J. und OSADA, S.: Kritik der Entstehungstheorie des Bronchialasthmatischen Anfalls auf Grund der Lungen-kreislaufstörung (Unter besonderer Berücksichtigung der Ähnlichkeit der Lungenvenenmuskulatur mit der Bronchialmuskulatur). Arch. Kreislaufforsch., *6*: 47, 1940.

TAKINO, M.: Der Lungenarterienstammreflex. Jap. J. Med. Sci., Part III, Biophysics, *9*: 1, 1943.

——: Reflex cardiac acceleration by the stimulating of the receptor area of the pulmonary veins and their vicinity in the atrium. Nihon Rinsho Shinzokekkangaku, *15*: 1, 1951.

——: The Theory of the Movement of Tension in Parasympathetic Nervous System. Dainippon Zoki Kenkyusho Publication, 1952.

——: The pulmonary artery reflex test and its clinical applications. Nihon Rynsho Shinzokekkangaku, *19*: 1, 1955.

TAKINO, M. and TAKINO, Y.: Allergy and Asthma. Maruzen Co., Ltd., Tokyo 1957.

——: Self-regulation of the parasympathetic nervous system based on variety of allergic phenomena and its relation to the parasympatheticus. Acta Neuroveg., Wien, *22*: 226, 1961.

TAKINO, M.: The difficulty in curative treatment of allergic diseases, especially bronchial asthma and its counter-measures from genetic point of view. Atti della Academia delle Science di Ferrara, *40*: 1, 1962–1963.

TAKINO, M. and TAKINO, Y.: Importance of pulmonary vagotonia as and indicator of the irritability of the parasympathetic and its relation to other organ vagotonia in allergic patients. Acta Neuroveg., Wien, *27*: 326, 1965.

TAKINO, M.: Patogenia del Asma Bronquial Basada en el Concepto de Vagotonía General y Vagotonia de Organo. Alergia, *18*: 137, 1971.

TANAKA, T., TZEN, M., ASAI, N., KAI, T., TANAE, E., NAKAGAWA, M. and SAGAWA, Y.: A morphological study of pulmonary vascular response to unilateral hypoxia in guinea pig. Acta Tuberc. Japonica, *16*: 21, 1966.

TERNI, T.: L'innervazione del pulmone. Minerva med., *21*: 2, 1930.

UNGAR, G. and GROSSIORD, A.: 1936. cit. from H. v. HAYEK.

UNVERRICHT.: 1934. cit. from K. KURE, and S. OKINAKA.

UYEDA, H.: Pulmonary circulation, Shinryo, *7*: 19, 1954.

VERSON, E.: 1868. cit. from W. S. MILLER.

WEIDMANN, H., BREDE, B. and BUCHER, K.: Die Lage der vagalen Dehnungsrezeptoren in der Lunge. Helv. physiol. pharmacol. Acta, *7*: 476, 1949.

WHITEHEAD, R. W. and DRAPER, W. B.: A respiratory reflex originating in the thoracic wall of the dog. Anesthesiology, *8*: 159, 1947.

WIDDICOMBE, J. G.: Regulation of tracheobronchial smooth muscle. Physiol. Rev., *43*: 1, 1963.

——: Respiratory reflexes. In: W. O. Fenn and H. Rahn's Handbook of Physiology. Sec. 3. Respiration, Vol. I (Wash. D.C.: Amer. Physiol. Soc.): 585, 1964.

YAGITA, M.: A histological study of sensory nerves in the lung and the visceral pleura. Nihon Geka Hokan, *23*: 569, 1954.

YANO, K.: Zur Anatomie und Histologie des N. phrenicus und des Nebenphrenicus. Folia Anat. Jap., *3*: 3, 1928.

MUSCULAR SYSTEM

AGOSTONI, E.: Action of respiratory muscles. In: W. O. Fenn and H. Rahn's Hand Book of Physiology. Sec. 3. Respiration. Vol. I (Wash. D.C.: Amer. Physiol. Soc.): 377, 1964.

ALEXANDER, H.: Überlegungen zur Frage der Lungenatelektase, unter besonderer Berücksichtung der Tuberkulose. Beitr. klin. Tbk., *104*: 422, 1951.

BALTISBERGER, W.: Glatte Muskulatur der menschliche Lunge. Zschr. Anat. Entwickl.-gesch., *61*: 249, 1921.

BAUDRIMONT: 1929. cit. from A. STURM.

BEHRENS, W.: Anatomischer Beitrag zur Frage der Atelektase. Schweiz. med. Wschr., *80*: 69, 1950.

BRONKHORST, W. und DIJKSTRA, C.: Das neuromuskuläre System der Lunge. Anatomische und physiologische Untersuchungen über die Lungenmuskulatur und ihre Bedeutung für die Klinik der Tuberkulose. Beitr. klin. Tb., *94*: 445, 1940.

CAMPBELL, E. J. M.: The Respiratory Muscles and the Mechanics of Breathing. Year Book Med. Publishers, Inc., Chicago, 1958.

CRAMER, H.: 1947. cit. from W. BALTISBERGER.

DALY, I. de B. and EULER, V.: The functional activity of the dog. Proc. roy. Soc., London, *110*: 92, 1932.

DUBREUIL, G. and LAMARQUE, P.: 1919. cit. from W. S. MILLER.

EBNER, v.: 1899. cit. from A. STURM.

ENGEL, S. and NEWS, G. H.: Musculature of the lung of children. Journ. Path. Bact., *49*: 381, 1939.

ENGEL, S.: Die Muskulatur der Lunge. Dtsch. med. Wschr., *73*: 382, 1948.

GEHLEN, H. v.: Der Acinus als elastisch-muskulöses System. Morph. Jb., *85*: 186, 1940.

HARKAVAY, J.: Pathologic changes of the alveolar passages in diseases of the lungs with special reference to the musculature. J. Path. Bact., *27*: 366, 1924.

HAYEK, H. v.: Muskulatur im Lungenparenchym. Zschr. Anat. Entwickl.-gesch., *115*: 88, 1950.

——: Die menschliche Lunge. Springer, 1953.

HUIZINGER, E.: Physikalische Atelektasen. Pflügers Arch. ges. Physiol., *238*: 709, 1937.

KÖLLIKER, A.: 1854. cit. from A. STURM.

——: 1881. cit. from A. STURM.

LUISADA, A.: Über Lungendynamik. Erg. inn. Med., *47*: 92, 1934.

LUSCHKA, H.: 1863. cit. from W. S. MILLER.

MACKLIN, C. C.: A note on the elastic membrane of the bronchial tree of mammals, with an interpretation of its functional significances. Anat. Rec., *24*: 119, 1922.

——: The musculature of the bronchi and lungs. Physiol. Rev., *9*: 1, 1929.

MASON, M.: 1933. cit. from W. S. MILLER.

MILLER, W. S.: The musculature of the feiner divisions of the bronchial tree and its relation to certain pathological conditions. Amer. Rev. Tbc., *5*: 689, 1921.

——: The Lung. C. C. Thomas, Springfield, 1947.

MICHELAZZI and FRANZESCHI: 1953. cit. from H. v. HAYEK.

MÖLLENDORF, W. v.: Lungenkonstruktion. Zschr. Anat. Entwickl.-gesch., *111*: 224, 1941.

NAGAISHI, C. and INABA, N.: Muscular System of the Lung. In: Nagaishi's monograph "The Structure of the Lung", Vol. II (in Japanese). Igaku Shoin Ltd., Tokyo, 1958.

NEERGAARD, K. v.: Neue Auffassungen über einem Grundbegriff der Atemmechanik. Zschr. Exp. Med., *66*: 373, 1926.

ORSÓS, F.: Die Gerüstsysteme der Lunge und deren physiologische und pathologische Bedeutung. Beitr. klin. Tbk., *87*: 568, 1936.

ORTH: 1887. cit. from A. STURM.

REINHARDT, E.: Beiträge zur Kenntnis der Lunge als neurovasculäres und neuromuskuläres Organ nach Beobachtungen an Lunge des lebenden Kaninchens. Virchows Arch., *292*: 322, 1934.

——: Lungenkreislauf und Lungenmuskulatur bei Atelektase und Emphysem. Verhandl. d. Dtsch. Ges. Kreislaufforsch., *8*: 173, 1935.

REISSEISEN, F. D.: 1822. cit. from A. STURM.

RINDFLEISCH, E.: 1872. cit. from W. S. MILLER.

SALFELDER, K.: Über Lungenmuskulatur. Vehr. dtsch. Ges. Path. 38 Tagg, 1954.

SCHULZE, F. S.: Die Lungen. In: Strickers Lehre von der Geweben. Leipzig, 1871.

SEEMANN, G.: Histologie der Lungenalveole. Jena, 1931.

STÖHR, P.: Lehrbuch der Histologie und der mikroskopischen Anatomie. Springer, Berlin, 1951.

SUNAHARA, S.: Clinical studies of the neuro-muscular system of the lung (in Japanese). Saishin Igaku, *8*: 2, 1953.

TROISIER, I., BARIÉTY, M. and KOHLER, M.: Histamine et pression intropleurale. C.R. Soc. Biol. Paris, *92*: 413, 1940.

VERZAR, F.: Regulation des Lungenvolumes. Pflügers Arch. ges. Physiol., *232*: 322, 1933.

VERZAR, F. and JEKER, L.: Die physiologischen Atelektasen der Lunge. Pflügers Arch. ges. Physiology, *238*: 379, 1937.

WILLIS, T.: 1676. cit. from W. S. MILLER.

PULMONARY PLEURA

AOYAGI, Y.: Diseases of the Thoracic Wall and Pleura (in Japanese). In: Japanese Compendium of Surgery, *15*: 107, Nihon Geka Zensho Kankokai, Tokyo, 1956.

BORST, M.: Pathologie der serösen Deckzellen. Virchows Arch. path. Anat., *162*: 94, 1900.

BRATIANO, S. I. and BRATIANU, C. S.: Absorption des graisses animales par la plévre. Compt. rend. Soc. biol., *98*: 461, 1928.

CROXATTO, O. C. and SAMPIETRO, R.: Pathology of pleural sclerosis. A study related to the loss of expansivity of the lungs and its treatment. J. Thoracic Surg., *21*: 259, 1951.

ENOMOTO, H.: Studies on the lymphatics of thoracic wall (in Japanese). Kaibogaku Zasshi, *3*: 1521, 1931.

FLEINER, W.: Die Resorption corpusculärer Elemente durch Lunge und Pleura. Virchows Arch. path. Anat., *112*: 97 and 282, 1888.

FUJIMORI, K.: Clinical studies on the absorption of the substances from the extrapleural dead space and the pleural space. Kyobugeka, *3*: 206, 1950.

GROBER, J.: Die Resorptionskraft der Pleura. Beitr. path. Anat., *30*: 265, 1901.

HAFFERL, A.: Anatomie der Pleurakuppel. Berlin, 1939.

HASZ, E.: Elastische Netzeder Pleura. Zschr. Anat. Entwickl.-gesch., *108*: 337, 1938.

HAYEK, H. v.: Die Pleura parietalis. In: Hayeks Monograph "Die menschliche Lunge". Springer, Berlin·Göttingen·Heidelberg, 1953.

HIRAKAWA, K.: Experimental studies on resorption, secretion and excretion. On the permeability of the alveoli of the lungs. Acta Schol. Med. Univ. Kioto, *8*: 279, 1925.

ITO, H.: Surgical treatment for pericostal tuberculosis (in Japanese). Nihon Gekagakkai Zasshi, *24*: 957, 1923 and *25*: 221, 1924.

——: Zur operativen Behandlung der Perikostal tuberkulose. Dtsch. Zschr. Chir., *185*: 124, 1924.

KARSNER, H. T. and SWANBECK, C. E.: The removal of particulate matter from the pleura. J. Med. Res., *42*: 91, 1920/21.

KIHARA, T.: The extravascular fluid passway system. Ketsuekigaku Togikai Hokoku, *3*: 118, 1950.

KLEIN, E.: The Anatomy of the Lymphatic System. London, 1873.

LANG, J.: Über eigenartige Kapillarkonvolute der Pleura parietalis. Zschr. Zellforsch., *58*: 487, 1962.

LETULLE, M.: In: Le poumon. ed. A. MALOINE, et FILS, Paris, 1924.

LOESCHCKE, H.: Experimentelle Untersuchungen über Saftstrom- und Resorptionswege. Virchows Arch. path. Anat., *292*: 281, 1934.

MAGNUS, G.: Über die Resorptionswegen aus serösen und synovialen Höhlen. Dtsch. Zschr. Chir., *182*: 325, 1923.

MILLER, W. S.: The lymphatics of the lung. Anat. Anz., *12*: 110, 1896.

——: A study of the human pleura pulmonalis. Amer. J. Roentgenol., *15*: 399, 1926.

——: The Lung. 2nd ed., C. C. Thomas, Springfield, 1947.

MONCKEBERG, J. G.: Über das Verhalten des Pleuroperitonealepithels bei der Einkeilung von Fremdkörpern. Zieglers Beitr., *34*: 489, 1903.

NAGAISHI, C.: Pulmonary circulation with reference to venous admixture. Japanese Circulation J., *20*: 1, 1956.

NAGAISHI, C. and MAEKAWA, N.: Histological studies of the intercostal lymph nodes in cases of pulmonary tuberculosis (in Japanese). Kekkaku Kenkyu, *3*: 13, 1947.

NAGAISHI, C. and SAGAWA, Y.: Influences of pleural scars on pulmonary function. In: Nagaishi's monograph "The Structure of the Lung (in Japanese)". Vol. II: 303, 1958.

NAGAISHI, C. and OKADA, Y.: Pulmonary Pleura. In: Nagaishi's monograph "The Structure of the Lung (in Japanese)". Vol. II, Igaku Shoin Ltd., Tokyo, 1958.

NAKAMURA, M.: Experimental studies on the communication of lymphatics between the lung and the thoracic wall in cases of pleural adhesion (in Japanese). Nihon Geka Hokan, *24*: 168, 1955.

NOTKIN, J. A.: Die Aufsaugung in den serösen Höhlen. Virchows Arch., *255*: 473, 1955.

OGO, M.: Pathological changes of the pulmonary lymphatics originated in the pleural adhesion (in Japanese). Nihon Geka Hokan, *11*: 939, 1934.

SAMPIETRO, R. and CROXATTO, O. C.: Pathology of pleural sclerosis. J. Thoracic Surg., *21*: 259, 1951.

SEKIGUCHI, K.: Pyothorax. Kyobugeka Sosho No. 14, Nankodo, Tokyo·Kyoto, 1951.

——: Some problems on the decortication. Nihon Kyobugeka Gakkai Zasshi, *3*: 247, 1955.

SINAPIUS, D. and VOLLHABER, H.: Zur Kenntnis der Pleuradeckzellen. Beitr. Klin. Tbk., *106*: 165, 1951.

TAKEDA, Y.: Pneumolysis in Cases of Pulmonary Tuberculosis. I. Extrapleural Pneumothorax (in Japanese). Kyobugeka Sosho 6, Nankodo, Tokyo· Kyoto, 1955.

TAKEUCHI, S.: Pathogenesis of pericostal tuberculosis and its radical operation (in Japanese). Nihon Geka Hokan, *19*: 1101, 1942; and Nihon Rinsho Kekkaku, *4*: 116, 1943.

TSUBOUCHI, M.: The structure of membrana cribriformis found in the subendothelial tissue of the pulmonary pleura and the peritoneum of human beings and mammals, and its significance. Kaibogaku Zasshi, *25*: 6, 1950.

WADSWORTH, T. W.: A mechanism maintaining the negative pressure of the pleura, and influencing absorption. J. Path. and Bact., *25*: 266, 1922.

WALTER, R.: Über die "Stomata" der serösen Höhlen. Anat. Hefte, *46*: 275, 1912.

YAMAMOTO, M.: Studies on the experimental incidence of pericostal tuberculosis. Nihon Geka Hokan, *25*: 495, 1956.

YANAGIHARA, M.: Histologic and pathohistologic studies on the structure of the pleura (in Japanese). Kyodai Kekken Kiyo, *7*: 148, 1959.

INDEX

B

C

D

E

J

K

L

M

R

S

T

U

V

W

X